TECHNICAL LARGE ANIMAL EMERGENCY RESCUE

TECHNICAL LARGE ANIMAL EMERGENCY RESCUE

Rebecca Gimenez
Tomas Gimenez
Kimberly A. May

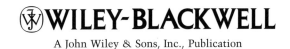

A John Wiley & Sons, Inc., Publication

Rebecca Gimenez, Ph.D., is a Major in the Signal Corps. US Army Reserves. She is the primary instructor for Large Animal Technical Rescue.

Tomas Gimenez, MVZ, DMV, is a professor emeritus in the Animal and Veterinary Sciences Department of Clemson University in South Carolina, and Safety Officer for the United States Public Health Service, National Defense Medical System, National Veterinary Response Team-2 (NVRT-2).

Kimberly A. May, DVM, MS, ACVS, is the Assistant Director of Professional and Public Affairs of the American Veterinary Medical Association.

Edition first published 2008
© 2008 Wiley-Blackwell

Blackwell Publishing was acquired by John Wiley & Sons in February 2007. Blackwell's publishing program has been merged with Wiley's global Scientific, Technical, and Medical business to form Wiley-Blackwell.

Editorial Office
2121 State Avenue, Ames, Iowa 50014-8300, USA

For details of our global editorial offices, for customer services, and for information about how to apply for permission to reuse the copyright material in this book, please see our website at www.wiley.com/wiley-blackwell.

Authorization to photocopy items for internal or personal use, or the internal or personal use of specific clients, is granted by Blackwell Publishing, provided that the base fee is paid directly to the Copyright Clearance Center, 222 Rosewood Drive, Danvers, MA 01923. For those organizations that have been granted a photocopy license by CCC, a separate system of payments has been arranged. The fee codes for users of the Transactional Reporting Service are ISBN-13: 978-0-8138-1998-3/2008.

Library of Congress Cataloguing-in-Publication Data
Gimenez, Rebecca.
  Technical large animal emergency rescue / Rebecca Gimenez, Tomas Gimenez. – 1st ed.
    p. ; cm.
  Includes bibliographical references and index.
  ISBN-13: 978-0-8138-1998-3 (alk. paper)
  ISBN-10: 0-8138-1998-9 (alk. paper)
1. Veterinary emergencies. 2. Animal rescue. 3. Domestic animals. I. Gimenez, Tomas. II. Title.
  [DNLM: 1. Animals, Domestic. 2. Emergencies–veterinary. 3. Rescue Work–methods. SF 778 G491t 2008]
  SF778G56 2008
  636.089'6025–dc22

                                                   2008001318

A catalogue record for this book is available from the U.S. Library of Congress.

Set in 9.5 on 12 pt Stone Serif by SNP Best-set Typesetter Ltd., Hong Kong
Printed in Singapore by Markono Print Media Pte Ltd

2   2009

Inside cover image: *Helping Hands, Helping Hearts*, by David J. Pavlak, was created to support the USRider Large Animal Rescue Endowment Fund at Eastern Kentucky University. For more information visit www.horseartgallery.com, or www.usrider.org.

This book is dedicated to the horse:
Who tolerates our predatory behavior while fated to carry us,
Who enabled our species to conquer empires and continents.
Who gives us the proverbial wings while on their backs,
Who teaches us patience and endures our mistakes.
The wind of the heavens in our faces blows twixt their ears,
May it ever be so.

Drs. Tomas and Rebecca Gimenez

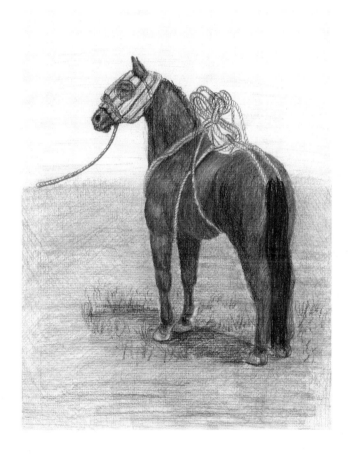

Table of Contents

Preface

TLAER AS A RESCUE SPECIALTY IS NEW

The public expects today's emergency response professional to have the knowledge and equipment to effectively respond to an increasing number of different situations (e.g., weapons of mass destruction, trench collapse, confined space rescue, domestic terrorism, agricultural bioterrorism, catastrophic natural disasters, hazardous materials). As the newest area in the fire/rescue professional's specialty cache of heavy rescue expertise, technical large animal emergency rescue (TLAER) methods encompass a wide variety of methods of manipulation and rescue tools to use to assist, shift, or lift an animal. Additionally, TLAER requires a good understanding of large animal victim behavior, particularly under the intense stress of the scene.

The goal for technical large animal emergency rescue is to remove a large animal from a hazardous environment without causing injury or death to the animal victim or to the rescuers. We believe this to be the first book for the professionals, drawn from a wide variety of groups, who may be involved on a TLAER scene. It is the hope of the authors that the material presented in this book will increase both the awareness of and surveillance by animal owners in order to prevent these types of incidents, as well as provide information on simple equipment and methods for emergency responders to use on scene.

The Word *Rescue*

In the animal protection and welfare worlds, the use of the word *rescue* has deviated from its original meaning and is commonly used to refer to animal starvation, neglect, and abuse scenarios that, unfortunately, are numerous. An Internet search of "horse rescue" yields a trove of organizations that provide rehabilitation to various animals, but none of these have training in TLAER techniques. There are numerous training courses for small animal handling, first aid, hoarding, cruelty investigation, etc. that do not exist for large animals. In many jurisdictions, large animal cruelty and neglect cases fall within the scope of animal control in coordination with local hooved animal protection societies or private "rescue" organizations. This occurs simply because the resources required to provide daily care for large animals are exorbitant when compared to the costs of caring for the small animals commonly seen in humane animal shelters. It is due to the expense that very few animal control agencies have facilities for quarantine or holding of large animals; they may have to refuse to respond to TLAER scenarios for this reason.

In this book, the word *rescue* is intended to refer to the technical aspects of heavy emergency rescue procedures, equipment, or methods that serve to lift, shift, or assist a large animal out of its predicament. No one incident scene is exactly the same as another, so this book attempts to provide general guidance and innovative ideas on response methodologies, rather than strict protocols. The responder will have to rely on his or her knowledge gained from this book as well as common sense to provide quality on-scene extrication leadership.

TESTED IN THE FIELD

The techniques presented in this book have been tested in the field, both on numerous actual rescue scenes and in multiple rescue training scenarios. Instructors have used large animal mannequins, plastic horses, and ultimately, live demonstration animals, to test the weight and variables specific to the large animal rescue environment (fractiousness, approachability, fear response, etc.). None of the information in this book is particularly new; rather, this book represents the first effort to collect all of the existing methodologies and philosophies in one usable reference. The book emphasizes, however, the importance of understanding large animal behavior as a crucial component of TLAER. Most of the techniques presented in this text have evolved over the years from field-expedient techniques and procedures used in live rescue; these techniques and procedures have been improved and refined by TLAER instructors and emergency response professionals. Demonstrations have been used as research and development methods. These demonstrations use trained animals (horses, dairy cattle, mules, and a llama) or untrained animals (horses, cattle) that have been sedated.

The Horse as a Model

In this book horses are used most commonly as models simply because they are most commonly involved in rescue efforts. However, these techniques, with minor modifications, apply to all types of large animals. Rescue is dangerous—period. Having a large animal victim involved raises the ante. This book emphasizes that large animal victims are unpredictable, strong, fast, fractious, and dangerous. Responders who prepare for the worst case scenario may be pleasantly surprised if the animals are docile and responsive in a way that does not further injure them and or a human. For each story of an animal panicking in those types of scenarios, there is a story about animals being trapped in barbed wire, hanging from bridges, trapped in mud or a carriage overturn lying quietly waiting for humans to help them. This requires trust in humans. For this reason, the chapter on animal behavior and perception is crucial to understand the animal's point of view.

CHANGING ATTITUDES

Large animal incidents are not rare, unusual, or freak accidents. The stacks of newspaper accounts, videotaped rescue attempts, written observer accounts by owners, and stories from veterinarians that the authors have collected over a 12-year period attest to the frequency of these incidents. Horror stories are recounted of well-intended rescuers being dragged, asphyxiated, crushed, injured, drowned, and dropped during attempted rescues in which the responders did not have the correct training. Many of these incidents are not reported because the owner or animal control officers write off the effort as a good try by well-meaning responders, not realizing that there are better ways to accomplish the mission. Recent students in TLAER-related courses have included professional and volunteer firefighters, technical rescue specialists, emergency medical services personnel, police officers, sheriff officers, emergency management personnel, public health officers, veterinarians, animal control officers, military special forces, and volunteer animal rescue humane groups. This book will detail simple procedures to be employed by these emergency first responders in what have become familiar, and unfortunately all too common, incidents.

Bring the Stakeholders Together

Over the last 12 years spent working on and observing documented emergency and disaster scenarios, the authors have noted that numerous rescues have required improved techniques on scene and that safety was often compromised. Most of the simple mistakes and safety offenses resulted from lack of communication between one group of people (emergency responders and law enforcement) who are knowledgeable about extrication, scene safety, and rescue, but not about large animals, and another group of people who do have knowledge about large animals (animal owners and veterinarians). Due to misunderstandings, the animal owner group may take a dim view of the methods and scene handling of the emergency responders or law enforcement and vice versa. In training and through educational materials, the large animal emergency rescue community has attempted to bring together these very diverse groups (emergency management, first responders, large animal owners and producers, veterinarians and staff, law enforcement) to discuss and improve all aspects of large animal emergency and disaster response.

Innovation Is Required

This book will discuss from basic to very advanced techniques of assisting large animals in an array of situations. But all incidents are different, requiring first responders to TLAER incidents to innovate based on their experience, training, and knowledge. Ideas and equipment are constantly improving and adapting to new technologies, so TLAER-related standard operation guidelines and protocols must be dynamic and flexible to add in new observations, equipment, and methodologies. Never say something cannot happen. For example, the author has documented in video and photography not one but two incidents of a two-horse bumper-pull trailer detached from the towing vehicle, resting on the back doors with the nose of the trailer pointed at the sky (with two live animals inside).

Prevention as a Theme

This book instructs the reader on response to incidents that have already occurred, not on methods of prevention or mitigation. However, large animal owners, employees, and professionals in those industries should have a grasp of the basics of TLAER methodologies relevant at the farm or facility level as part of their planning efforts to minimize the effects of disasters and the occurrence of emergencies within their areas of responsibility.

Prevention of incidents is an all-hazards approach to animal ownership that, if each individual owner and facility ascribed to it, would minimize calls to emergency services for many types of rescues. Providing prevention education to owners on a local, statewide, and national basis should be a focus of veterinary and cattle associations, saddle clubs, Pony Clubs, Future Farmers of America, and 4-H clubs; in association with emergency responders, these educational efforts could mitigate significant hazards and encourage local networking of an animal preparedness and response plan. In this vein, in 2006 the first U.S. national legislation to support the idea of animals being addressed as a crucial part of community disaster response planning was enacted.

Large Animals Are Different

Many governmental agencies lump all animal issues under one heading. The equipment and resources necessary to react to a large animal incident is orders of magnitude larger than that needed for small animal incidents. Although many of the methods discussed in this book are certainly applicable to small animal scenarios, generally small animal rescues will be very capably covered by the local animal control in a jurisdiction. However, very few animal control offices will have the resources to correctly deal with the scenarios described in this book.

A fundamental problem with large animal emergency response is that in many jurisdictions, animal control either is not able to do the large animal work (due to local guidance, lack of experience and training, or lack of facilities), or they respond to large animal neglect, starvation, and abuse cases but do not have the equipment and training to properly respond to TLAER rescue scenarios. For TLAER cases, animal control calls other emergency responders. In many communities with these challenges, there may be large animal neglect organizations that can set the standard for a relationship with animal control and can provide support in the form of transportation, TLAER equipment, and even aftercare facilities for large animals. For example, the Palmetto Equine Awareness and Rescue League is a 501(c)3 organization in South Carolina that has forged this relationship with the animal control officers in their region, providing transportation for large animals, specialty resources, trained TLAER volunteers with equipment, and even quarantine facilities for large animals to the animal control agencies in their jurisdictions.

WHY SO MANY ACCIDENTS?

Large animals are becoming increasingly common as companion animals in urban environments. Accidents involving large animals, especially horses, are becoming more common as people begin to live in more urban environments, purchase a diversity of livestock to include exotics for their farms, and travel across the country with their animals for show, breeding, and recreational purposes. Many owners may not know how to properly maintain, drive, and use farm equipment, trailers, and large farm vehicles or how to build and maintain safe fencing and facilities. Some people are not prepared and get lost out on the trail; others treat their large animals as pets; still others allow their animals to be trapped or injured on poorly maintained property. The lack of a basic evacuation plan plagues the large animal-owning public just as it does other groups who live in identified hazard zones (for natural and human-caused disasters). People in general are entering into much more personalized and close relationships with their animals; thus, euthanasia is not always an option. And even if the animal is severely injured, recent advances in veterinary medicine can often save it, and the owner will be willing to pay for it.

WHO KNEW?

When the 911 call comes for help in an incident involving a horse trailer or an overturned transport loaded with cows or pigs, emergency responders at the scene are expected to know how to handle a large animal incident in a safe and efficient manner. The public assumes that emergency responders will know something about large animal handling and extrication techniques when they call for assistance. However, informal surveys of the law enforcement community and fire services by the author has revealed that approximately 5% of emergency responders know something about handling large animals; even fewer report feeling comfortable actually handling a large animal on an incident scene. Certain local areas are fortunate to have a greater percentage of responders with animal experience and confidence, but generally there is a lack of experience in responders. Reflective of society, many emergency responders were raised in an urban environment and know very little about large animals.

Another common misconception is that a veterinarian or his or her staff will know more than a firefighter about how to save a horse or cow in some of the most common entrapments. Entrapment and rescue is a specialty of the fire and rescue services; they study and train for these eventualities. While in veterinary school, most students receive minimal to no training in technical large animal emergency rescue, disaster triage, or advanced handling of large animals. It is expected that if their interest is large animals, students will get that experience before coming to veterinary school or soon after they leave. Even subjects as common as the response to cast horses or downed cattle are rarely taught in veterinary school. The student is expected to learn those techniques in collaboration with a sponsor during a residency or internship. Over the last 12 years, the author has had numerous licensed veterinarians and certified veterinary technicians relate tragic tales of animals in scenarios (from the very easy to the very difficult) where the animal was lost or suffered severe iatrogenic injury due to lack of knowledge of better equipment and techniques.

This focus is changing. As of 2006, six veterinary schools in the United States have provided ongoing training to interested students in any aspect of technical large animal rescue. University of California-Davis had the very first veterinary emergency rescue team program in the early 1990s; Louisiana State University has offered training to individual students in aspects of rescue and use of slings; University of Florida initiated the VETS program in 2005; and North Carolina State University, University of Pennsylvania-New Bolton Center, and Tuskegee Universities have offered three-day short courses in the subject. The American Association of Equine Practitioners has recently promoted disaster preparedness education through student chapters at the veterinarian schools, bringing in nationally known speakers to increase awareness of disaster considerations. The American Veterinary Medical Association has promulgated numerous educational products for members and their clients through its disaster programs.

Improve the Standard of Care of Large Animal Victims

A basic presumption in this book is that a large animal emergency scene should be treated like any other extrication scene, including implementing incident command, scene safety and security, coordinating mutual aid, transportation assets, and professional (veterinary) support. A risk assessment and incident action plan should be made and followed. Few law enforcement or emergency medical personnel know how to work safely around large animals in rescue scenarios or how emotionally sensitive and medically delicate these animals can be; thus, veterinary support is crucial to the success and safety of the scene. Persons on scene with large animal experience should be employed as advisors or even as part of the incident operations team to help keep emergency responders safe around the animal. Review of videotaped rescues (as commonly shown on TV and privately loaned) and photographs have revealed numerous lapses in attention to patient care protocols, victim safety, and personnel conduct on scene. The techniques in this book illustrate examples of techniques used to accomplish moving the animal both vertically and horizontally, as well as approach and extrication concerns.

Fire and rescue and emergency medical support response personnel may not realize that they can apply some human rescue techniques to free these large, dangerous, terrified, and unpredictable animals. The same ideas of primary triage, first aid, medical support during the extrication, and packaging for transport to definitive care apply to large animals as well as humans. Despite strict standards of care in human extrication, on-scene treatment, and transport, it is far too common to see animals treated like a carcass—dragged by their neck, head, or legs. Such "rescues" are performed with the best intentions to help the animal, but are the direct result of lack of knowledge. The authors argue that a live animal victim (especially someone's pet or family member) should be offered a higher standard of care than a carcass!

The use of the techniques presented in this book requires the development of specific patient care protocols, standard operating procedures, and a rescue team trained to the existing standard in the use of this equipment. Professionals in emergency large animal critical care should be educated in the very latest technology and equipment available to them for use in everyday on farm scenarios, as well as emergency and disaster situations. Most of the principles, equipment, and techniques used in human rescue can be applied to large animal rescue.

Improve the Safety Margin for Responders

A review by numerous emergency rescue professionals of well-intentioned large animal rescue attempts worldwide, as commonly shown on TV and in private videotapes, have identified many critical responder safety offenses. These offenses are made by veterinarians, professional emergency responders, volunteer rescuers, owners, law enforcement, pilots, and the general public on scene. Many TLAER scenarios occur in concert with confined space, trench, hazardous material, mud, and swiftwater or floodwater concerns and require that the incident commander acknowledge and respond to these hazards. Improved procedures and effective alternatives to complete a successful technical rescue of large animals are available to responders and are outlined in this book. These techniques emphasize safety, planning, use of locally available equipment, incident management, training, responder safety, and understanding the behavior of large animals.

Use the Right Equipment

In many rescues, responders demonstrate a consistent lack of knowledge of the simple equipment and techniques that are commonly available to conduct TLAER rescues in an efficient manner. The equipment specific to each of these technologies is generally affordable and locally available, making it easy to collect into a large animal emergency rescue cache for a local fire and rescue squad, private veterinary practice or school, zoological park, or regional equine response unit. Some of the specialty equipment is not available for purchase and may require collaboration with a local fabricator, especially a welding shop. Although a number of items are designed specifically for large animal rescue, generally there is no need to reinvent the wheel.

Prioritize the Rescue

This book stresses at all levels the importance of selecting the appropriate rescue technique as part of the planning consideration on scene. There are many alternatives available to the animal owner and rescue team that are low-tech, lower risk, and much safer than using cranes, helicopters, or extreme rescue techniques to release animals from their entrapment. Specialty techniques exist for the removal of large animals trapped in mud, ravines, broken through ice, trapped in floodwaters, fallen into holes, and even downed from exhaustion or starvation. These options include the use of simple nylon webs (i.e., backwards drag, forward assist, horizontal or sideways drag, Hampshire slip), and they increase in complexity through the vertical lift systems (modified simple vertical lift web sling, air-assisted mud rescue, rope hauling and anchor systems, tripod and A-frame) to the transport of downed animals on a Rescue Glide sked. Only rare scenarios will require the highly technical, expensive, and high-risk involvement of a helicopter (usually due to extreme topography or flooding).

TLAER TRAINING PHILOSOPHY—A TIERED APPROACH

Awareness Level

For Awareness level training, a plastic horse or jointed large animal mannequin should be used to practice the basic methods and techniques of large animal rescue. It is a common problem that students will treat it like a plastic horse, and they don't expect it to move or kick. The larger stuffed or plastic mannequins attempt to simulate the weight of a horse, and some are jointed to simulate the movements of legs and neck for manipulation with webbing, rope systems, and restraint. The greatest benefit of mannequins is that they may be placed in practice scenarios that more closely simulate very difficult reality scenarios, where a live demonstration animal should never be placed. However, mannequins do not give students an opportunity to realize the strength and speed of a live animal in these scenarios. These mannequins are also excellent for trained teams of personnel who want to practice extremely

difficult scenarios on a training basis or to perform research.

Operational Level

For Operational level training, an introduction to basic containment, haltering, leading, restraint, and loading of live animals is a crucial part of any would-be rescuer's resume and should include many types of large animals. Students should not be allowed to become complacent around quiet or well-trained demonstration animals; these animals occasionally kick, bite, or react poorly despite their high level of training and normally quiet demeanor. The closer training is to reality, the better the students will react in a real situation—and it teaches them safety. It also will humble them. Many students initially become impatient and try using brawn to intimidate or force animals to do something instead of figuring out a better method. All prey animals only get more "hyper" and reactive when force is applied. *Note:* Anyone involved in this level or higher training should have a signed liability waiver.

Technical Level

For Operational and Technical level training, live animals should be used wherever possible to simulate as much as possible the reality of the worst case scenario. As students graduate to the technical levels, untrained animals may be introduced to practice advanced containment, leading, restraint, and loading of live animals. Simple procedures such as the forward assist should be attempted with untrained animals so that students learn about the normal reactions of unsedated, untrained animals.

USING LIVE ANIMALS FOR DEMONSTRATIONS

The authors feel strongly about the benefits of using live animals in demonstrations for students. The authors do use plastic horses, wooden horses, and even a plastic, realistic-weight mannequin to introduce the concepts of hands-on application of rescue equipment to students and to demonstrate safe handling behavior. Over the years, the authors realized that using these mannequins are excellent for Awareness level training and for extreme practice scenarios where a trained team must try to rescue a dummy horse from difficult circumstances. (The Fire Service uses a tiered training structure of Awareness, Operational, and Technical level training that the authors have tried to mirror in training courses.) However, after an Awareness level introduction of the basic concepts, the authors found that, both for safety reasons and to prevent complacency, students need to interact with a living, breathing, opinionated, and responsive animal to reinforce that the animal handling part of the rescue is often the most important element of the rescue effort.

Sedation

There are certain demonstrations that will always require slight sedation to maintain safety for the animal, in particular the Rescue Glide demonstration, often completed by the students as part of a night search and rescue scenario. With veterinary oversight, sedation for training scenarios can be used; however, even sedated animals can kick and bite as a side effect of the drugs. It is also possible to use untrained animals for these demonstrations if a veterinarian is part of the team and can administer a safe level of sedation. This will allow students to get close to the animal to perform a hands-on rescue training demonstration.

SUGGESTED TRAINING PROGRAM FOR DEMONSTRATIONS

Training animals to act as demonstrators for technical large animal emergency rescue training starts with imprinting at birth and continues with everyday training and handling. There are numerous excellent natural horsemanship teachers and clinicians (Pat Parelli, John Lyons, Clinton Anderson, Linda Tellington-Jones, On Target Training, etc.) available to animal owners. All of these animal/people training techniques and methods emphasize positive responses, encourage the building of a inter-species communication system, and use low stress and minimal force when training the animal.

The authors have found that application of these techniques is useful to prepare the animals for the introduction of unusual requests, such as asking the animal to lay down in front of crowds of students, perform vertical lifts without sedation, and allow various webbing configurations to be placed on their bodies. Without the cooperation of these animals, most of the photographs and contributions to TLAER knowledge presented within this volume would not have been possible. The authors consider these animals to be their close family members.

Training Demonstration Animals

When training demonstration animals, remember that everything is a learning experience. The trainer should try to document in writing (training journal) and photos the animal's special accomplishments out on trail rides, learning sessions, and doing things that seem to just be waiting to be done, such as learning to step up onto platforms, learning to stand quietly while other horses are running and jumping, and learning to lie down on command. The more exposure to unusual circumstances that the trainer can provide to a young animal, the more reliable the animal will be in a rescue demonstration situation. Learning to teach a horse to lie down is not unusually difficult; it requires patience, good communication, trust, and repetition on the human's part. However, asking a horse to lie down in front of 40 people, in the dark, and under strobe lights with a generator running—now that is much more difficult!

Teach animals to interact positively with humans at liberty in the round pen, lead them behind vehicles, pony behind another horse, and improve their general ground manners and on-halter respect. They should learn to negotiate many obstacles: getting up on a bridge or stairs, going over plastic when asked, and backing into their stall on command. These are daily requests of the young horse, and they get used to the idea that things that are abnormal for most horses are "normal" for them. From foalhood, teach them to lie down and even to allow you to turn them all the way onto their backs, then over to the other side. This teaches them that humans are not going to hurt them, even in their instinctually most vulnerable position. This training is supposed to be fun for both animal and human; they should get lots of scratching and petting for being quiet and calm.

Expose the horses to things as youngsters that they will see in their "job," for example, taking them to the lake to explore the mud and paw at the water. Eventually, this leads to going in the water to swimming depth together, following their buddies. Horses especially love nothing better than cool water after a hot and sweaty trail ride. The trainer wants his or her animal to be unafraid of water, crowds, loud noises, fast-moving flags, obstacles, vehicles, and other animals.

Natural horsemanship is a big part of daily life on the farm; try to incorporate the ideas and playtime into everything done with the animals so that they start to view humans as fun and interesting instead of boring and associated with work. Anything humans can think of that is different and will expand their animals' exposure to new situations and experiences (safely) should be tried. Lead them under scary overhead objects, take them to shows to get used to gobs of people moving and talking around them. One of the hardest things for most people is letting the horse think for itself, while giving it time to work out the right thing to do. This includes liberty work, yielding to direct and indirect pressure, learning to come to the trainer, all interspersed with a lot of on line work and games.

TRAINING MAKES FOR SUCCESSFUL RESULTS

On over 230 occasions since 1995, training scenarios based on the author's experiences with real life rescues have been used, along with the author's animals, to train professional emergency responders and veterinary personnel and to research new methods and techniques. Live demonstration animals (horses or a llama) have been used to demonstrate webbing configurations, the various sling systems, and the Rescue Glide and have been used in simulated or live practice helicopter sling loads. Most of these demonstrations do not require sedation for the animals. In each scenario, a trained demonstration animal is secured in the equipment by students. The "load" is then pulled by rope systems and is lifted by crane, a winch system with A-frame, or helicopter out of the training scenario's rescue environment (i.e., swamp, ravine, hillside, snow, or other significant terrain feature).

Each of these training scenarios has been successful, and there have been no injuries to demonstration animals or personnel.

INTO THE FUTURE

It is the sincere hope of the authors and collaborators of this book that the methodologies and equipment presented here will be used and improved by responders in the field, who will in turn provide feedback to the authors for dissemination in future editions of this text. As the ever-evolving field of specialty equipment and techniques in TLAER changes and educational opportunities become available, readers are encouraged to correspond with the authors regarding their suggestions and documentation of rescue efforts.

Dr. Rebecca Gimenez
Dr. Tomas Gimenez

Acknowledgments

No project of this size and scope is possible without the love and support of a broad section of colleagues, friends, family, and wonderful TLAER students who have eagerly contributed their experiences and knowledge from numerous life paths to this book. The initial concept of this book was to involve a wide cross-section of people in the animal industries who are interested in TLAER efforts and specifically to shine the spotlight on those that have moved the basic concepts of rescue of large animals from dreams to reality. The TLAER course needed a text to pull all the ideas from so many people together for the first time.

The people who set the stage for furthering of this technical form of specialty heavy rescue have come in the form of animal disaster response volunteers, animal hobbyists, veterinary professionals, firefighters, and emergency response teams worldwide. Lastly, there are those who have set the challenge for the animal industry to come up with better ways to address the technical and logistical issues associated with these 50–8,000 kg individual or mass casualty (disaster) animal victims, in coordination with other agencies and volunteers. Their combined interests and willingness to ask the hard questions in order to improve the standards of care have provided impetus to all of us.

I have tried to include the main people who supported me in this effort, but I am sure that I have forgotten someone; that is my fault alone. Numerous owners, various emergency responders, humane officers, and professionals in the veterinary fields have contributed their suggestions, ideas, and hard experiences to this collection over the years. Their names and faces may be lost to history, but I have tried to bring their contributions into an organized framework with this book. I hope that this effort will stimulate more ideas within this technical area of specialty heavy

rescue. After all, these efforts are for those who are mute and depend on us to assist them.

Thank you for writing the Introduction, Dr. Richard Mansmann. By sharing your knowledge and expertise you were my inspiration for making TLAER as a specialty come out of the shadows into the light of legitimacy. You were doing and preaching disaster medicine long before it was a cool buzzword. Similarly, Dr. Mellissa Nixon, you were a legend in the arena well before I met you on-line, then in person. Your introspection and guidance brought focus to the purpose and importance of this effort.

Thank you to the people who promised to leave me alone to write the text and refused to tempt me with offers of horseback trail-riding and glorious repasts on gorgeous days: Susan Melvin, Kris Yon, Kathy Powell, Dr. Kat Dooley, Sharri Harris, Dr. Mary Gabriel, and Becky Tolson. For offering to join me for coffee to discuss the effort, I thank Dr. Todd Linscott.

I offer my thanks to my outstanding contributing authors for their successful effort to herd large cats; Dr. Kimberly A. May, Dr. Janice Baker, Dr. Kathleen Becker, Lt. (Ret.) Jeff Galloway, Dr. Tomas Gimenez, Bob Mauck, Tori Miller, Dr. Lisa Murphy, Dawn Slessman, and Jennifer Woods. I hope that my humble efforts to edit and bring a similar style to your chapters is appreciated; the content you brought to this text is cutting edge in so many ways.

I thank my mentors from the U.S. Army at Ft. Bragg, North Carolina, who provided encouragement during my active duty tour from January to December, 2005, to finish the book in time: Major Mellissa Stanfa-Brew, Master Sergeant Donald B. Ross, Colonel Theresa Sullivan, Command Sergeant Major William Franklin, and Al Bazzarre. I thank my mentors at the 359th TSB, Ft. Gordon, Georgia, who supported continuing my Reserve military career while juggling the writing of this text: Brigadier General Geoff Freeman, Command Sergeant Major Jennifer Dettorty, Staff Sergeant David King, Lieutenant Colonels Janice Haigler, Scott Wisnieski, and Walter Milne. As I write this preface I am preparing for a deployment tour to Operation Iraqi Freedom. I hope my efforts will make you proud.

For supporting me with mental health through walking workouts and weight loss efforts between writing sessions I thank Ree Cooley, MSG Donald Ross, Nicole Walukewicz, Katelyn Johnston, Sharri Harris. Here I stand 56 pounds lighter despite the thousands of hours in front of the computer!

Thank you Ree Cooley for taking wondrous care of my "children," the nine horses, llama, cat, dogs, tegu, and snakes that I had to leave at home while I traveled for speaking and teaching engagements or served at Ft. Bragg. You are always there with new ideas and encouragement.

For their constant encouragement, technical advice, editing, and assistance I thank Janice Baker, Slim Ray, Pat Gillespie, Becky Kalagher, Helen Keulemans, Bill Slusher, Mark Cole at US Rider, Inc., Paul Baker, SGM (Ret.) Ronald Biggs, Ree Cooley, Tanya Rayes, Tori Miller, Marietta Gambrell, Harold Martin, Mary Durnin, Nicole Walukewicz, Dr. Mary Gabriel, Dr. Keith Stafford, and a Wilde Yankee Rose. I know there were times you thought that I was changing my name to Tom Sawyer, but together we got the fence painted! I prefer to think of it as excellent delegation skills.

For transcribing tapes of our lectures and editing assistance, I thank Nichole Walukewicz, who came into my life at the right time to assist me with documenting the technical details of the book. I thank Pat Belskie for devoting many hours to proofreading all the text. Isn't it amazing how experiences of a previous chapter in your life came to fruition in this book? Thank you for scanning all those pictures, Sharri Harris. You are always there for me when I think that I cannot get it done. Your encouragement is always valuable, and your friendship through all the challenges was solid. I offer a huge thank you to Erica Judisch, my contact at Wiley-Blackwell; your hands-off approach worked.

Thank you to my wonderfully supportive parents Carolyn and Michael Durak, who alternatively pulled and pushed me through the first 17 years of my life and since then have served as a touchstone for advice and guidance. Dad, your artwork is fantastic, and I am proud to include it here.

For their technical advice and artistic contributions to the book I thank CPT Mark Mellott, Pat Gillespie, Becky Tolson, and my main artists, Michael Durak and Julie Casil. You made it come alive! Multiple photographers sent pictures for inclusion in the book, but particularly Tori Miller and Axel Gimenez are to be thanked for their time and excellent attention to detail. I wish that I could have included everything in the stories and pictures that I've received over the years.

To my sweet husband Tomas, thank you for supporting me through all the trials and tribulations of generating and finishing this worthwhile project. May our efforts be of assistance and usefulness to new generations of emergency services personnel, owners, and veterinary practitioners who value the lives and dignity of these animals with whom our lives are intricately woven.

I was once asked by a student why I am so passionate about conducting training to potential animal emergency responders from all walks of life and varieties of experience. My response at the time was: I am just trying to make things better for the animals. If, 50 years from now, the concept of a technical specialty in the area of large animal rescue is a mainstream thing, like the concept of paramedics for humans is today, then I will have rightly completed my life's work for the greater good. This would be my legacy to the world of animals. Let me go to no heaven without them.

For you—you know who you are. You give me the breath of life.

No acknowledgement would be complete without thanks to our demonstration animals that have made it possible for us to experiment with better methods and equipment. From the time they came out of the placenta they patiently allowed us to lay them down, flip them over, tie them up, and hang them from various appliances.

And finally a thanks to you, dear reader, for your interest in this worthwhile subject. I hope that future editions of this text will be improved with your suggestions and comments.

Rebecca Gimenez
Pendleton, South Carolina

Contributors

Dr. Janice L. Baker
Vass, NC 28394
stormyjb@earthlink.net

Dr. Kathleen Becker
President
Hast, Inc.
Floyd, VA 24091
becker@hast.net

Jeff Galloway
President
Emergency Training Systems, Inc.
Clarkrange, TN
jpjgalloway@aol.com

Dr. Rebecca M. Gimenez
Rebecca.gimenez@us.army.mil
Pendleton, SC 29670

Dr. Tomas Gimenez
Primary Instructor
tlaer@bellsouth.net
Pendleton, SC 29670

Dr. Richard Mansmann
Director, Equine Health Program
University of North Carolina College of Veterinary Medicine
Chapel Hill, NC
ccep@mindspring.com

Bob Mauck
Diversified Business Services, Inc.
DeMotte, IN
bob.dbsinc@mchsi.com

Dr. Kimberly Ann May
Assistant Director of Professional and Public Affairs
American Veterinary Medical Association
kmay@avma.org

Dr. Lisa Murphy
Assistant Professor of Pathobiology and Toxicology
University of Pennsylvania College of Veterinary Medicine
    at New Bolton Center
Kennett Square, PA murphylp@vet.upenn.edu

Dawn R. Slessman
Director
Nature's Way Animal Rescue
Bristol, IN
nwar@verizon.net

Jennifer Woods
Primary Instructor, Consultant
Reflected J Livestock /J Woods Livestock Services
Blackie, Alberta. Canada
livestockhandling@mac.com
www.reflectedjlivestock.com

Statement of Humane Treatment

None of the animals used in training courses, laboratories, or demonstrations were subjected to pain or distress. Photographs of many of the scenarios, procedures, and methodologies in this text are of these animals that are the personally owned "family members" of the authors. No animals were used in training scenarios that could potentially cause pain, injury, or distress. Only trained demonstration animals were used in training courses, laboratories, and demonstrations.

Mild sedation was used in some scenarios to prevent any possible distress from the procedures or to prevent the animal possibly injuring itself and was administered by a licensed veterinarian in each case. The animal's well being and level of comfort was constantly monitored during all training exercises and demonstrations, often by multiple humane officers and veterinarians.

Introduction

Dr. Richard Mansmann

Technical Large Animal Emergency Rescue is a specialty function within a new branch of veterinary medicine called Disaster Medicine. In veterinary emergency medicine and critical care, the situation involves one patient and that veterinary practice and its staff. In Disaster Medicine there is usually more than one patient; but more than one veterinarian is needed to have a reasonable outcome. Much of Disaster Medicine response success is related to pre-hospital planning and work. And these responders, including the veterinarian, need training in triage and specialty techniques needed to resolve the local emergency or very large disaster. In Santa Barbara, CA in the mid 1980's, my colleagues and I would get called for horses fallen over cliffs, stuck in ravines, trapped in trailer accidents or fires. Not only were we being called to assist with the horse's health issues created by the emergency or disaster, but also to figure out how to extricate these animals from these unusual natural and man-made situations. We were being looked to as the sole problem solver; but it was obvious to us that we needed additional help, training and skills in these circumstances. It was up to those of us that were interested to devise new ways to assist individual large animals trapped in what were at times dangerous and outrageous circumstances. Over the intervening years, many people have devoted countless hours of research and development to solving the difficult management, equipment and technique problems of assisting large animals in numerous scenarios. I am now honored to be asked to write the introduction to this first book on the subject of Technical Large Animal Emergency Rescue which introduces many of the ideas of Disaster Medicine while emphasizing what individuals can do on an emergency scene to assist large animals.

At that time, the California Veterinary Medical Association also was thinking of ways to help their clients during disasters. The original ideas of Disaster Medicine for humans was related to the global nebulous threat of the atomic bomb but now was being expanded to include assisting with locally common problems. What we veterinarians did was to begin organizing interested horse owners at evening educational meetings and discussing ideas of how we could work together to help our fellow horse owners in a disaster situation. The group called themselves the Equine Assistance and Evacuation Team and began working with local emergency management and emergency services personnel.

Like almost any other area, the impetus to disaster planning came in the form of a real disaster to bring organization to true fruition. In 1990, the Painted Cave Fire struck the area and left 300–400 horses homeless while killing 25 horses. The homeless horses were sheltered at the Earl Warren show grounds for up to three weeks and the necessity of applying the theoretical planning of the previous 5 years to the reality of the situation was obvious. After that summer, planning became in earnest and the Santa Barbara Humane Society stepped in to help the organization with funding for the equipment, meeting sites, and paddocks for displaced animals. This was a model situation and we knew that other communities would benefit from hearing our story and solutions. The Santa Barbara Humane Society sponsored the First International Conference on Equine Rescue in Santa Barbara, CA in 1993 and the Second International Conference on Equine Rescue in Southern Pines, NC in 1995. People from all over the world who were interested in sharing their ideas and learning from each other about disaster and emergency response brought their knowledge into these forums, and professionalism grew. Coincidently, Hurricane Andrew struck south Florida in 1992 and created a whole new level of challenge and emphasis on disaster planning for humans and animals within the United States.

I was involved in some of the early thinking in disaster planning for horses, but other people were instrumental, too. Mr. Clark Beckstead, a farrier from Santa Barbara, CA who single-handedly first started organizing people that day to take care of the horses in the Painted Cave Fire. Mr. Don Cole, the executive director of the Santa Barbara Humane Society made many things happen for the local horse owners to enhance the EAET with equipment, facilities and continues to support local disaster planning to this day. Without Dr. Sebastian Heath's ideas and encouragement, a lot of our ideas would have gone for naught. Dr. Heath's programs at Purdue University with veterinary students and his dealings with the state of Indiana gave him excellent insight to help organizations and individuals deal with the aftermath of Hurricane Andrew. He subsequently joined forces with FEMA to create online independent study courses to train responders in aspects of disaster planning for animal communities and individuals.

Other states have seen the wrath of natural disasters and subsequently have become more involved with disaster planning for animals and their agriculture industries. Florida, North Carolina, South Carolina and newly affected states like Alabama, Mississippi, Louisiana, and Texas are coming on board due to the seriousness of their disaster potential and reflect an important emphasis at all levels on the need for mitigation, planning and an organized response as part of the Incident Command System. Planning and prevention are historically not attractive items for large animal owners or the public to consider or fund; but no state, locality or individual is immune. This book does not go into detail on prevention but offers enough actual scenarios to stimulate the reader to draw conclusions for their individual situations. The cohesive notion that humans might not evacuate a disaster zone without consideration of their animals' welfare began to surface in the 1980's for state, federal and non-governmental organization (NGO) planners to consider. The importance of this effect on people was reflected in new legislation promulgated in 2006 to require pets and animals to be included in community disaster planning at all levels.

Each reader of this book should think in terms of what is their plan for their own animals, and coordinate with the emergency management and response professionals in their community. Disaster and emergency planning begins fundamentally with the individual owner and it works better from the bottom up, not the top down. Then expand that planning into a Neighborhood Watch type program. You will not get all your neighbors to participate, but those who feel it is important will bring their own skills, facilities and equipment assets to the effort. For instance, if one person has a larger barn, then they could store a hay supply for 7 days for the neighborhood's horses. Or neighbors could get together and purchase a few large tanks so that fresh water will be available for all the neighbors' horses for 7 days. Making the decisions of evacuation (who goes, who stays, how horses are to be moved, where they will go, and are horses broke to load) are critical pre-disaster assessments for everyone, as was witnessed in the various hurricanes and wild fires of the past decade. At the very basic level, having a local cache of simple but effective rescue equipment that allows volunteers to be able to respond to the everyday emergencies such as trailer accidents, minor or major chemical spills, or barn fires is much more important and commonplace than a catastrophic hurricane disaster. Local efforts and education within your own county and livestock / horse organizations is a critical starting point for an all-hazards approach to planning. A natural outgrowth would be more organized approaches to seemingly simple emergencies, like helping a neighbor and their veterinarian to get a colicky horse successfully trailered to a veterinary hospital with on-board fluid therapy. This would be an exciting addition to pre-hospital care of equine patients. A good Neighborhood Watch type program could coordinate this effort and become a major asset to the regional tertiary care equine hospitals. It would increase positive hospital stay outcomes and reduce owner costs. Including those regional tertiary veterinary caregivers in the neighborhood planning discussions would be helpful to owners and help animals, too.

Certainly, this book will bring forth new ideas and techniques and serve as an excellent resource for owners, veterinarians and emergency personnel and these emerging ideas and techniques will expand over time. I hope you read this book and put some parts of it into action planning once you set it down. Use it as a reference, contribute your ideas and successes on scene to future editions. You may find that by practicing the techniques and adopting the philosophies offered in this text, your attitudes change and make your perspective more of an all-hazards assessment. My hope is that as aspects of Large Animal Disaster Medicine begin to grow more rapidly, the teaching of this new specialty will spread; first locally, then nationally and internationally, and eventually that it will be taught at the veterinary colleges.

Over the years my dream of increasing the stature and professionalism of Equine Disaster Medicine has thought that the major future champions and supporters should include organizations like the US Cavalry Association. The Cavalry certainly learned and have had experience in all kinds of emergencies and disasters, providing major movements and training related to horses and serious situations from Valley Forge to Petersburg in the past to Afghanistan today. As an example, that organization could make available to animal owners throughout the US many of their time-honored skills that are swiftly being replaced by modern mechanical military machinery, offering a way that the US Calvary could continue its tradition not only in the memories of a few older people, but be brought forth to become part of active success stories amongst horse owners today and in the future.

Enjoy this book and put this information into action to help horses!

Richard A. Mansmann, VMD, PhD
Director of the Equine Health Program
North Carolina State University
College of Veterinary Medicine
Raleigh, North Carolina

TECHNICAL LARGE ANIMAL EMERGENCY RESCUE

1 Historical Overview and Development

Dr. Rebecca Gimenez

INTRODUCTION

Animal emergency rescue, and disaster medicine in general, are being taken more seriously by the veterinary, medical, and emergency response communities. Historically, animals were left to fend for themselves in large-scale disasters, while human welfare was the priority. Recent surveys have shown that the human–animal bond is strong enough to cause many animal owners to refuse to evacuate their homes without their pets in a disaster. Following recent natural disasters, animal owners expressed great frustration at being unable to rescue stranded animals or enter declared disaster areas to check on the welfare of their animals. Over the years, with the involvement of humane and veterinary organizations, formalized plans and protocols for providing animal rescue resources and access at the local, state, and federal level have been promulgated (Figure 1.1).

ANIMALS AND DISASTERS—A HISTORICAL PERSPECTIVE

Animal Welfare in the Nineteenth Century and the Birth of the Animal Welfare Movement

Humane welfare groups initially concerned themselves with large-animal cruelty, abuse, and neglect issues. Most of the early humane societies were formed to assist horses, livestock, and draft animals, not for companion animals such as the dogs and cats that are their focus today.

Horses and oxen were the main methods of transportation of goods and people in the early nineteenth century, but they were often subjected to abuse and neglect at the hands of drivers who did not own the animals. Coach and draught horses were frequently neglected or abused due to prevailing attitudes and lack of education.

The honor of being the first person in the world to champion a law relating to the fair treatment of animals went to Richard "Humane Dick" Martin of the United Kingdom, who brought an ass (donkey) into the courthouse to allow the magistrate to view its wounds and ensure that the offending owner was fined. This brought vast publicity to the plight of animals, ironically in a time when children were often more poorly treated and abused than working animals. Richard Martin's Act, passed on July 22, 1822, allowed prosecution for cruelty to farm animals.

The organized animal welfare effort began in the United Kingdom with the Society for the Prevention of Cruelty to Animals (SPCA) in 1824. The first years of the SPCA in England were shaky at best, until Queen Victoria awarded it "royal" status and the organization became the RSPCA in 1840. It is now arguably the most prestigious and active humane organization in the world, and its model has been copied in dozens of countries. Due to the RSPCA's efforts to improve harness horse welfare, a quick release mechanism was designed in 1874 that allowed rapid disengagement of a horse fallen in the traces. This principle is still used today by drivers, yachtsmen and the U.S. military.

A charter for the proposed American Society for the Prevention of Cruelty to Animals (ASPCA), modeled on the RSPCA, was brought before the New York legislature by Henry Bergh and was passed on April 10, 1866; nine days after it was passed, the first anti-cruelty law to animals in the United States was passed, with the ASPCA granted the right to enforce the law. At Bergh's death in 1888, 37 states (of the existing 38 in the Union) had passed animal cruelty prevention laws, with humane societies and animal shelters opening across the United States. One of the ASPCA's most

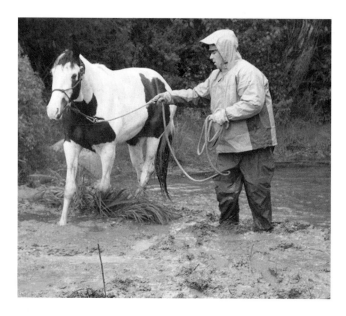

Figure 1.1 *A responder practices leading a horse through mud while escaping a flooded barn scenario. Personnel who have experienced large animal emergency scenarios agree that basic handling skills and understanding of behavior are crucial to safety and success. Courtesy of Claudia Sarti.*

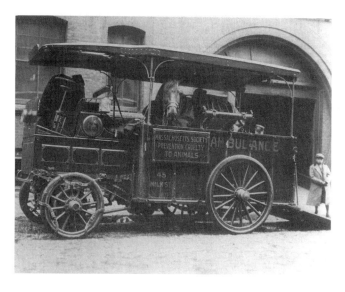

Figure 1.2 *An early motorized MSPCA ambulance for large animals featured a slinging device to hold animals that were too weak to maintain a standing position during transport for veterinary treatment. Courtesy of Massachusetts Society for the Protection of Animals.*

significant early contributions was providing fresh drinking water to the cart and streetcar horses in Manhattan. In 1867, the ASPCA operated the world's first equine ambulance for injured horses and by 1875 had created a crude sling for downed horses to be lifted in a stall for treatment.

Shortly after the ASPCA was established, the Massachusetts Society for the Prevention of Cruelty to Animals (MSPCA) was formed in March 1868. The MSPCA was actually founded when a Boston lawyer, George T. Angell, heard about a horse race in which two horses, each bearing two riders, were raced to their deaths over 40 miles of rough roads. His high-profile protest of the race drew local citizens together, resulting in the provision of newsletters and educational materials to the public and direct assistance to animals. In 1890, the MSPCA published and distributed over 2 million free copies of the first American edition of *Black Beauty*, written by Anna Sewell, to raise public awareness of cruelty to horses.

Also based on the RSPCA's model, the Society for the Prevention of Cruelty to Animals-Australia (RSPCA-Australia) was formed in Victoria in 1871. Other SPCAs formed in Tasmania (1872), New South Wales (1873), South Australia (1875), Queensland (1883), and Western Australia (1892). The first paid inspector was appointed in 1883, with honorary inspectors appointed throughout the country. The 1885 Annual Report of RSPCA-Australia recorded that educational literature was being distributed to owners, drivers, and farriers. The regional SPCAs were awarded royal status in 1956, and they combined to form the RSPCA Australia in 1981.

Harvard University's veterinary hospital was opened in 1884, with horses making up the majority of its caseload. With the assumption that horses would no longer be necessary as cars became more available and affordable, the hospital closed in 1904.

The Early and Mid-Twentieth Century—Floods, Wars, and the Equine Ambulance

In Australia early laws were more concerned with damage to animals as property, but the 1901 Animals Protection Act (APA) was specifically aimed at preventing cruelty to animals. The 1925 amendment to the APA gave legal status to the RSPCA-Australia and specific powers to its officers.

In 1910, the MSPCA purchased the first motorized horse ambulances (Figure 1.2) with sling support systems, including one with a trailer (Figure 1.3).

In 1917, the MSPCA opened the first permanent animal shelter at Nevins Farm in Methuen, Massachusetts, to care for retired police horses and other working animals. It remains the centerpiece of their large animal work today.

The American Humane Animal Emergency Services (Red Star) provided services to war animals beginning in 1916. During World War I (1914–1918), the secretary of war officially requested the American Humane Association take over the war animal relief effort in the United States. They raised money for supplies and ambulances for horses, as well as volunteer veterinarians and assistants. The entry of the United States into World War I in 1917 tipped the balance in favor of an Allied victory. Long before the United States sent its men into the struggle, it had sent another resource—its

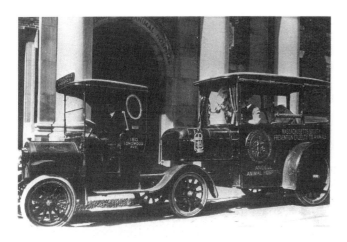

Figure 1.3 *This early motorized MSPCA equine recovery vehicle featured one of the first trailers as the ambulance. In an era where the abuse of children was still not receiving significant notice, public support for improving large animal welfare was very vocal. Courtesy of Massachusetts Society for the Protection of Animals.*

horses and mules. The United States was called upon to supply the Allied forces with cavalry remounts and working horses, exporting nearly a million horses to Europe. When the American Expeditionary Force entered the war, it took with it an additional 182,000 horses. Of these, 60,000 were killed, and only 200 were returned to the United States. World War I used horses in great numbers for noncavalry purposes. It is estimated that some 6 million horses served, and considerable numbers of these were killed in the line of duty.

In one year, 1918, British veterinary hospitals treated 120,000 horses for diseases. Like human combatants, horses required ambulances and field veterinary hospitals to care for the sick and injured. Motorized horse ambulance vans were used as equine ambulances on the western front.

The Boston Molasses Flood of January 15, 1919, involved large animals by pure chance, at a time when the use of mechanized transportation was increasing. A tank holding over 8.7 million liters (2.3 million gallons) of molasses ruptured, resulting in a molasses wave 7.5 m (over 24 ft) high that traveled at 56 kilometers per hour (35 miles per hour) through the North End of Boston. The wave overwhelmed a livery stable and several horses owned by the city, which were hitched to municipal carts, at the North End Paving Yard (a department of public works municipal yard) located just 25 meters (82 feet) from the molasses tank. Approximately 20 horses were killed in the flood, some immediately from the molasses wave; others were trapped in the viscous fluid as it quickly hardened. Humane and police officers dispatched the trapped animals that evening (Puelo, 2003). This local disaster helped focus the public's attention on the welfare of large animals in emergencies.

The great Mississippi flood of 1927 was the first disaster that involved humane officers and volunteers from animal protection and welfare societies across the United States. The Mississippi River and its tributaries flooded Arkansas, Illinois, Kentucky, Louisiana, Mississippi, and Tennessee with up to 10 meters (30 feet) of floodwaters. This was the first massive-scale disaster animal rescue effort, and although poorly organized, clearly indicated the public's support for assisting animals trapped by natural and human-caused disasters.

During World War II (1939–1945), animal protection reached a fever pitch on the war front as well as at home. In 1939, the RSPCA published a pamphlet, "Air Raid Precautions for Animals," and sold more than 100,000 copies. Due to the demand for the pamphlet, five subsequent editions were published. After one bombing blitz, three horses were found by humane officers, unhurt but trapped in their stable. To free them, a building was demolished in the East End of London. Thousands of dollars were raised for the horses at war and were sent by animal societies around the world to purchase blankets and veterinary supplies. This effort was based on the 1914 Geneva treaty called the International Red Star Alliance. This was the first treaty intended to foster international cooperation on behalf of sick and wounded war animals and secured neutrality for those providing assistance to the animals in times of war.

Advances During the Late Twentieth Century—The Birth of Organized Response Efforts

The Humane Society of the United States (HSUS) began in 1954 with an animal welfare education mission, and it is currently considered the lead nongovernmental organization in the United States championing the response to animals in disasters.

The Veterinary Academy on Disaster Medicine was begun in 1983 by founding members, including Dr. Robert Shomer, VMD (elected first president), and Dr. Ole H.V. Stalheim, DVM, PhD (first secretary). This organization is now known as the American Academy on Veterinary Disaster Medicine and serves to distribute information about animal disaster medicine to veterinary staff (AAVDM, 2002).

In 1985, volunteers from across the country, animal control, and other rescue groups joined the Humane Society of Missouri (HSM) employees in a daring rescue of 55 horses at Creve Coeur Stables, saving these horses from drowning after the Missouri River levy surrendered to floodwaters. A few years later, the HSM worked 24-hour operations to help thousands of pets displaced by the great flood of 1993. The Mississippi and Missouri rivers overflowed their banks in Illinois, Iowa, Kansas, Minnesota, Missouri, Nebraska, North Dakota, South Dakota, and Wisconsin; this was considered to be the worst U.S. disaster since the great Mississippi flood of 1927. Animals were rescued from abandoned homes and dangerous environments by trained teams of field rescuers, and temporary foster homes were found while the displaced owners rebuilt.

In 1988, the University of California-Davis School of Veterinary Medicine's Veterinary Emergency Response Team (UCD-VERT) was organized. Students, faculty, and staff were trained in the use of technical equipment to rescue animals and worked with local and state humane organizations and government agencies to practice mock disaster drills.

In 1991, a prototype Anderson Sling was developed to fully and comfortably support the weight of a horse, developed by UCD-VERT advisor Dr. John Madigan and the late Mr. Charles Anderson (founder of Care for Disabled Animals). That same year, the team was called to rescue five mules and a horse trapped in the Sierra Mountains. All of the animals were successfully airlifted 4 miles to solid ground, representing a breakthrough in large animal rescue equipment.

In 1999, the UCD-VERT team responded to a call to assist with the helicopter lift of five horses in a flooded North Carolina disaster zone following Hurricane Floyd and brought large animal rescue to the international stage on Cable News Network (CNN). This team has continued their research into new technologies for equine rescue.

A disaster animal rescue team (DART) for horses and livestock was developed after Hurricane Andrew in 1992 in Florida, and similar teams for companion animals (including horses) were developed in affected states after Hurricanes Floyd (1999), Katrina (2005), and Rita (2005).

In 1993, a group of veterinarians with an interest in disaster medicine and a concern that animal issues during national disasters were not being sufficiently considered approached the American Veterinary Medical Association (AVMA) for assistance. As a result, the AVMA negotiated an agreement with the Office of Emergency Preparedness of the U.S. Public Health Service (USPHS). With the signing of a Memorandum of Understanding in May 1993, veterinary services became incorporated into the Federal Response Plan for disaster relief as part of the National Disaster Medical System (NDMS). The NDMS system was developed to provide supplemental medical care to victims of catastrophic disasters in the event state and local resources are overwhelmed and federal assistance is required. Federal recognition of the need for animal care provided the framework for veterinary professionals to be organized into Veterinary Medical Assistance Teams (VMATs) that would respond to the needs of animals during a disaster in the same way that disaster medical assistance teams provide medical aid to human casualties of disasters. VMATs remain the only response teams recognized in the National Response Plan (NRP) that provide veterinary medical treatment and address animal and public health issues resulting from natural, human-caused, or any other type of disasters. VMATs are available to assist the United States Department of Agriculture in the control, treatment, and eradication of animal disease outbreaks. VMATs are deployed in response to an invitation from the affected state after a disaster has been declared and a request for federal assistance has been submitted and approved. If a state alone requests a VMAT, the state is financially responsible for the response effort (AVMA, 2002). The World Trade Center disaster (September 11, 2001) was the first time that VMAT teams were deployed to support the dogs of the Federal Emergency Management Agency (FEMA) Urban Search and Rescue task forces. Since that time, the teams have regularly worked together on training and actual missions. As of 2008, VMAT teams officially changed their name to NVRT (National Veterinary Response Teams).

In the United States, Dr. Richard Mansmann, with the Santa Barbara Humane Society (California), was instrumental in promoting the First and Second International Conferences on Equine Emergency Rescue held in the early 1990s in California and North Carolina. These conferences brought the leaders in the large animal (specifically equine) disaster medicine area together from across the country and internationally to share their ideas and methodologies; the presentations were published in an international veterinary journal to increase the awareness of these issues. Since that time, there has been an expansion of published large animal rescue techniques and information within the veterinary and emergency response literature, culminating in this text.

The MSPCA Animal Disaster Relief Fund was established in 1993 to aid with protection and rescue efforts for animals around the globe. In 1995, the MSPCA launched the Equine Ambulance Program under the direction of founders Joe Silva and Roger Lauze to establish one of the first training programs in equine rescue and emergency transport. To date, the program has trained more than 4,000 people around the globe (Lauze, 2006). Also in 1995, the MSPCA developed the first Rescue Glide, changing the way recumbent (downed) animals were transported. With this "equine stretcher" came a streamlined way to allow recumbent horses (who previously may have had no chance of survival) to be transported to a veterinary hospital. Today the Rescue Glide concept and modifications of the original design are used around the world.

In 1994, Trail Riders of DuPage, Illinois (TROD), developed and presented their Equine Rescue Techniques course under project leader Kandee Haertel. Since that time, TROD has educated hundreds of local emergency responders in surrounding jurisdictions on basic to intermediate catching, leading, loading, and handling skills, particularly with horses as a model. This course was designed for first-response emergency personnel to get didactic and practical training with horses and develop confidence about safe horse handling (Haertel, 1999).

The TROD course is very specific: response to traffic accidents involving a loaded horse trailer. By keeping the focus narrow, it became applicable to all fire and police districts, and students received a reference manual for on-scene use. The training begins with basic catching, haltering, and leading techniques and continues with each student leading an excited horse through an obstacle course. These skills help the student deal with dangerous and challenging scenarios, such as a horse loose by the side of the road (Figure 1.4). Using the safe leading methods and principles of leverage that they have already been taught allows even the smallest and physically weakest student to maintain relative control of the situation and get the animal to move where it is wanted. This is an excellent example of a local citizen group providing a necessary instructional resource to emergency response professionals, providing expertise that they cannot get elsewhere.

Code 3 Associates of Erie, Colorado, has been providing education and animal disaster relief services throughout the United States since the mid-1990s with a mobile animal command center. Founder Nan Stuart stated that their mission is not only to respond to disasters, but also to educate and train local organizations in disaster preparedness and response for animal issues. Code-3 annually offers several large animal rescue courses nationwide, such as the Technical Animal Rescue and Big Useful Livestock Lessons, and is actively involved in large animal cruelty investigations training for animal control or humane officers. Any type of natural disaster can elicit Code 3's response by request

through the state to provide emergency veterinary services. Their vehicle, Big Animal Response Truck, is a 70-foot tractor trailer featuring a mobile field hospital and surgical suite for small animals, as well as emergency gear and first aid supplies for large animals, portable livestock corrals, water rescue gear, and one week's supply of food and water for humans and animals. During transport, the unit houses a truck and a two-horse trailer that are wheeled out for local use. In the 1990s, Animal Planet network and the American Humane Association teamed up to sponsor a similar educational and response vehicle in the form of a mobile command center that could deploy to disaster zones.

In the mid 1990s, the Felton (California) Fire Protection District's Large Animal Rescue Program came under the direction of firefighters CPT John Fox and his wife Debra. Together, they wrote the curriculum for Large Animal Rescue and submitted it to the California State Fire Marshal in 2003 to provide train-the-trainer concepts to emergency responders in their state. They were the first to provide actual hands-on large animal rescue training specifically tailored to emergency responders and to apply many of the concepts of human heavy rescue to large animals (Figure 1.5). Their training emphasizes the use of backpacks pre-rigged specifically with special equipment for technical large animal emergency rescue (TLAER). John and Debra Fox have pursued research and development of life-size horse models and even a close-to-live-weight, bendable-limb, plastic mannequin named Lucky for very realistic scenario trainings (Figure 1.6). Their team responds to several large animal incidents a month within a four-county area due to extreme geography and a high-

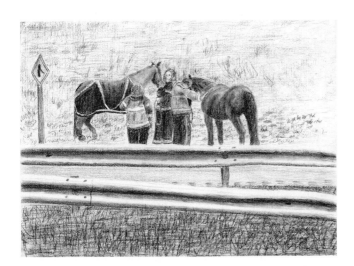

Figure 1.4 *One of the most challenging places to handle large animals is along the side of an active road. Handlers should keep animals away from the active scene but close to each other, encourage relaxation by providing forage or allowing animals to graze, and consider secondary containment. Courtesy of Julie Casil.*

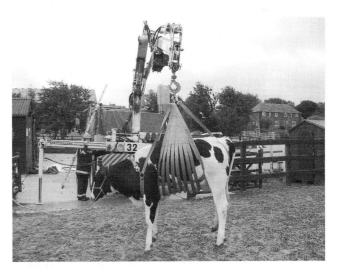

Figure 1.5 *TLAER students in the United Kingdom learn vertical lift techniques with an unsedated dairy cow demonstrator. Interested firefighters participate in a multiday course that teaches animal handling skills as well as technical aspects of equipment to be used on the animals for various scenarios. Courtesy of Paul Baker.*

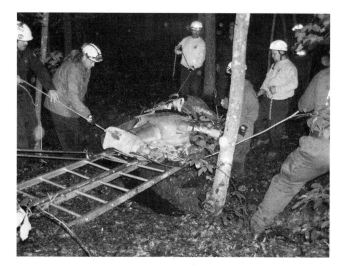

Figure 1.6 *Large animal mannequins may be used for advanced operational and technical level training scenarios, such as in this Winston-Salem Rescue Squad night field rescue training, which used Lucky the Horse Rescue Mannequin. In the scenario, the "animal" was moved on a Rescue Glide by personnel several hundred meters through deep woods, across this creek, and up a steep bank into the waiting equine ambulance. Courtesy of Tomas Gimenez.*

density local horse population. Their large animal training course has been offered all over the West Coast, and they continue to provide leadership in their state and nationally addressing these issues.

In 1995 communications between Dr. Venaye Reece (with Clemson Poultry and Livestock Health) and Shawn Jones (of the Charleston County Emergency Preparedness Division) emphasized the need for an organized large animal rescue team (LART) in the state of South Carolina. At the same time, Dr. Tomas Gimenez was developing an applicable workshop for veterinarians at Clemson University in South Carolina. The first Technical Large Animal Rescue course was held in August of 1997 at the Berkeley County Fire Training Grounds in Moncks Corner, South Carolina. Under the direction of Chief Ricky Metzler, the squad designed a heavy rescue truck that included a 10-ton extensible crane, with large animal rescues in mind. Working with the Low Country Saddle Club, various business and individuals around the area contributed funding for equipment. Large animal rescue Special Operations Groups for responders and dispatch centers were developed and implemented with success. With the creation of the County Agriculture Animal Response Teams (CART) with funding from the Department of Homeland Security (DHS), the LART has acquired training aids to teach local responders the basics of large animal rescue under the direction of the Regional Animal Services Advisory Group for Charleston, Berkeley, and Dorchester counties. In addition to the LART and CART, the Regional Advisory Board is in the process of developing a DART program using citizen emergency

response team members with additional training to assist in animal missions such as establishing pet and livestock shelters, evacuation and repatriation of owner's animals, and operation of animal recovery centers and field hospitals.

The Early Twenty-First Century—The Age of National Animal Disaster Preparedness

The large animal industries have undergone radical changes over the last centuries due to the vertical integration and corporatization of many of the commercial food animal (pig, cattle, poultry) industries; as a result, today's equine industry is largely recreational.

Humane organizations and veterinarians have worked together in many countries over the last century on slaughterhouse reforms to make the process of animal slaughter (including transportation to slaughter) more humane. Public transportation using horses (e.g., carriage companies in cities) has become better regulated to prevent overwork and injury of animals, including the use of a quick-release device to disengage a fallen horse from the harness at the carriage. (*Note*: This snap shackle is best known in the yachting industry today but has come back to large animal rescue in the form of the quick-release device described in Chapter 16.) As of this writing, humane education and rescue work is ongoing and increasing in most developing countries where large animals are still primarily used for work and as beasts of burden.

The ASPCA's educational efforts have culminated in a regular television program, *Animal Cops*, on the Animal Planet network, which brings the reality of horrific animal neglect, abuse, and the occasional need for technical rescue of animals into the living rooms of the public.

The first TLAER training at a state fire academy was a two-day course in horse rescue offered at the South Carolina State Fire Academy, as part of the Southeastern Fire School 2000. Since that time, numerous other states have brought this type of specialty rescue training to their emergency response professionals.

In 2000 the HSUS and FEMA signed a historic agreement as part of Project Impact, an initiative designed to help communities change their approach to disasters by building "disaster-resistant communities" through public–private partnerships. HSUS agreed to provide technical expertise, develop methodologies, and assist communities and individuals to develop effective disaster plans that address the needs of animals (small and large) and their owners. HSUS publishes owner guidelines for disaster preparedness for horses, and another for livestock, that are available free as client education brochures for veterinarians, animal control officers, and humane societies to distribute.

In a statement of understanding, the American Red Cross recognizes HSUS as the nation's largest animal protection organization responsible for the safety and well-being of animals, including disaster relief. On November 13, 2000, the HSUS signed a partnership agreement with FEMA to include animals in emergency management planning.

The ASPCA's New York State Disaster Response Services hosted the first ever Large Animal Rescue Summit at Cornell University's College of Veterinary Medicine on May 16, 2005. Speakers and responders from across the country came together to share expertise in large animal technical rescue and to discuss national standards in personnel, training, equipment, techniques, and response. Representatives from Southampton Fire Brigade (United Kingdom), Code 3 Associates, Days End Horse Farm Rescue, State Animal Response Team (SART) for New York state, the American Association of Equine Practitioners (AAEP) Disaster Committee, Equine Emergency Response Unit (EERU), Hast PSC, MSPCA-Nevins Farm, and Technical Large Animal Emergency Rescue, Inc. attended. Demonstrations of progressive large animal rescue and transport equipment and several equine ambulances were available in the parking lot for discussion and sharing.

By 2000 the TLAER course had evolved into a two-day workshop, including significant hands-on practice with live animals for the students and live animal demonstrations in mud rescue, crane-operated vertical lifts, and a night operation featuring use of the Rescue Glide with a live "patient." That year, Dr. Gimenez provided the first class in TLAER at the South Carolina Fire Academy. During the summer of 2001, the South Carolina LART performed the first practice helicopter sling loads of live animals on the East Coast, accomplished with the Georgia Emergency Management Agency and a Georgia State Patrol Bell UH-1 (Huey) helicopter. In coordination with the South Carolina Veterinarian's Office, an exercise was conducted with members of the South Carolina Army Air National Guard from McIntyre Air Base and a Sikorsky UH-60 (Black Hawk) helicopter.

The AAEP created an equine emergency task force in 2001 and two years later published an "Emergency and Disaster Preparedness Guidelines" booklet. These guidelines explained the role of veterinary practitioners in disasters, provided standardized advice for local practitioners to get involved with their community planning and preparedness and educate their clients, and included a list of resources. The task force was converted to a standing committee that continues to advise the AAEP on future concerns and directions related to emergency and disaster preparedness issues.

The first cross-training event between state, federal, and Department of Defense (DoD) assets in both the veterinary and medical arenas was the "One Medicine" exercise in December, 2002. This joint NDMS/VMAT, Special Medical Augmentation Response Team–Veterinary, and USPHS training was held in Raleigh, North Carolina. The North Carolina State University College of Veterinary Medicine (NCSU-CVM) hosted livestock handling and foreign animal disease courses for Special Operations Response Team DMAT-1, North Carolina, and included training provided by the Military Police K-9 units and Special Operations Forces from Ft. Bragg, North Carolina.

In December, 2003, a full-day large animal disaster response hands-on lab was held for attendees to the "National Multi-Hazard Symposium: One Medicine Approach to Homeland Security," also in Raleigh at NCSU-CVM. It included training in basic handling and restraint of food animals and horses in disaster scenarios, basic management of animals in disasters, and basic recognition of foreign animal disease lesions. Attendees were familiarized with dairy cattle, beef cattle, horses, pigs, sheep, goats, and poultry.

In 2004, the UCD-VERT team released their large animal lifter/extractor, a prototype simplified sling device for raising cattle, horses, or other large animals for short vertical lifts. This sling was a modification of the old figure-eight cotton rope or webbing sling that was initially promoted by the University of California at Davis-College of Equine Health and HSUS.

In 2005 the Veterinary Emergency Treatment Service (VETS) was founded and sponsored by the University of Florida College of Veterinary Medicine (UF-CVM) under the driection of John Haven. The UF-CVM is a partner agency of Florida's SART. The SART is part of the state's Strategic Plan and assists the State Emergency Operations Center in Emergency Support Function 17, the emergency support function for animal and agricultural issues in Florida. With a mission to provide veterinary care during a disaster or emergency response, VETS comprises teams of trained individuals specializing in companion, livestock, and equine veterinary medicine and surgery. The VETS program is envisioned to provide basic- to moderate-level animal care from mobile treatment facilities, which include diagnostic equipment and medical and surgical instrumentation and supplies. The teams coordinate with local practitioners, the Florida Veterinary Medical Association, the Florida Association of Equine Practitioners, and emergency response agencies in order to support practitioners in reestablishing veterinary service to the community. The UF-CVM facility provides definitive care for affected animals in the absence of functioning local veterinary care facilities.

Other training groups have emerged recently with focus on specific aspects of large animal or equine emergencies. In 2005, the EERU began offering a Basic Equine Awareness and Rescue course to emergency responders in the Kansas City, Missouri, area. Emergency Training Systems, Inc. of Clarkrange, Tennessee, provides courses in barn fire prevention and evacuation techniques of horses from burning barns, including hands-on and demonstrations with live animals and smoke, to owners of large animals.

As of 2006, the UK Fire Service estimated that it rescues in excess of 10,000 animals a year; approximately 10% of these are large animal rescues. The increased training in methodologies and equipment, as well as advisor assistance on scenes, has improved their success rate in the three counties that feature this program from 4%–10% to almost 96%. United Kingdom fire brigades have been called to assist with a wide variety of animals, including giraffes and elephants. Rural units are "regularly called to incidents involving large farm animals, e.g., cattle, horses, pigs, etc." (General Risk Assessment, 2005).

Police and fire services in the United Kingdom are improving their methods of dealing with emergencies involving horses following a reporter's 2006 investigation. In several incidents, owners raised concerns over a lack of protocol to help on-scene officers get in touch with appropriate animal welfare and veterinary responders. This was due to the centralization of police control rooms and the loss of the dispatchers' familiarity with the area and available local resources. The British Horse Society began working with the Association of Chief Police Officers and the Chief Fire Officers Association to agree on a new set of national equine emergency guidelines. Representatives from the British Equine Veterinary Association, RSPCA, and International League for the Protection of Horses lent their expertise to developing guidelines and initiating discussions for dealing with horses in distress (Horse & Hound, 2006).

In response to recent disasters and the need to include the topic of animals in disaster planning, the state of Virginia appointed a task force to investigate the issue. The task force recommended that the Virginia Horse Council appoint a representative to the Virginia Disaster Animal Care and Control Committee to keep the horse industry involved in the development of a statewide disaster plan.

LESSONS LEARNED

Lay Volunteer Concerns

When most large animal rescues were performed by humane society volunteers, lay persons, and animal owners in the United States, there was a tendency to self-deploy to local emergencies, as well as regional and national disasters. The response to Hurricane Andrew in 1992 by animal rescue organizations demonstrated that the vast number of volunteers attempting to assist with field animal rescues did not have the proper training to handle animals or to safely perform technical rescues. This led to serious concerns by emergency management officials over the involvement of animal rescuers on disaster and emergency scenes from the perspective of scene safety and security. As of this writing, updates to the NRP, the laws concerning pets and large animals in disasters, and other operational planning considerations for animals are being made.

Immediately, the national organizations made efforts to coordinate and provide training to their volunteers, emphasizing certification before responders could be deployed to disaster zones. Over the years, training in technical aspects of large animal emergency rescue has relied on the fire service models for safety, call out, and efficiency: the National Incident Management System (NIMS) and incident command system (ICS). Through the leadership of national animal welfare and veterinary organizations, large numbers of volunteers have attended professional fire service-related courses in subjects including agroterrorism, technical animal rescue, swiftwater and floodwater rescue, ICS, disaster animal response team training, and have received CPR and first-responder certifications.

Veterinary Leadership

Communication between veterinary practitioners and professional emergency rescuers is crucial. Integration and coordination on a regular basis is critical for smooth disaster response on both sides (Kellogg and Ho, 2002). These events and training opportunities increase the networking and distribution of information to team members across fields of expertise.

In addition to sponsoring the VMATs, the AVMA provides the veterinary profession with disaster resources in the form of online databases, educational materials, and continuing education opportunities. The mission of the AVMA Committee on Disaster and Emergency Issues (AVMA CDEI) is to address the veterinarian's role in emergency and disaster issues; address the impact of disasters on animal health, public health, and the veterinary profession; develop guidelines for veterinarians in disaster situations; and help develop AVMA policy regarding disaster and emergency issues that affect the veterinary profession.

National Animals in Disaster Summit. In response to the problems encountered during the response to Hurricanes Wilma, Katrina, and Rita in 2005, the AVMA sponsored the 2006 National Animal Disaster Summit. An invitation-only event, attendees included representatives from federal agencies (including the DoD and USPHS), humane organizations, state governmental agencies, charities, animal-related groups, VMATs, veterinary associations, and the AVMA CDEI. Participants took part in breakout sessions to identify and resolve major roadblocks in disaster response efforts.

In response to the recommendations from this summit, the AVMA established a National Coordinator, Disaster Preparedness and Response position to foster cooperative efforts among stakeholder groups and assist in the development of disaster assistance plans.

Humane Organizations

National Conference on Animals in Disaster. Hosted by the HSUS and sponsored by a variety of animal rescue organizations, the annual National Conference on Animals in Disaster (NCAD) welcomed approximately 700 individuals, including veterinarians, VMAT members, emergency response professionals, state veterinary medical officers, state veterinarians, USPHS personnel, DHS delegates, U.S. Army personnel, non-governmental and private organization representatives, and animal care and control professionals. Dedicated to learning from the 2005 hurricanes, the 2006 NCAD included a focus on animal disease/avian influenza preparation and resource typing as part of the Department of Homeland Security's NIMS and the NRP.

GETTING ORGANIZED

Disaster Response at the National Level

On October 6, 2006, President Bush signed into law the Pets Evacuation and Transportation Standards Act (PETS). The PETS Act is an amendment to the Robert T. Stafford Disaster Relief and Emergency Assistance Act and requires state and local preparedness offices to take into account pet owners, household pets, and service animals when drawing up evacuation plans. Offices that fail to do so would not qualify for grants from FEMA. Although the PETS act does not apply to horses or cattle because they are not considered companion animals or pets, it is a significant step forward in involving all animal owners in evacuation planning and personal responsibility for their pets.

State and Local Animal Response Teams

The first SART was founded in North Carolina after Hurricane Floyd in 1999, during which the lives of more than 3 million domestic and farm animals were lost. Many could have been saved by a coordinated emergency response plan. The SART in North Carolina is based on the principles of the ICS and involves a coordinated effort of over 30 government and animal organizations. Using ICS as a set of core principles, SART develops units for addressing all aspects of animal disaster response. Today, many states have adopted the North Carolina model to develop their own SART teams. The SART structure is based on the county large animal response team (CART) concept. CARTs are under the jurisdiction of the county emergency management, and include animal control officers, cooperative extension, sheriff's personnel, veterinarians, forestry officers, animal industry leaders and concerned citizens.

LOCAL RESOURCES IN DISASTER RESPONSE TRAINING

Specialty Rescue Training

The unfortunate prevalence of large animal emergencies (e.g., horses and cattle trapped in mud, floodwaters, or highly inaccessible areas) has allowed research and development of new techniques to decrease stress and iatrogenic injuries while rescuing large animals from these predicaments. Expertise in the technical aspects of large animal emergency rescue is a skill area that did not receive much attention from the emergency response and veterinary communities until the late 1990s.

In improving the standards of large animal technical rescue, the leaders of this field have attempted to apply the lessons learned in the great advances of human rescue (technical and specialty) to these animals. Training in these techniques is now being offered by several groups and Eastern Kentucky University to professional emergency responders (firefighters, law enforcement, emergency medical services, animal control, etc.), veterinarians, and technicians. The purpose of training courses is to introduce concepts applicable to safe and effective methods among these groups of people for use in the field.

A grassroots effort by a variety of people from emergency services, animal owner volunteers, and veterinary academia has been providing organized large animal rescue training to emergency personnel in many countries since the late 1980s. A select few are highlighted in this chapter as examples of how to get personnel trained and how to approach the relationship with local agencies; there is no way to include them all. It is hoped that sharing the basic facts about these pioneering efforts at promoting the field of large animal rescue will stimulate new areas of interest and networking around the globe.

Training First Responders

For many years the Farm Medic course has trained fire, rescue, and emergency services personnel in the proper techniques of dealing with agricultural emergencies. Students become familiar with emergencies involving grain bins and silos, agricultural chemicals and pesticides, dangerous large animals and farm equipment from the human emergency perspective. Extrication techniques from manure pits, equipment, and facilities are reviewed and demonstrated but may not necessarily address large animal handling or involvement (Figure 1.7).

Training Veterinarians

Veterinarians interested in obtaining education and expertise in disaster response and wilderness medicine can receive training in many ways. Many veterinary conferences include disaster response lectures in the

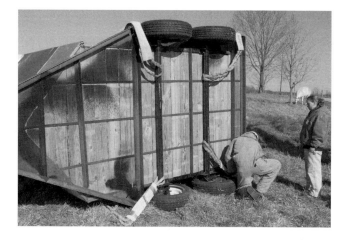

Figure 1.7 A variety of equipment for manipulating the weight of an overturned trailer with animals inside is available to responders and is based on the same equipment used for human extrications: cribbing, cutting tools, webbing, and rope systems. A collection of TLAER equipment should be made for teams to use on scene. Courtesy of Axel Gimenez.

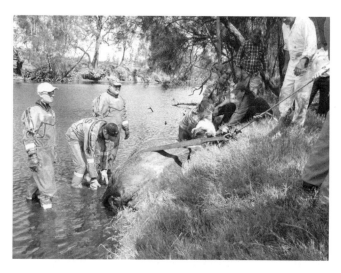

Figure 1.8 A mix of technical rescue, livestock handling, and general medical skills is commonly brought together in these incidents. Here, a cow went into a billabong and was unable to get out of the mud after suffering hypothermia, even though the water was relatively warm. Special Operations teams and a veterinarian were deployed. Courtesy of Steve Cliffe.

continuing education curriculum. Veterinarians may obtain ICS training through online venues or in association with local first responders and may gain technical large animal rescue expertise through courses such as Large Animal Rescue and TLAER.

Training the Lay Public

The lay public can receive training in disaster response through avenues similar to those of veterinarians and first responders. In response to increased public interest in disaster response, many organizations have begun tailoring their programs for animal owners.

GETTING INFORMATION OUT

Animals as victims of emergencies and disasters are rarely considered or discussed in mainstream training books, standard operating protocols (SOPs), or other materials used as references or taught by the fire service or other emergency responders. Although some of this information may exist in one form or another in veterinary resources, it is not easily available to emergency services personnel and is not commonly taught in first-responder schools. Several professional training teams and organizations that have been providing workshops and courses in various aspects of large animal emergency and disaster rescue are discussed here.

Numerous governmental, veterinary, and humane organizations have produced educational materials for animal owners and emergency managers related to animal disaster and emergency planning at the local and state level. As an example, the California Animal Response Emergency System, administered by the California Department of Food and Agriculture, was created

to work with the Office of Emergency Services as a coordinator for animal issues and animal emergency planning across the state. They provided a template plan for each county to assist with developing their own county plan for animal disasters and emergencies, similar to the SART/CART model developed in North Carolina.

CONCLUSIONS

The field of large animal disaster and emergency response is a rapidly evolving area. Recent natural and human-caused disasters have dramatically increased the demand for information, SOPs, and training in the field. Veterinary professionals, first responders, and animal owners have recognized the value of being prepared and will serve as primary driving forces for great strides in advancement in the field (Figure 1.8).

ACRONYMS USED IN CHAPTER 1

AAEP	American Association of Equine Practitioners
APA	Animals Protection Act
ASPCA	American Society for the Prevention of Cruelty to Animals
AVMA CDEI	American Veterinary Medical Association Committee on Disaster and Emergency Issues
AVMA	American Veterinary Medical Association
CART	County animal response team
CVM	College of Veterinary Medicine

DART	Disaster animal rescue team
DHS	Department of Homeland Security
DoD	Department of Defense
EERU	Equine emergency response unit
EMS	Emergency medical services
FAEP	Florida Association of Equine Practitioners
FEMA	Federal Emergency Management Agency
HSM	Humane Society of Missouri
HSUS	Humane Society of the United States
ICS	Incident command system
LART	Large animal rescue team
MSPCA	Massachusetts Society for the Prevention of Cruelty to Animals
NCAD	National Conference on Animals in Disaster
NCSU-CVM	North Carolina State University College of Veterinary Medicine
NDMS	National Disaster Medical System
NIMS	National Incident Management System
NRP	National Response Plan
NVRT	National Veterinary Response Team
PETS	Pets Evacuation and Transportation Standards
PHS	Public Health Service
RSPCA	Royal Society for the Prevention of Cruelty to Animals
SART	State animal response team
SOP	Standard operating protocol
SPCA	Society for the Prevention of Cruelty to Animals
TLAER	Technical large animal emergency rescue
TROD	Trail Riders of DuPage
UCD-VERT	University of California-Davis School of Veterinary Medicine's Veterinary Emergency Response Team
UF-CVM	University of Florida College of Veterinary Medicine
VETS	Veterinary Emergency Treatment Service
VMATs	Veterinary medical assistance teams (see NVRT)

WEBSITE RESOURCES

American Academy on Veterinary Disaster Medicine: http://www.cvmbs.colostate.edu/clinsci/wing/aavdm/aavdm.htm

American Association of Equine Practitioners Emergency and Disaster Preparedness Resources: http://aaep.org/emergency_prep.htm

American Veterinary Medical Association Disaster Resources: http://www.avma.org/disaster/default.asp

ASPCA Disaster Preparedness Resources: http://www.aspca.org/site/PageServer?pagename=disaster

California Animal Response Emergency System: http://www.cdfa.ca.gov/ahfss/ah/disaster_preparedness.htm

CIDRAP Overview of Agricultural Biosecurity: http://www.cidrap.umn.edu/cidrap/content/biosecurity/ag-biosec/biofacts/agbiooview.html

Code 3 Associates: http://www.code3associates.org

Community Emergency Response Teams Homepage: http://www.citizencorps.gov/cert/index.shtm

Emergency Training Systems: www.emergencytrainingsystems.com

Equine Emergency Response Unit: www.eeru.org

Federal Emergency Management Agency: www.fema.gov http://aaep.org/emergency_prep.htm

Felton Fire Protection District Large Animal Rescue: http://www.feltonfire.com/lar.html

Hast, PSC: http://www.hast.net/

Humane Society of the United States' Disaster Center: http://www.hsus.org/hsus_field/hsus_disaster_center/

National Disaster Management System Homepage: http://www.oep-ndms.dhhs.gov/index.html

National Incident Management System Integration Center: http://www.fema.gov/emergency/nims/index.shtm

State Animal Response Teams: http://www.sartusa.org/

Technical Large Animal Emergency Rescue: http://www.tlaer.org

Trail Riders of DuPage: http://www.trod.us/index.htm

University of California-Davis Veterinary Emergency Response Team: http://www.adjective.com/htdb/disaster

US Department of Health and Human Services' Disasters and Emergencies Resources Page: http://www.hhs.gov/emergency/index.shtml

US Search and Rescue Task Force: http://www.ussartf.org/index.html

USDA: http://www.usda.gov

Veterinary Medical Assistance Teams: http://www.vmat.org/

2 Purpose of Technical Large Animal Emergency Rescue

Dr. Rebecca Gimenez

INTRODUCTION

Domestication and the encroachment of human society on animal habitats have caused many animals to become dependent on humans for their existence and welfare. As a society, humans exercise great compassion toward animals and will even risk life-threatening conditions to help them without regard for the consequences. As a result, many untrained but well-intentioned rescuers are injured or lose their lives each year trying to help animals in need of assistance. Rescuing large animals or wild animals can be particularly dangerous; even professionally trained emergency responders have been severely injured or have died attempting to assist large animals in trouble (Figure 2.1).

The emergency or first responder with awareness of technical large animal emergency rescue (TLAER) methods will have increased knowledge and skills to assist large animals in emergency situations. More importantly, their understanding of behavior and responses of those animals will help prevent injuries to human responders and bystanders at the scenes. Although this text covers a wide variety of issues and methodologies relating to large animal emergency rescue, readers are encouraged to participate in hands-on practice using these methods or attend training courses to raise their knowledge to an operational or technical level.

THE "PERFECT" RESCUE

Extricating an animal successfully out of its predicament is not the "perfect" rescue—getting it out efficiently and professionally with no injury to the animal victim or human rescuers is the "perfect" rescue. No two TLAER incidents are the same; a successful TLAER plan considers factors unique to the animals, the situation, and the environment. Standard operational guidance should be referred to for an incident. Responders must implement commonsense TLAER solutions based on their knowledge of restraint, animal behavior, the available equipment, and personnel. Professionalism on the TLAER scene includes attention to safety and security, operational personnel with TLAER training, planning (incident action plan) and organization (incident command system, or ICS). It is important to raise the standard of care to avoid iatrogenic injury to or death of the large animal victim.

Why TLAER Is Necessary

The most common questions asked by professional emergency responders and those within the veterinary community might be:

- What is the purpose of TLAER?
- Why is this knowledge applicable to my jurisdiction?

In most cases, the owner and multiple bystanders will try to help the animal despite a lack of training in TLAER equipment and techniques. This is such a new area of specialty rescue that many emergency responders are not aware of the progress in methodology and procedures available for a successful and safe response to these scenarios. Due to a lack of training and equipment, it is not uncommon for people to get injured and for the animal victim to be further injured, or even killed, by well-intentioned but uneducated rescuers.

Aren't the owners responsible for their animals and the incidents that might occur with their large animals? Animals are considered property by law. Thus, the owner is responsible both legally and financially for the animal's well-being and upkeep and has a moral and

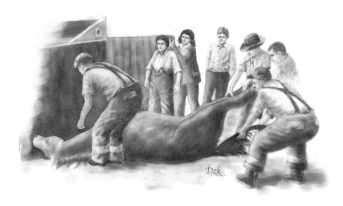

Figure 2.1 *These responders are attempting to help the horse out of the trailer, but are risking their personal safety. Even sedated and exhausted, animals can still kick. The spring-loaded ramp presents a risk of injury. There are too many people in close proximity to the horse, resulting in a risk of injury and interference. Dragging the animal on the pavement and using the legs as handles presents high risks of injury to the animal. Courtesy of Michael Dzurak.*

ethical duty to the animal as imposed by society. However, large animals cannot be picked up and carried out of their predicament as a small animal can. TLAER commonly involves the use of heavy equipment and heavy-duty specialty webbing and rope systems that most owners do not have on site, and it requires an emphasis on understanding behavior.

Fifty years ago, owners of large animals called a farmer or friends in their area to bring tractors or other heavy equipment, and they attempted to extract the animal on their own. The percentage of successful rescues is as poor now as it was then, even in the best of scenarios. Modern owners rarely have access to equipment or the handling skills to accomplish a rescue attempt, but they have probably seen rescue scenarios on TV and believe that the fire department will rescue their animal. The public calls 911 emergency response for almost any type of incident and expects their paid public servants to be able to respond and successfully solve the problem.

The status of animals has evolved as our society has grown to place more financial and sentimental value on individual animals. Fifty to 100 years ago, animals were commercially valuable, and very few were considered members of the family. In today's society, the average value of an unregistered beef cow is $500–$800; registered stock may be valued at $2,000–$15,000 per head. The average value of an unregistered horse is $1,500–$2,000, and registered stock average $2,000–$5,000 per head. There are many animals valued in excess of $50,000. Even "backyard" horses may be purchased for $1,000–$10,000. The sentimental value of these animals can be very high, and it is not unusual for owners to spend thousands of dollars on surgery and rehabilitation for their animals. A breeding pair of show-quality alpacas might be as valuable as $80,000.

Some racing or breeding livestock and horses may be sold or syndicated for millions of dollars. Horses and other breeding and show animals can be insured, and some are valued in excess of $1 million. Responders should remember that a large animal's sentimental value as a pet or companion may be considered to be priceless to the owner. Specially-trained animals (e.g., handicapped assistance and service animals, mounted police animals) are valuable beyond price to their owners and partners.

Owners of large animals often forget how intimidating animals can be to other people, because they routinely assess their animal's behaviors for a variety of signals. Most firefighters and police officers have little to no experience handling large animals and no knowledge of animal behavior in stressful situations (Nixon, 2006). Providing hands-on experience and didactic awareness of TLAER methods allows the professional emergency responder to be in better control of response to TLAER incidents.

Large Animal Incident Frequency

Another question might be how many actual incidents of this type occur in communities across the globe, or more importantly, how many might be expected in a local community. Many wonder why the local animal control cannot handle these incidents.

The author searched for information on vehicle wrecks involving large animals, expecting the data to be more robust since road accidents are usually reported through law enforcement or the fire service. Research revealed that there is currently no centralized database of incidents involving large animals in any country, and on-road accidents involving animals are sporadically reported. One commercial swine producer reported having over 1,200 trucks on the road each week in the United States, with an average of 12 overturned trucks per year (Woods, 2006a). One large horse show in Ohio reported an informal count of over 1,400 horse trailers coming through the gates in a two-day period (Keulemans, 2006). Other large livestock and horse shows commonly report 600–1,000 individual animals attending their events, and some county animal control offices get over 2,000 calls per month. The author has gathered information on over 200 horse trailer accidents and 60 livestock hauler wrecks over a five-year period in the United States, gleaned from Internet accounts and newspaper reports (Gimenez and Gimenez, 2006b). Another researcher has a database of livestock hauler wrecks and accidents in North America (Woods, 2006a), while U.S. Rider maintains records on incidents and calls for service (Cole, 2006).

The only data available outside of these sources is based on anecdotes, accounts by veterinarians, professional emergency responders and lay volunteers, newspaper reports, and Internet searches. The volume of large animal incidents is large enough to justify an awareness level of training in most communities, and areas with a large concentration of these animals necessitates more specialized operational and technical level training.

CONSEQUENCE MANAGEMENT

Whether it is an emergency, accident, act of terrorism, or other incident, the public expects emergency management to respond and deal with the situation in a proper manner. When the public calls 911 (United States) or 999 (United Kingdom), they expect emergency responders to respond regardless of the nature of the situation. That expectation has grown over the last 50 years to include large animal incidents because many owners do not have the equipment or knowledge to effectively and safely extricate the animal.

Natural phenomena and occurrences such as blizzards, hurricanes, tornadoes, and earthquakes have occurred for millions of years on Earth. It is the human tendency to build permanent structures and maintain our valuables in the path of such natural occurrences that has made them truly human-caused disasters.

Progression of the TLAER Response

The response to human-caused incidents or small-scale emergencies generally begins with a 911 (or 999 UK) call to the local emergency response dispatch center. For emergencies involving animals, calls are occasionally made directly to a local veterinarian or to the local animal control officials.

Emergencies involving large animals most commonly fall into the arena of the professional emergency responders who routinely respond to such incidents as overturned trailers on surface roads and interstates or loose animals in neighborhoods or on roads. Training for these types of situations has been sporadic, with several groups across the United States offering training at various levels.

Who Will Respond?

At most traffic accident scenes, the first responder to arrive is a law enforcement officer. Depending on circumstances, fire services, emergency medical services (EMS), and other rescue personnel may be dispatched (see Chapter 12). Most emergency responders have received extensive training in how to assist human victims, but very few are familiar with how to help or even handle an injured or trapped animal. Most firefighters are volunteers who may have little to no experience with handling large animals, making handling of a frightened animal not only difficult and dangerous, but also potentially lethal.

Many large animal incidents occur near or on roads and require state patrol or sheriff/police traffic control at a minimum. If the incident involves a wrecked vehicle, the fire department and police will respond to provide life-safety supervision, and EMS will also respond in case rescuers are injured.

The fire service is called to the scene in almost any emergency situation, and their leadership, teamwork, safety and risk assessment skills will be invaluable on scene. Animals can be financially very valuable and represent both life and property, both of which the fire service is sworn to protect. In addition, the fire service brings pieces of equipment and methodologies to the scene that may be easily converted to large animal use. Many fire departments have highly trained specialty rescue teams that may have equipment and training to deal with entrapment, confined spaces, trench rescue, and vehicle extrication—all scenarios common on TLAER scenes.

Police, sheriff's deputies, and highway patrol officers are rarely trained in extrication and removal methods unless they have years of experience or prior service in the fire/rescue/EMS arenas. Their primary concern and responsibilities are to protect public safety. They are experts at setting up a safety zone around the incident and providing scene security.

EMS and paramedics are highly trained in life-saving first aid and first responder scenarios for people. These professionals can easily be trained to assess basic clinical parameters of the large animal (heart rate, pulse, temperature, etc.) and can be of help to the veterinarian on scene or by stabilizing a victim until the veterinarian arrives. Responders can increase the quality of triage and pre-hospital care to the large animal patient by using standardized patient care protocols developed on a local basis and based on a combination of veterinary and emergency response knowledge (see Chapters 17 and 20).

Common sense dictates that extricating a human victim from a car by placing a rope around their neck and pulling is unacceptable. Despite the anatomical similarities between the neck of humans and that of animals, the neck is a common anchor point for rescues. Although inappropriate for large animal rescue, this technique is commonly emphasized in the media. Similarly, many televised "heroic" animal rescues depict the animal being dragged out of the entrapment by the neck or limbs. The head, neck, and legs of a large animal should not be used as "handles."

Manipulation of large animals is possible and safest using the torso as an anchor point for various webbing appliances (see Chapters 15 and 16). Large animals can be herded, led individually with halters, contained with portable fencing, and transported en masse by trailers (depending on species and their familiarity with humans). In general, this text will emphasize avoiding the extremities as handles or anchors to pull an animal out of entrapment, instead using the larger surface area and skeletal support of the torso to reduce injury and increase success.

Animals can and do sustain serious and sometimes iatrogenic life-threatening injuries in TLAER incidents. Animals have died due to asphyxiation during rescue attempts, particularly if their heads and necks are used as anchor points for ropes. As an example of an inappropriate rescue deemed a "success," a pregnant Arabian mare fell into an ice-covered pond; the videotaped rescue effort showed responders lassoing the mare's neck from the bank 20 meters away. The rope was attached to a winch and the horse pulled out of the hole onto her side, then winched across the surface of the ice kicking violently. When the animal reached the bank, it stood and was led away by an animal handler. Such rescues are performed with the best intentions to help the animal, but are the result of lack of knowledge and training. This book offers learning points based on numerous scenarios, including correctly and incorrectly executed rescues (see Chapter 22).

TLAER CAN BE DANGEROUS TO RESPONDERS AND VICTIMS

In the early 1990s in the United Kingdom, large animal rescues that were successful (i.e., did not maim, severely injure, or kill the animal victim) were estimated to be 4%–10% out of an estimated 6,000–10,000 annual total (small and large) animal rescues. Approximately 10% of these rescues were estimated to involve large animals. With the addition of animal rescue advisors trained in TLAER techniques, the percentage of successful rescues has been raised to 96% (P. Baker, 2006). Although the percentages of injured, killed, or iatrogenically injured animals during rescue are unknown and not officially tracked in the United States or other countries, many professionals estimate low success rates for large animal rescues. Few rescuers discuss the unsuccessful rescues or botched attempts (Baker, 2006).

Sometimes a situation arises on TLAER scenes when there is no time to do things the "correct" way. An example would be an overturned gooseneck trailer in an accident with two or three horses inside, trapped in lateral recumbency, and the living quarters smoldering. If the animals are not removed from the trailer quickly, they will probably die from smoke inhalation or fire. At this point, using a tail tie and pulling on the rear legs, although not preferred methods, may be the best option given the situation. These methods may injure the animals, but they may save them, and responders must manage the risk (Fox, 2006). Experience and veterinary knowledge are the best teachers when determining if the animal must immediately be removed or if the animal can wait to be rescued after careful planning.

In the United Kingdom, recorded injuries to police officers from animals (data includes both small and large animals) included one fatality, 178 major injuries, and 192 hospital stays longer than 3 days in the period 1999–2002 (HSE, 2003).

A study utilized Census of Fatal Occupational Injuries files from the U.S. Department of Labor for the years 1992–1997 to tabulate human workplace fatalities associated with animals. During the six-year time period, 350 workplace deaths were associated with animal-related events. Cattle and horses were the primary animals involved, and workers in the agricultural industry experienced the majority of events. Exotic animals, primarily elephants and tigers, were responsible for a few deaths. A small number of workers died of a zoonotic infection (Langley and Hunter, 2001).

Zoological records provide further insight to the dangers of handling any type of animals. As of 2001, there were 183 Association of Zoos and Aquariums–accredited zoos and aquariums in the United States. A survey of human injuries from animal attacks, whether offensive or defensive in nature, ranged from simple abrasions and lacerations to fractures, amputations, and death.

INCREASINGLY DISTRIBUTED CONCENTRATIONS OF ANIMALS

Over the last 50 years, there has been a trend toward increased concentrations of large animals in urban and suburban areas. This increases the risk of incidents during transport or due to unsafe environments. Many people have large animal pets or horses literally in their backyard, and it is not uncommon in some communities to have zoning that allows two to four horses on one-quarter to one-half acre. Norco, California; Wellington, Florida; and Alta Loma, California are good examples of horse-related communities where there are literally thousands of horses. In many of these equine-focused communities, there are urban trails through the housing areas that lead to show and recreational facilities for horses. In Rancho Cucomonga, California, the township actually owns two horse show facilities as well as maintains the trails through the housing areas. The close relationship that owners will have with their individual animals in these living conditions will be very different from a ranch owner who runs 2,000 horses and 4,000 cattle on a huge ranch in the Southwest.

An example of the worst-case scenario in an area with a high population of large animals occurred in South Dakota in January 1997. Twice in a seven-day period an Arctic cold front moved over the state. The governor closed the interstate highways for public safety. More than 36,000 head of cattle were reported to have perished; many died from hypothermia, but starvation and dehydration claimed large numbers of unreported cattle and other large animals. Roads were still blocked or covered 15 days after the storm ended, due to 6.5–14 m (21–46 ft) vertical drifts blocking the highway. Three people died while trapped in vehicles along the highways. Livestock losses, damaged buildings, and feed shortages occurred in an area called the "red zone," a concentrated area of 4,722 cattle operations, 1,200 sheep operations, 1,000 hog farms, and 515 dairies along the northern third of the state. This storm caused a minimum of $29,527,562 in damages and cleanup efforts (SD OEM, 1997).

WHAT DOES IT TAKE TO MOTIVATE?

Instructors and TLAER responders report some frustration in their attempts to arouse the interest of emergency responders in this new specialty area of heavy rescue. Sometimes it takes a highly visible or heavily publicized incident to motivate professional responders to get involved in training and preparedness for these incidents. In the author's state (South Carolina), an accident on the interstate in 1999 at the Broad River Bridge on I-20 killed the passenger in a truck and severely injured the driver when the truck and trailer slammed into a bus that was stopped in traffic from a previous accident. One horse was killed in the wreck, and a second was euthanatized due to the severity of its injuries. The response time for the veterinarian and the firefighters was prolonged due to the stopped traffic and lack of police escort. For many hours the accident blocked traffic as emergency responders tried to determine what to do with the live horses and how to get to the injured animal(s). Ironically, the accident occurred approximately two miles from the South Carolina Fire Academy, which subsequently hosted the first Fire Academy TLAER training course in 2000.

In other areas, it may take an emergency or disaster that is well publicized by the media to inspire interest in TLAER training. The live coverage of the 2006 Preakness Stakes and the injury of favorite Barbaro brought the concept of equine ambulances and urgent large animal care into the public's living rooms. Similarly, live coverage of field rescue teams helping small and large animals from the flooding and devastation of Hurricane Katrina prompted the Pet Evacuation and Transportation Standard legislation in 2006 to address animals in the planning and preparation stages of disasters. Awareness is a powerful motivator. For example, the Atlantic coastal states have been proactive compared to interior states when it comes to natural disaster preparation for animals due to their seasonal risk of hurricanes. However, the jurisdictions where animal emergency response awareness, training, and team formation have improved are irrespective of geography and climate; it is the passionate focus of people on the issues that allow the development of these ideas.

DISASTER DEFINITION

Natural phenomena and occurrences such as blizzards, hurricanes, tornadoes, and earthquakes have occurred for millions of years on Earth. These natural occurrences become human-caused disasters when they impact human-built structures and communities. While disasters are not the focus of this book, the intricate interrelationships that occur with emergency management results in a marked similarity between emergencies and disasters. Some information on the subject of disasters from the TLAER perspective is justified. Natural disasters are not unusual; they happen every year, somewhere in the world. Local responders should not wait for the disaster to happen to start planning for animal issues.

The number of disaster declarations (460) in the United States from 1990 to 1999 was approximately double that of the previous decade and all preceding decades for which there are records; $25.4 billion was spent in comparison to the $3.9 billion (current dollars) spent in the 1980s. In the years 1998–2000 alone there were 186 declared disasters.

Events that some people might not consider to be a disaster can ravage the large animal industries. Hyperthermia and dehydration due to drought and heat extremes have caused significant losses in the cattle industry in 1977 (725 cattle died), 1995 (10,000 beef feedlot cattle died), 2006, and 2007. In one heat wave, the rendering of dairy carcasses in Wisconsin per week increased from 400 to 15,000 (Heath, 1999). In 2005, over 10,000 livestock were lost to one wildfire in the western United States. Preventing the interruption of power to commercial poultry and swine facilities is a constant concern of producers, who want to prevent massive losses due to hyperthermia.

Noninfectious hazards to animals during and immediately after disasters include traumatic injuries, aspiration pneumonia, toxic- and sewage-related gastroenteritis, and stress-induced illness. These appear to be more common than the much feared but less commonly reported infectious hazards. Traumatic injuries to large animals were common in Hurricanes Andrew (1992) and Fran (1996) and were caused by flying debris or direct injuries from scattered obstacles after the winds died down. Lower limb injuries were the most common injury in horses after Hurricane Andrew (Heath, 1999). Hurricane Katrina added weight to the argument for evacuation due to hundreds of large animal drownings.

Only one infectious hazard has affected animals significantly since 1975. Following flooding of the Red River, morbidity and mortality due to western equine encephalitis were observed. There is little scientific evidence to link natural disasters to consistent and significant increases in the occurrence of infectious diseases (vectorborne animal diseases, anthrax, cryptosporidiosis, etc.) in animals. In some cases, the risks actually decreased in disaster zones (Gilchrist, 2000; APHIS, 2002; Watson et al, 2007).

Disasters are amalgamations of numerous smaller incidents that overwhelm the ability of normal emergency response jurisdictions to deal with the situation in a timely and efficient manner. They require additional resources from the region, province, state, or federal government. Catastrophic disasters often overwhelm the resources of the state or province level as well, requiring augmentation by federal and national resources. The declared disaster area after Hurricane Katrina (2005) was 233,000 square kilometers (90,000 square miles). Single emergencies do not overwhelm local resources, and there is usually a much quicker response time (a timeline measured in minutes to hours versus hours to days).

In disasters, as in emergencies, the professional emergency responders place first priority on human victims.

Technological Disasters

According to the Federal Emergency Management Agency, technological disasters include electrical blackouts, hazardous material (HazMat), nuclear emergencies, and domestic terrorism. The close relationship between animal owners and their livestock or pets has been documented and suggests that providing care for animals in disasters should be an integral part of providing care for humans (Monti, 2000; Heath, 1999).

Responsibility for Large Animals

Disasters are made up of many different types of incidents and quickly overwhelm the systems that are in place to assist both owners and their animals. They emphasize the value of educating owners and owners' taking personal responsibility for their animals. Animals are owned property as well as being living things, and it is the responsibility of the owner to evacuate the animal and provide normal care and prevention from injury. In disasters, often response time may be measured in hours to weeks. Many disasters (hurricanes, flooding, wildfires) give owners, volunteers, and professionals time to prepare for their response, while others (earthquakes, chemical spill) will impact without warning. Responsibility for assisting animals often falls to volunteers because the full-time emergency responders will be helping people.

The logistics (personnel, equipment, and support systems) effort is often the most challenging part of a disaster response. As many disaster responders will agree, response to disasters is 90% logistics and 10% action. Administrative and planning functions must be in place to do the job in a timely and efficient manner. Good disaster preparedness planning extends to the emergency arena and should be an integral part of emergency planning. The persons and organizations that respond, and the response time, are important factors to consider—human victims are the first

priority. In disasters, the paid and volunteer emergency responders (fire, EMS, and rescue) are going to be primarily involved with human concerns. There are numerous nongovernmental organizations available that focus their efforts on animal disaster response; this grassroots effort has matured over the last 20 years. This book is not intended to be a disaster response guide, but rather should increase awareness of the issues surrounding large animal sheltering, evacuation, and technical rescues that make up a large part of disaster planning and response.

OWNER STATUS

The owner must make the decision as to disposition of the animal by rescue or euthanasia, and in unusual cases may refuse treatment for the animal on the scene. In some jurisdictions, the animal control officer could charge the owner with neglect and force the owner to surrender the animal, allowing the officer to take over and make legal decisions about the disposition of the animal. In disasters the owner will not be present, and a decision must be made how animals will be dealt with on scene.

ANIMAL PARAMEDICS

The human medical community recognized years ago the need for professionals who could provide medical care within a short period of time, termed the "golden hours," after an incident in the absence of an emergency physician. A comparable system for large animal emergencies is not present in most countries (including the United States). Several hours may elapse before a large animal receives emergency medical attention by a professional (veterinarian) after an incident. Furthermore, as is the case with physicians, veterinarians are not commonly trained to be first responders. In addition to having a skill applicable to an emergency situation (firefighting, human medicine, veterinary medicine, etc.), the first responder must be able to speak and understand the emergency language and protocols of the ICS, understand how to perform triage, and must also be able to participate in a safe manner to avoid injury (see Chapter 5).

As of 2007, Eastern Kentucky University is developing an "ani-medic" program modeled after the Swedish (Helsingborg) program, which has been in existence for over 20 years. The purpose of this program is to combine the knowledge and experience of human paramedics and emergency medical technicians (EMTs) with that of the veterinary community.

THE MEDIA EFFECT

Incidents involving animals rapidly gain attention in the news media, including television and newspapers.

For example, it is not uncommon to see three or four news helicopters hovering over an incident where rescuers are freeing a horse stuck in mud or ice, streaming the video live to their audience. Popular TV networks are always on the lookout for homemade videos of animal incidents to run on animal rescue programs.

Many well-intentioned but untrained rescuers use the media coverage as an example for how to perform a large animal rescue. However, the techniques employed in the rescue may not be correct; the fact that the victim survived the rescue procedure does not mean that the rescue was adequate. It is important to remember that these videos are shown for entertainment, not educational, purposes. Televised rescues may be edited to make them appear more entertaining or suspenseful. Others are edited to omit the death of the animal after the rescue and leave the public with the impression that the methods demonstrated were correct and acceptable.

Well-meaning owners, emergency responders, and veterinarians often use the head and neck to manipulate the animal. The extremities are not intended for use as a "handle" for rescues. In fact, using the extremities will negate any benefit of the animals' muscle power that could have been used to assist in the rescue. When a large animal feels traction on its head, one of its basic instincts is to pull back against the pressure; this reaction is called the opposition reflex; It means that the animal is not assisting, and may be hindering, its own rescue (see Chapter 4). Most people have seen roping of animals on TV, movies, or in the rodeo, but they do not understand that the intent of roping is to stop the animal from moving, not to asphyxiate (strangle) it. There are very few exigent situations in TLAER that will require such desperate measures as roping an animal and pulling it by the neck or other extremities.

WHO SHOULD GET INVOLVED

Veterinarians and their staffs, paramedics/EMTs, firefighters, police and sheriff's officers, animal control officers, mounted police officers, military special operational units, Department of Natural Resources officers, humane societies and animal rescue organizations, as well as individual owners, all have a vested interest in learning how to properly employ TLAER techniques. These techniques are commonly applicable to daily on-farm emergencies as well as emergency and disaster scenarios.

WORKING TOWARD A SOLUTION

Concerned local citizens should introduce themselves to the personnel in the local jurisdiction emergency management/operations center and state animal and emergency organizations. A good local emergency response will require a variety of skills offered by experienced large animal professionals, including veterinary staff, animal control officers, humane personnel, emergency responders, and rescue professionals. This book discusses response to emergencies with large animals, not the mitigation and prevention phases, which are covered in other literature.

Getting "plugged in" to the ICS system is the first step for increasing the visibility of and involvement in this type of rescue specialty. It is rare for animal emergency response units to be part of the normal dispatch system linked to 911. Local volunteers should build a working and training relationship with the emergency responders in their area and be aware of the needs of the individual stakeholders. Encouraging cross-training with other emergency professionals and volunteers within the local area, which may include volunteer organizations, horse rescues, humane organizations, and others. To be effective, mutual aid agreements, memorandums of understanding or agreement, and other paperwork should be completed. Interested volunteers should consult with their local office of emergency management to learn how to proceed.

RESPONSE PRIORITY

The priority for professional emergency responders should always be the safety of humans. In local emergency incidents featuring a response that occurs in minutes to hours, it is rare for organized animal rescue volunteers or TLAER-trained teams of personnel to be involved from the beginning. (Recent reports from large animal rescue and TLAER-trained teams have emphasized their increased success on scene.) A solution is to increase the communication and involvement of local animal rescue and welfare organizations. Although animal rescue volunteers and groups are available to assist with animals impacted by disasters, the effort may be delayed for days to weeks, depending on the number of humans impacted by the disaster, because the priority for resources and rescue efforts must rightfully go to the human effort.

Responders must learn to use field expedients (resources and equipment employed in emergency situations) and improvise on the scene; they might have to learn to work with an individual or be placed on a team. A mixed group of technicians, veterinarians, fire rescue, etc., with a variety of specialties and opinions on scene will need to work together to answer the following questions:

- What is more valuable, the life of the animal or the life of the human bystander who attempts to help?
- How many humans are going to become involved if the animal is not rescued?
- Should professionals try to rescue the animal?
- What are the pros and cons of this course of action?

This becomes a risk assessment process that the local department must make.

In some cases, departments have responded to animal incidents as training and practice scenarios, taking their time to benefit from the training value of the incident (see Chapter 5).

IT'S NOT JUST ABOUT THE ANIMAL

The purpose of TLAER is not only to assist a large animal victim without harming it, but also to prevent death or permanent injury to human rescuers and bystanders. Animal rescues are often made by first responders trying to prevent injury to people who may attempt to rescue the animal themselves. For example in December, 2004, the Poudre Fire Authority in Colorado responded to rescue two Canadian geese trapped on the surface of a frozen lake with their legs stuck in the ice. Saving geese or other animals is not a priority of the fire department, but saving human life is. To prevent well-intentioned bystanders on the scene from venturing onto the surface of the ice to try to rescue the geese, the shift battalion commander deployed the surface ice rescue team to successfully rescue the geese.

WHO SHOULD PERFORM TLAER IN THE COUNTY?

Officers and agencies often split the responsibility for animals in their jurisdiction; the animal control officer may address animal issues during normal business hours, but the after-hours responsibility may fall elsewhere. Who addresses road hazards such as cattle or horse loose in the road? Does the same individual or group address trailer accidents? Within the local jurisdiction, there should be a standard operating protocol to determine the realm of an individual's or agency's responsibilities in these areas and to respond to specialty issues.

Any approach to planning for emergencies and disasters potentially affecting large numbers of livestock (pigs, goats, sheep, dairy and beef cattle, llamas, alpacas, emus, horses) must consider maintaining public health standards, safeguarding the human food supply, assuring the safety of disaster personnel, preventing foreign animal disease (FAD), employing large animal emergency rescue techniques, and the using of humane euthanasia.

An Ideal Example

An example of valuable planning and mitigation steps for minimizing the effect on commercial food animals in a flooding scenario would include making certain that a county or other jurisdiction has a plan for assisting farmers in the loading, transport, and early delivery to slaughter or alternate facilities for large animals in

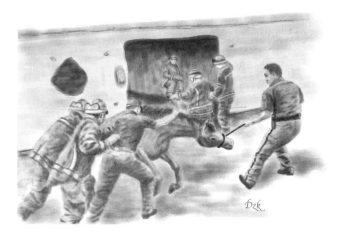

Figure 2.2 *The design of this overturned six-horse trailer allowed the first horses to escape when rescuers removed the dividers and the rear door. The other horses panicked when cutting equipment was used to access the roof. The injuries they sustained required euthanasia. Courtesy of Michael Dzurak.*

100 and 500 year floodplains. It would include coordination with the land use and zoning boards to prevent or discourage the building of food animal facilities in those floodplains.

Make a Decision

In past disasters, many jurisdictions responded too late and with poor preparation and training (Figure 2.2). This increases the risk of death and suffering of large numbers of animals, injury to rescuers, higher carcass recovery costs, biological HazMat concerns, and possible compromise of public health and safety. Some agencies fail to realize that animal disasters are also human disasters; others prepare well and promote coordination that allows an excellent response. The ice storm that hit North Carolina in 2002 was anticipated; the response plan included properly allocated resources and coordination between agencies and was effectively handled by farm owners and disaster personnel within the state. Similarly, a minor hurricane that hit that state in 2003 provided an excellent snapshot of the high level of preparation by the state animal response teams (SARTs) in coordination with over 100 other agencies in North Carolina (McGinn, 2004).

Ask the Tough Questions

Is the jurisdiction prepared to handle a wide variety of scenarios, which might include a 200-cow dairy farm destroyed by a tornado, a large 50-horse facility in the path of a chemical leak from a nearby railroad tanker car, or a 500-pig farm in the path of a flood? Do law enforcement, animal control, and fire department personnel have basic training to accomplish catching, handling, restraint, and containment of large animals? Are vehicles and trailers available from local owner volunteers to transport large animals? If not, are there contracted volunteers who can provide those services on short notice? What is available in the county and state? Are there mutual aid agreements with other jurisdictions? What events (hazard analysis) can be anticipated in the area? Are earthquakes, nuclear accidents, chemical spills, tornados, or hurricanes possible? Or are wildfires, structure fires, ice and snow, droughts, or flooding of more concern? What are the secondary hazards that will be associated with the primary hazard event? What veterinary resources are willing to volunteer to assist on the scene?

Coordination Is Key

Evaluate the emergency response plan for the state and county: Has it been updated recently? Has anyone practiced the plan in that jurisdiction? What logistical resources are prepositioned for animal response? Do personnel have ICS training? Does the state have a Good Samaritan law that can be applied to animal rescue, and does it pertain to "an injured or displaced animal at the scene of an emergency on or adjacent to a roadway, or to a sick, injured or displaced animal during the pendency of a disaster" (Florida Statute 768.13 (3)) in the law? There may be other laws that need to be updated or revised to address companion animal and livestock involvement in incidents and disasters.

Have agencies or personnel in appropriate positions in the jurisdiction provided training in mitigation and preparation for large animal owners in the area? Mitigation efforts are permanent changes or improvements intended to lessen the severity of damage during an incident or disaster. What other resources are available, keeping in mind that professional emergency response personnel will be preoccupied with human issues during the disaster and probably will not be available.

Has anyone coordinated with other agencies to make sure they realize how important animal issues are to their planning and mitigation efforts? Does every farm owner have a personal emergency and disaster plan in writing? Is there shelter room for large animals in addition to dogs and cats? Large animals require more room, resources, and feed; this must be coordinated well in advance to work properly (see Chapter 3).

Document Everything

Are there large animals in the jurisdiction? It does not have to be an agricultural or rural area to have backyard horses, goats, pigs, emus, llamas, alpacas, and cattle. Are there food animals in the jurisdiction? This may include poultry (turkey, quail, chicken, etc.), which are technically not large animals. Some of these production facilities may be readily visible, while others may be backyard operations behind fences or woods where no one would notice their existence. Good coordination with the state, local, and county agencies (Department

of Agriculture, animal control, sheriff's department, humane society, county extension service, 4-H clubs, etc.) will allow a more coordinated response. Consistent and compatible documentation and computer software further enhances the cooperative effort.

Mapping and Global Positioning Satellite/Geographic Information Systems. The use of global positioning satellite and geographic information systems (GPS/GIS) technology allows accurate mapping for planning and response purposes in disasters as well as emergencies. Maps can be produced with overlays of all animal facilities, proximity of those facilities to watercourses, manmade landmarks (railroads, highways, buildings), and other terrain features. Coordinated tabletop exercises, such as those held at the North Carolina Department of Agriculture and Consumer Services, allow rapid assessment and response. With just one click, a ring quarantine of areas affected by FAD can be imposed, evaluation of natural hazards in floodplains can be evaluated, and proximity of facilities to a chemical spill can be determined. This gives emergency managers the tools they need to conduct pre-assessments and plan their response, even as ground teams are gathering and transmitting data (McGinn, 2004).

Practice and Planning. Setting up possible scenarios within the county or local jurisdiction to test how personnel and agencies react to these situations is an excellent forerunner to preparedness. These exercises improve documentation methods and mapping and planning skills and increase interaction with other agencies to solve specific problems as they arise. Following the exercise, debriefing and documentation of the training exercise allow analysis and revision. Many counties now include animals in their semiannual training exercises, and there are even computerized scenarios available to practice natural and manmade disaster response.

MAINTAINING PUBLIC HEALTH STANDARDS

It can be very difficult to maintain clean food and water for humans and large animals in a disaster environment. Important measures include minimizing the number of animal carcasses, reducing contamination by waste products, and preventing spoiled food products from getting into water sources and the environment. During Hurricane Floyd, over 28,000 pigs drowned in North Carolina, and many of their carcasses floated downriver. The state response to this scenario was expensive, and consumed time and resources that could have been more efficiently spent elsewhere. Since that time, the North Carolina SART has provided leadership nationally in prevention of these scenarios by encouraging disaster planning and mitigation by commercial growers (McGinn, 2004).

Recovery of carcasses before they affect the environment is vital to protecting public health following a disaster. There should be prior coordination with local commercial animal growers for equipment, personnel, and training. This may include heavy equipment, trucks and trailers, boats, and HazMat personal protective equipment (PPE). Bacterial (e.g., *Staphylococcus* spp., *Streptococcus* spp., coliforms, etc.) and viral (e.g., rabies) infections resulting from animal bites and contact are not uncommon as both domesticated and zoological animals can serve as reservoirs. Many zoonotic diseases are transmitted by bites, and symptoms can range from localized swelling and infection to septicemia and multiple organ infection. Measures to prevent bites include wearing gloves; appropriate use of physical, mechanical, and chemical restraint; and protective clothing.

Protecting public health also requires protecting first responders and volunteers. All personnel must be immunized appropriately. Regular health checkups are recommended to identify individual health concerns. Responders and volunteers should be trained in zoonosis prevention and proper personal hygiene techniques. Food and water provisions for emergency and disaster workers must be appropriately maintained. Daily safety briefings should be conducted to ensure awareness of hazards in the field environment on disaster and large emergency scenes.

Safeguarding the Human Food Supply

Despite an increasing respect by humans for the place of animals in society, responders must understand that protecting the quality of the food supply remains a higher priority than the life of individual animals. This is especially true in a disaster situation (see Chapter 3). Food animal products are shipped nationwide and internationally, and contaminated food can have a widespread effect on human health. Livestock that are exposed to unknown chemical or biological contaminants in hazardous materials or floodwater scenarios, or simply allowed to wander the neighborhood in search of clean water and foodstuffs during a disaster, cannot be allowed to become part of the food chain for people. Live animals exposed to these scenarios must be properly identified. Veterinarians must be consulted to devise a time line to allow metabolic elimination of any contaminants or to recommend and perform euthanasia.

Chemical and biological contaminants can enter the animal's tissues through the skin, mouth, or mucous membranes (see Chapter 19). Safeguarding the food supply is a primary concern of the Department of Homeland Security and the U.S. Department of Agriculture due to its potential vulnerability to terrorism. Veterinary personnel and animal owners should be

trained to recognize unusual symptoms in their species of concern and should be aware of the proper reporting procedures if they suspect a disease.

BETTER METHODOLOGIES

Large animal emergency rescue techniques have been expanded greatly since the 1980s. Special techniques have been developed for the rescue of large animals trapped in mud, ravines, floodwaters, holes, and downed from exhaustion or starvation and are the focus of this text. However, these techniques require training and the use of modified equipment to protect the rescuers and raise the standard of care for the animal victim.

Humane Euthanasia

A variety of physical methods of field euthanasia have been used over the years by well-meaning volunteers and professional responders in situations involving large animals. There are a limited number of euthanasia methods that are approved by the American Veterinary Medical Association.

Humane methods of euthanasia for individual and potentially large numbers of animals must be a part of training for emergency responders and veterinary personnel who intend to participate (see Chapter 13). Commercial food animals exposed to hazardous material (i.e., floodwaters) should not enter the food chain for people. Large numbers of food animals kept in standard facilities may not be able to be transported, removed, or shipped early to slaughter before a disaster. Volunteers and responders should understand that providing humane euthanasia is more humane than death due to drowning, starvation, dehydration, or predation.

Proper field euthanasia requires knowledge of the anatomy and physiology of each animal species to be euthanatized. Chemical (e.g., barbiturate overdose) euthanasia may not be practical in field situations or disasters where dozens, hundreds, or thousands of animals must be destroyed. Barbiturate euthanasia solutions are controlled substances and are subject to Drug Enforcement Agency regulations. These solutions are not often available in sufficient volume to provide euthanasia for large numbers of animals. Humane physical methods of euthanasia (proper for each species) must be taught by veterinary personnel to volunteers from each participating group, and the proper equipment must be on hand. This may include a projectile weapon (e.g., pistol or rifle), captive bolt device, and/or properly sharpened knives to induce pneumothorax and exsanguination after use of the captive bolt.

Encourage Mitigation and Planning

At the community level, owners should be educated about disaster and emergency planning for their animals and facilities. Owners should have written personal emergency preparedness plans that are updated regularly. Trucks, trailers, and other necessary equipment should be well maintained, including annual evaluation and cleaning of flooring, brakes, lights, and electrical systems. All animals should be trained to lead and to load readily into the trailer. A priority system may be necessary, allowing animals to be evacuated based on value and ease of transport. Animals should be evacuated to a predetermined shelter or facility that is out of the affected region or projected path of any storm or fire. Several possible disaster evacuation routes should be planned to allow for road closures or blockages. Hay, feed, and fresh water stored in sturdy and secure containers should be available for quick loading into the trailer. A file folder of documentation, identification photos, and health records for all animals should be kept in the trailer at all times. A first aid kit should always be in the trailer. In addition, a National Oceanic and Atmospheric Administration–approved weather radio should be kept with the emergency supplies.

Decontamination of Large Animals

Working animals are often expected to work in areas where their human counterparts are protected from air pollutants by masks or PPE. Minimizing the risk to these valuable animals is crucial to the response effort (Murphy, 2004). Proper decontamination of police and military working dogs and privately owned horses is not a scenario that many jurisdictions have considered. Areas with mounted patrol and police horses should include animal decontamination as an alternate and more advanced scenario when practicing weapons of mass destruction decontamination scenarios (see Chapter 19).

Standard decontamination protocols involve establishing hot, warm, and cold zones (see Chapter 19). The problem of decontaminating large animals is complex. Contaminated human victims are often decontaminated in decontamination tents, where they disrobe, wash thoroughly, and don clean clothing. Of course, this approach is not feasible for large animals.

The situation may require establishing HazMat triage and decontamination zones for large numbers of affected animals. Decontamination options include using a portable tank of decontamination solution with a pump after hosing down the animals with large volumes of plain water, or temporarily submerging large numbers of animals in a pond of decontaminant solution.

Developing issues associated with large animal decontamination methods include identifying safe decontamination solutions, restraint during the decontamination procedure, and methods of catching the effluent (Murphy, 2004). Another issue that arose during training sessions was the fearful reaction

demonstrated by the animals in response to the PPE and the use of high-pressure hoses.

Other considerations unique to large animal decontamination include the withdrawal times necessary before food animals should be allowed to enter the food chain. Proper identification of treated animals is important, especially if withdrawal times are required.

Maintaining a secure decontamination area is critical to successful decontamination. Concerned owners may attempt to violate the zone boundaries to reach their animals; this can present severe health and security risks.

Prevention before Decontamination. The emphasis for decontamination efforts has to be placed on preventing the spread of the contaminant, particularly for biological hazards and FAD transmission. Prevention efforts on commercial food animal farms are intensive and include restricted access, using PPE while handling animals, and bathing upon entry to and exit from each animal facility before going to the next. Zoos, horse ranches, and small cattle farms are different; they encourage public participation and interaction and may experience high human and animal traffic through the area.

FOREIGN ANIMAL DISEASE

The introduction of a FAD into the United States could produce devastating agricultural and economic losses. The most obvious losses would occur in the agricultural sector, resulting from the loss of animals due to culling. Foreign trade would be negatively impacted, and local tourism would cease due to travel restrictions and public panic.

When the United Kingdom suffered an outbreak of foot and mouth disease in 2001, the country suffered severe economic losses that will continue to impact the economy for years to come. The damages extended beyond the loss of animals; the tourism industry was negatively affected, and travel restrictions resulted in severe damage to local economies. Approximately 6.5–10 million animals had to be culled by responders to effectively eradicate the disease, involving over 70% of livestock farms in the country. Foot and mouth disease is a disease of split-hooved ruminants (e.g., cattle, sheep, goats, and pigs), but many horses and other animals were euthanatized because the owners could not provide proper care due to quarantines and travel restrictions. The horse industry was negatively impacted due to travel restrictions and monetary losses from cancelled horse shows.

Although foot and mouth disease is not zoonotic (a disease that is transmitted from animals to humans), the human impact was also costly; the affected animals were the farmers' livelihood, and the emotional toll of the animals' deaths was devastating. An outbreak of foot and mouth disease in the United Kingdom in 2007 is being responded to at this writing.

Computer simulations have shown that a FAD could spread rapidly if introduced into the United States health certificates are currently required whenever livestock and horses are transported over state lines. There are several states (Florida, Arizona, Wyoming, Georgia, and California) that the author has found to be consistent about checking for proof of negative Coggins test and health certificates for horses. However, most states are less diligent in their surveillance of transported horses and more concerned with monitoring the transportation of cattle and other livestock. Although horses are not affected by foot and mouth disease, they can serve as fomites and physically transfer the virus on their hair or hooves. If foot and mouth disease were introduced into the United States, it is possible that the virus could spread across state borders more easily on horse trailers than on livestock trailers due to less stringent enforcement of animal health regulations for equine species.

Mass Carcass Disposal

In the case of a mass animal casualty disaster or FAD that necessitates the culling of a large number of animals, logistical challenges to mass carcass disposal would include geography, climate, expense, and laws. The terrain of the affected area may be unsuitable for burying carcasses due to the presence of rock or a low water table. Experience in previous outbreaks has shown that mass incineration or burning is expensive and slow, while burial requires a large area and significant equipment. Recent advances in mass euthanasia and composting efforts have shown promise, but do not present a panacea for these issues.

ACRONYMS USED IN CHAPTER 2

EMS	Emergency medical services
GIS	Geographic information system
GPS	Global positioning satellite
HazMat	Hazardous material
IAP	Incident action plan
ICS	Incident command system
FAD	Foreign animal disease
PPE	Personal protective equipment
SART	State animal response team
TLAER	Technical large animal emergency rescue

3 Incident Prevention and Evacuation Planning

Dr. Rebecca Gimenez

INTRODUCTION

Preparedness for emergencies and disasters involving large animals must begin at the local level and be a cooperative effort. Animal and facility owners should take responsibility for their animals, and emergency services and management personnel should preplan for evacuation and sheltering considerations of large animals. Planning for an all-hazards approach will ensure that worst-case scenarios and a variety of incidents are simulated and evaluated to expand the awareness of the community to these hazards. This chapter is not intended to be an inclusive effort, but to increase awareness of some of the considerations that communities may take in their planning efforts.

Prevention includes all the efforts taken at the local level by the owner and the animal community to educate the animal industry, animal owners, and emergency responders about the issues related to technical large animal emergency rescue (TLAER). Extending preparation to include training of emergency response personnel in basic animal handling is suggested (Figure 3.1).

How Bad Can It Get?

Owners should consider the hazards that may affect their facilities. For example, they should determine how facility operations and animal care would be affected by loss of power for one or more days. The effects of weather should also be considered; for example, maintaining the provision of fresh water, feed, and care for the animals in freezing temperatures without power should be included in the planning phase. In areas at risk of wildfire, the emergency plan should address the possibility that an immediate evacuation may be necessary. Local emergencies and disasters of this type are very common and provide a stimulus

for responsible animal owners to thoroughly consider the aspects of planning that are important to their farm or animal-related business.

Self-reliance is a critical part of TLAER planning and emergency management policy; it is the owner's responsibility to develop a plan to take care of his or her family and their animals. Facility owners that board animals should understand that the animals' owners will look to them to be responsible for taking care of their animals during an emergency or disaster.

When disaster planning fails, human and animal lives are at risk. In 2002, a 500-year flood event occurred in Europe that overwhelmed the zoo in Prague, Czech Republic. Several animals drowned. Other animals died when they breached the zoo property and were sacrificed when they could not be recaptured. International media attention was gained when the zoo's most famous inhabitant, Kadir, the bull elephant, was destroyed when he could not be rescued from the rising waters.

An investigation revealed that although the zoo had a 100-year flood plan, this was a 500-year flood that was not predicted in time to adequately warn the zoo officials. The water rose much higher than expected, but the staff and volunteers were able to get approximately 1,200 animals to safety in a period of 12 hours. The successful rescue efforts included the vertical lift of a rhinoceros, an impressive feat, coordinated with the local fire department.

PREPAREDNESS BEGINS AT THE LOCAL LEVEL

Regardless of the size of the facility, owners should have an evacuation plan for every conceivable emergency. Examples include barn fires, wildfires,

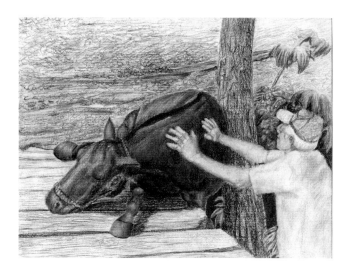

Figure 3.1 *This horse was trapped between a tree and a bridge in its home pasture for over six hours before responders arrived. This scenario illustrates that even unanticipated situations can be resolved with proper training and execution. A veterinarian was called to the scene immediately and treated the animal for shock and other injuries, while responders successfully extricated the animal with fire hose webbing. Courtesy of Julie Casil.*

earthquakes, mudslides, blizzards, chemical spills, and high wind events (tornado, hail storms, hurricanes). There are two levels of disaster preparedness for each facility: personal preparedness and business preparedness. Personal preparedness involves the creation of a family disaster plan. Business preparedness consists of resumption and contingency planning for the business.

Facility owners should be encouraged to write down their plan and practice it. In general, a properly developed emergency and evacuation plan can be successfully applied to many other scenarios. Being proactive will minimize the amount of time and expense required to restore operations, preserve animals and valuables, and minimize stress. Practicing the plan improves efficiency, response time, and safety.

Owners should be encouraged to be proactive in emergency and disaster prevention, planning, and response. In 2002, a veterinarian informed the author that he was on one of the field rescue teams that attempted to help 350 cows from multiple farms in North Carolina following Hurricane Floyd. The cattle were standing on the last piece of high ground for miles, and the water continued to rise. Responders were able to rescue some smaller calves with boats, but the remaining cattle drowned or were euthanized.

Proper planning includes establishing predetermined meeting places and multiple evacuation route options from the facility and the area. If evacuation is not possible, the disaster plan should include a means of sheltering in place.

THE PLANNING CYCLE

The planning cycle of the Federal Emergency Management Agency (FEMA) includes recommendations that owners and emergency management personnel identify potential hazards, perform risk and vulnerability assessments, and assess capabilities and resources. These efforts will allow personnel to make informed decisions regarding the proper course of action in response to each hazard. The plan should evolve and change dynamically based on new information, review, and testing. The plan should also be updated regularly in response to changes in staff (names or numbers), animals, or other factors affecting the facility.

Evacuation Planning Is a Process

Facilities should post an evacuation plan where everyone can see it and read it easily. The planning process is as important (if not more important) than the plan itself, involving all affected people as a team in generating the plan (family, employees, friends, boarders, etc.). This cooperative process ensures commitment by everyone to the effort. This kind of training and preparation makes employees and family members more self-reliant, efficient, and confident if a disaster or emergency occurs.

According to a study, approximately 30%–50% of pet (cat and dog) owners leave their pets behind during evacuations, even with advance notice to leave (Heath, 1999). However, Heath noted that 50%–70% of these same owners attempted to later "rescue" their animals, breaching security barriers to provide food or attempt to bring the animals out of the affected area. Even under mandatory evacuation orders, some owners will not leave their animals; as observed during and after Hurricanes Katrina and Rita in 2005, refusal to evacuate may pose life-threatening consequences.

The Emergency Management Cycle

The emergency management cycle consists of four phases: mitigation, preparation, response, and recovery (Figure 3.2). The length of each phase may vary with the type of disaster or emergency, and events in one phase may overlap those of the previous phase.

Mitigation includes the permanent changes made to minimize the effect of a disaster. Examples include installing sprinkler systems and passive heat detectors or using nonflammable materials to build a livestock barn.

Preparation consists of the steps involved in readiness for disasters and emergencies. This phase occurs when the local area is under the watch and warning phases and facility or farm owners implement their plans. Steps include creating the family and facility evacuation plans, videotaping or photographing all assets and safely storing the tapes or photographs, obtaining and maintaining insurance (including flood

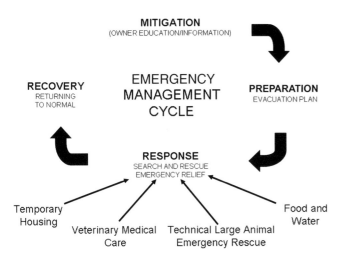

Figure 3.2 *The emergency management cycle depicts the stages of mitigation, preparation, response, and recovery. Each phase may overlap with the previous or subsequent phase, depending on the situation.*

insurance, where applicable) on the property, backing up computer records, and making copies of identification records, registration papers, and photographs for each animal or lots of animals.

Between the preparedness and response phases is the incident or disaster itself. The disaster often overlaps with the response phase, as plans are implemented during the disaster.

The *response* phase is the period during and immediately following a disaster. During this time, emergency assistance is provided to victims of the disaster and efforts are made to reduce further damage.

Recovery is the fourth and final phase of the emergency management cycle and continues until all systems have returned to normal or near-normal operation. The purpose of short-term recovery is to restore the operation of vital support systems. Long-term recovery lasts until the entire affected area returns to its previous conditions or undergoes improvement; this may go on for months or years. Cleanup, carcass removal, emergency repairs, and rebuilding all take place within this phase.

Planning Methods. There are three methods for development of a disaster plan for animals (Heath, 1999). Planning in the absence of an immediate threat is the preferred method, because it provides unhurried time to thoroughly consider the plan and identify resources. A common method for planning takes place immediately following a disaster. Planning during the actual disaster is a necessary but biased method that is followed by another large contingent of the public. The latter two methods are associated with higher risk of failure due to inadequate or improper planning and implementation.

Domesticated livestock depend on humans to provide for their daily needs. When humans domesticated animals and placed them in confinement for convenience, the animals' skills and instincts that kept them out of danger were blunted. However, vestiges of those instincts remain, and the survival instincts may surface at times of stress. The urge to flee in panic may take over and can make handling the animals more dangerous. In the wild, animals find the safest place to get out of the storm, flee the wildfire, or endure the blizzard. Domesticated animals may be placed at higher risk of injury during disasters because they may be trapped by stalls or fences. Proper planning accounts for the physical and behavioral factors that affect implementation.

Identify Hazards

Facility owners should identify all possible hazards that can realistically occur in their area. The facility should be closely evaluated for the hazards specific to the facility, such as obstructed exits, improperly functioning equipment, and machinery hazards. Multiple evacuation routes should be planned. An adequate amount of good-quality equipment should be available, and arrangements should be made to enable the transportation of all animals.

Requirements for Sheltering

Disaster management essentials include having a first aid kit (one for animals, one for humans), identification of all animals (e.g., with microchips), and up-to-date preventive care (vaccination, deworming, equine infectious anemia screening, etc.) as recommended by the veterinarian. Animals may need to be taken to a local public evacuation shelter or legally cross state lines in a major evacuation; adequate preventive care ensures that animals are protected from infectious diseases when they are exposed to unfamiliar animals at these facilities. Owners may lose track of their animals during a disaster, so identification is crucial. After every major disaster, there have been documented cases of animal theft from shelters, the evacuation area, and the owner's unprotected facility.

Properly identified animals are more likely to be reunited with their owners. Methods of identification include brands, microchips, neck bands, tags, etched or branded hooves, and non-water-soluble body paint. Many dogs and cats that are rescued after a disaster are stray or abandoned animals, but there are very few cases where horses are abandoned or stray prior to a disaster. Commonly, however, large animals may be left behind because the owner was unable to catch, transport, or find a place to house the horses or livestock for the duration of the disaster.

Evacuation Drills

Even a well-designed preparedness plan can fail if not rehearsed. Regular (e.g., every six months), unannounced evacuation drills familiarize personnel and animals with the procedures and reduce the risks of failure. The time of day and the requirements of the drill should vary (see Chapter 10).

Simple Prevention. Examples of prevention are included in each chapter of this book, but they are intended only as introductions to the phase of the emergency and disaster planning cycle being discussed. A short list of simple prevention methods at a local facility or farm might include the following:

- Prohibit smoking and alcoholic beverages within 250 feet of the facility.
- Ensure all staff, employees, and family members are familiar with the emergency and disaster plans and how to enact them.
- Ensure that several days' supply of feed, water, supplements, and medications are stored for each animal being evacuated or sheltered in place.
- Identify and make arrangements with sheltering facilities ahead of time. Overnight or short-term boarding facilities outside the area at risk are preferred. The contact information should be kept with the identification and other important papers. The average cost for housing at evacuation facilities is approximately ≤$25 per day per animal.
- Train animals to load easily and safely in transport vehicles under varying conditions (e.g., dark, raining, windy, etc.).
- Use permanent identification (e.g., freeze brands, implanted microchips) for every animal.

CHAOS, CONFUSION, AND COMMUNICATION

In some disasters, the impact of the event can be overshadowed by the chaos and confusion that occur afterward; disasters may not seem significant until they directly impact one's life (Figure 3.3). For example, the worst damage from Hurricane Floyd occurred from flooding in rural counties with large concentrations of food and companion animals. Losses included 28,000 swine; 2.9 million poultry; 680 cattle; and smaller numbers of horses (Ferris, 2000). Due to excessive flooding, families that evacuated and expected to return within 48 hours after the storm were not able to return home for weeks. A similar event occurred after Hurricane Katrina in September 2005.

Logistics (Personnel, Equipment, and Supplies). Following Hurricane Floyd (1999), the outpouring of public support to help animals resulted in tons of

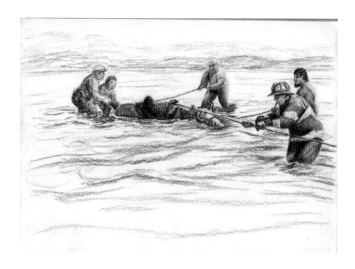

Figure 3.3 *A horse being ridden across a flooded river to drive cattle trapped in the flood became mired in the river's muddy bottom. The animal was assisted by personnel on scene, using the saddle as a field expedient forward assist. However, owners with livestock in the path of natural disasters and local emergencies should have a better plan than riding through a flooded area to move them. Courtesy of Julie Casil.*

donated pet and livestock feed that overwhelmed the available storage facilities and distribution personnel. Over 800,000 kg (880 tons) of pet food were distributed over a three-month period after the disaster. A fund was set up to manage the monetary donations and expenses associated with the disaster (Ferris, 2000).

Numerous volunteers self-deployed to the area to assist the rescue efforts. However, the majority of these volunteers were inadequately trained, unfamiliar with the emergency management system in place, and unequipped for their tasks. As a result, the demand for resources was increased. Inadequately trained personnel are at risk of sustaining injury and compromising the safety and health of animals and other rescue personnel (Ferris, 2000). The state animal response team (SART) model was developed in 2000 specifically for planning, preparedness, response, and recovery from animal emergencies in North Carolina. The team operates under the state's Emergency Management System (EMS). At the county level, there are county animal response teams (CARTs) to assist with local animal rescue planning. This model for animal planning and coordination has been successfully duplicated across several U.S. states since that time.

Get Out Early

Due to the manpower and transportation resources necessary to evacuate large numbers of animals, evacuation should be performed as early as possible in the case of wildfires, flooding, and hurricanes. Prearranged evacuation resources, such as borrowed trailers or arranged transportation, should be incorporated into the emergency/disaster plan. Animal owners should consult with their local emergency management service about planning for animal emergencies and disasters in their area. When watches or warnings have been issued, careful monitoring of the situation (on the Internet, radio, or television) is recommended.

In 1988, the Northern California 49er wildfires featured the largest-scale evacuation of a variety of livestock, horses, llamas, and other animals (including pets) to date. Local volunteers played a vital role in the success of the evacuation. Their efforts were most effective during the voluntary evacuation period, when it was safest for both humans and animals to be transported (Heath, 1999; Nixon, 2006).

EVACUATION PLANNING FOR OWNERS

Owners should be encouraged to ensure that adequate space is available to transport animals and the ability to acquire the necessary supplies on short notice. A four-horse gooseneck trailer loaded with four horses and the equipment necessary for their care may limit the space available for the transport of pets, humans, and their associated equipment and supplies. More than one trip to evacuate may not be possible due to weather, road, or traffic conditions. Predetermined evacuation sites (including alternate sites) and driving distances should be included in the plan. The evacuation plan should include a specific checklist of tasks specific to the facility or farm that must be performed prior to evacuation (e.g., turn off the power, unplug all appliances, etc.). Human and animal first aid kits should be readily available. A National Oceanographic and Atmospheric Administration-approved radio is recommended for monitoring the situation.

The value (actual market value and/or sentimental value) of the owned animals should be determined, and a prioritized list should be generated to ensure that the most valuable animals are evacuated first. The individual needs of each animal should be considered; horses that are difficult to load in a trailer or that appear more susceptible to health problems when stressed may need to be placed lower on the priority list to ensure the most efficient evacuation possible. A minimum of a three-day supply of hay, feed, and water should be stored and transported with the animals.

A well designed hurricane evacuation plan was successfully enacted by a local veterinarian in 2003 in Florida. Arrangements were made for a horse van to evacuate horses to Georgia when a hurricane watch was issued. Animals and their supplies were loaded and moved from the area prior to inclement weather and mass evacuation conditions. Owners shared the horse transportation costs (Merrick, 2004).

Sheltering in Place

There are some emergencies and disasters in which large animals cannot be evacuated from the area before the hazard. In some population centers of the United States, animal owners are advised to plan for sheltering in place. An example of this is southern Florida, where the evacuation routes may be clogged due to heavy traffic.

Many owners are unsure if they should leave horses turned out in fields during disasters or confine them in stalls. The decision should be based on the facility environment; there are perils associated with each option, and owners should make the decision based on which option presents the lowest risk of injury. In general, livestock should be kept outside in the largest, adequately fenced pasture available. Horses will find cover in a copse of trees if necessary, but normally will stand in the middle of the field with their hindquarters to the wind. The muscles of the hindquarter provide the most protection from flying debris. However, fields may not be the optimal housing arrangement if there are dead or fallen trees, unsecured farm equipment, or inadequate fencing in the area. Horses have been electrocuted by fallen power lines, struck by lightning, crushed by flying vehicles and equipment, or lacerated severely by flying debris.

Horses trapped in barns may be at increased risk of injury due to flying debris, fire, or building collapse. Ice and snow storms may seem to be examples of emergencies where animals should be brought inside for protection, but snow loading on roofs can collapse them. Veterinary medical assistance team (VMAT) and the Humane Society of the United States (HSUS) field response members deployed to Mississippi and Louisiana following Hurricane Katrina in 2005 observed and reported there were no barns left standing after the hurricane, and all animal facilities they visited were destroyed.

Do the Math

If an owner must evacuate his or her animals 10 or 100 km to safety, and three round trips are required to evacuate all of the animals, 60–600 km must be driven to accomplish the evacuation. Planning multiple trips to accomplish evacuation can be risky; weather or traffic conditions may prohibit returning to the facility for remaining livestock. Owners and animals stranded during an emergency or disaster present logistic difficulties for responders and may consume vital resources during the rescue effort.

IDENTIFICATION OF ANIMALS

Lessons from Hurricane Andrew (1992) and more recent disasters (Hurricanes Floyd and Katrina) included the importance of permanent identification for all animals. Locating animals, establishing rightful ownership, preventing animal theft, and eliminating confusion are facilitated by proper, permanent identification.

Permanent identification provides the additional benefit of traceability during disease outbreaks. Brucellosis and tuberculosis in cattle have almost been eradicated over the last few decades through the use of animal tracking systems. According to Dr. Valerie Ragan, "Without identification, everything else is untraceable and untrackable."

Brands, tattoos, and ear tags are common methods of permanent livestock identification that have been used for hundreds of years to confirm ownership or identify individual animals. Responders should document any identification methods used on animals and plan a method for tracking animals found in the field as to found location, markings, and condition.

Color
Color is one of the most easily observed characteristics of an animal, but can be subject to differences in interpretation and name by observers. Coat color can change with age, hair growth, and exposure to sunlight. In addition, "a horse's color can be changed by the use of dyes and coloring agents by the unscrupulous." (Metcalf, 2004).

Natural Markings
Natural markings are another visually observed characteristic on animals and may include hair whorls, focal muscle defects (also called Allah's thumbprint, Prophet's thumbprint, or Devil's thumbprint), special patterns of white hairs, unusual coloration, lightning marks (irregular white markings on the legs that do not contact the hooves), or ermine and halo effects. Most of these do not change with time, but not all animals have distinguishing markings. Often unique to the animal, some markings may be altered by the use of hair dyes or coloring agents.

Acquired Markings
Acquired markings include visually noticeable scars, tattoos, or brands that are unique to the animal. Lip tattoos, as performed on racehorses, may become illegible as the horse ages and can be altered.

Hot branding induces a permanent scar on the hide of the animal that is commonly used in livestock, but it is painful to the animal. The procedure generally requires anesthesia in horses. Traditional brands identified the owner, but not individual animals. To identify an individual, a system of numbers and characters is necessary. Hot branding of the hoof is an excellent and painless way to identify a horse, but the brand eventually grows out as the hoof grows.

Freeze branding is a popular and painless method of marking an animal that destroys the ability of the hair cell to produce pigment. Thus the hair grows in white and gives adequate contrast on most hide colors to allow reading the mark from a distance. Responders can list the brands of animals found in the field. Because freeze brands are difficult to alter, they may discourage or prevent theft.

Photographs
Photographs provide a quick method to allow an owner or shelter manager to document an animal; however, matching the owner to the animal may still be difficult if the animal's appearance has changed due to weight loss or injury. Photos can be retouched.

Identification Bands or Tags
Neck collars, bands, or chains are common temporary methods of identification for animals brought into shelters or veterinary facilities. Ear tags are commonly inserted in the ears of livestock but must be matched to the owner's documentation for identification of a particular animal; this can be difficult to achieve in a disaster situation.

Pastern or fetlock bands for horses and other animals can be effective means of identification. Rescuers in the field can place the bands on the pastern or above the fetlock and mark the band with the grid coordinates of the site at which the horse was found, as well as any other necessary information. Testing by the authors has found that permanent ink on these bands was intact and legible for two months. Placement of bands on cattle and some other livestock can be more difficult, because the animals are not accustomed to handling.

Blood typing and DNA
Blood typing and DNA analysis are suitable for parentage testing, genetic screening of diseases, and are the most individual methods of determining the exact identity of the animal. Due to the associated expense and time required to perform these tests, they are not practical or useful for identifying individual livestock in a disaster or emergency situation.

Microchips
Microchips are passive transponders known as radio-frequency implantable devices (RFIDs). They are activated by a frequency-specific reader that displays alphanumeric characters unique to that microchip. RFID readers are becoming commonplace across the United States (Cordes, 2000).

Equines. Over 100,000 equids in the state of Louisiana have been implanted with microchips; this effort has been credited with reducing the number of equine infectious anemia–positive horses in that state. Following Hurricane Katrina, the presence of implanted microchips facilitated reuniting horses with their owners. At the time of this writing, only four horses (out of hundreds rescued) had not been reunited with their owners (Culver, 2006). Microchips are practically impossible to remove once implanted and stay with the animal for life, improving the chance of recovery in the case of theft.

The placement of microchips in the nuchal ligament of the horse is relatively easy to perform, with minimal discomfort to the animal. A microchip is unique to the animal in which it is implanted, and allows shelter managers or veterinarians with readers to determine the owner of the animal. Following microchip implantation, the animal must be registered in a database; failure to register the microchip complicates the identification process. The standardized location for a microchip in an equid is in the nuchal ligament on the left side of the neck, halfway between the ears and the withers and approximately 1 in. (2.54 cm) below the origin of the mane hairs. This is the only implantation site approved by the U.S. Department of Agriculture (USDA) and the Food and Drug Administration for use in equids. Other animals have specific approved implantation sites, which are described below. Tissue migration has not been a concern since antimigration caps were added to the transponders in 1989 (Cordes, 2000).

Agricultural Animals. The implantation site for the bovine, ovine, porcine, and caprine, or other species used for meat production, is subcutaneously at the base of the left ear on the scutiform cartilage. Implanted food-producing animals should be marked with an external identifier to indicate that a microchip is present so that it can be recovered at slaughter. Local trade or government guidelines must govern the use of implanted microchips in food-producing species as their use may not be permitted in some situations. Alpacas and other camelids are implanted subcutaneously midway on the left side of the neck or on top of the head behind the left ear.

U.S. NATIONAL ANIMAL IDENTIFICATION SYSTEM

In the interest of protecting animal health and as a foundation for the nation's agricultural infrastructure, the National Animal Identification System (NAIS) has been proposed and is being implemented in the United States. The NAIS is a voluntary state–federal–industry partnership that involves premises registration as well as identification and traceability of individual animals. Similar identification systems exist in the European Union, Canada, and Australia. The NAIS will include camelids, cattle and bison, commercially raised cervids, equids (horses, donkeys, and mules), goats, poultry, sheep, and swine.

Horses probably move farther and more frequently than other species. Some food animal species, such as pigs and poultry, are transported only once or twice in their lives, when they are moved as young or to be slaughtered and processed. Cattle may be transported several times (e.g., from the cow-calf operation to a sale facility, then to a feed lot, then to slaughter). Show animals and breeding stock often travel more frequently.

Tracking animal movement effectively can be a daunting task due to the number of animals that are transported on a daily basis. In case of a disease outbreak, such as the multistate equine herpesvirus type-1 (EHV-1) outbreaks of 2005–2006, tracing the outbreak to its source can be difficult. As an infected animal is transported to multiple facilities for shows or similar events, the other animals housed at each facility may be exposed and infected. As those animals are transported to other facilities or events, the number of potentially infected horses can increase exponentially. For example, the author's horses are transported over state lines approximately 50 times per year; this presents a significant risk of infection and disease transmission if the horses are commingled with other animals at each housing facility.

Premises Identification Number

Show facilities, sales facilities, and veterinary clinics can be registered with a premises identification number (PIN) under the NAIS. To track large numbers of animals, animal health officials must know where the animals are born and where they are moved. Therefore, identifying locations that manage or hold animals—referred to as premises—is the starting point of the NAIS. Each premises is identified with a unique seven-character identifier, or PIN.

The NAIS assigns each farm, ranch, auction barn, fair, and animal handling or show facility with a PIN based on the 911 address and Global Positioning Satellite coordinate of the facility (see Chapter 12). The PIN stays with the facility or land for as long as it is used as an agricultural or livestock facility; the information is not specific to the person or company that owns it.

Sites of animal commingling, such as show and race facilities, sales barns, and veterinary clinics and hospitals, should be registered with the NAIS. An infected animal at this type of facility could theoretically expose hundreds of other animals to infection. In some cases, the entire facility may be quarantined to prevent further spread of the disease. This situation occurred numerous times during the EHV-1 outbreaks (2005–2007) in Florida, California, Virginia, Maryland, Kentucky, Ohio, Pennsylvania, New York, Michigan, Connecticut, and Oregon.

Program Purpose. The primary intent of the NAIS is to facilitate epidemiological investigations. The ability to track animal movement allows more rapid detection of the source of the outbreak. This is especially important in surveillance for equine viral arteritis and foreign animal diseases (FADs) such as foot and mouth disease (FMD), African horse sickness, piroplasmosis, and glanders. Exposure to these diseases, coupled with poor epidemiological tracking mechanisms, has the potential to cause panic and severe losses within the agriculture industry.

The NAIS is expected to be a fundamental tool for implementing animal health monitoring and surveillance programs. State and federal animal health officials will be able to access a centralized NAIS database to ascertain a herd's health status and issue intra- and interstate animal movement certificates.

The system is designed to allow animal health officials to identify all animals and premises that have had contact with a foreign or domestic animal disease of concern within 48 hours after discovery, limiting the scope of such outbreaks and ensuring that they are contained and eradicated as quickly as possible.

The NAIS (USDA, 2004) is intended to enhance the efforts of veterinarians by

- improving FAD surveillance, control, and eradication,
- facilitating epidemiological investigations,
- improving biosecurity protection of the livestock population,
- distinguishing vaccinated from unvaccinated animals during USDA disease control and eradication efforts,
- furnishing official identification for interstate and international commerce,
- accurately identifying blood and tissue specimens for laboratory diagnostics and registration of purebred animals,
- tracking the health status of certified herds,
- enabling regionalization and risk assessment in support of international trade,
- establishing uniform identification methods for each species, and
- tracking and recording the performance characteristics of individual breeding animals.

Sick or exposed animals should be identified, tracked, and quarantined as early as possible in a disease outbreak situation. As an example, over 300 horses per day cross the state line into Florida; this represents almost 110,000 horses a year crossing the border of one state. Horse trailers regularly travel thru 3 to 6 states in one day. Given these statistics, the potential risk for spread of an infectious disease in livestock is very high.

Participation by Industry

Facilities involved in the agricultural industry but that do not house livestock or horses are encouraged to register with a non-producer participant number. This includes farriers, mobile veterinary clinics, feed stores, breed registries, identification providers, and others. A 7-character alpha-numeric identification unique to that facility is assigned. Individual animals are assigned

a 15-character number, called an animal identification number (AIN). For groups of animals, such as flocks of poultry or litters of piglets, a lot number is assigned.

The NAIS is a voluntary program for horse owners, but it is highly recommended by veterinarians and agriculture officials. Each state implements the system within its borders. One roadblock to implementation of the NAIS is the concern about the confidentiality of the system's information database. In its current form, NAIS information will be part of a confidential database free from public disclosure laws. Proprietary data is not included in the PIN or AIN for USDA or any other agency; only information for disease monitoring and tracking are linked to the PIN and AIN.

BIOTERRORISM

Veterinary resources can be used to prevent as well as respond to a bioterrorism incident. Veterinarians receive advanced training in the treatment and diagnosis of animal diseases, many of which are zoonotic (passed from animal to human). Five of the six Category A potential agents of bioterrorism (Centers for Disease Control classification), and more than 50% of Category B agents, are zoonotic diseases (CDC, 2007).

Veterinary hospitals stock supplies necessary for the recovery phase, including atropine, oxygen, antibiotics, and surgical and medical supplies. Veterinary resources should be included in any local and regional planning for these types of events (Anderson, 2002).

Laws such as the Public Health and Security and Bioterrorism Preparedness and Response Act of 2002 protect the U.S. food supply from terrorist activity. The Animal Health Protection Act of 2002 (Public Law 107–171; Farm Security and Rural Investment Act of 2002, 116 Stat 134) repealed previous animal health and quarantine laws and strengthened the secretary of agriculture's authority to control and eradicate disease. The Animal and Plant Health Inspection Service National Animal Health Emergency Response Plan for a foreign animal or highly contagious animal disease forms an operational annex to the National Response Plan (NRP) (Johnson, 2002).

Agroterrorism Vulnerability

Agroterrorism is defined as "the use of a biological, chemical, radiological, or other agent against either the pre-harvest or post-harvest stages of food and fiber production to inspire fear or cause economic damage, public health impact, or other adverse impact." (LSU, 2004)

In the United States in 2006, the commercial food animal population consisted of approximately 97 million beef cattle, over 9.1 million dairy cattle, 6.2 million sheep, 62 million hogs, and 9.6 billion poultry (National Agricultural Statistics Service, 2007). At 200 billion dollars, the agriculture business is the largest in the United States; approximately ≤$55 billion are contributed to the U.S. economy in farm-related exports, constituting 9.7% of the U.S. gross domestic product and generating cash receipts of ≤$991 billion. One in eight Americans works in an occupation directly supported by the agricultural industry, reflecting the importance of the stability of the agricultural economy.

The infrastructure of agriculture is inherently vulnerable because it is so large and covers so much territory. Visitors are commonly allowed on farms, with the exception of most commercial poultry facilities. Wildlife often have free access to pastures and serve as reservoirs of infectious diseases. Biosecurity measures have become high-priority issues in agriculture; this is especially true for poultry and swine farms because of their intensive concentration of animals (LSU, 2004). For example, the exotic Newcastle disease outbreak in California in 2002 cost the country approximately ≤$175 million, and negative trade restrictions additionally affected California and the U.S. poultry industry. The introduction of a FAD would be expected to cause a cascade effect of negative consequences: animal loss, loss of genetically valuable breeding stock, reduction of consumer confidence in food safety, increased food prices, and restricted movement of animals (LSU, 2004).

The United States is the largest producer of food and agricultural products in the world; there are over 500,000 farms and over 6,000 meat/poultry/egg product production establishments. However, most cities have approximately a five-day food supply cache. The average "farm to fork" distance traveled by food animals is 1,300 miles over their lifetime (LSU, 2004).

Cooperation between Human Medical and Veterinary Medical Communities

The threats of bioterrorism and agroterrorism emphasize the importance of communication between the human medical and veterinary medical communities in ensuring national security. Both communities play important roles in the mitigation and response effort, and the unification of efforts, expertise, and resources facilitates these roles. Five of the six Category A high-threat pathogens and 76% of the 156 pathogens associated with emerging diseases are zoonotic.

The National Multi-Hazard Symposium: "One Medicine" Approach to Homeland Security was convened in 2003 in Raleigh, North Carolina, to increase collaboration between the human medical and veterinary medical communities in the area of national security. Recommendations produced by this conference included: development of critical public health infrastructure and core capacities to ensure that communities and states can detect and eliminate infectious diseases; integration of human and animal surveillance, detection, preparedness, and response systems; assessments of food and water to include evaluation of

production, processing, and distribution; performance of comprehensive risk and vulnerability evaluations to mitigate current threats; research of pathogens and hazards that can impact human and animal populations in order to develop effective diagnostics, vaccines, and therapies.

The U.S. National Strategy for Homeland Security, under the Uniting and Strengthening America by Providing Appropriate Tools Required to Intercept and Obstruct Terrorism (USA PATRIOT Act; 107th Congress, 1st session, HR 3162 RDS 24 Oct 2001), identifies agriculture as one of the critical infrastructure components that must be protected. In this act, these components are defined as "those systems and assets, whether physical or virtual, so vital to the United States that the incapacity or destruction of such systems and assets would have a debilitating impact on security, national economic security, national public health or safety, or any combination of those matters."

Vulnerabilities in the food chain provide opportunities for bioterrorism and agroterrorism. The World Health Organization has urged governments to draw up contingency plans to protect their populations against these risks. If contamination of the food supply occurred at a slaughterhouse or food-processing facility, widespread dissemination could pose a significant national risk (WHO, 2002).

In April 2007, the Executive Board of the American Veterinary Medical Association (AVMA) approved the formation of a 13-member One Health Initiative Task Force, composed of veterinary and human medical professionals. The task force is charged with identifying areas of joint agreement between the human and veterinary medical fields; identifying needs for increased collaboration; and developing strategies to address challenges and increase cooperation between the medical professions. In June 2007, the House of Delegates of the American Medical Association adopted a One Health resolution in response to the increasing need for collaboration, and it is working with the AVMA in the initiative.

CHEMICAL, BIOLOGICAL, RADIOLOGICAL, NUCLEAR, AND EXPLOSIVE HAZARDS

The original impetus for drawing veterinary resources into the integrated local and state response were models predicting workforce needs for chemical, biological, nuclear, radiological, and/or explosive (CBNRE) events. Numerous computer exercises and conferences had predicted and demonstrated the need for integrating the veterinary community, whose emphasis and training in public health can augment the expertise of the human medical community (McGinn, 2004b). The 2004 National Animal CBNRE Summit was held in conjunction with the 2nd Annual National Multi-Hazard Symposium to facilitate and encourage communication among federal, state, and local animal response agencies and associations with an interest in animal issues, protection, and decontamination (Murphy, 2005).

In cases of foreign animal disease introduction, United States Codes 8305–8310 authorizes the U.S. secretary of agriculture to

- prohibit or restrict interstate movement of farmstock
- quarantine, treat, or destroy animals
- declare an emergency
- approve compensation for destroyed animals at fair market value
- stop and inspect, without warrant, movements of animals
- enter agricultural properties without warrant
- cooperate with other agencies in the control and eradication of disease
- acquire property, employ a person, make a grant, or enter a contract
- conduct any inspection/investigation to gather and compile information
- create and insure loans to established farmers

FAD AND BIOSECURITY

Prevention for farm owners begins with attention to a biosecurity program. The transport and distribution of large animals often involves hundreds or thousands of kilometers from point of origin to the sale point or slaughter; this makes it important for all animal industry personnel to educate themselves about FAD. This chapter introduces some of the ideas related to FAD prevention and transmission.

Methods for reducing the chance of disease spread include cleaning and disinfecting equipment and vehicles (trailers) between loads of animals and separating feed and water sources. Others methods include testing and screening, selective purchasing from proven clean herds or flocks, isolation and quarantine, vaccination, monitoring and evaluation, and cleaning and disinfection of facilities. Animal owners should contact their veterinarian immediately when a suspicious disease or unusual symptoms are displayed by animals. Biosecurity programs on commercial animal facilities include using sign in/sign out logs, restricting access to the facility, excluding wildlife and free-roaming pets from the facility, keeping feed covered, and providing for appropriate disposal of dead animals.

FAD Investigation

FAD investigations are conducted when a private veterinarian or concerned farmer or animal owner contacts the state or federal officials with a FAD concern. After examination, an epidemiologic investigation and collection of samples for diagnostic testing are performed. The case is assigned a number from the USDA

for tracking purposes. Strict adherence to biosecurity methods is followed from the beginning of the investigation; investigators burn or disinfect their clothing and other fomites as they leave the premises. Specific examination and sampling protocols are in place for the investigation and epidemiologic tracking of FAD. Reaction to a proven FAD may include:

- increased awareness about the FAD
- slaughter of infected, recovered, and contact animals
- disinfection of premises, disposal of carcasses, and litter
- control of human and animal movement, vector control, and herd or flock emergency depopulation measures

The potential emotional toll and zoonotic concerns for the animal owners and professional personnel responsible for enforcing the protocols should be addressed in the emergency management plan. Debriefing and counseling may be necessary during and following the response and relief efforts.

ANIMAL DISEASES AFFECTING HUMANS

Domestics and wild animals can be sources of human illness. Diseases transmitted between animals and humans are called zoonoses. Most are preventable with attention to proper hygiene (including washing hands after handling the animal) and preventing exposure to bites or injury. There are many zoonotic diseases that are not foreign animal diseases, but which must be cautiously evaluated in TLAER-related incidents. The veterinarian is the most qualified professional on the scene to assist emergency personnel with the evaluation of these hazards.

Rabies is an example of a zoonotic disease and is also one of the most feared diseases. The virus attacks the nervous system of mammals when the saliva of a rabies-infected animal is transmitted through a bite or open wound. Rabies is a rare disease, but people in rural settings are at greater risk than those in urban settings because of increased risk of exposure to wild animals. If someone is bitten by any animal, the animal should be examined by a veterinarian and the person should seek immediate medical attention.

Rabies is an example of a zoonotic disease that disaster and emergency workers might encounter, also one of the most feared because it can be fatal in humans. Other zoonoses include animal pox (e.g., monkeypox), ring worm (dermatophytosis), Newcastle disease virus, histoplasmosis, roundworms, hookworms, toxoplasmosis, cryptosporidiosis, and insect-borne animal diseases such as Rocky Mountain spotted fever, ehrlichiosis, and West Nile virus infection, or equine encephalitis.

RABIES IN LIVESTOCK

Equids and other livestock suspected of having rabies must be carefully handled to prevent exposure of attending personnel (veterinarian, staff, owner, etc.). Horses or other livestock displaying signs compatible with rabies (fever, lack of appetite, lameness, colic, facial nerve paralysis, weakness, restlessness, progressing to lack of coordination, self-mutilation, aggressiveness, vocalization, drooling or paralysis) should be examined by a veterinarian immediately.

Protocol for Euthanasia of a Potentially Rabid Large Animal

When local practitioners discover a possible rabies case, they must notify their state veterinarian's office, county animal control office, and county health department immediately.

Suspected Rabies Case—General Handling Precautions

When an animal is suspected of having a rabies infection, there are some precautions to take.

- The animal should be isolated by direction into a safe and secure enclosure, such as a round pen or stall. If this is not possible, or the animal is loose, see the procedure for darting described below.
- Avoid contact with the animal directly. If the animal must be handled for the euthanasia procedure, all personnel should wear gloves and take precautions to prevent contact with the animal's saliva and mucosal surfaces or secretions. It is preferable that personnel in direct contact with the animal have undergone pre-exposure rabies vaccination.
- Personnel should wear full coveralls with long sleeves, boots, and double gloves. Only saliva contains the virus; clothing that touches these fluids of the animal should be sanitized with bleach and all facilities cleaned thoroughly. Blood and urine do not contain the rabies virus.
- Photographic and/or video documentation of the horse's behavior prior to euthanasia should be taken and submitted to the state veterinarian for assistance with diagnosis and history.

Quarantine of Other Animals on Property

Other mammals (dogs, cats, horses, etc.) with or without proof of rabies vaccination should be isolated on the property and quarantined in accordance with the rabies control officer (state department of health) in consultation with the state veterinarian's office.

Immobilization

Chemical immobilization is indicated to prevent aggressive biting, kicking, or exposure during euthanasia of the animal. Administration of injectable agents with a syringe by hand should be attempted only with extreme caution and preferably be given through a protective barrier (e.g., in the rump muscle from the other side of the overturned horse trailer wall, or using an extensible jab stick while the animal is distracted).

Chemical immobilization can also be accomplished by use of a carbon dioxide (CO_2) dart pistol, CO_2 dart rifle, blow dart, or bang/jab stick. Only personnel trained in the use of chemical capture equipment should be allowed to attempt this method. Due to the volume of drug needed, multiple darts given in rapid sequence should be used.

Drugs and Dosages

A veterinarian must be consulted and administer or observe the administration of drugs to euthanatize an animal. The following drugs have been effectively used to immobilize a rabid large animal. Individual and species-specific resistance to these drugs must be considered.

- Xylazine hydrochloride
- Ketamine hydrochloride
- Detomidine hydrochloride
- Pentobarbital sodium (euthanasia solution)
- Succinylcholine (may be used intramuscularly only for rapid induction of recumbency, and must be followed immediately by intravenous [IV] euthanasia solution or it is considered an inhumane method).

Physical Immobilization

Physical immobilization should be used after the animal is chemically immobilized to ensure safety for personnel humanely euthanatizing the animal with IV euthanasia solution. The legs should be roped and tied using a slip knot around the pasterns of both front and back legs (a cane or boat hook may be used to slide the ropes around the legs). The ropes should be secured to the closest possible secure anchor (heavy vehicle, post, tree, etc.). Personnel should remain behind the back of the downed animal to minimize the chance of injury.

A makeshift halter may be placed on the animal by roping the head to secure it, and the head and neck should be stretched if possible; this increases accessibility to the jugular vein.

Euthanasia

The veterinarian should draw and retain a blood sample prior to euthanasia to facilitate differential

Continued

diagnosis of other neurological diseases. The euthanasia solution should be administered intravenously from a safe position by the horse's shoulder. A "buddy line" should be placed to allow someone to safely pull the veterinarian away from the animal if it struggles. Field euthanasia with a firearm/captive bolt is not indicated because it will destroy the brain and make laboratory diagnosis difficult.

Submitting Sample for Diagnosis

The entire animal should be transported to the state veterinary diagnostic laboratory for identification and diagnosis of the case. In the event that rabies is diagnosed by examination of brain tissue, the local health department will investigate and consult with individuals who may have been exposed to the rabid animal and help determine if human postexposure rabies treatment is necessary.

Rabies cannot be diagnosed through blood, saliva, or urine tests or by any other means in a living animal. The only way to obtain a definitive diagnosis is by examining the patient's brain tissue after death. A special stain can identify Negri bodies (clusters of the rabies virus) in affected brain matter. Contact with brain, lymph nodes, and nervous tissue, which may contain significant virus levels, should be avoided. Virus may be shed in saliva a few days before clinical symptoms occur (the exact duration of viral shedding by horses is unknown).

Tetanus is considered a zoonotic disease because the natural reservoir of the tetanus-causing organism (*Clostridium tetani*) is the intestinal tract of herbivorous animals, especially horses. The bacterial spores remain in the soil, street dust, or fecal material and can infect humans via skin wounds. The case fatality rate (the percentage of those showing signs of disease that die from the disease) for tetanus can be high; therefore, all personnel handling large animals (owners, responders, emergency services personnel) should be properly immunized.

Leptospirosis can be transmitted to humans through contact with infected urine or water contaminated with infected urine. Carriers include domestic animals, rats, and wild rodents. Signs of leptospirosis in humans include high fever, headache, and muscle aches. Severe infection may result in liver or kidney damage.

Carcass Disposal

After Hurricane Floyd (1999), the carcasses of approximately 28,000 drowned hogs entered the North Carolina river system when the floodwaters washed them out of submerged confinement facilities. The cleanup effort required the presence of contractors, veterinarians, and health officials, and was associated with significant cost (McGinn, 2004b). In addition, the public health concerns arising from contamination of the rivers delayed the return of people moving back into their homes even after the water had receded. The mosquito population increased significantly due to the continued presence of standing water, and extensive mosquito control measures were implemented.

As a result of the disaster, the state of North Carolina developed provisions regarding carcass handling in mass animal fatalities.

CARE IN LESS-THAN-OPTIMAL CONDITIONS

Scope of care in medicine refers to the range of services that can be provided by a human medical or veterinary medical professional. It is defined by the education and qualifications of the professional, as well as the legal limitations determined by local, state, and federal laws. The scope of care provided by a veterinary technician differs from that provided by a licensed veterinarian. In some states, there are also legal differences in the capabilities of a registered veterinary technician and an unlicensed assistant. An individual licensed in one state may not be able to legally provide that same level of service when responding to a situation in another state. It is each individual's responsibility to fully understand his or her legal scope of care when assisting animals.

In the excitement and chaos of an emergency or disaster, the rules do not change regarding the scope of care or standards of care in providing veterinary treatment. A veterinary technician or veterinary student is not qualified to perform surgical procedures, diagnose conditions, or prescribe medication. For example, following an ice storm, phone lines are nonfunctioning and an owner cannot move his or her vehicle and trailer. A friend's horse boarded in the barn is demonstrating signs of abdominal pain (colic), and the veterinarian cannot be contacted. Another boarder, or the barn manager, administers an injection of pain killer, which appears to resolve the condition. This is a common occurrence and is often associated with minimal consequence. However, potentially fatal complications such as clostridial infection, intra-arterial injection, or anaphylaxis can occur. By assessing and treating the horse, the individual who administered the medication diagnosed a disease, prescribed a medication, and administered the medication to the animal; these procedures are considered to be within the scope of practice of a veterinarian. If complications arise, this individual may be charged with practicing veterinary medicine without a license and may be held liable for damages.

In some states, implied consent or Good Samaritan laws may apply in situations where the owner or the owner's authorized agent is not available to give consent for treatment or euthanasia. In this situation, it is implied that the owner would consent to procedures and treatment necessary to save the animal's life or temporarily relieve suffering. Good Samaritan laws may also offer some protection against liability if the individual providing care is practicing within their usual scope of care. Good Samaritan laws are usually applied in situations such as providing care to an injured horse or other animal on a roadway. Implied consent laws apply when an animal is presented to a veterinarian operating in his or her usual or assigned environment, such as his or her own clinic or a recognized animal treatment station in a large-scale disaster. Since these laws can differ between states, it is essential that responders in a disaster or emergency be aware of the laws in that state and abide by them.

During Hurricane Katrina, numerous licensed veterinarians self-deployed to the disaster from other states to assist with animal care efforts. Several individuals disregarded state veterinary licensing requirements and laws in their efforts to provide care to animals in need. These individuals were turned away by federal and other official organizations, which required proof of licensure. Practice owners are legally responsible for the patients in their practice and the safety of their employees, and employment of an unlicensed veterinarian is associated with legal and ethical risks.

FIELD EXPEDIENCE

Field expediency is characterized by creativity and resourcefulness in adapting available materials to solve the problem at hand. A field expedient may be a piece of equipment, a method, or a natural or manmade resource that is adapted for use or used in an emergency situation. Natural resources can sometimes be used to the advantage of the rescue or response effort, especially in disaster scenarios. An example of a natural expedient is the persistence of freezing temperatures associated with a blizzard. In January 1997, the state of South Dakota was subjected to back-to-back Arctic air storm fronts. Approximately 36,000 head of cattle died. Temperatures maintained well below freezing for an additional month; the carcasses of the cattle were frozen, minimizing the health risk and allowing responders to address surviving humans and animals instead of expending resources collecting and rendering carcasses.

TLAER constantly strives to minimize "reinventing the wheel" in response methods. Methods for confined space and trench rescue of large animals are similar to those applied when rescuing human victims from these situations. In turn, some methods developed for TLAER have benefited the human rescue environment; for example, the Rescue Glide has been used for transporting morbidly obese humans. Similarly, the technique of pumping air into mud surrounding the limbs of an entrapped large animal has also been used to extricate humans from viscous mud. Many of these methods began as field expedient solutions and have evolved into protocols and equipment for recommended use.

Decontamination of Large Animals

Early efforts to determine methods of decontamination for large animals faced logistical difficulties when adapting human decontamination systems. Challenges included difficulties in individual handling of some animals and species, addressing the identification of displaced animals, and developing protocols for the decontamination of large numbers of animals (Hamilton, 2003). The identified need for improved response and handling training in hazardous material (HazMat) and decontamination techniques resulted in a large multistate exercise held in South Carolina in 2005, "Operation Bitter Almond," which included a live large animal (one horse). Later that year, VMAT-2 hosted the first joint field trial exercise (FTX) specifically intended to develop and practice techniques for decontamination/HazMat for live large animals (simulated police horses and a llama) and live military working dogs. This FTX involved the teams VMAT and special medical assistance team-veterinary (SMART-V) at Ft. Bragg, North Carolina, (see Chapter 19). Since this time, numerous exercises and training scenarios have been held across the country.

SHELTER CONSIDERATIONS

A large-animal shelter should be established by knowledgeable and trained veterinary personnel under the National Incident Management System (NIMS) model. Large animal sheltering requires significantly more logistical considerations than for those of small animals and pets; however, expertise is available (Culver, 2006a; Bevan, 2005). Recent large-animal sheltering efforts and lessons learned after the 2005 hurricanes are included in this chapter. The reader is encouraged to consult with other resources, particularly the HSUS Disaster Animal Response Team (DART) training course for expertise in this focus area of TLAER and disaster response (Culver, 2006b).

Animal Health History, Examinations, and Identification

Each animal should be examined at a triage site in the intake area. Particular attention should be paid to hydration status, cuts and abrasions, hoof/foot health, eye and ear health, oral injuries, vomiting and diarrhea, respiratory disease, and evidence of internal or external parasites.

Animals should be bathed and decontaminated upon entry to the shelter area if the animal has been in contact with contaminated floodwater, chemical agents, etc. Liquid dish soap removes petroleum and some other toxic chemicals, but care should be taken during its use on sensitive species (e.g., horses.) Personnel bathing animals should wear protective clothing, gloves, and a face shield, or goggles with a surgical mask, to avoid mucous membrane contact with droplets and splashes that may contain toxic materials. Many large animals (cattle, llamas) may not allow individual bathing, and it may be necessary to place these animals in stocks or a head gate to allow thorough bathing. Other animals may require additional personnel for adequate restraint during bathing and decontamination (see Chapter 19).

Intake shelter personnel should ask if the animal has been in the custody of the owner or was picked up on a field rescue. If possible, owners should be asked about the animal's health and vaccination history, current medical needs or chronic health problems, and usual temperament (if known). All information gathered should be documented.

A health record for each animal should be created and updated as needed. Identification information for the animal should correspond to that of the owner, so that animals and their owners can be reunited. Owned animals should be clearly marked as "owned" and not "abandoned" to reduce the risk of error. Photographs should be taken from front, back, and both sides of the animal, with special attention to markings or other identifying marks (scars, whorls, etc.). A band or collar (leather or nylon, not choke chains) labeled with readily legible identification information should be placed on each animal. Ideally, all animals should be given microchips at intake to the shelter to facilitate tracking and identification (Nixon, 2006).

Pens, cages, and stalls should be clearly labeled so that newly arriving personnel are easily apprised of the health status, nutrition needs, and temperament of sheltered animals.

Animals arriving without owners should be scanned for microchip identification. At this time, not all scanners are capable of reading all microchip frequencies; the animal should be scanned with each type of microchip scanner before being declared microchip-free. Animals without microchips should be checked for other forms of identification, such as a brand, tag, or tattoo. Tattoos and brands may correspond to registration numbers, and this information should be used to trace the animal, if possible (CDC, 2006).

ANIMAL INDUSTRY RESPONSIBILITIES

Local owners and animal industry representatives should realize most emergency responders are not proficient in basic techniques for large animal handling, leading, and restraint. Owners can assist their local professionals in emergency management by helping them develop a crucial skill best learned through hands-on practice and familiarization. This can be achieved with a workshop session and is an investment of time and effort that may provide a valuable payoff in the future when the owner's animals require assistance.

In some areas the firefighters have initiated this type of training; for example, the animal rescue advisors in Hampshire, United Kingdom, initiated a handling course for firefighters and emergency personnel. This program is expected to expand throughout the United Kingdom (P. Baker, 2006). The large animal course for firefighters includes familiarization with pig, sheep, horse, and cow handling and facilities in an intense week-long course.

Large Animal Handling Workshop

Regardless of the animals' monetary or perceived sentimental value, a local animal community needs to be able to assist animals. Despite the industry, discipline, training, or performance goals of each animal owner, it is important to teach first responders to competently aid animals in emergencies. Prevention and preparation are the most important components of any effort. Firefighters may be unfamiliar with animal behavior and the effects of physical injury, stress, and fear. Hosting a basic handling skills workshop can be a rewarding activity to bring local large animal owners together with their local emergency management personnel to build a lasting and beneficial working relationship.

The Target. Local emergency response professionals include fire department personnel, police officers, sheriff's deputies, state highway patrol, county emergency management, public health officers, and the rescue squad. Local animal control officers and humane society volunteers can also benefit from workshop sessions. Forest rangers and park police should also be included if the area is near a state or national forest.

Considerations for Inexperience. Proper animal handling skills are often based on familiarity and experience; people raised in urban environments may be uncomfortable or fearful when exposed to large animals. In addition, stereotypes of animal behavior may be fostered by portrayals in the media. If first responders are fearful of the animals, their ability to safely and efficiently rescue and handle the animals is reduced. Fear can also result in attempts to overpower the animal and may hinder the rescue effort.

Animal behavior can be markedly affected by an emergency or disaster situation. Normally, calm horses may become fractious when separated from herd mates or when exposed to unfamiliar surroundings, sights, sounds, or smells. Experienced animal handlers often encounter difficulties in adequately restraining horses under these circumstances, and inexperienced handlers may be unable to control the animals without assistance.

Tasks that appear basic to many horse owners, such as catching, haltering, leading, and loading, can be challenging for those without knowledge of the equipment and safety procedures and horse behavior.

Many animal owners are unaccustomed to catching or leading their animals under less-than-ideal conditions. Wind, darkness, rain, smoke, fire, heavy snow, and passing traffic can be terrifying for animals in emergency or disaster situations.

Firefighters and law enforcement personnel may have already been exposed to a worst-case scenario on a TLAER scene: the emotionally invested horse owner who might have been inconsolable, angry, guilty, terrorized, or fearful. As a result, they may conclude that all animal owners are emotional and illogical. To overcome these misperceptions, encourage interactions between owners and responders during the planning and preparation phases when stress and emotions are not hampering communication. Encourage a team approach, where animal owners and responders can mutually instruct each other in their respective fields. This is often a relationship that takes months or even years to build with responders (Figure 3.4).

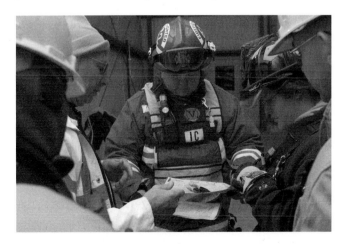

Figure 3.4 *The incident commander (IC) on an emergency scene is directing operational personnel in preparing a search and rescue operation after a local flooding event. Although human victims are the primary focus early in an event's rescue and recovery phase, there is a place for large animal field rescue response if there is a local plan with trained personnel available. Courtesy of Axel Gimenez.*

Get Responders to a Workshop. To invite responders to a workshop, visit the local departments during the day when a paid person might be available, or make an appointment to visit the chief and contact the county emergency management office. Many unpaid volunteer departments have a weekly or monthly drill schedule (often on the weekend or an evening during the week). Try to find an emergency response person who also owns livestock or horses; he or she may be more open to setting up a training event. Send out personalized, handwritten invitations with a flyer about your event, and follow up with e-mails and phone calls to make sure invitees preregister. Explain that a simple introductory course in handling, leading, and catching horses and other large animals might be a two- to three-hour lesson at the minimum. It may be necessary to explain that proficiency in these skills cannot be gained in minutes. A five- to six-hour course is preferred for further polishing their skills.

What to Bring. Encourage students to bring their firefighting or police duty uniform (bunker gear, helmet, etc.), but to wear comfortable clothing for the workshop. At one point during the handling, students should put on their gear and watch the reactions and altered behavior of the animals in response. Emphasize the importance of calm behavior and talking to dispel fear in the horses they are trying to catch.

Teaching Plan

Take it slowly. Remember that years of experience are necessary to be truly comfortable and proficient in animal handling. A series of short lectures and example scenarios followed by demonstrations will allow most students to grasp the concepts involved. The techniques and concepts should then be applied using live animals. Low instructor/student ratios, such as two students per animal/human instructor team, is preferred.

An adequate foundation might involve several hours in one module, increasing in difficulty once those skills are mastered, similar to the Trail Riders of DuPage's model (Haertel, 2000) below.

Basic Module. This module should include the following: a review of the senses (vision, smell, hearing, touch), defensive reactions, herding instincts, and social structure from the horse's point of view; the parts of a halter and lead rope; how to approach a horse; how to put a halter on a horse; how to contain uninjured horses in an enclosed area without having to catch each horse individually; suitable fencing for horses (both temporary and permanent); when, where, and how to safely tie horses; safe stocking densities (safe number of horses in a confined area) to prevent injuries; safety around horses (including where not to stand); applying an emergency rope halter and leading an animal from one place to another.

Allow the students to observe several horses in a paddock or round pen and explain the animals' body language and behaviors with each other (biting, kicking, driving, alpha dominance, etc.). This module should include hands-on work with gentle, older, and generally nonintimidating animals, one person and one horse at a time. Take into account that many fire and emergency personnel may not realize that size is not always indicative of temperament and ease of handling and that breed-related differences in temperament may play important roles in an emergency situation.

Intermediate Module. The intermediate module should include a review of social structure and offensive reactions from the animal's point of view; offering grain to catch animals; how to lead a horse (to include turning, circling, and backing it); where to stand when a horse gets excited and tries to run away; and how to use eye pressure (direct eye contact with the animal), terrain, or bystanders to assist in driving a small group of horses into a contained area. This module should include some work with gentle but young or excitable animals that are more intimidating than those in the first group.

Review the use of a Judas animal to encourage the other(s) to be caught. A Judas animal is a relatively dominant animal in the group that can easily be caught and led; due to the social nature of most livestock species, other animals will follow the Judas animal into an enclosure, where they can be more easily caught and restrained.

Advanced Module. This module should include a review of physical restraint techniques (shoulder, nose twitches); properly tying a horse to solid objects and knots for tying; how to prevent injury from an aggressive horse; how to catch a group of horses using multiple personnel; how to restrain a frightened horse on a lead rope; how to load and unload a horse in a trailer (beginning with a stock trailer, then progressing to smaller trailers). This module should include some work with young, less-trained, excitable, and very intimidating animals in small groups. More advanced skills would include leading animals from a moving vehicle, leading animals through an obstacle course, then through a chute of waving objects with people forming the walls.

Basic Learning Points. These modules should make the responders aware of the following concerns:

- Lead rope: Do not hold it at the clip to prevent constraining the head and to prevent getting a hand or fingers trapped; do not wrap lead rope around hands or arms; use at least 1 m of rope to create leverage; use a 3 m or longer lead rope.
- Body language: Slow, quiet, low movements are better than fast, loud, and high.
- Standing: Locate yourself to the side and next to the shoulder; allow the horse to move in a circle; be quiet with voice and body movements; keep yourself between the horse and potentially frightening objects; let the horse graze if possible, to keep it occupied.
- Leading: The body follows the nose; untracking or pushing the shoulder to get the horse to move forward if unwilling; safe distance between horse and human.
- Tying: Not too close to objects; good ground surface; very solid object, not to a movable or unhitched vehicle/trailer; leave enough room between horses; tie off up high, and do not leave excessive lead rope hanging.
- Loading: Emergency professionals should use a stock trailer for loading, as two-horse trailer loading is a very advanced maneuver.

Teaching Pitfalls. Volunteer instructors should receive prior instruction and practice together before the event to be as professional as possible. Disorganization, lack of professionalism, and discord decrease the efficacy and credibility of the course. Consider using a portable hands-free microphone for the lead instructor to keep everyone on task.

Consider a liability waiver for all involved in the course. Standard waivers are available or can be created with the input of a lawyer and the insurance carrier. Equine liability waiver signs on the property do not fully protect the facility owner or instructor. Do not include any known dangerous animals, kickers, or biters in the group of animals selected for the student practice sessions.

Don't be upset or disappointed if very few students show up for the first course. If their experience is rewarding, the students who do attend will recommend the course to others, and interest and attendance will increase in subsequent sessions.

SEARCH AND RESCUE EFFORTS

Search and rescue (SAR) is a specialty rescue interest that requires attention to a variety of technological skill sets that are outside the scope of this book. The details of professional SAR efforts are well-covered in mounted, helicopter and un-mounted SAR texts and resources elsewhere. However, TLAER responders are urged to consider the importance of this function within their jurisdictions for both human and animal scenarios.

As an example of the value of an organized search and rescue effort, one owner offered her story (Askew, 2001).

A herd of horses was given access to a 41 acre pasture overnight, usually returning to the barn at daylight for grain. The following morning, all but one had shown up for breakfast. The owner grabbed a halter and searched the most obvious places for the missing mare. The search area was increased to include an additional 150 acres when survey of the property did not reveal any open gates or damaged fences.

When the owner's search on a four-wheel all-terrain vehicle did not locate the mare, neighbors and the sheriff's department were contacted. The search intensified, with walking searches and aerial surveillance with a plane. Horse owners within a two-mile radius were contacted, and the horse was officially reported as missing or stolen, while the owner immediately checked local horse sales and informed the local and national equine-interest media. The horse was added to the "missing or stolen" postings for horses, and news of her disappearance spread. The owner devoted several hours each day learning about branding, microchips, tattoos, border patrols, and the cycle of horse sales and theft.

Two months later, her husband noticed coyote activity near a big ditch on the farm. He investigated further and found a deep hole camouflaged by brush and weeds. This hole was over 2 m (6 1/2 ft) deep, and a hoof was visible at the bottom. The owners and other searchers had walked within a few feet of the animal many times without knowing they were close to the mare. The mare was confirmed dead, and a backhoe was called to fill in the cave and bury the mare's body (Askew, 2001).

An analysis of this incident reveals the importance of effective grid search planning and coordination with local law enforcement, mounted patrols, and search volunteers. All possible and seemingly impossible locations must be searched intensively and in an organized manner.

MAKING AN IMPACT FOR OWNERS AND VOLUNTEERS

After a disaster, everyone wants to help. They are willing to give time, money, and effort as the devastation unfolds and in the aftermath. The horse-owning and veterinary communities can help in many different ways, from donations in cash, in-kind donations of equipment, supplies, and professional expertise, and volunteering time and effort (Figure 3.5). In the last

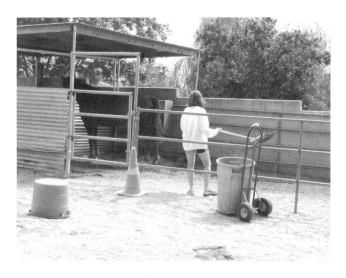

Figure 3.5 *The most valuable and useful donation of volunteer effort in a disaster or sheltering situation of large animals may be those who assist by cleaning stalls and cages, working the third-shift feeding or medicating the animals, or performing data entry and answering telephones. These are the unsung heroes after each disaster and provide a valuable service to the recovery effort. Courtesy of Tomas Gimenez.*

decade, outstanding improvements in planning for animals in disasters have occurred nationwide. Learning the many lessons from those recent responses will allow veterinarians, volunteers, and owners to make a better impact in the future on all phases of the disaster response.

Understand the Big Picture

How big is the disaster? Hurricane Katrina created 90,000 square miles of disaster area that included deep swamps, agricultural land, quaint towns along the beach, and major urban areas across five states (Florida, Alabama, Mississippi, Louisiana, Texas). Hundreds of thousands of people had to evacuate and make heart-wrenching decisions about what to take with them. How do people define what is valuable to them when faced with a looming disaster and only a few hours to react and escape? Fortunately, most large animal owners were able to evacuate their animals prior to the storm. When Hurricane Rita struck less than one month later on the Texas coast, many thousands of horses and livestock were evacuated along routes to the west and north in advance of the severe weather.

The animal issues in a large-scale disaster can be divided generally into two main groups: individual animal rescue, transport, and sheltering and concerns for public health and food safety. These two areas overlap in many ways. Displaced or stranded animals need to be rescued or captured, then decontaminated, provided with food, water, and shelter, and given veterinary care if needed. Large numbers of loose animals or animal carcasses can create a significant public health risk.

Self-Deployed Volunteers and the Law. Most veterinarians and their support staff who aren't involved in community disaster planning look at disaster response from the point of view of individual animal care. They may self-deploy and volunteer their veterinary expertise to affected areas to help save the animals. Despite their good intentions, they often have minimal to no training in response, search and rescue, and the emergency management/incident command system. The lack of familiarity with the procedures increases the risks of liability and conflict with responders and may decrease the safety and efficacy of the response effort. When there is a massive influx of self-deployed and largely untrained responders, often it becomes necessary for emergency managers to restrict all access to the area to prevent additional problems. There are valid reasons for these restrictions. As a part of good risk management, human responders should be provided every safety and preventive medicine methods, including vaccination, safety equipment, personnel accountability, clean food and water, nonhazardous places to sleep and rest after work cycles, etc. Awareness of these issues has grown throughout the veterinary community, and past disasters have allowed emergency managers to learn from others' mistakes and improve their coordination and posture for response.

Meanwhile, organizations and leaders with veterinary public health responsibilities are taught to approach these situations in terms of masses of animals, fair damage assessments, and preventive medicine. Rescuing animals is not their priority; the emphasis of these organizations is to protect public health. Bystanders may get the impression that these organizations do not accomplish anything because their efforts are not as visible as those made by field rescuers. Regardless of where responders and volunteers feel they are best suited to fit into the overall response, everyone involved needs to understand the big picture, be willing to assist with the overall plan, and acknowledge and accept the roles of the individuals and organizations involved in the response effort.

Prepare and Educate Locally First

The most important thing responders can do to help in a disaster is to become knowledgeable in the language of disasters. If trained in the incident command system (ICS) and the NIMS, they will be able to help implement the local, state, and even federal animal disaster plans. There are numerous free basic courses on emergency management, community planning, and disaster response and relief. There is also training available for emergency responders in search and rescue, animal sheltering, community planning, TLAER, funds and donation management, agro-terrorism, HazMat, weapons of mass destruction, public information, and field medicine of working dogs and patrol horses.

Remember, veterinary skills alone are not enough to effectively help in an emergency or disaster. One must understand both responder qualifications and limitations, then make the effort to get regular training and consider joining an official response group that will be activated. Persons without knowledge in these areas may be refused entry to affected areas. Volunteers should be patient and wait until there is an official call for outside volunteers, then respond in an organized manner.

Neglect and Abuse Cases. In each disaster, animal groups report finding starvation and neglect cases that were occurring well before the event. These cases need to be well documented (photographs or video and a written description of the case) if possible so that future prosecution can be initiated through animal control or humane agencies. Large animals trapped in stalls or small paddocks with no food can lose up to 10 pounds a day and approximately one point on a body condition score (BCS) scale (Henneke et al., 1984) in 12–14 days. For example, if a horse with a BCS of 2 (out of 9) is found 6 days after the disaster, animal neglect should be suspected and investigated. If a horse with a BCS of 2 is found 24 days after the disaster, it may indicate that the horse was thin (BCS 4/9) prior to the disaster. If the horse is a 6 on the BCS scale at 24 days after the disaster, the horse was likely obese (8/9) before the disaster. Most dogs and cats that are left behind are considered abandoned unless there is significant evidence of ownership (microchips, collars), whereas most livestock are usually considered to be lost or misplaced.

Triage Is a Skill. Practice triage skills with members of the local TLAER team. Providing euthanasia is one of the most difficult jobs for veterinarians, animal rescue professionals, and volunteers. Some animals are injured beyond repair by the disaster itself, and others become extremely ill or die from preexisting conditions, complications, or diseases that develop secondary to wounds, injuries, or stress. In a disaster environment where transportation and medical care resources may be severely limited, veterinarians must conduct field triage and may have to make hard choices regarding treatment and euthanasia. Conditions that in normal circumstances might have a chance of being surgically or medically corrected (colic, botulism, broken bones, etc.) may not be possible to correct immediately after the disaster, when communication and transportation resources are minimal and treatment options are severely limited by time and resources.

Getting the Resources. Animal-related response resources are typed by FEMA and NIMS. The type definitions provide emergency managers with the information they need to request and receive the proper resources required during a disaster response effort.

Typed definitions for 120 response resources have been completed to date and are continuously updated, revised, and expanded. Resources are classified by *category* (which refers to function) and *kind* (including teams, personnel, equipment, and supplies). Information about their level of capability is referred to as *type*, which is a measure of minimum capabilities to perform the function. Type I implies a greater capability than Type II. For example, animal resources are categorized as Animals and Agricultural Issues. For the large animal sheltering team, the "kind" is *team*. Personnel requirements for Type III consist of a 2-person team to support local efforts to set up a small animal shelter, whereas Type II requirements increase to a minimum of a 5-person team to set up a shelter. Type I personnel requirements consist of a 22-person team to set up and run a shelter.

Don't Add to the Problem

When public sanitation and sheltering abilities are overwhelmed, an influx of volunteer relief workers can increase the burden on already limited resources. Food, water, sleeping accommodations, medical care, and restroom facilities must be provided for response team members. It may take days to mobilize, transport, and set up an entire deployed unit, even if the supplies and personnel are waiting in staging areas near the disaster site. In the first hours after the disaster, urban search and rescue teams conduct human rescues; lower priority is placed on animal lives at this time. Experience shows that teams must be organized, with the necessary resources to meet the needs of responders, before they can be deployed. Volunteers should respond from outside the disaster area only when requested and activated by an organized agency that has legal access to the affected area. In the event of a catastrophic-scale disaster, several days may elapse before a request is made; patience is necessary during this time. One of the desirable qualities of a potential team member is the insight and self-discipline to know when not to rush into a situation.

Most animal organizations away from the disaster zone will have a high demand for volunteers in local shelters to assist individuals who are relocated from the disaster area by providing for their animals' needs. In addition, unowned or surrendered animals from the disaster zone are usually transported to other facilities for adoption. Thousands of evacuees from Hurricanes Katrina and Rita surrendered their pets to animal shelters because they did not feel they could afford them or did not have a place to keep them.

Don't Break the Law. Examples of questionable practices during recent disasters have included veterinary students or technicians performing tasks that should be performed by graduate veterinarians; animal rescue groups competing in unethical manners for donations; and well-intended, nonlocal veterinarians providing preventive services at no charge, thus taking away income and business from functional veterinary practices in the area. Veterinary licensing laws still apply in disaster situations, and the importance of proper procedure and attention to veterinary ethics should not be overlooked.

Rethink the Term *Heroic*

In Hurricanes Katrina and Rita, the media focused on some people who bypassed accepted procedures and entered restricted areas without permission from the proper authorities. They were depicted as "dedicated rescuers" and "heroic citizens;" despite the positive outcome of their efforts, the media coverage of these individuals erroneously promoted the idea that circumventing accepted and proven systems was acceptable.

The floods from Hurricane Katrina overwhelmed the organized EMS and official SAR teams' ability to provide assistance in a timely manner. There is no question that thousands of people and animals were saved by citizen-volunteers who were helping as individuals and not part of an organized, official team. However, the response effort is best served when all individuals coordinate with and work within the established EMS and ICS.

Self-deployed volunteers unassociated with organized rescue teams can present problems to the existing system. Entering a dangerous area to rescue a person or animal sometimes leads to a "rescue the rescuer" situation. Well-meaning, inadequately trained people may put themselves in harm's way to help save a person or animal and must be rescued themselves when problems occur. Thus, a simple primary rescue, best handled by trained professionals, becomes a secondary rescue and diverts time and resources from other response efforts. The personal risk of rescuing animals should be considered when deciding whether or not to attempt an animal rescue. Unsafe or illegal actions should not be encouraged.

Volunteer Motivations

Following a disaster, some volunteers may feel that their skills and knowledge are "wasted" if they are spent performing tasks such as feeding, cleaning cages (or kennels or stalls), or other routine chores. They may have expected that their time would be spent rescuing animals, which is often perceived as a more glamorous duty. These misperceptions are best addressed by adequate communication; no task is menial during a response effort, and each individual should be willing to assist in whatever capacity necessary to provide for the animals.

During many disaster response efforts, animals have been stolen by otherwise well-meaning individuals who feel that they can provide a better home to the animal than its current owner. Others are intentionally stolen because of their value. While this has been relatively rare with horses, it has occurred.

Build on Skills and Interests. Responders do not have to be on site in a disaster area to assist in the response effort. In Hurricane Katrina (2005) and every other disaster the last 15 years, VMATs, HSUS DARTs, and other animal groups (animal controls, humane societies, volunteer organizations, pet rescues) have become adept in setting up staging areas early in the response effort. Efficient systems have been developed for the collection, organization, and distribution of large numbers of in-kind donations of animal food, supplies, equipment, tack, and other items that people consider that disaster victims and their animals might need.

Some individuals may be most useful to an organized group by using their home computer to enter donations in a database or provide coordination for distribution of supplies to shelters. Others can coordinate press releases, take photographs for documentation purposes, or assist in coordinating volunteer duties. State and national animal organizations' member databases may be used to disseminate information, press releases, and relevant information. This is an often overlooked yet vital aspect of volunteering for disasters.

The response effort is facilitated by the rapid distribution of accurate information. Addresses of staging areas, mailing addresses for response groups, contact e-mail and phone data, and wish lists of donated items should be released in a timely manner to the proper authorities, organizations, and individuals. This may require a staff of personnel dedicated to answering phones, checking e-mails, and maintaining accurate records; the staff can be located away from the disaster zone, thus allowing potentially limited resources to be used for deployed members.

Animals arriving by means other than approved emergency management agencies must be tracked, triaged, decontaminated, and provided access to veterinary medical care. Establishing a central database for all animals entering the shelter maximizes the chances of reunification with their owners and facilitates relocation efforts. Following Hurricane Katrina (2005), the staff at The Horse (www.thehorse.com) created a database for horse owners that had left the area but were concerned about finding their animals. This information was provided daily to animal rescue groups such as HSUS in the field by fax or e-mail, allowing them to check those homes for the status of the animals and arrange rescue if necessary. The database was later incorporated into other pet-loss databases to expand the possibility of owners finding their lost animals.

Plug into the Existing Plan

Volunteers should coordinate with and plug into the existing system of incident management at the local level. There is little need to reinvent the system, and many communities have established, written emergency plans that include plans for animals. The plan should be evaluated regularly and updated as needed. County and state animal response team (CART, SART) models are working very well for many communities. Some states also have very strong state veterinary and agriculture/animal health offices that are providing leadership for these efforts.

Official teams (such as NVRTs) respond to requests for assistance made through official channels and do not sanction "free-lance" activities by individuals. Individuals who take the initiative to become involved without being part of an official team deployment do so without the benefit of liability protection and are not authorized to represent any organization to the media. While they may seem restrictive, these guidelines are intended to prevent conflict.

Understanding Limitations. Veterinarians must be licensed in a state to practice veterinary medicine. On occasion, the state veterinarian will enter into an agreement that allows licensed veterinarians from other states to practice within strict limits during the response to the disaster. If this agreement is not made, veterinarians from other states could be prosecuted for practicing without a license.

Entering people's properties even with the best of intentions is dangerous and might be illegal. It is illegal in some states to enter a house to assist pets; because the pets are considered the property of the owner, removing them from the house may be considered theft. Removing a horse from a property requires complete documentation so the owners will know why, when, and where the animal was transported. If the animals have access to food, fresh water, and adequate shelter, it may be advantageous to leave them on the property and deliver hay as needed.

Cash and In-Kind Donations

To help restore the local economy as quickly as possible, cash donations to the charities involved in the animal rescue effort should be encouraged. The purchase of supplies and equipment from local sources increases the flow of money into the recovering economy of the devastated area. Within days, businesses that are able to reopen will do so, and many supplies will be available for purchase.

In-kind donations of supplies can be beneficial if they provide items that cannot be readily obtained in the affected area but can result in logistical difficulties. After Hurricane Katrina, several tractor trailers fully stacked with over 15,000 kg (33,000 lb) of animal supplies were delivered to animal-sheltering facilities. However, the personnel necessary to unload the tractor trailers were not available at the time, and the fully-loaded trailers were locked and left in place. Several hundred worker hours were required to unload (by hand), inventory, and pack for distribution all of the donations in the trailers. Many of the items (such as bags of horse feed) were discarded because they had been exposed to heat extremes for prolonged periods of time and were no longer useful or safe. In most circumstances, cash donations are preferred because they can be used where and when needed, are more easily stored, and do not require large numbers of personnel to manage.

ACRONYMS USED IN CHAPTER 3

AIN	Animal identification number
BCS	Body condition score
CART	County animal response team
DART	Disaster animal response team
EHV-1	Equine herpesvirus (type 1)
EMS	Emergency management services
FAD	Foreign animal disease
FEMA	Federal Emergency Management Agency
FTX	Field training exercise
HazMat	Hazardous materials
HSUS	Humane Society of the United States
ICS	Incident command system
IV	Intravenous
NAIS	National animal identification system
NIMS	National incident management system
PIN	Premises identification number
RFID	Radio-frequency implantable device
SAR	Search and rescue
SART	State animal response team
TLAER	Technical large animal emergency rescue
TROD	Trail Riders of DuPage
USDA	United States Department of Agriculture
USA PATRIOT	Uniting and Strengthening America by Providing Appropriate Tools Required to Intercept and Obstruct Terrorism
NVRT	National Veterinary Response Team

4 Understanding Large Animal Behavior in TLAER Incidents

Dr. Rebecca Gimenez

INTRODUCTION

The psychological aspects of the technical large animal emergency rescue (TLAER) should be taken into account for both the victim and the rescuers. A terrified large animal can injure or kill a human and should be approached with preparation and proper caution. Understanding their behavior patterns and herd instincts and using calm and quiet handling are vital. Accidents with large animals occur when the animal reacts with fear or panic, when male animals use dominance aggression on a human, and when a female animal's maternal instinct for protecting her young overrides her normal fear of humans. "Danger is inherent in handling large animals," according to Grandin (1999).

Understanding the different behaviors and responses of these animals is important in helping responders predict how the animal might react on an incident scene. The animal handler's knowledge of methods or techniques to decrease fear and distress of the large animal victim may be the most important skill that defines success on TLAER scenes. Gaining a basic understanding of large animal senses, normal behavior, and behavior under stress is best accomplished by training and hands-on practice, just as any other skill set is attained (Figure 4.1).

A human cannot sneak up on a prey animal; it will smell, see, or hear them without fail. These animals are supremely outfitted by nature to sense their environment and react quickly. Although animals cannot understand human spoken language, their senses of touch, hearing, vision, and smell are several hundredfold more sensitive than those of humans. Consequently, the use of human facial expressions, body language, tone of voice (talking or yelling), noises (sirens, extrication tools), smells (sweat, smoke from bunker gear and gloves), and touch (calm stroking or nervous patting) will determine if humans are perceived as threats or sources of reassurance by the large animal victim.

To inexperienced people, large animals can be very intimidating. It is logical that these animals can be dangerous if not handled properly (Figure 4.2). Inexperienced individuals may have the tendency to walk up quickly and pat an animal on the face; however, this is not advised. The nervous patting indicates to the animal that the person is anxious, and the head-on approach may be interpreted by the animal as aggression. When possible, experienced large animal handlers should be used to contain and handle large animals.

SENSES OF MAMMALS

Rescuers should be aware that animals perceive what is going on around them and feel pain. In general, the senses of prey animals are heightened and superior to those of humans, especially the senses of smell and hearing. The anatomy of a prey animal can tell the rescuers much about the approach and handling techniques that will increase their success. In this chapter a horse skull is used as a model, but the functional anatomy is similar for any prey animal.

Receptors

Thermoreceptors. As indicated by the name, thermoreceptors detect changes in temperature. There are two types of thermoreceptors; those that detect cold temperatures and those that respond to warm temperatures.

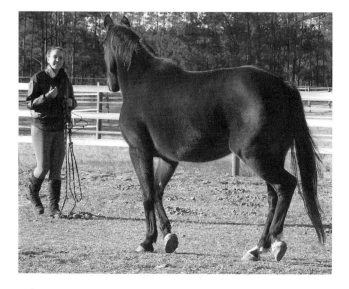

Figure 4.1 *A friendly approach toward a horse includes having the animal walking calmly, with head and ears up, toward the animal handler, who is backing up slowly with the halter and lead rope ready. The animal handler should focus on approaching the animal at the shoulder, grooming the animal with his/her hand, and gently slipping the lead rope around the neck prior to placing the halter. Courtesy of Tori Miller.*

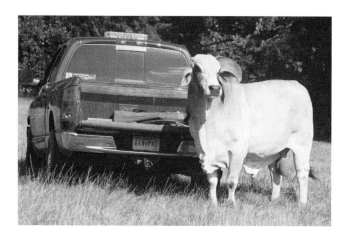

Figure 4.2 *Where are the responders? At a rescue extrication training event in South Carolina, this 1,000 kg (2,200 lb) Brahma bull walked up to investigate the events, and all of the responders got into their vehicles for safety. The owner demonstrated that the bull was friendly and caught and contained the animal to prevent further interference. Courtesy of Tori Miller.*

Mechanoreceptors. Mechanical forces are sensed by mechanoreceptors, which provide information to the animal's brain based on changes in the pressure or movement of fluids. Mechanoreceptors are involved in detecting touch, monitoring body position, and sensing sound and motion. Examples include the inner ear and vestibular apparatus, which detect fluid changes that trigger receptors that enable the animal to maintain its balance relative to the gravity of the earth. The middle ear contains mechanoreceptors that allow mammals to hear, or perceive sound.

Chemoreceptors. Chemoreceptors react to chemical stimuli in the environment. Examples of chemoreceptors include the taste buds and the olfactory receptors. Other chemoreceptors, such as the carotid and aortic bodies, react to the level of carbon dioxide in the bloodstream.

Proprioceptors. Proprioceptors sense changes in the tension of the muscles and tendons and position of the joints. Responses to stimulation of proprioceptors allow the maintenance of balance, body position, and normal movement.

Nociceptors. Nociceptors are pain receptors; they detect physical or chemical damage to the tissues. The activation of these receptors can lead to reflexive responses intended to protect the tissues from further damage.

The Phenomenon of Sensation

In large animals as well as humans, specialized sense receptors collect information from the environment and stimulate the nerves to send impulses along sensory fibers to the brain. There, the cerebral cortex forms a perception that is projected to the brain so that the animal "sees" or "hears" or "smells" its environment.

Sensory impulses are caused by mechanical or chemical stimulation that induces a change in the receptor cell's membrane potential, causing the generation of electrical currents in the nerve. If it reaches a threshold potential, an action potential is generated and travels down the nerve to the central nervous system (brain and spinal cord). The animal's sensations depend on the region of the cerebral cortex receiving the impulse. The cerebral cortex projects a sensory sensation back to the region of stimulation, where the animal experiences the sensation of pain, heat, taste, etc. This is the same system used by the human body.

Sensory adaptation is the adjustment of the animal's sensory receptors to repetitive stimulation. Receptor membranes become less responsive to a stimulus when the animal has become accustomed to it. This is partly how animals can be adapted to block their instinctual aversion to having humans ride and handle them. Through desensitizing the animal to certain things in their environment, a human can accustom (or "train") animals for driving, riding, and other similar activities. Mounted police in particular use these concepts to desensitize horses to vehicles, loud noises, gunfire, crowds, and other stimuli that would otherwise induce a fearful response that may interfere with the officer's ability to perform his or her job.

Sensing Temperature Changes

Temperature change (hot and cold) is indicated by thermoreceptors distributed throughout the skin and internally so that the organism can maintain homeostasis of body temperature. The skin of an animal (including humans) is the largest organ in the body. A few degrees above or below the optimal range can have serious consequences. The thermoreceptors do not require conscious awareness to function. Neural processing by the brain of the input from the thermoreceptors induces behavioral responses to restore or maintain body temperature. Examples of behavioral responses include finding shade or a cool pond during the heat of the day or huddling together in cold temperatures.

If animals are not able to physically avoid heat or cold (i.e., trapped in a trailer, ravine, or mud), their bodies will attempt to correct the problem by panting (exception: horses cannot pant) to cool themselves or shivering to warm themselves. Responders should make an effort to use decontamination procedures on rescued animals to remove mud or ice that may prevent the animal from regaining normal body temperature (see Chapter 19). Similarly, animals trapped in a trailer or under sedation lying on the pavement in the middle of summer can easily overheat (Figure 4.3). A stationary trailer in direct sunlight rapidly achieves high temperatures inside that can become life threatening; responders have used water fire extinguishers to cool these animals or the trailer around them. Rubbing the hair coat of an animal covered with snow or ice may be harmful to the animal because the air spaces between the hairs creates an insulating effect; if the air spaces are exposed, wet and cold can reach the once-insulated skin, and the animal will be chilled by cool ambient temperatures.

The Sense of Touch and Pressure

The free ends of sensory nerve fibers are the receptors for sensations of touch and pressure and are found in the skin. In humans, there are special receptors for sensing light touch and texture (called Meissner's corpuscles) that are abundant in hairless portions of skin (lips, fingertips). Animals have similar distributions of sensory organs across the skin of their bodies, along with corpuscles in the deeper subcutaneous tissues that sense heavy pressure and vibrations. Animals are much more sensitive to vibrations than humans; therefore, vibrations of the ground produced by the movement of heavy equipment may induce a fearful response in animals.

Animal handlers should avoid touching the face, head, and ears of large animals, as these are sensitive areas that are protected by many animals. Some animals become desensitized to handling these areas, and others may enjoy it; when on scene, responders should

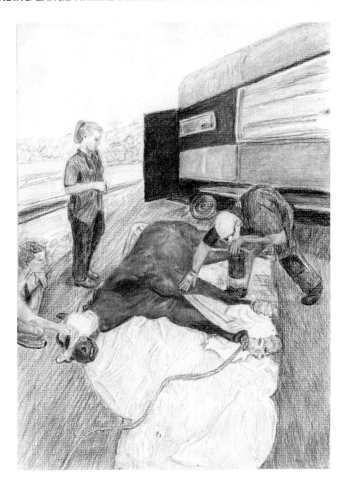

Figure 4.3 *A horse lying on the pavement after being pulled through the escape door of a trailer beside the interstate demonstrates how sedation can frustrate rescuers who do not have an alternate plan for transport of the animal. Additionally, concern for the animal's exposure to sun and heat from the asphalt should be addressed. Courtesy of Julie Casil.*

assume that the animal will be headshy (see below) and avoid handling the areas. Flat-handed slaps on the shoulder or rear may also be interpreted by horses as aggressive gestures. Responders should groom the animal with their hands, using circular massaging strokes (Figure 4.4). Grooming behavior is common in cattle and horses and makes them more relaxed.

Proprioception

Proprioception is the detection of body position and movement. This sense is mediated by stretch receptors (muscle spindles) and Golgi tendon organs.

Stretch receptors provide information about length and tension of muscles and tendons. The muscle spindle (located in the skeletal muscles) stretches when the muscle is stretched, triggering sensory nerve impulses that travel to the spinal cord and motor nerve fibers leading back to the same muscle. This "stretch reflex" produces muscle contraction that opposes the overlengthening of a muscle.

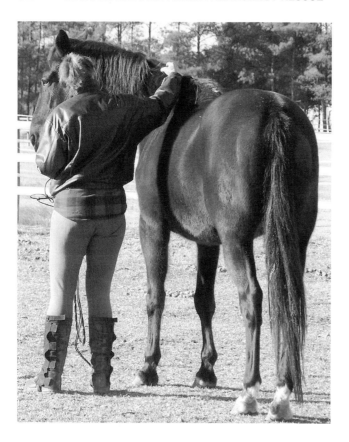

Figure 4.4 *This person has approached the horse at the shoulder in a safe position and is performing a grooming maneuver in preparation for lifting the lead rope around the horse's neck. Courtesy of Tori Miller.*

Golgi tendon organs, located within the tendon fibers near the site of tendon attachment, are stimulated when muscle tension increases. They initiate a "relaxation reflex" in the muscle to maintain posture and protect muscle attachments from being pulled away from their insertions by excessive tension.

Animals that are in unusual positions for rescue may not be able to prevent overstimulation of these structures and may develop muscular or postural abnormalities. Similarly, an animal that has been hanging from an extremity or even from a sling may appear to be walking abnormally when first set down or may allow its body to drop all the way to the ground. The posture will be corrected within seconds to minutes in healthy animals. The head and neck in particular should be supported in a normal position during lifting or manipulation of the animal because they are sensitive and heavy.

Pain Sensation (Nociception)

Pain reception provides protection to the animal as it grows and learns, and it is very similar to human pain regulation. Tissue damage triggers pain receptors to communicate to the brain that whatever the animal is doing is painful and should be avoided. This is the way

animals learn to avoid leaning against a barbed wire fence, being kicked, or touching an electric fence. The pain sensors can be stimulated by changes in temperature, mechanical force, and chemical concentration.

Pain receptors are the only receptors in viscera that provide sensation and are most sensitive to certain chemicals and lack of blood flow (ischemia). The sensations of visceral discomfort may be displayed as referred pain. For example, horses may roll violently with "colic" from various abdominal or nonabdominal causes, all of which are commonly interpreted as abdominal pain.

Pain and nerve pathways are made up of two main types of pain fibers—acute and chronic. Acute pain is the sharp pain that animals feel when kicked or bitten; carried by fast-conducting nerve fibers, the acute pain ceases when the stimulus is removed. Chronic or aching pain is carried on slow nerve fibers and may continue for some time after the stimulus stops. Pain impulses generally are processed in the spinal cord and ascend in tracts to the brain, where they pass through the reticular formation before being conducted to the thalamus, hypothalamus, and cerebral cortex. Humans process pain in a similar manner.

The regulation of pain impulses is handled in the brain. The animal's awareness of pain occurs when pain impulses reach the thalamus. The cerebral cortex "judges" the intensity of the pain and locates the source. The brain sends impulses to release pain-relieving substances, such as enkephalins (similar to morphine) and serotonin (which stimulates other neurons to release enkephalins). Endorphins are examples of pain-relieving, mildly sedating substances produced by the brain. This may explain why an animal trapped in a trailer wreck or under a tree might not struggle. Similarly, this mechanism may be involved in the response to intense physical pressure, as observed in animals in a sling or when using a twitch; the animals may appear sedated or relaxed, and many slung animals will collapse in the sling. This does not mean that they cannot react.

Special Senses

Senses with receptors located within the large, complex sensory organs in the head include smell (olfaction), taste (gustation), hearing (audition), and sight (vision). These senses are crucial to the animal's ability to locate food and water, detect and avoid danger, and find offspring and other herd members (Figure 4.5). Animals are very protective of their heads because they instinctively know that a blinded or otherwise sensory-deficient animal is less likely to survive in the wild. Horses that exhibit the resultant avoidance behavior are often called *headshy*. It is generally recommended that handlers assume an unfamiliar animal is headshy, and contact with the horse's face or head should be limited to the minimum amount of contact necessary to place a halter and adequately restrain the animal.

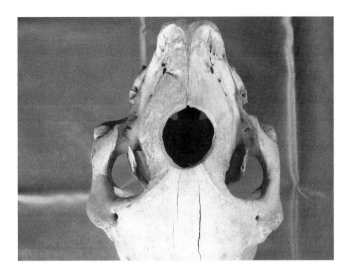

Figure 4.5 *This photograph of a horse's skull shows the parts of the head that are involved in the special senses. Courtesy of Tomas Gimenez.*

Olfaction. Prey animals rely on their sense of smell (olfaction) to find food, discover predators, find mates, and identify each other. Omnivores such as pigs have a highly developed sense of smell and are commonly trained in Europe to find truffle fungi (a delicacy) under the soil. Prey animals have to lower their heads to the grass to eat. The skulls of prey animals are elongated to allow the eyes to be above grass level while grazing, and their eyes are placed farther to the sides of their skulls to enhance peripheral vision; these are adaptations to allow them to survey their environment as they eat and enable rapid detection of predators. However, the high, lateral placement of their eyes does not allow them to see the food they eat; therefore, they use their lips, vibrissae, and their sense of smell to determine and select their food.

A large portion of the animal's brain is devoted to the sense of smell. This sense is mediated by the olfactory receptors in the olfactory organs of the head, where chemoreceptors are stimulated by chemicals dissolved in liquid. These function together with taste receptors and aid the animal in food selection or avoidance. The olfactory organs consist of the olfactory receptors and the supporting cells in the nasal cavities, including the ciliated neurons that increase surface area and make their sense of smell extremely sensitive compared to that of humans. Nerve impulses travel from the olfactory receptors through the olfactory nerves, olfactory bulbs, and olfactory tracts to the interpretive centers in the limbic system of the brain. Unusual smells such as sweating; nervous humans; blood; and smoke are quickly identified as unusual and something to either avoid or investigate.

Research suggests that mothers imprint on the smell and look of their young as much as the offspring imprint on their mother. Neural pathways in the brain encourage the use of postures and communication that allow the young to recognize their own mothers, even in a herd of hundreds. If mother and offspring are separated or fearful, the young will make separation calls (high pitched whinnies, bawling) to alert the lactating mother. The limbic system in the mother's brain processes memory and pattern recognition (the smell and look of their young) and is stimulated by these sounds to find her offspring. Humans or other animals that interfere with the reunion may be at increased risk of injury.

Animals are able to communicate over long distances with their sense of smell. For example, on the ranges in Wyoming there are accumulations of horse manure deposited by numerous stallions; depositing manure is a stallion's way of marking its territory or challenging another stallion's territorial claim. Animals can actually sense the sex, health status, and stage of estrous by smelling the animal's manure or urine.

Using Olfaction On Scene. The "nose" of prey animals is not limited to the nostrils, or external nares. The nasal passages extend from the nostrils almost to the base of the brain. The proximity of the olfactory receptors to the brain demonstrates the sensitivity and importance of rapid sensation, processing, and response. Unfamiliar smells, such as smoke, perfumes, and soaps, may elicit nervous or fearful responses from prey species. Anxious, sweating humans may produce odors that mark them as predators.

The firefighter attired in smoke-penetrated bunker gear or hazardous material (HazMat) gear approaching an animal will often elicit a nervous or fearful response, even from normally calm and accepting animals. Animals don't comprehend that the apparent predator poses no threat. A horse on a trail ride may react to a hiker with a backpack or a biker on a mountain bike the same way—by going on alert, then trying to escape.

This principle also applies to the smell of blood and smoke. Animals are suspicious of unusual smells and are likely to become agitated. The smell of blood may elicit a dramatic, fearful response.

The animal's excellent sense of smell may also be used to the responders' advantage. Loose animals may be moved into safe areas or enclosures by coaxing them with feed or forages.

Gustation. The animal's sense of taste, or gustation, is mediated by chemoreceptors called taste buds located in papillae of the tongue. The taste buds consist of receptor cells and supporting cells. Receptor cells have taste hairs sensitive to particular chemicals dissolved in water or mucous. Chemicals bind to receptor sites on the surface of taste hairs, triggering impulses to the brain. The concentration and type of chemicals determine whether the taste is perceived as pleasant or unpleasant. In prey animals the sense of taste is inexorably linked to smell, especially since they cannot see their food as they eat it.

Throughout its life, an animal learns to associate taste and smell so that they do not make the mistake of eating something poisonous or unpleasant more than once. A pig's tongue contains 15,000 taste buds; by comparison, the human tongue has 9,000 taste buds. However, food can be an excellent facilitator for catching loose animals of all kinds. Beef cattle are often familiar with range cubes, available in most farm supply stores, that can be spread on grass or pavement, and horses can often be coaxed with sweet feed.

Audition. The ears of prey animals are typically very large and are located high on the head to maximize their ability to detect sound. The external ear acts to focus and amplify even the slightest sounds and convey them to the ear canal. Prey animals do not have to move their heads to move their ears; many muscles function to turn the external ears in many possible directions. The external ears can be moved synchronously or independently. The sense of hearing of animal species is highly sensitive, and it allows them to detect sounds that are out of the range of human sound perception. If the sound is alarming or unidentified, the animal will turn its entire head to fixate on the source of the sound and try to visually identify the source. The ability to rapidly change ear position to localize and detect sound is well preserved despite domestication, and it is not lost except in cases of severe exhaustion or shock.

The mechanics of the sense of hearing is similar in all mammals. The external ear (pinna) collects sound waves created by vibrating objects or voices and channels them to the ear canal. Sound waves alter the pressure on the tympanic membrane. The pressure waves are conducted to the middle ear (which lies inside the temporal bone), where the auditory ossicles (malleus, incus, and stapes) further conduct the wave to the oval window of the inner ear. Within the cochlea of the inner ear, the different frequencies of vibrations stimulate different sets of receptor cells. Auditory impulses travel into medulla oblongata, midbrain, and thalamus and are interpreted in the cerebrum as "hearing."

Sounds on an Incident Scene. Responders should use a silent approach to the scene (consider turning off the sirens) because sirens can induce fearful responses in the human and animal victims. The strobe and warning lights should be used because animals acclimate to them very quickly, and they improve scene safety. Responders and bystanders should be encouraged to remain calm and quiet on scene. When people are excited, angry, or afraid, they tend to speak in loud voices. Similarly, high-pitched, nervous voices may induce fearful responses in animal victims. Animals interpret this as fear and may demonstrate a stress response.

To ensure awareness and not startle the animal, handlers should start by using a low, rhythmic voice, allowing the animal to become accustomed to an approaching human. A responder nearing a horse 40 m (131 ft) away in an overturned trailer can start to interact with it at that distance. Responders should try to cultivate that tone of voice because it works very effectively with animals in crisis.

Vocalization. Although not a true "sense," animal vocalization is a specialized body response to stimulation of the senses. Vocalization is rarely used as a method of communication among prey animals. From an evolutionary standpoint, it is unwise for prey animals to call attention to themselves. Instead, a complex language of body movements, which include subtle movements of the legs, ears, eyes, and neck, has evolved to allow these animals to communicate with others of their species. By reading the body language of the lead animal, an entire herd of feral, semiferal, or domestic horses can run and turn in unison to avoid an obstacle. The normal vocalizations of prey animals are soft sounds, such as low wuffles, nickers, grunts, moos, and humming (llamas). When cattle or horses bellow or whinny frantically, it is usually because they have been separated from their young or their herdmates. When cattle and horses are alarmed or trying to warn other herd members of a possible threat, they snort loudly by forcing air out through their nostrils (McDonnell, 2003). It is possible for prey animals to scream, but this vocalization is usually expressed only in extremely aggressive situations (fighting stallions or llamas) or extremely painful and fatal scenarios (such as predator attacks). Prey animals can be in severe pain and not vocalize; they instinctively sense that vocalization increases their risk of attack by predators. Responders cannot rely on noise, or lack of it, to determine if an animal is in pain.

Vision. The most prominent features of the heads of most prey species are the eyes and their size and placement. The eyes are placed on the sides of the skull and high on the face away from the muzzle and nose. Due to the ridges created by the frontal and lacrimal bones and zygomatic processes, most prey animals (camelids and swine are an exception) cannot see directly in front of their heads (Pasquini et al., 1995). Touching a horse in the center of its skull (between the eyes) may elicit escape behavior because the horse does not see the hand as it touches the skin. These animals also cannot see directly behind them because the muscles of their hind end obstructs their view; however, just a slight turn of the head allows them to see what is behind them.

Most domesticated large prey animals are herbivores and spend 18–20 hours a day eating grass (except swine, which are omnivorous). During the evolution process, the eyes of prey species moved away from the nostrils and widened in placement on the skull, enhancing the animals' peripheral vision and facilitating the detection of predators or other threats. Prey species rely on sensitive vibrissae hairs on their muzzles and skin and an extremely well-developed sense of smell to select their food. In contrast, the eyes of predators such as humans, dogs, and cats are set more closely on the face, in close proximity to the nostrils, to facilitate the use of stereoscopic (binocular) vision.

Eye placement in prey animals gives them a visual field approaching 360 degrees. The horizontally lengthened pupil allows a wide lateral sweep of vision (Figure 4.6). They can move their eyes independently, and each eye sees 180 degrees on each side. Prey animals are particularly sensitive to movement that might appear in the monocular field of vision on either side of the head; this is similar to human peripheral vision, but it is more highly developed. Monocular vision is less focused than binocular vision; typically, the animal will raise its head and turn to look directly at the object of its concern to allow viewing the object with binocular vision.

Stereoscopic (binocular) vision gives animals depth and distance perception, but only in a small area directly in front of their skulls. This occurs because the eyes form two slightly different retinal images that are superimposed and interpreted by the brain as a three-dimensional image, but this phenomenon occurs only in the area directly in front of the animal where the monocular fields of the eyes overlap. Binocular vision provides some depth perception when both eyes are looking directly ahead, but it is inferior to the clarity and perception that humans enjoy. Animals may raise

or lower their head to try to focus their binocular vision while trying to make a judgment about the object in question.

A study from the University of Wisconsin (Carroll et al., 2001) reported that horses' vision is either achromatic (white and shades of grey) or desaturated dichromatic (pastel blue or yellow). Other large prey animals may have similar vision. There is evidence to support some color vision in prey animals, but it is not the spectrum of colors detected by some carnivores and primates. The large eyes of prey species capture more light, increasing their ability to see in low light conditions.

A mammal's retina contains visual receptor cells called rods, which are responsible for black and white vision in dim light, and cones, which are responsible for color vision. Certain animal species have better color vision than other species, but it is generally poor in large domestic and exotic animals. However, since their visual receptor rods contain the visual pigment rhodopsin, in dim light their eyes function much better than those of humans. Many mammals have a reflective retinal layer, called the tapetum, that allows light to reflect inside the eyeball, thus increasing their ability to gather faint light in the dark. This tapetal layer is responsible for the green or yellow reflection that is seen in photographs of animals or when lights shine into animals' eyes.

Vision on the Scene. Concern is often expressed that colors of jackets or clothing will scare the animal, but the importance of personnel safety should override this concern. All personnel on scene should wear something that will make them readily visible, such as reflective gear in bright orange or lime green colors like those worn by road construction crew members or emergency responders. A large number of animal incidents occur close to roads, and wearing reflective materials minimizes the chance of a secondary incident, such as a responder being struck by a vehicle.

In general, animals are more concerned about the body language of the approaching humans than the colors and styles of their clothing—within reason. A firefighter wearing bunker gear and a self-contained breathing apparatus will likely be unsuccessful in catching a loose horse. Similar results would be expected when a responder in HazMat gear attempts to approach a loose animal. If a person approaches an animal slowly yet confidently, avoids directly approaching the head, avoids direct eye contact, and talks in low, soft sounds, the likelihood of success is greater than if he or she walks directly toward the animal in a crouching position making direct eye contact. Predatory body language exhibited by humans results in the same flight response that would be observed in response to an animal predator. Although most prey animals will become accustomed to continuously flashing lights

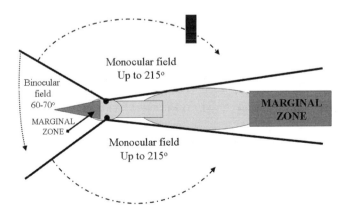

Figure 4.6 *The vision zones of the horse are similar to other prey animals, with a large monocular field on each side of the head and binocular vision for depth perception in front. Slight head movements to either side allow the animal to see behind itself. Courtesy of Rebecca Gimenez.*

and strobes, flash photography and flashlights may startle animals, especially in confined spaces. In addition, the noises generated by the cameras may further startle the animal.

Controlling Movement. On a scene, there may be an opportunity to control the movement of prey animals by using their sense of vision to the advantage of the responder. The responder should understand that stationary objects such as parked fire trucks or heavy equipment may be difficult for the animal to distinguish and thus be intimidating, but a small flapping movement, such as plastic waving in the breeze or flapping flags, can be terrifying to the animal. Once an object is perceived in the monocular field with one eye, the animal will bring the head around to look directly at the object of interest with its binocular vision. Sometimes they will raise and lower their heads to get a better picture and may appear surprised (as though the image jumps at them when it comes into focus). Other unusual aspects of their vision are that they cannot visually assess the depth of a puddle or distinguish the "holes in the floor" effect of a black and white tiled floor, lines painted on a road, or hoses strewn across the yard. To them, the holes appear deep, and the animal may refuse to cross the obstacle. However, terrified and running animals may not see actual holes in the ground until it is too late, and it is not uncommon for horses and cattle to fall into the holes and sustain severe injuries. "The rider's grave is always open" says an old Arabian proverb.

Cattle guards use these characteristics of large animal vision to prevent animals from crossing roads. By creating the impression of deep holes with a grate, most large animals will not attempt to cross the cattle guard. They can be dangerous traps, however, because curious animals may explore by pawing at the "hole" they see, unintentionally risking entrapment of a hoof in the spaces of the grate. However, the knowledge of large animals' aversion to contrasts provides a safer alternative to cattle guards; by painting parallel white lines across the lane, the animals interpret the contrast between black and white as holes and will not cross the marked lane. A series of cut lengths of fire hose or planks arranged in parallel approximately 15 cm (6 in.) apart and a minimum of 2 m (6.6 ft) wide across an egress point may deter prey animals from attempting to cross and allow redirection.

Similarly, the use of fladry is based on a centuries-old technique used in Poland, where a barrier of light rope with hanging streamers prevented wolves from approaching sheep and vice versa. This method is excellent for funneling or driving animals into containment areas. A successful improvisation of this method uses videocassette tape (pulled from the plastic cassette case) strung at a height of approximately 0.9 m (3 ft) between trees to make an enclosure or funneling lane; because animals are apprehensive of the rolling and flashing movements of the tape as it reflects light, they will not approach the barrier. Similarly, the white electrical tapes available on rolls from hardware or farm stores make excellent funnel and enclosure material; if it can be electrified, its efficacy as a barrier is increased. It is stronger than videocassette tape or surveyor's tape, but it will break if the animals run into it.

Some cattle and horses are sensitized to electric fences (hot wire). These fences are often marked with orange surveyor's tape, and many animals will not approach a barrier marked with this tape, even if it is not electrified. However, once the animals discover that the barrier is not electrified, a barrier of this type is no longer effective. Most domesticated animals are used to enclosures of some form and will respect the tape barrier if they are moving slowly and have time to accommodate to the enclosure.

THE ADVANCE

Animals are more aware than humans of the pressure zones around their bodies. When a person advances toward an animal from the front, the animal may interpret the movement as an aggressive approach and may attack if cornered, or turn and run away if it perceives the human as the aggressor (Figure 4.7). The only time this frontal approach should be used is when protecting an injured person. A barrier should be in place between the large animal(s) and humans at all times, especially in confined spaces such as overturned liners (Woods, 2006a).

Horses and cattle usually greet each other nose to nose, as a way of identifying each other. These animals are curious about the smell of a new person and should

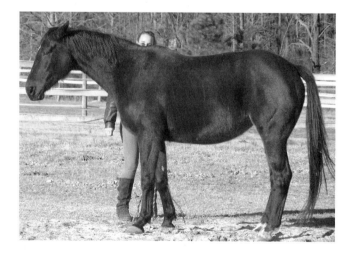

Figure 4.7 *An animal with pinned ears and aggressive body posture is showing antagonism to the animal handler, who should be wary. Uncastrated male animals of all large animal species tend to be aggressive and can be extremely dangerous; a knowledgeable handler is required for these animals. Courtesy of Tori Miller.*

be allowed to sniff the animal handler in a passive manner. Animals that are new to each other will usually establish dominance within seconds of greeting, and this may include aggressive behavior. Animal handlers should attempt to keep all animals being led separated from other animals to prevent this reaction. Llamas will approach to sniff noses, then sniff each other's perineum. In general, other species of animals are very disconcerting to horses because of their unusual smells and behaviors. Mixed shipments of different species can be difficult to contain for this reason.

Domesticated horses are accustomed to being approached on the left side at the shoulder. Military tradition guided the instruction of horsemanship and riding for the last 4,000 years. This military tradition was based on carrying a sword in a scabbard on the left hip because soldiers were right-handed (militaries consider everyone right-handed for uniformity purposes); thus, soldiers mounted from the left to avoid interference from the scabbard. Despite the fact that very few horses or riders use a sword today—unless participating in a reenactment of an historical battle—the approach and handling techniques used today are still based on this ancient tradition because those riders taught the next generation of riders. Most horses can (and should) be trained to accept handling on both sides, but on a rescue scene, the rescuer's default approach to the horse should be from the left whenever possible.

Catching the Animal

When attempting to catch a horse or other livestock that can be haltered and led, the handler should approach at the left shoulder, holding the lead rope in the hand nearest the animal, with the halter in the opposite hand (Figure 4.8). The handler should speak to the animal gently, in a soft voice, and carefully observe the animal's body language. Offering a treat or forage may facilitate the process. If the animal starts to move away, the responder should slow his or her movements further or move backward, away from the animal. If the animal is cornered or feels threatened, it may try to turn its hindquarters toward the handler and kick, or spin and attack. If there are several animals, be aware that they may crowd the handler. Horses can become aggressive toward handlers or other animals when feed or treats are offered and may crowd the handler, increasing the risk of injury.

It is recommended that the responder approach the animal from the side, where the animal's monocular vision can detect the approaching person. Predators tend to attack the back or hind legs of their prey; a human approaching from the rear may be regarded as a predator. Responders should remember that these animals cannot readily see someone or something approaching them, especially from the rear. Sneaking up on a prey animal is very difficult unless the animal is trapped (in a trailer, in a well, or ravine), and it will

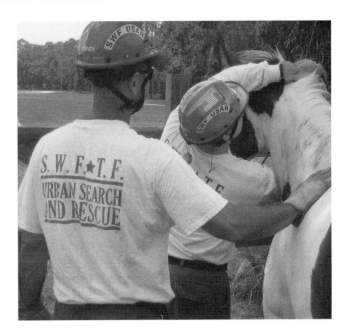

Figure 4.8 *Any basic large animal training provided to local emergency responders should include practice in approach, haltering, and leading of horses, as well as containment of groups of animals and other large animal species. Courtesy of Tomas Gimenez.*

cause them to be apprehensive of the animal handler. For example, the sudden appearance of a responder's head above or in close proximity to an entrapped animal's head may elicit a strong fear response. Prey animals are instinctively suspicious, and they may panic when trapped because they are denied the option of a flight response. In these situations, talking softly before appearing in the animal's line of sight can prevent or lessen the fearful response and decrease the risk of injury to the animal or responders.

Once the handler is touching the animal, they should stroke it gently on the neck and slowly place the free end of the lead rope over the neck. The handler should be standing alongside the animal's neck. The halter should be placed on the horse by bringing it upward onto the nose and fastening the poll portion over the head and behind the ears. A halter should never be forcefully pulled over the face and ears of an unfamiliar animal. The free end of the rope should be folded and held, rather than wrapping it around a hand or fingers, to prevent serious injury (such as broken or dislocated fingers). Gloves may be worn to protect the hands from rope burns (Figure 4.9).

Getting Close Enough to Touch

In order to extricate an animal from its entrapment (trailer, mud, ravine, etc.), rescue personnel will have to get close to the animal to place webbing or slings. If a responder must get close to the animal, he or she should approach at the shoulder (see Figure 4.10), then strive for body contact with it. Although it may seem

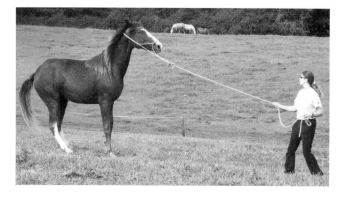

Figure 4.9 *The use of a long lead rope allows the animal handler to stay with an animal that is fractious and upset while maintaining a safe distance. Courtesy of Tori Miller.*

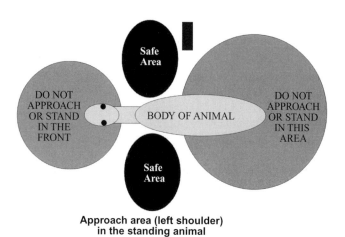

Approach area (left shoulder)
in the standing animal

Figure 4.10 *The zone around the rear end and the marginal zones at both ends are to be avoided. Approach an animal at the shoulder, on the left side if possible, and use the correct, calm body language and voice to encourage the animal to remain calm. Courtesy of Rebecca Gimenez.*

more logical to increase one's distance from an animal, proximity actually increases safety. The energy (and severity) of a blow from a kicking limb increases as the distance from the kicking animal's body increases; therefore, a responder in close proximity to the animal's body is exposed to less potentially injuring energy than one that is farther from the body. This is the same principle used by boxers to minimize the severity of punches—if they grab and "hug" the opponent closely, a blow does not hurt as much because the opponent can not get as much leverage and energy into it.

If possible, personnel should keep one hand on the animal, grooming it softly, and feeling for any changes in tension in its body. Prey animals, even young ones, are stronger, faster, and bigger than a human. A person should never get between a large animal and a heavy, immovable object (horse trailer, wall, gate, tree, etc.); if the animal panics and attempts a flight response, the person could get crushed by the animal. Placing equip-

ment on a cow trapped in a concrete septic tank is difficult without getting into the tank itself, but the chances of getting stepped on, crushed, or gored (if it is not a polled breed) are too high to risk it. Horns, hooves, and heads can be used as very effective weapons by a fearful animal, and responders should devise a method for getting the equipment on the animal from above (see Chapter 15).

Responders should avoid giving the animal swing room to get leverage with a kick, and personnel should be reminded to keep heads and extremities out of harm's way while attempting to put any equipment on the animal. Use an extension of the arm, such as a cane or hook, to manipulate rope, webbing, or objects around the animal (see Chapter 15).

The animal handler and the operational personnel who are placing the webbing or equipment on the animal will be focused on their efforts; thus, each operational person should have a safety buddy who is responsible for pulling their partner out of the danger zone or pointing out possible dangers while the rescuer is working. Intense concentration on tying knots, performing tasks, handling animals, and performing other demanding tasks decreases awareness of potential dangers; the safety buddy allows the responder to concentrate on the tasks while protecting his or her safety.

Unless working with a very cooperative animal (e.g., exhausted or injured), responders should not get close to an unsedated animal. In the agricultural industry, anecdotes are retold of mules that can stand on two limbs and still kick with another limb, or the horse that appeared to kick the brush out of someone's hand without making an apparent movement, or the dairy cow that must be milked with a foot tied up for safety or a pressure bar across the spine to prevent kicking.

Injury Statistics. An examination of 78 accidents related to horseback riding found that 76% of all injuries did not occur during the active phase of riding, but in the time preceding and following the riding phase (Rathfelder et al., 1995). Attention to proper technique (e.g., not wrapping ropes or reins around any body part) and wearing proper personal protective equipment (e. g., boots, helmets, gloves) when handling large animals can prevent injuries on a rescue scene and should be encouraged. Injuries are commonly sustained while performing an apparently simple task such as leading a horse, because the potential dangers are often underestimated. In 8 of the 78 accident cases, inappropriate grip of the reins or halter rope while leading a horse or pony resulted in an avulsion injury to a finger or thumb (Regan et al., 1991). Similarly, seven cases of severe digital injuries were caused by the habit of entwining reins around the fingers, and up to 12% of all injuries might have been prevented if adequate footwear had been worn (Chitnavis et al., 1996).

In a comprehensive review of equestrian activity–associated injury studies, the most common location of horse-related injuries is the upper extremity (24%–61%), followed by injuries to the lower extremity (18%–40%, with 25% suggested as the most accurate figure). The head and face sustain 20% of horse-related injuries. The most common type of injury is a soft tissue injury (up to 92% of cases included soft tissue injury alone or in combination with other injuries), followed by fracture (up to 73% in some studies, approximately 40% in most studies), and concussion (estimated to be 10%–15% or less). Concussion and fractures more frequently required hospitalization. The most common injury to leave residual impairment is injury to the central nervous system (e.g., from head or spinal trauma). In mortality studies from Australia and the United States, head injuries caused the majority of deaths (78% and 60%, respectively), followed by chest injuries (9%; Bixby-Hammett and Brooks, 1990). A review of 637 horse-related injuries in 581 stable and stud workers in a representative sampling of thoroughbred stables in Japan reported that the principal mechanism of injury was kicks, which accounted for 39.2% of all injuries and included 11 serious and 1 lethal visceral (internal organs) injury. In this study, the upper half of the body was more frequently involved than the lower half, and ribs and the bones of the hand and foot accounted for more than half of 148 total fractures. These findings are distinct from those in horse-riding injuries reported in the literature and emphasize the importance of developing preventive strategies specifically for workers in horse stables (Iba et al., 2001).

Recent studies have supported the increased risk of injury associated with horse-related activities. Horseback-riding–related injuries cause an estimated 50,000 emergency room visits each year (Carrillo et al., 2007). Multiple, severe injuries often occur (Carrillo et al., 2007). In a retrospective review of 151 patients admitted for trauma sustained while riding, chest (54%), head (48%), abdominal (22%), and extremity (17%) injuries were observed. Victims were injured when they were thrown from or fell off a horse (60%), crushed by a falling horse (8%), kicked (8%), stepped on (4%), and by other mechanisms of injury (13%). Rider inexperience played a role in only 5% of cases, reinforcing the fact that even experienced horse handlers can be severely injured (Ball et al., 2007). All deaths (10 victims, or 10%) in the study were the result of head injuries, further reinforcing the importance of appropriate head protection when riding or handling horses.

One study used the Census of Fatal Occupational Injuries files from the U.S. Department of Labor for the years 1992–1997 to describe the events surrounding human workplace fatalities associated with animals. During the six-year time period, 350 workplace deaths were associated with an animal-related event. Cattle and horses were the animals primarily involved, and agricultural industry workers experienced the majority of events. Exotic animals, primarily elephants and tigers, were responsible for a few deaths. A small number of workers died of a zoonotic infection (Langley and Hunter, 2001).

ANIMAL BEHAVIOR UNDER STRESS (RESCUE CONDITIONS)

Many animals may have to be driven into confinement, especially if they have space to run. A truly frightened animal may crash through wooden fences, jump over cars, or even hurtle itself off a cliff. Understanding why animals take actions that are often misinterpreted as stupidity is crucial to an animal handler's success on scene. For the animal, these are very basic motivations and behavioral traits. Animals tend to associate a specific fear with a specific place and/or object. Their place associations are very strong and long-lasting (Grandin, 2004). *Thinking* is not simply reacting on instinctual and behavioral patterns or classical conditioning; it is defined as applying previously learned information to new situations. Large animals are capable of thought; however, when the animal is fearful, it is more likely to react instinctively.

Basic Behavioral Traits of Large Animals

Dr. Robert Miller, a leading equine behaviorist, states that horse enthusiasts need to understand the 10 basic traits of the horse based on its anatomical, physiological, and behavioral characteristics. These traits shape how the animal perceives the world and reacts to its environment. Every horse shares these 10 traits, and humans who understand these concepts of horse behavior will be safer when working around horses. These concepts can be extended generally to other prey species to better avoid danger around the animals on scene. The 10 traits described are flight (the natural instinct to flee from real or imagined danger); perception (vigilance and awareness of their surroundings); response time (the ability to perceive stimuli and react in a very short period of time); rapid desensitization (the ability to ignore frightening but harmless stimuli with repeated exposure); learning (the ability to learn rapidly); memory (the ability to form lasting attitudes based on experiences); dominance hierarchy (as herd animals, the need to seek leadership); control of movement (the ability to exert dominance by controlling the movement of peers); body language (the ability to read subtle cues in body language); and precocity (prey species are neurologically mature at birth and can be imprinted) (Miller et al., 2005).

Handle the Individual

Animals are individual in their reactions, and two animals presented the same stimulus are not likely to react in the same manner. In addition, stressful situations may induce unexpected behavioral reactions. The normally docile pony may become frantic in a trailer wreck, while the champion racing Thoroughbred may be quiet and lay still during a trailer overturn and subsequent rescue. Some animals seem more trusting of people and appear to understand that the humans are trying to help them (Fox, 2006). In a rescue situation, any breed or species of large animal can react in a way that is the opposite of what might be expected under normal circumstances. Breed biases exist that propagate the belief that the "hot" horse breeds (e.g., Thoroughbreds and Arabians) are more likely to become frantic or dangerous during strange and scary situations, but these behaviors are primarily due to the breeds' heightened sensitivity (Stafford, 2006).

The Flight Reflex

Prey animals are flight animals and wanderers; they rely on their speed, senses, and heightened awareness to detect and escape perceived or real threats. When approaching loose or trapped animals, animal handlers should do everything they can to avoid being perceived as a predator. Animals that have experienced negative scenarios with humans can be expected to avoid and run away from well-meaning responders. Chasing large animals should rarely be an option; prey animals instinctively react to subtle body language cues, and it is very unlikely that a responder will be able to outrun a large animal (Figure 4.11).

The fight or flight response is an evolutionary mechanism that has dictated the prey animal's response to the environment and predators for at least 160 million years. Most large animals are prey species, and their instinct has taught them for those millions of years that the best chance of survival in a danger situation comes from flight. If forced or cornered, they will fight with teeth, hooves, and/or horns. This basic response pattern is common to all prey animals (herbivores in particular), and remains instinctive despite 6,000 (horse, llama) to 10,000 years (cattle, goats, sheep) of domestication (0.009% of their evolutionary development in years).

Prey animals are delicately sensitive to movement in their monocular field; if a threat is perceived within their flight zone (personal space), they may quickly move to increase their distance from the potential threat and reestablish their flight zone. Once they have reached a safe distance, the animal will stop and turn its body, eyes, and ears toward the perceived threat and view it with binocular vision. Sudden movement increases the risk of flight from a prey species: for example, a tractor parked in the middle of a field incites a lesser fear and flight reaction than does a piece of paper or plastic bag blowing across a parking lot or road. Anything that moves on the horizon within their visual zone is initially interpreted as a predator.

Evolution has selected for speed in horses; slower animals were more likely to be killed by predators. From an evolutionary standpoint, the increasing speed of predators resulted in selecting for increasing speed in the prey animal, as well as other behaviors to increase the safety of the prey species (herding, circling with horns displayed outward, kicking, etc.). This relationship is exemplified in the evolution of the cheetah and the Thomson's gazelle of Africa. As the cheetah's speed increased over millions of years, so did the speed of its main prey (the Thomson's gazelle). These basic rules of evolutionary biology are also found in the prehistoric horse; as a small mammal, predation pressure favored the selection for traits that we now see in the large, fast animal of modern times.

Despite the relative lack of predation pressure on most modern horses in stable settings, humans have tended to genetically select for the same characteristics that drove their evolutionary development: speed, size, and athleticism. In other domestic livestock species, humans have consistently selected genetics for calm behavior, larger size, and superior meat or milk characteristics. Although these animals are domesticated and have accommodated to human behavior—through desensitizing processes—it does not mean that the flight or fight instinct has been eradicated.

Predictably Unpredictable. The large animal victim's behavior is predictably unpredictable, and their reaction times are much faster than those of the human handler. Handlers and operational personnel should use caution in safety procedures on scene even around a seemingly quiet animal, because the unexpected can

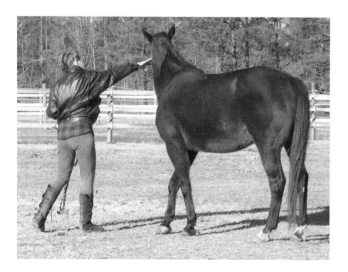

Figure 4.11 *While the handler is attempting to catch the animal, he or she should not chase it if it pulls away (as this horse is doing). The animal's body language indicates flight, and chasing or trying to grab it at this point will only make it more likely to run. The handler should stop, back up, and try enticement again. Courtesy of Tori Miller.*

always happen. All animals are different, and what may be safe with one horse or herd of cattle might not work with another. For safety's sake, humans should assume the animal is going to react quickly to the stimuli with which it is presented. In addition to the inherent risk of the rescue operation itself, the rescuer should never assume that the victim will be cooperative. When a large animal is scared, struggling, or fighting, it is literally fighting for its life and may injure a human who gets in its way by using its legs, feet, teeth, or body as weapons.

Some clothing and objects may frighten large animals, especially flapping jackets, umbrellas, and crinkling plastic raincoats. Equipment and noises may spook the animal as well. Bystanders and other rescue workers on scene should not approach the animal without asking or warning the handler. Studies of trauma patients have described patterns of injuries sustained from unfortunate encounters with large animals. A retrospective review was performed on charts collected over five years (1998–2002). Most of the accidents involved a horse known to the patient. The most common mechanism of injury was falling from a horse; however, being kicked was correlated with a more serious injury. The most frequent injuries were abrasions and contusions (39%), followed by lacerations (32%), and fractures (29%) (Ueeck et al., 2004).

Lying Quietly Trapped. A large animal will not move once it becomes trapped and determines that it cannot move, but as soon as it senses freedom, it will try to leave that environment. It may attempt to go through or over humans, exit through a hole too small for its body size, or scramble. This is instinctive behavior, and not a reflection of the animal's temperament or its bond with humans. By putting their weight on the animal's neck and tipping the animal's nose up and away from the ground, rescuers may adequately restrain a recumbent animal. Gentle stroking and calm voices may also help relax the animal.

The animal might be stimulated by something as simple as opening a window or bumping the sides of the overturned trailer. The weight and strength ratios between the victim and the rescuer are several fold in favor of the victim. Struggling animals can be impractical to restrain due to the violent force of their efforts. Responders should always stay in a safe position and ensure they have an escape route around large animals.

The Opposition Reflex

The opposition reflex is the tendency for prey animals to fight, push, or lean into pressure put anywhere on their body. A halter or rope is for guidance and control, but not as an anchor point for pulling on the animal. Anything placed around or on the head or neck should not be used for an anchor point. In response to pressure

(pulling) on the head and neck, the immediate reaction of an untrained animal is to heave its entire body backward so violently that it can flip over and break its neck (Gimenez, 2006a), fracture a leg, sustain a basilar skull fracture or other cranial injury (Stafford, 2006), or break the pelvis when it hits the ground or other solid object (Gimenez, 2006b). For example, in South Carolina a calf and cow jumped out of a trailer traveling at 80 kph (approximately 50 mph) when the back was left open and survived the incident. A well-meaning person lassoed the cow around the neck and tied it to the guardrail. While this person was busy catching the calf the cow pulled back on the rope, tightening the noose and asphyxiating itself.

Alternatively, after fighting the pressure and being unable to escape, prey animals will exhibit "sulking" behavior, where the animal does not appear to respond to stimuli. This is a dangerous time to approach the animal because it may unexpectedly come out of this state into a frantic struggle. This can endanger the rescuer as well as hinder rescue efforts.

The best strategies for an efficient and effective large animal rescue are to determine techniques that allow the animal to help itself, providing an "engine" to push itself out of the entrapment with the guidance and assistance of the human rescuers (Figure 4.12). The opposition reflex ensures that the animal will balk at first, but pressure around its chest will cause the animal to relax, then move forward. The forward assist (see Chapter 15) is the best example of this concept; by putting a sling around the animal's body, the animal can still move its head and neck to balance itself and move the legs to walk or power out of the entrapment scenario (Fox, 2005).

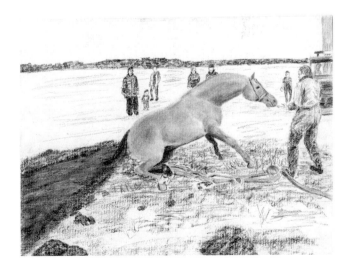

Figure 4.12 *This horse was pulled out of a ditch using webbing in an appropriate manner, but now the rescuer is too close to the animal and is pulling it by the head; this prevents the animal from participating in its own rescue and maintaining its balance. Rescuers should not stand directly in front of an animal or pull an animal by its head. Courtesy of Julie Casil.*

Evolutionary Pressures

In her *Equine Ethogram*, Dr. Sue McDonnell documented for the first time all of the simple to complex behaviors demonstrated by equines in their native and domesticated environments (McDonnell, 2003). These behaviors are derived from evolutionary pressures placed on these prey animals that formed their instincts, and they are crucial for animal handlers to be aware of on scene.

The importance of the correct body language and patience on scene was demonstrated at a HazMat/decontamination training event in North Carolina in 2003. A VMAT member illustrated the value of equine body language by her ability to approach a loose Arabian horse with a halter and lead rope while in full HazMat gear with a respirator. She took 10 minutes to do it, quietly walking around the paddock to let the horse get used to her, and talking to him. It proved the point that a soft approach using proper visual and verbal cues increases the chances of catching an animal. In some situations, however, spending 10–20 minutes attempting to catch an animal may not be practical or possible.

The Alarm Reaction. When the head of a prey animal is up, with its eyes and ears focused on a person or an object, and the animal is snorting, this is a demonstration of the alarm reaction in that animal. This is part of their flight or fight mechanism. In addition, the animal communicates that fear to the other members of the herd.

Fear. Agitation in animals must be treated as equivalent to fear. High-pitched noises generated by equipment or vehicles, sudden movements of people or gear, and distress calls from other members of the herd will activate sympathetic nerve circuits that result in high levels of attention and agitation, followed by fear. Fear is a very strong stressor in animals as well as humans, and it is measurable by scientists because the hard wiring of the nervous system is well documented. Habituation and desensitization can allow animals to become calm, but are difficult to induce on scene. Bad experiences may create a permanent fear memory that is not erased (Grandin, 2004). The best illustration of this is the difference in response to handling between dairy cattle and beef cattle. Dairy cattle are handled daily; therefore, their attitude toward people can be very positive. Beef cattle rarely get handled except for management procedures (castration, dehorning, vaccination, deworming, etc.), and these procedures are usually performed in a head-gate where the animal cannot escape (Figure 4.13). As a result, these animals tend to be more fearful and resistant of human handling and restraint. The handler must keep in mind that the fear memory of these animals may be complex.

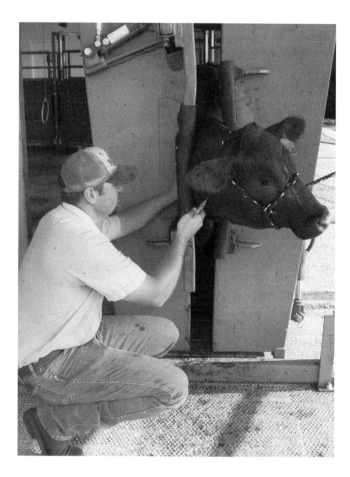

Figure 4.13 *A cow in a head gate demonstrates the industry standard for restraint for these large animals. Courtesy of Carla Huston.*

Curiosity. Novelty is a stressor. Paradoxically, it is also very attractive to animals; they are curious and fascinated by new things and places (Grandin, 2004). Animal handlers and operational personnel should attempt a gradual introduction to new aspects of the scene (equipment, harnesses, slings, loud noises.) The animal should be allowed to approach and investigate on its own and accommodate to the new stimulus. According to Pat Parelli (2004), "The opposite emotion of fear, is curiosity." If the animal handler can get enough trust from the animal to get past their instinctive fear, the animal will become curious.

An example of using an animal's senses and curiosity that can be used to the benefit of the rescuer is that horses can smell a treat in a pocket from 10 m away. Any kind of treat to offer, even empty candy wrappers, may work to entice the animal to the rescuer. Real grain or alfalfa hay is best if available, but even a little bit of sand or pebbles rattling around in the bottom of a can is a sound they may associate with grain. This strategy will often work for cattle, llamas, pigs, sheep, or goats if they have ever been accustomed to being fed.

Herding Instinct. Instinct tells prey animals that if they are alone, they are at risk of predation. Thus, herbivores are gregarious. One of their strongest instincts is to stay with the herd. Statistically, this minimizes the chances of predator attack and increases the number of eyes, ears, and noses available to detect predators. This strong instinct can be used to the responders' benefit by introducing a Judas animal of the same species to attract loose animals to a contained area or portable fence trap. The Bureau of Land Management uses trained Judas horses to help capture loose mustangs, and this technique has been used to successfully capture entire feral horse herds (see Chapter 7).

Dominance Hierarchy. Herding animals exhibit strong dominance hierarchy systems in which one animal is the boss, or alpha animal, with authority, and the subordinate animals are ranked by factors including age, sex, body size, strength, athleticism, and temperament (Figure 4.14). This can be observed in cattle by removing a mature cow from the herd for a period of time and then releasing her back into the herd. Whichever cows were immediately below her in rank will challenge her, seizing the opportunity to move up in the hierarchy. They will body-slam her, butt her, shove her, and then relentlessly pursue her to cement their newfound dominance; alternatively, she will meet them head on and reassert her dominance and stature in the hierarchy. In contrast, releasing a group of yearlings who have established order of dominance within their own group, but who are all younger than any cattle in the larger herd, will produce minimal struggles (Durak, 2006). The young animals are inherently placed in lower positions within the hierarchy.

In the wild decisions for the entire herd are made by the alpha animal; the remaining animals follow by instinct. Human animal handlers must learn to establish themselves as the alpha leaders in order to get respect from the animal and reduce the risk of being trampled or attacked. This can be learned only by hands-on practice with large animals. The follower instinct can be used to the responder's advantage when moving an entire herd by catching and leading the alpha animal and allowing the rest of the herd to follow. However, the dominance hierarchy can also be a hindrance to the rescue effort when a group of animals is placed in a small space (e.g., trailer, emergency paddock); dominant animals may injure or kill smaller or less-dominant ones (McDonnell, 2003).

Adaptability. Adaptability is the ability to adapt readily to different conditions and can be an advantage for rescuers. This characteristic is best exemplified in prey animals by horses allowing humans to ride on their backs. It is this trait that will allow responders in numerous situations to safely handle and manipulate animals, even without sedation. However, even a gentle animal can revert to the feral state quickly; they are "hard-wired" to rapidly respond and react to stressors. Pat Parelli (2000) says, "Inside every gentle horse is a wild animal, and inside every wild horse is a gentle one." Animals' responses are not symmetrical; an animal may allow approach or equipment to be applied on one side of its body, but not the other. A horse may accept the sight of a bicyclist passing on its left, but be startled when he sees the same bicyclist pass on its right. Ideally, animals should be desensitized by getting them accustomed to handling or stimuli on both sides of their bodies.

Prey animals seek comfort, not praise. There are many equid clinicians who teach owners natural horsemanship methods—how to play with their horses in a manner similar to the horse's normal interactions with herd mates and rewarding the animals by removing a pressure, not by giving praise or food as a reward (Parelli, 2000). On scene, removing the pressure of many human eyes staring at the animal or returning the animal to a herd situation would be good examples of providing comfort to the animal to allow it to relax and calm down.

Reading Body Language

When humans get scared or panicked or are in a hurry, animals sense this from the body language of the humans, and they may quickly become nervous. Large animals are also sensitive to the body language of other prey animals as well, and one excitable animal in a herd can whip the rest into a fractious frenzy. Confidence is part of a good animal handler's body language and develops with experience. Prey animals are adept at recognizing different and extremely subtle body languages; in their herd society, body language is very important. The way people hold their heads, their hands, and position their bodies all hold important

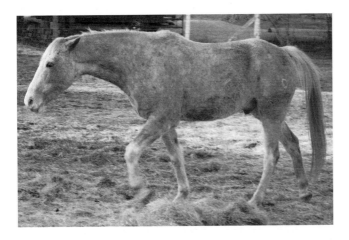

Figure 4.14 *A horse showing aggressive posture including pinned ears flattened onto the neck, lowered neck, and forward movement in an intimidating manner. Courtesy of Rebecca Gimenez.*

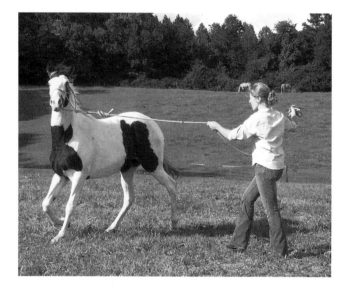

Figure 4.15 *The body language of this horse shows it is about to rear and fight the restraint of the halter and the directions of the handler. A 15 ft (4.5 m) lead rope allows the animal handler to be far out of the way of the feet when this occurs and gives the handler leverage to stop the animal's movement. Courtesy of Tori Miller.*

clues for animals about leadership (or lack thereof). Large animals may take advantage of hesitation or fear on the part of humans, assuming the human to be more afraid than the animal itself (Figure 4.15). The knowledge that its handler is frightened only escalates the animal's anxiety.

The body language of healthy prey animals, and particularly horses, as a person is approaching them is not that difficult to read: anytime the animal handler can see the rear end of the animal, it is neither paying attention to them nor giving them respect. However, in rescue scenarios the handler must evaluate many other options—the animal may be exhausted, sick, debilitated, or in shock. The animal may be trapped and unable to move. Another possibility the handler must consider is that the animal has run as far as it could to the end of its flight distance and is now considering fighting with teeth and hooves as the human approaches within the critical distance.

Animals anticipate the actions of humans that approach them. If given the correct nonaggressive body language they will often allow handlers to touch them. The handler should start touching the animal in the least intimidating area, usually at the shoulder. Animals are often very protective of their heads, and may be sensitive (and dangerous) around their hindquarters. The best chance of getting close to an animal is to approach it and establish contact at its shoulder in front of the withers. It is safest to always approach the animal from the side, preferably the animal's left side, speaking in soft, soothing tones. Prey animals can hear sounds before they can see the source of the sound. Because they cannot see well directly in front

or behind them, staying to their side near their shoulder is the safest position.

Sensitivity to Visual Cues and Facial Expressions. It should be impressed upon rescuers that prey animals are receptive to human facial expressions. Intense focus tends to bring a person's eyebrows closer to each other, a frown to the mouth, and to pull the shoulders forward; the animal may read this body language and facial cues as predatory. If the rescuer's face is open and smiling, with open posture—shoulders back and face up—the animal is less intimidated. Eye contact can be interpreted as aggression, and direct eye contact should be avoided.

Large animals pay attention to visual cues. For example, in documentaries of herds of horses or cattle running across the hills, the animals remain closely gathered and move in unison without vocal communication. When the lead animal readies to make a turn, it turns it's ears, eyes, and head in that direction; the rest of the herd follows that cue and makes the turn with the leader. These cues are almost imperceptible to humans, but animals learn them from birth. Young animals run with their mothers and learn to follow the movement of the other herd members—a crucial skill in the wild.

Specialized Behaviors

Herbivores have specialized behaviors that assist them with detecting predators, especially their tendency to scan their environment while chewing their cud or between bites of grass. Prey animals do not put their heads down to graze and keep them down; instead, they lift their heads and look around every 30 to 120 seconds.

The instinctive fear of being trapped or caught unprepared to run away is demonstrated in the horse's evolutionary development of a stay apparatus in the hindlimb that allows it to sleep while standing up. It is very rare for all of the animals of a herd to lay down at one time and truly relax. Normally, one animal will stand guard for predators. When horses lie down, it is usually for a short time, and adult animals rarely lie in complete lateral recumbency. (Exceptions are cattle and camelids, which lie down in sternal recumbancy to chew their cud.) However, a recumbent adult animal that allows an unfamiliar person to approach without getting up may be severely injured, trapped, or dying.

Large animals are often reluctant to pass through tight spaces or go underneath structures or objects, and some cattle and horses will refuse to go through such areas. Horses are rarely willing to be led through these types of obstacles, and most cattle will not lead in these situations. Animals should be led or driven through areas that appear open and nonconfining (like a funnel of cattle gates). If forced to lead an animal out of a trailer or overhead obstacles, the handler should stay to the side of the animal to avoid crushing and injury if the animal suddenly surges forward.

Although animals understand the concept of personal space among herds or flocks (primarily with respect to flight distance), they may not acknowledge the personal space around a human handler. This is especially true of horses that have succeeded in exerting dominance over their handlers. "Horses are just like attorneys, always re-negotiating the contract," says Mike Kinsey (2003). Handlers should attempt to maintain a meter or more of space between themselves and the animal to minimize the chance of being trampled or injured. This spacing with a longer lead rope also gives the animal handler leverage to prevent the animal from escaping (Figure 4.16; see Chapter 6).

As animals pass from dimly lit to brightly lit areas, or vice versa, it may take a few minutes for their eyes to adjust to the change. Asking an animal to enter a dark trailer on a bright day may induce a fearful response because the horse may perceive the darkened trailer as a deep hole. The animal should be allowed time to adjust, regain focus, and judge the distances and obstacles it needs to negotiate. Animals are sensitive to differences in contrast and notice dichromatic (two-color) components that may create a visual illusion of changes in the ground (Grandin, 2004). Cattle have depth perception, but must move their head down to use it. Shadows look like holes for these reasons, and animals will usually avoid these areas. An animal that is allowed to calm down and adjust to the situation will usually be able to navigate the obstacles around it.

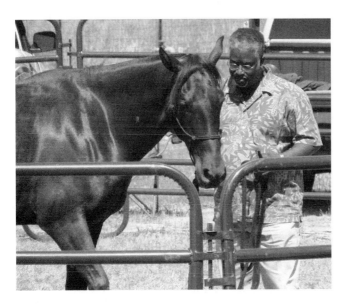

Figure 4.16 *When the animal has been successfully caught and haltered, responders should keep 1–1.5 m (3.3–5 ft) of lead rope between themselves and the animal to give them greater leverage if the animal fights restraint or panics and attempts flight. The handler should be positioned near the animal's shoulder when leading it. Courtesy of Tomas Gimenez.*

HOW DANGEROUS CAN IT BE?

Large animals can and occasionally do kill humans, including people who work with them on a daily basis. They can kick hard enough to crush organs, split skulls, and break bones. Most people are aware that animals can kick and that they should not go near the rear end of the animal. From 1990 to 2006, over 65 people were killed by elephants; in 2005 a handler with 15 years of experience was crushed by 3 elephants being loaded onto a transport trailer. Elephants are capable of reaching out with their trunks to grasp objects with tenderness or crushing force. Elephants can trample a human with their feet or use their tusks and skull to press someone's body against a wall or the ground.

An animal's front end can also injure or kill a person. Horses have powerful jaw muscles and necks and can exert enough power to grab and lift an adult person off the ground. During a four-year prospective study of 40 patients who presented to a hospital with bite injuries from mammals (including from horses and donkeys), the researchers noted that 70% of injuries were characterized by the tearing away or separation of (avulsion) of tissue (Ullah et al., 2005). Cows, sheep, deer, and goats do not bite for defense purposes, but every large animal species can and will do so. Pigs, alpacas, camels, and llamas can bite and cause severe wounds. Cattle and goats can use their horns and heads to gore and crush opponents, and even a hornless cow can swing her head and shove a human to the ground.

A Double-Edged Sword

Experience and exposure to large animals are two factors the professional responder must consider. Expertise with large animals is a function of experience, but experience does not always teach a person expertise. (Gimenez, 2006b) The best way to increase one's experience level with large animals is to contact local producers or ranchers and ask them to train responders with hands-on basic defensive safety pointers and handling of a variety of large animals. This knowledge will give responders a greater respect for the size and fear responses of animals and some of the basic skill sets required to assist with animal rescues.

In several studies, the statistical risk of serious injuries when handling horses was not associated with level of experience or expertise, but was a function of cumulative exposure to horses. This suggests that horse owners tend to become complacent or less careful around these animals (Exadaktylos et al., 2002). In Greece, where horses, donkeys, and mules are still used in agriculture and horse riding is a popular leisure activity, researchers collected information on 244 equestrian-related injuries that occurred during farming, equestrian sports, or horse racing. Fractures accounted for 39.0% of injuries in horse racing and 30.5% in farming; head injuries accounted for approximately

50% of injuries among farmers. Farming injuries were more serious, with 25% requiring hospitalization. The conclusion of the researchers was that "equestrian-related injuries are a serious but underappreciated health problem and merit targeted prevention efforts for each category affected." (Petridou et al., 2004).

Inexperienced large animal handlers are subject to injuries because they may underestimate the speed and strength of these animals. Increasing the experience level and handling skills will keep animal handlers safer on scenes with large animals and is crucial to any coordinated response. Handlers with minimal experience tend to be more easily and seriously injured, but more experienced handlers are not immune from injury.

Statistics Don't Lie

This book presents many ways to build a safety margin into various types of emergency scenes with large animals present. There is a good reason why humans are inherently intimidated by a 1,100–2,200 lb (500–1,000 kg) prey animal. Large animals can be dangerous, especially when they are fighting to protect their lives. Humans tend to anthropomorphize relationships with animals, and this can lead to underestimation of risk. Many horse and livestock owners will assert that it is only a matter of time before a person choosing to work with horses and livestock will be injured. It has been shown that a person's own horse is most likely to be the source of injury, because the owner may develop overconfidence, which can lead to complacency and inattention to safety.

Numerous studies available in the scientific and medical literature emphasize the dangers of working with large animals. Assessments included patterns of injury, specific injury mechanisms, and species-specific injuries. In one study, 79 patients (55%) were injured by horses, 47 patients (32%) by bulls, 16 patients (11%) by cows, and 3 patients (2%) by wild animal attacks. The predominant species-specific mechanisms of injury were falls (horses), tramplings (bulls), and kicks (cows). Bull and cow encounters usually resulted in torso injuries (45% and 56%, respectively). Multiple injuries occurred in 32% of patients (Norwood et al., 2000). Similarly, in Turkey, of 113 patients hospitalized for large animal-induced injuries, 30% (33) had sustained abdominal injuries and 63.6% required surgery. One patient died (Ok et al., 2004). Over a six-year period, 134 patients were admitted to another hospital for large animal-related trauma. The most common mechanisms of injury included animal kicks (39 people) and animal assault (42). The authors mention the importance of education to prevent these types of injuries (Busch et al., 1986).

Horses can be particularly dangerous when handled on the ground. Over a five-year period in British Columbia, Canada, 1,950 hospital admissions were due to equestrian-related injuries; of these, 15 died (0.7%). The author concluded that if an equestrian presents to a hospital, the severity of the injury often requires admission. Statistics of injuries include being knocked down, trampled, and kicked by horses (Sorli, 2000). In another retrospective study of all human fatalities involving horses used for work and recreational purposes on farms and ranches between 1975 and 1990, records from the Office of the Chief Medical Examiner of Alberta, Canada, revealed that 38 people were involved in horse-related fatalities and that 22 of them died of head injuries. All 38 deaths were classified as accidental (Aronson and Tough, 1993).

In Switzerland over an 18 month period, 80 equestrian injuries presented, and of these 17 (21%) were unmounted equestrian patients admitted to the Level I trauma center. Nine (53%) suffered facial injuries, 5 were referred to plastic surgeons, and 3 of the 5 underwent maxillofacial surgery. The authors concluded that equestrians may underestimate the risk of severe injuries due to kicks from hooves while handling horses and that direct trauma to the face is mainly associated with handling horses, not riding them (Exadaktylos et al., 2002).

A study in eastern Ontario, Canada, reported that common patterns of injury from farmers working with cattle included lacerations, bruises, and crush injuries (Brison and Pickett, 1991). A retrospective assessment of ocular (eye) injuries in 11 patients admitted for cattle horn injuries revealed that 7 had open globe (ruptured eye) injuries with vitreous hemorrhage. Only 3 patients regained good visual acuity. The conclusion of the study was that the majority of eye injuries led to permanent visual impairment (Goldblum et al., 1999).

Veterinarians are not immune to injuries. A survey of American Veterinary Medical Association members (large animal and small animal practitioners) revealed that 64.6% had sustained a major animal-related injury. The reported mechanisms of injury included animal kicks (35.5%), bites (34%), crushing (11.7%), scratching (3.8%), and other causes (e.g., pushing, goring, head butting, trampling, and falling on the veterinarian) (14.9%). Cattle were the most common species involved (46.5%), followed by dogs (24.2%) and horses (15.2%). Days lost from work secondary to animal injury averaged 1.3 days (range, 0–180 days) in 1986 and 8.5 days (range, 0–365 days) over the veterinarian's career (Landercaspar et al., 1988).

A comprehensive survey of 315 members of the American Association of Zoo Veterinarians was undertaken to identify the frequency of injuries. Significant findings included major animal-related injury (61.5%), back injury (55%), necropsy injury (44.1%), adverse formalin exposure (40.2%), animal allergy (32.2%), zoonotic infection (30.2%), and insect allergy (14.2%). Zoo veterinarians with more years of experience were more likely to receive major animal-related injury and associated hospitalization, back injury, and lost work time associated with back injury. The conclusion of the authors was that the frequency of injuries reported demonstrates a greater need for comprehensive health and safety programs for zoo veterinarians (Hill et al., 1998).

Exposure Frequency. Exposure to large animals seems to be the best indicator of the chance of injury—the more exposure to these animals, the greater the risk of injury to the person. This may simply be a reflection of the time of exposure or may be due to complacency working around these large animals. Animal handlers may also be harmed on the job due to injuries inflicted by animals; dangers related to the facility, work activities, equipment, and weather extremes. Traumatic or venomous attacks by animals can result in fatality. Attention to safety measures is of critical importance in the field of animal handling (Langley, 1999).

Weird accidents can and will happen, and may not be the result of the actual rescue scene; handlers can be injured after the animal has been caught and is being led to safety. Some large animals will kick and bite each other if the handlers allow them to get too close; the urge to fight may overwhelm the animals' fear and create additional danger. A handler may be injured when a horse attempts to evade the threat of another horse and unintentionally knocks over or tramples its handler. In discussing the unique risks of partnering with a horse, Sorli points out ". . . that one member of the team is non-human, weighs upwards of 1,100 lb (500 kg), wears metal shoes, has teeth that can inflict injury to unmounted persons, moves at speeds up to 65 kph (40 mph), elevates the rider 3 m above the ground, and can change direction and speed (accelerate or decelerate) in less than a second." (Sorli, 2000).

Built for Acceleration

The musculoskeletal system of the large animal is a marvel of biomechanically efficient engineering and natural design. The long leg bones in the hind end of the animal make up a system of levers coupled with a muscular "spring" that pushes the entire 1,100 lb (500 kg) animal ahead; it is the "drive axle" or "motor" that drives that animal forward. When reacting to fear, some horses can reach 70 kph (43 mph) in only a few seconds. Human reaction times are much slower, and a handler in front of a horse is at risk of injury. A cow can run almost as fast as a horse. Cattle, llamas, emus, camels, and goats are also capable of jumping obstacles.

Certain breeds of horses (stock type horses) are capable of amazing acceleration rates. Their muscle types and development permit quick sprinting movements, faster than other breeds of horses in the first quarter of a mile. Other breeds, such as Arabians and Thoroughbreds, are recognized for having the endurance for racing 1 to 2 miles (1.6–3.2 km) on the flat (typical horse racing events) or completing 100 mile (161 km) endurance races in one day. All prey animals can move quickly, and the argument about whether to chase is a moot point; any large animal (even a young one) is capable of outrunning a human. Instead of chasing the animal, responders should encourage it to come to someone with feed, or incorporate the assist of a Judas animal, or attempt to contain the animal.

On emergency scenes, the animal may be trapped where it cannot run away, and its biomechanical force will be transferred to the animal's attempts to free or protect itself. The powerful blow of a horse kick can deliver more than 10,000 Newtons (the force of approximately 1 metric ton) to a person's body; this is enough force to bend a coin in your pocket at the point of impact and to cause major soft tissue damage, bone fracture, and devastating injuries to the abdominal organs. Other large animals can be just as lethal with their hooves. One study found that hoof kick injuries to unmounted children represented 30% of the total injuries and was the most severe equestrian-related injury, when ranked with a severity score. These injuries ranked second in severity to pedestrians struck by vehicles and received higher severity scores than all-terrain vehicle, bicycle, and passenger motor vehicle crash injuries (Jagodzinski and DeMuri, 2005). In a study of 262 equestrian-related injuries in children at a hospital in Germany, accidents from handling horses were of special significance. Patients were kicked by the hooves (11.8%), stepped on by the horse (3.8%), or bitten (7.3%). Horse kicks caused life-threatening head injuries in 41.6% of the cases, and 1 patient died (Giebel, Braun, and Mittelmeier, 1993). Furthermore, an examination of 78 accidents in horseback riding found that 76% of all injuries did not occur during the active phase of riding, but in the time just preceding and following the activity (leading, loading, handling) (Rathfelder et al., 1995).

Take the Time

Patience with horses and livestock is the key to gaining their trust and respect. Human predatory tendencies to move hurriedly can make animals untrusting of the intention of the human. Handlers should always work with calm and deliberate movements around animals; losing their temper or taking out their frustrations on the large animal victim will make an already unsafe situation worse. "What most people think is slow is fast," says Jennifer Woods (2006b). A large animal rescue scene is not the place to be in a hurry or on a time schedule. Decreasing the stress placed on the animal increases the speed of the rescue and reduces the risk of injury to the animal victim. Panic reactions (fast movements, unexpected motions, loud noises, fear smells) by people on the scene may amplify the animal's fear response and distress.

The animal handler in particular should know something about the behavior, restraint, and safe handling of the particular species in trouble. This person can help the animal to relax and cooperate by using appropriate approach, greet, interaction, and body language. Lower stress techniques will result in lower stress for both animals and people. Personnel on scene should be reminded to avoid raising their voices, flapping their arms, or yelling at animals. All livestock and horses must be worked by calm, slow, and sensitive handlers to get their cooperation. Often called low-stress stockhandling methods, using body language and understanding of the flight zones of animals will ensure cooperation more efficiently than yelling and using whips or sticks. The only time a person should strike an animal, raise his or her voice, or use an electric prod is in self-defense if being attacked. Responders should not chase livestock with vehicles (Woods, 2006a).

An example is the 2 a.m. call from frightened urban dwellers about 13 loose longhorn cattle in Greenville, South Carolina. The animals had gotten out of their fenced pasture and were roaming through a nearby suburban area. After fixing the fence and putting alfalfa hay in the pasture, responders strung white electric fencing strands between trees to make a long funnel back to the gate. The officer at the gate had instructions to stand back and wait until all the cattle got through and then shut the gate. The cattle were slowly driven through the middle of the neighborhood right into the readily visible funnel. As the animals approached the gate, the officer turned on a flashlight. Fearful of the light, the cattle panicked and scattered throughout the neighborhood. When responders returned at first light, half of the cattle were in the fenced pasture, and the rest were standing outside the pasture gate.

To drive loose animals to containment, find an animal handler with a low-pitched voice and calm body language. Horse and livestock handling skills are not something learned in three days at a clinic or workshop; these are skills that must be cultivated and practiced. Horse and livestock owners who practice these skills will improve their rapport with their own animals. Responders should always have an escape route planned and should stay alert to all that is going on at the scene. Providing forage or allowing the animal to graze will decrease its stress level. However, the animal will still react to a stimulus, and responders should be prepared if the animal suddenly moves without notice (Woods, 2006b).

THE APPROACH

Pulling together these concepts of sensation and reaction mechanisms, consider an approach toward an animal loose on the interstate (the animal is represented by the black spot in the center of Figure 4.17;

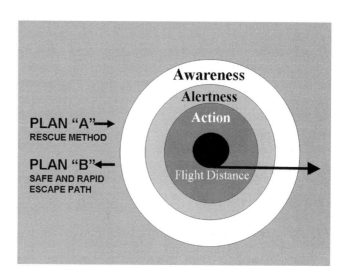

Figure 4.17 Action, alertness, and awareness zones show the responder how an approach toward an animal will affect the movement and apprehension of the animal being approached. Courtesy of Rebecca Gimenez.

Grandin, 2004). The animal might be a llama, cow, horse, or emu. As the rescuer approaches the animal, he or she will pass through three invisible zones around the animal: the awareness zone (white), the alertness zone (light gray), and the action zone (dark gray). What kind of action should be expected from the animal depending on the approaching animal handler's body language and position?

Have an Approach Plan

As direct line thinkers and predators, human nature determines that we must catch the animal. This predatory thinking can be detrimental to the situation. If animal containment is desired, driving them through a portable fencing funnel to a pasture or cutting the fence on the interstate and driving them into a backyard as a more confined area may be good options. Humans cannot outrun or outdodge a prey animal but can outplan and outsmart them by using the animal's behavior and instincts to the rescuers' advantage.

Safety should always be considered, and there should be an escape plan. If an animal's body language indicates aggression, responders should have a plan established that will protect them. Start asking questions: Is there a rapid, safe escape plan for personnel? Is there a buddy system?

Awareness Zone

The awareness zone shown in white (Figure 4.17) is the safest zone—the rescuer is farthest away from the animal. The rescuer will know he or she is within the awareness zone when the animal has smelled, heard, or seen him or her; it is aware through some sense that an intruder is there. Normal reactions to this phase of the approach might include flicking the ears toward

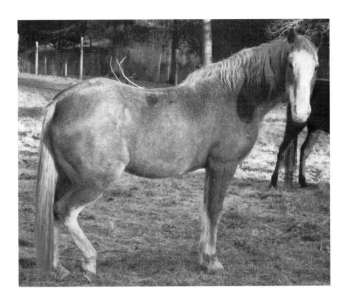

Figure 4.18 *A calm horse is standing still with a hind leg cocked in a resting position indicating relaxation, and the head is looking at the photographer in a friendly, interested manner. With enticement and the correct body language, this horse should be easily caught. Courtesy of Rebecca Gimenez.*

the person or raising the head, using the senses to gain information about the intruding animal handler (Figure 4.18). Remember that on emergency scenes, one or more of the animal's senses may be impaired (blocked vision, muffled sounds, overwhelmed sense of smell).

To understand these zones, consider a situation familiar to most people: a person visiting a stranger's house. There is a dog in the yard, and it sees a stranger exit a car and enter its awareness zone. As the person moves forward, the dog looks straight at him or her with both eyes. This is considered "on alert" in predators such as dogs and cats. At this point, most humans are wary of the dog and become cautious. The dog may growl or bark as the person approaches the house, indicating that the person is within the dog's alertness zone. If that person keeps walking to the door, they will have entered the action zone, and the animal may attack.

In emergency or stressful situations, many humans disregard these zones. Their urgency and willingness to assist an animal in distress drive them to rapidly cross the awareness and alertness zones. By slowing their approach and spending time in the animal's alertness zone, they may observe and evaluate the animal and allow it to relax and become accustomed to their presence. When the rescuer then enters the animal's action zone, the risk of an aggressive response is reduced (Parelli, 2005).

The radius of the awareness, alertness, and action zones depends on the species, level of agitation, and the individual animal. An example to consider is a 20 year old pony that is well-adapted to being ridden by children. It may be that when the rescuers enter the awareness zone—approximately 100 m (330 ft) away— the animal's attitude remains positive and relaxed. Alternatively, other animals in that exact scenario may be frightened by the approaching humans. Some animals have a small action zone radius, while others have a larger radius. The animal's flight distance is also affected by injuries, handling history, general temperament, and level of fear. It is impossible to accurately predict what that particular animal is going to do in a particular situation, despite familiarity with the animal involved.

Alertness Zone

When the rescuer enters the alertness zone, the animal will attempt to turn to face the human. Prey animals will try to gain information by turning their ears, eyes, and nose toward the rescuers. In rescue scenarios trapped animals may not be able to face the rescuer. The animal(s) may be trapped in a trailer where they cannot see humans, but they can hear and smell. An animal trapped in a hole may be unable to turn its head and will try to look up. Prey animals are instinctively alarmed by stimuli above them (because that is where an ambush often originates in the wild). Being in this position can be stressful to the animal; in their attempts to turn, and upon stimulus, they may scramble and further injure themselves. This is where a soothing tone of voice will assist the animal to relax and serve as an introduction for the animal handler.

The Action Zone

Once a person enters the action zone, several responses may be elicited; animals may stand still, run away, attack with the front or hind end, rear up on their hind limbs, or move to the side. Alternatively, the animal may be severely injured or debilitated and unable to flee (Figure 4.19).

Flight distance is the distance to which a threatened animal will run until it feels safe. This escape mechanism allows it to react immediately to fear-inducing scenarios, then evaluate the stressor from a safe distance. When spooked, animals will attempt to reach their flight distance even when restrained by a halter and lead rope. As an example of flight distance and adaptation, pronghorn antelope in the western United States will run away from humans to a distance of approximately 300 m (990 ft), then turn to look at the humans; the animals have learned that the average hunter is accurate at 100 m (330 ft), somewhat less accurate at 200 m (660 ft), and very rarely can hit an antelope at 250–300 m (825–990 ft). As long as humans remain 300 m away, the pronghorns appear to ignore them. Equally, they appear to ignore vehicles moving closer to them unless the perceived predators get out of the vehicle.

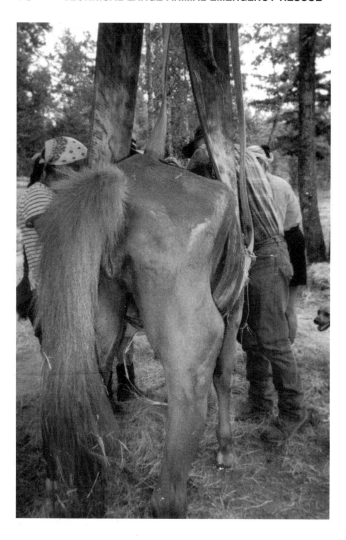

Figure 4.19 *This neglected horse's body condition score is considered extremely emaciated. Equine abuse/neglect organizations and animal control commonly respond to these types of cases in all communities, and many of the animals will be recumbent and unable to stand. Courtesy of Karen Zajicek.*

Critical distance is the distance at which an animal that perceives no escape route will attack. For large and wild animals, that distance might be much farther away from the animal than humans tend to acknowledge. Attacking a human is a last resort for many species, but more common in others, especially lactating females and intact males. The maternal instinct can be very powerful and make an animal aggressive. Intact male animals (bulls, stallions, etc.) tend to be more aggressive than females of the same species. In addition, they are usually larger and more intimidating. Those working with cattle need to be aware of their posture. The rescuer should avoid leaning forward when offering a cow a pan of feed. This may be interpreted by the cow as a challenge, and she may drop her head and charge. If an animal feels trapped, it will be more nervous and may become aggressive. Tight spaces and those with overhead cover may worsen the animal's perception that it is trapped.

ANTHROPOMORPHISM

People can become emotionally attached to animals and may keep them close to their homes and families. Those without firsthand knowledge of this human–animal bond may not understand an animal owner's emotional reaction to the situation. Anthropomorphism, or the practice of assigning human emotions and value systems to animals, is common in animal owners. According to the HSUS in 2005, 37 million cats get a Christmas present, and many owners clothe their animals, including horses. Over 10 million dogs sleep in their owner's bed. According to surveys, 46.9% of horse owners consider their horses to be family members; 39.1% consider them to be pets/companions; and only 5.7% view them as property (American Veterinary Medical Association, 2002.) Despite the animal's size, many horse owners become very bonded to their horses. Time spent caring for something is closely connected to the degree of affection we develop for it.

The real miscommunication is the failure of humans to recognize that each species of animal has its own language, emotions, and interactions. From a scientific standpoint, it is improper to anthropomorphize animals. Many animal lovers agree, but for another reason—they know that animals have their own set of needs and desires. Although a clean living space, food, and water provide for the animal's basic needs, studies have shown that prey animals need interaction with their own kind, especially since they are herd animals. Animals can have emotional and psychological disorders. As an example, early zoo designs were infamous for inducing stress and abnormal behaviors in the animals by depriving them of beneficial interactions with others of their own species. Anxiety and stress can be fatal, but animals respond to antidepressants and other medications, further proving emotional similarities between animals and humans.

If humans are to learn to communicate effectively with animals, humans must learn their language (Parelli, 2005). Animals may not be capable of speaking a language that is easily understood by humans, but they share the same basic emotional needs. Animals are different by degrees, not in the mechanisms or design. In the area of "natural horsemanship," where humans are learning to use body language and leadership to communicate with horses, better communication is becoming more commonplace. It takes years of effort to learn and understand the fine details of this communication method, but the basics can be learned by anyone and applied to rescue scenarios.

BIOCHEMICAL SIMILARITIES

Humans may consider themselves superior to animals, overlooking the fact that our bodies are equipped with the same fundamental biochemical and emotional processes. The complexity of human society and the utilization of animals for labor, food, fiber, and recreation tend to encourage this belief. Attributing emotions to animals raises ethical and philosophical debate; such awareness might imply a necessity for us to handle them with more care and respect, or even as equals. Until the late 1970s, the physiological and sociological scientific tools needed to investigate these questions were not available. Current biological and behavioral research studies in primates and other animals are elucidating the answers to many of these questions. Responders should understand that anthropomorphism is not necessary because the emotional and behavioral response mechanisms of animals are similar to humans.

Fear

The most primitive and fundamental emotion in all mammals is the hormonal reaction to fear. It is also the most powerful emotion studied in all animals, because it directly affects the survival of the animal. Fear is developed in the reptilian part of all mammal brains; this area also regulates heart rate, breathing, and flight responses. True fear is not processed by the higher-functioning areas of the brain; it is hardwired in the spinal cord of prey species and induces the rapid response of flight. Invertebrates, such as octopi, can change color when angry and fearful; they become flushed, similar to humans. Large animals such as horses, cattle, and llamas respond to fear by adopting the flight or fight reaction; the sympathetic nervous system releases epinephrine to increase the heart rate and breathing rate and prepare the muscles for their flight. From an evolutionary standpoint, a quick, reflexive reaction to anything that scares the animal allows it to escape that stressor and survive to reproduce.

When animals behave as if they are afraid, it is not a casual fear. It is a perception of a life-or-death situation. In humans, this type of fear response produces a flushed face, racing heart, rapid breathing rate, and tensed muscles. Fear for animals is either black or white; there is no gray area.

Attack Behavior. Attacking humans or other predators is not normal behavior for cattle or horses, unless protecting their offspring or challenging other herd males. (The common exception is dogs; horses, cattle, and llamas do learn to attack dogs, including coyotes, when teased or threatened; Figure 4.20). In wild mustangs or feral cattle, aggression is normal behavior for intact males fighting over the right for the herd, but very few prey animals will fight to the death. Most commonly, they will test the strength and mettle of their opponent; the weaker animal will run away to fight another day.

Aggressive behaviors in prey species are unusual, but may be exhibited by a mother protecting her offspring

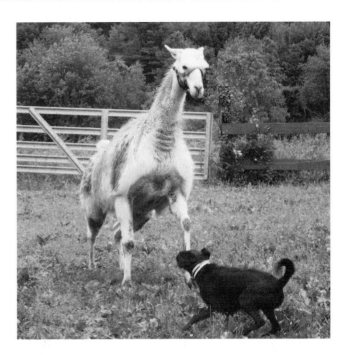

Figure 4.20 *Once a perceived predator enters the action zone of an animal, the prey animal may choose to attack instead of running away, as this llama demonstrates. Courtesy of Tomas Gimenez.*

or an injured animal protecting its life. When animals fight the animal handler by rearing, pawing, lunging, and pulling away, these behaviors may be aggressive responses, but are most often defensive behaviors driven by fear. The animal handler should try to reduce pressure on the animal by stepping farther away to allow the animal to calm down. Approach and retreat methods work well with prey animals. Animals that have endured abusive or minimal handling by people will be more difficult to handle than animals used to gentle and frequent contact with people.

Society

Mammals have amazing evolutionary adaptations to the ancient reptilian brain, including larger brain size; multiple layers of processing neurons; and the abilities to learn, to teach their young, and live in social groups. Complex societies (harems, herds, crowds, flocks, communities) demand a certain amount of give and take to encourage cooperation, which enhances survival of group members and increases their opportunities to reproduce and contribute their genes to continue the species. One animal (often female) is the alpha, making the decisions (e.g., when to eat, when to drink, where to graze, where to seek shelter from the approaching storm). In wild horse, cattle, and buffalo societies, the herd has a strict hierarchy that determines the order in which herd members eat or drink, as well as where they sleep (McDonnell, 2003).

Social Stress. Emotional stress is applied in social societies (herds, flocks, groups) and is introduced at a young age. Animals must learn socially acceptable behaviors as well as ways to reduce stress and earn acceptance. There are reward and punishment systems in animal societies as well as in our own. Prey animals adopt a gregarious herd strategy. These behaviors build lifelong or temporary social covenants between members of the herd, which are important to long-term survival when watching for predators, raising young, etc. This natural tendency can be helpful with cattle, for instance, if personnel will take advantage of the fact that cattle will be more relaxed—even in an enclosure—if they can stay with their group. Isolation leads to panic.

Research has revealed that the human traits of friendship, gentleness, and kindness can eventually win out over aggression, bullying, and cruelty. In all mammalian animal societies studied, mammals appear to make "friends." They have their preferred play and grooming buddies. The practice of reciprocity for favors (e.g., food, grooming, protection, social obligations) is followed by many large animal groups. Young animals "smile;" this is called a play face and is characterized by open eyes, a lowered head, play body position (the animal's front end is lowered while the rear end remains up), and upturned lips. It is a communication with facial expression that universally signals a willingness to play to most mammals (especially the young). Most prey animals do not have the facial musculature necessary to adopt the wide variety of obvious facial expressions of which primates are capable, but this does not mean that they lack emotion or do not react to stress.

Loyalty. Elephants are known to override their drive to feed to stay with an injured or dying herd member. They have been documented on video rescuing young that have become stuck in the mud. In the group effort, each elephant performs a separate task, such as building a ramp, lifting the baby, driving off predators, guarding the herd, etc. This is performed using vocal communication outside the auditory range of humans. Wild and domestic cattle often demonstrate herd protection behaviors when approached by predators, forming a ring with their heads and horns pointing outward. If they are able to surround a dog or coyote in an open field, they will form a ring around the individual to attack it with their heads. Wild horses have been documented to present the same herd ring formation, with young animals in the center and their hindquarters pointing out to allow them to protect themselves—and the herd—with their hindquarters.

LEARNING FROM ANIMAL BEHAVIORAL RESEARCH

Field research has provided excellent insights into handling live animals on large animal emergency scenes.

As an animal scientist with a doctorate, and a highly functioning autistic person, Dr. Temple Grandin has written several books providing excellent insight into animal perceptions and reactions. She is internationally known for her efforts to improve humane methods of animal slaughter, transport, and processing. The information she has learned from this lifetime of research with livestock and horses transfers directly to handling large animals on emergency scenes.

If humans are to eat a balanced diet containing meat protein, there is a need for a slaughter industry for commercial food animals (chickens, cattle, pigs, etc). However, ethical consideration for their dignity as beings able to feel pain determines that they should die humanely. It is irrational and financially detrimental for producers to hurt, injure, or stress the animals before sending them to slaughter; these animals represent a large investment of money, time, and effort. Historically, animals were stressed or injured due to a lack of understanding or education regarding animal well-being. The industry has a vested interest in making the slaughter process safer and calmer for the animals: when an animal is slaughtered in a relaxed, nonstressed manner, the result is a product with superior taste, higher value, and less waste. Every time a cattle prod is used, it causes a bruise on the meat that must be excised and discarded. Scientific studies have determined that a minimum of 30 minutes is required for stress hormone cortisol levels to return to baseline if humans are yelling at cattle during processing (Grandin, 1999).

Dr. Grandin's insight is responsible for dramatic improvements of the humane slaughter industries in the United States and internationally, and they should be applied to rescue TLAER scenes. For example, many slaughter facilities previously had straight lanes with tight corners to funnel cattle from trucks to the kill floor, and the animals were driven down the lanes by yelling or cattle prods. Dr. Grandin observed that cattle in curved chutes (where the animals can not see what is in front) tended to move forward on their own and recommended that facilities modify their chute systems. New facilities implement these approaches to the process of loading, transport, and slaughter, improving the humane treatment of commercial food animals. Over 70% of slaughter facilities in the United States— and now internationally—use Dr. Grandin's designs and methods. Employees are taught to minimize distractions for animals such as wind, waving or fluttering plastic, sudden transitions to darkness or light, or banging chains. Although they may appear minor to humans, these stimuli will stop or slow the forward movement of the animals. Similarly, responders should be reminded that these stimuli may have similar effects on animals being led from overturned trailers (see Chapter 21), burning barns (see Chapter 10), or other situations (Grandin and Johnson, 2005).

In addition to the natural tendency for cattle to move around gentle curves discovered by Grandin, two other tendencies that could be used to the rescuers' advantage in working with cattle are that they prefer to move up a slight incline rather than down and they move toward light. This is best demonstrated by moving cattle through a lane of panels toward an apparent "opening." This is a challenge if the lane leads into a darkened cattle trailer, but those working with cattle on scene need to be aware of these natural tendencies and, when possible, use them to the rescuers' advantage.

For example, in 2005, 12 miniature bison got loose in a Baltimore, Maryland, suburb approximately 10 km from their pasture. The local responders' original containment plan was to drive the bison into a fenced tennis court, which worked well. The owner parked the transport trailer outside the fence approximately 15 m from the gate, and responders attempted to use a line of people as a funnel while driving the entire herd onto the trailer. Although this approach may be successful with tame species, it was unsuccessful in this situation, and the bison scattered. Eventually, the responders moved the trailer to a corner of the tennis court and cut the fence. They herded the animals across the tennis courts with plastic chairs, and eventually were able to successfully load the animals in small groups.

Bison present a unique challenge in these situations. Unlike domesticated animals, they do not respect barriers. Few obstacles can stop them, and they are very difficult to keep quiet and calm. In the video of this incident (broadcast live nationwide), one officer was knocked over, but was uninjured. Based on the common observation that "bison that are fed will stay inside one strand of barbed wire; otherwise, the Great Wall of China will not hold them," they are easy to bait with grain or forage into containment (Woods, 2006b). Putting alfalfa hay or grain in the trailer may attract the animals to the trailer, but may be less effective if a small trailer is used. One problem with this technique is that the first animals to reach the hay stop to eat, and there may not be enough room for the rest of the group to load.

ZOOLOGIC EXOTIC LARGE ANIMALS

There are very few scenarios in which emergency responders with minimal training in exotic large animal rescue and restraint would be called to assist with exotics and zoological specimens. However, sufficient numbers of escaped animals (e.g., lions, tigers, zebras, gorillas, ostriches, elephants, buffalos) and wild animals (e.g., elk and moose) occur across the country to merit their inclusion in this book. Additionally, many of them are transported in unmarked trailers through our locales. As with any species, it is recommended that potential rescuers visit a farm that raises that species to learn how to handle them. Practice in handling and learning about the animal's normal habits and behaviors leads to expertise. Going to the zoo to watch the animals is generally not sufficient for training, because there is always some degree of separation from the public. The experience of walking up to an ostrich whose body is at human height and whose head is 2 m (6.6 ft) in the air makes a responder realize the intimidating size, strength, and speed of these animals.

Significant numbers of exotic animals, including large, hooved prey animals, are housed in towns and cities around the world. Private collectors and breeders, backyard enthusiasts, zoos of all sizes, and private hunting ranches may have many varieties of exotic animals in their collections. Escaped animals, especially in the face of a disaster, may present challenging public safety concerns to the jurisdiction in which they are present. Wild animals are potentially extremely dangerous and unpredictable, and a team effort is required to safely resolve the situation.

Remaining quiet around zoologics is even more important than with domesticated prey animals; alternatively, white noise from a radio can lessen the effect of some sudden noises. Wrestling, roping, darting, or shooting an animal as seen on TV are drastic actions that excite and fascinate people but should be minimized on a rescue or recapture scene. In many cases, with some time and patience, the animal can be slowly encouraged to move back to its original living site (Kiessler, 2004). Fences may be cut to create a place to drive the animals, field gates may be opened to drive the animals off the road, or chutes made of portable fencing material may be used to drive them to a safe area or onto a stock trailer.

Similar to domestic prey animals, wild animals and zoologics may become fractious and disoriented when escaped from their enclosures, and they will usually seek shelter and food away from humans. Often the easiest plan is to make the home enclosure quiet and allow the animal(s) to return. In disasters, this may not be a viable alternative, so careful planning will be required to safely recapture the animal.

Minimize Human Injuries and Death

Injured persons will detract from the time and effort to complete the animal rescue or capture, and these exotic large animals are capable of injuring or killing a person. As in all other rescue scenarios, human safety is the first priority (Kiessler, 2004). Animal handlers should obtain training and experience in handling exotics before attempting to assist with these rescue situations. Small antelopes, goats, and wild deer are significantly stronger, faster, and more reactionary than domesticated goats and sheep. These animals are well known for redirecting their fear and frustration into aggression, and they may attack a well-meaning human with their horns or may run over them.

Containment Options

When attempting to corral or drive animals, responders should always be aware of their body position and possible cover (e.g., trees, vehicles, big rocks) behind which they may hide if the animals don't behave as expected or desired. Rescuers should avoid recapture of animals in areas with physical hazards to the animal (e.g., holes, poor footing) or where sudden stop syndrome (fractured neck) can occur when stressed animals run blindly in their fear into immovable objects (Kiessler, 2004).

Never overestimate humans' capabilities or underestimate the nature of the animals. In addition, the environmental dangers while trying to contain or drive loose animals should be considered. Falling trees, wind, downed power lines, rising flood waters, mud slides, holes, and poor footing are among the perils that can endanger rescuers as well as the animals (Kiessler, 2004). Portable fencing may work to move or drive some species, especially if responders move very slowly and are very quiet. However, most zoologics will not remain inside a portable corral that is too small.

Capture myopathy (also called white muscle disease) can cause immediate or delayed death in a prey animal that is stressed, overheated, or pushed (chased) too hard by well-meaning rescuers (Figure 4.21). Hyperthermia is indicated by open-mouthed breathing and panting (otherwise not seen in prey animals) (Kiessler, 2004). Humans are too close and stressing the animal if the animal begins pacing up and down a fence; this reaction indicates that rescuers are inside the action zone of the animal's flight distance. The exception to this rule is ratites (ostrich or emu); they very commonly

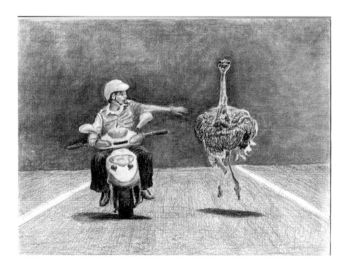

Figure 4.21 *Prey animals should not be chased by people in motorized vehicles, on horseback, or on foot. Ostrich in particular, can achieve speeds of up to 40 mph (65 kph) for short periods, and if stressed by the chase, can die from capture myopathy. Most other large animals and exotics can outrun a human. A better strategy for containment should be devised. Courtesy of Julie Casil.*

pace up and down any obstacle (such as fences) in their way. This can be used to the rescuers' advantage to drive them into a funnel along the fence and into containment.

Zoologic Animal Behavior

The basic nature of the individual animal is going to make or break the recapture effort and will determine the strategy used to attempt to recapture it. Every species has special considerations for approach, handling, and containment. If at all possible, a person with experience with these exotic large animals should assist on the scene. Some animals are high-strung and nervous; others are docile and easily approachable. The attitude of the animal is easily determined by approaching and retreating from the animal a few times; once inside the action zone, the animal will move.

Do not allow anyone to approach the animal until the plan is made and everything is ready. If their flight distance is penetrated to the point where the animal perceives that it has no method of escape, then the critical distance has been reached and the animal will switch its response from flight to fight and can become overwhelmingly aggressive. All prey animals have a herd mentality and may find their way back to safety in the original pen or close to similar hooved animals (Moxley, 2004).

Transporting Zoologics

Zoologics and exotics are commonly recaptured in a zoo environment and, after tranquilization, are carried in cargo nets made of webbing by many people. The cargo net provides many handles, but it does not prevent someone from being kicked or gored by thrashing horns and hooves. The cargo net also allows easy manipulation around corners and through narrow openings (Kiessler, 2004). Using a Rescue Glide or similar plastic sled (see Chapter 11) should be considered for moving recumbent or anesthetized zoologic large animals, as well as carcasses, in a more professional manner.

Co-locating and Sheltering Groups of Large Animals

In general, the rules for keeping groups in a small area or putting strange animals together are similar to those for other large animals.

- Animals of the same species should be kept together. (There are few exceptions to this rule, and experienced handlers can advise the rescuers.)
- Males should be separated from female animals, juvenile animals, and other males.
- Horned animals should be separated from nonhorned animals; horns can be dangerous weapons that induce severe injury or death in less-protected species.

- Allow much more space than you would anticipate the animals to need so that omega animals lower in the pecking order can avoid the alpha and aggressive animals. Provide a place for omega animals to escape aggressive animals.
- In sheltering situations for herds of animals, always put one more pile of hay and one more feeder than the number of animals; also, provide more than one source of water. Provide shade, windbreaks, and places to hide from aggressive animals (e.g., brush piles or trees).

SPECIAL COMMENTS ON LARGE ANIMAL SPECIES

Hooved Ungulate Zoologics

The ungulate species include the Perisodactyla, with odd numbers of toes (e.g., horses, zebras, wild horses, asses, rhinos, hippo), and the Artiodactyla, with even numbers of toes (e.g., giraffes, pigs, deer, sheep, goats, cattle, antelopes, camels, llamas, alpacas). These are herbivorous prey mammals that characteristically move in herds.

Sheep and Goats

These ruminants are used to being herded and are normally passive, but they can escape by climbing, jumping, or crawling under obstacles. Although these animals may be of a size that can be manually manipulated, sheep should not be lifted by their fleece or horns. Pulling on the wool or fleece of sheep may cause bruising to the underlying skin and degrade the quality of the wool. Goats and sheep may charge when afraid. Rams and goats jump up as they charge the person, and can inflict significant injury. Even small horns can be extremely dangerous. Goats and horned sheep are known to gore by swinging their heads and hooking the individual, potentially causing severe injury to both skin and internal organs. Sheep will instinctively gather into a group, sometimes so tightly packed that the individuals in the center may suffocate. Loose herds of these animals are easily worked by trained herding dogs and professional handlers, but they can be easily spooked into a stampede.

Cattle

A quick look at the industry containment standards for cattle reveals sturdy 2 m (6 ft) fencing with 15 cm (6 inch) diameter posts buried in concrete to a depth of 1 m (3 feet) and steel construction of head gates and corral panels. By comparison, improvised confinement equipment may be ineffective. One veterinarian told the author of a farmer's containment facility that had not been well maintained; the bull whose head was locked into the head gate walked away with the entire steel head gate hanging on its neck.

Cattle use their heads as weapons whether or not they are horned. Horns are incredibly dangerous weapons; long or short, the animal knows how to use them for defense and aggression. Cattle will swing their large heads and use their weight to shove other animals out of their way, or lower their heads and menace an approaching dog, human, or object. Cattle tend to use their heads for protection and aggression much more than other large animals. Cattle use their heads intentionally to make other cattle move and as an offensive weapon to gore and crush. Cornered cattle are capable of using their powerful heads and shoulders to lift a gate or panel off its hinges (Durak, 2006).

The original phrase *cow kick* was first applied to dairy cattle when being milked. When a cow kicks, they usually swing laterally (to the side) at a 90-degree angle from the hip, not behind them like a horse. Cows tend not to kick with their feet backward, although they are capable of doing so.

Cattle have a lower center of gravity and normally move more slowly than horses; this may lead inexperienced responders to develop a false sense of safety around these animals. Excited cattle have been known to jump 2 m (6 ft) high fences and crush various contrivances intended to contain them, including cars, gates, barn walls, and fences. Cattle weigh as much as horses, move as quickly, and can jump much higher than most people would estimate.

Beef cattle and dairy cattle are very different. Dairy cattle are handled on a regular basis, usually twice daily, and are accustomed to people. They are groomed, fed, milked, and regularly moved from place to place. However, beef cattle are rarely handled by people except for procedures such as vaccinations, de-worming, dehorning, and castration. They are handled by running them through a cattle chute and trapping them in a head gate. Because their interactions with humans are less frequent and more likely to be associated with discomfort, beef cattle have a heightened sense of fear in response to the presence of humans.

Bulls, like most male mammals, have natural instincts of aggression that require respect and extreme caution. Although dairy cattle are usually gentle, dairy bulls are often dangerous and aggressive (Woods, 2006a). Bulls tend to be larger than cows and can be recognized by their larger musculature, body frame, and pendulous scrotum. Bulls should only be approached by experienced livestock handlers when possible. Experienced handlers will usually search for an indirect method to restrain or catch a bull.

Swine

Pigs encountered on a TLAER scene should generally be considered dangerous. Their low stature is deceiving—handle them with respect and caution (Woods, 2006a). Pigs are smart, low to the ground, very strong, and have large teeth. Very few are halter-trained to lead, and most are very difficult to restrain. Pigs' ears are not appropriate handles. Pet pigs can grow to enormous sizes approaching 770 lb (350 kg), but they are more commonly 165–605 lb (75–275 kg). Market-size hogs (approx. six months of age) that would be encountered in an overturned slaughter trailer are approximately 165 lb (75 kg); adult sows approach 550 lb (250 kg), and boars can reach 770 lb (350 kg). Even if responders are handling pigs respectfully, they will squeal when touched, or just because they want to. This can look bad to bystanders who will assume responders are injuring the animals.

Pigs are very sensitive to environmental temperatures and can die of heat stress, frostbite, or hypothermia. Pigs have very little hair on their bodies and cannot sweat, so they should not be chased. In addition, they are difficult to chase and should be driven in slow motion, allowing them to find their way (Woods, 2006a). Portable fencing is a good method of gently guiding market-sized hogs into containment. It is difficult to tell if a pig is injured unless it is very obvious.

Often, the only handholds available on a small pig are its legs, but it may bite if held by the front legs; it should be restrained by the back legs. This will result in marked struggling and open-mouthed, loud squealing. Pigs are capable of squealing at volume levels up to 135 decibels, which is louder than the supersonic Concorde. Hearing protection should be considered for all rescuers.

Remember that a pig in a backyard is probably a pet, and it may best be handled by enticing it with food. Pig boards or similar equipment (e.g., emergency medical service backboard, folding chair) should be used to protect the rescuers' legs while driving a pig; this prevents hands and legs from getting bitten. Pig boards are commonly used in commercial swine facilities. Pigs do not readily step up or down, so any ramps used to load them should not be steep (Woods, 2006a).

The most effective method for catching pigs individually is to slide a rope, chain, or a catch pole cable into its mouth and around the top jaw (snare). The pig will immediately squeal and back up, allowing the animal handler to back it into a trailer, paddock, etc. However, if the pig has been snared once, it may not allow it to happen again. The snare should not be excessively tight; it is possible to actually tear the cartilage of the animal's nose. Putting a snare, collar, or loop around a pig's neck is not recommended. The anatomy of the pig's head and neck does not create a place for the snare (or loop or collar) to catch, and it will slide off over the animal's head.

Common Swine Response Scenarios. Most first responders will never enter commercial facilities with thousands of pigs unless required for depopulation purposes (due to eradication efforts associated with foreign animal disease situations). The most common scenarios involving pigs are pet pigs that get loose in the neighborhood or a livestock trailer that rolls over on the interstate (see Chapter 21). Animal control officers commonly respond to calls to catch a loose neighborhood pig. Pigs can make good pets in the proper situation. Like dogs, they are intelligent and can be trained to be aggressive and protect the property. Others may have them on a farm, possibly as a companion for another animal.

Camelids (e.g., llama, camel, alpaca)

Llamas are very curious, always interested in new things, and intelligent. These South American camelids can weigh from 250 to 400 lb (113.6–181.8 kg) and are formidable opponents if upset. Llamas can be very intimidating to novice handlers. They can be very aggressive; one veterinarian related that a great number of injuries to their employees were due to llama kicks or bites. Alternatively, stressed llamas become passive and may refuse to move, lying in a kushed (sternal recumbent) position (Nixon, 2006). Alpacas are very valuable for their fleece, slightly smaller than llamas, and less aggressive; but camelids can be flighty, and should be driven slowly as a herd—or, more easily—led with feed or alfalfa hay into containment. Camels are much larger than llamas or alpacas and wield the same formidable weapons with greater reach. Their bites and kicks commonly maim or kill handlers in countries where they are used as work animals or for entertainment. Only experienced animal handlers should be allowed to approach and handle camels.

Most camelids are minimally tolerant of being handled. Many are not affectionate and may resent human contact; it may hurt their sensitive skin to be brushed and handled. Pulling on their fleece can cause severe skin bruising. Due to their fleece, camelids are very sensitive to heat, especially when they have a heavy coat. In warm weather they should be removed from an overturned trailer as soon as possible and given shade to recover, or thoroughly hosed down, to prevent heat stroke. Many llamas, camels, and alpacas are accustomed to being haltered and led like horses, and can be led on surfaces (slick floors, tight spaces) that are impossible for cattle and horses to negotiate. Camelids will often lie down (kush) while being transported in a vehicle or when they are stressed. They may refuse to move. Unlike a blindfolded horse, a blindfolded llama or alpaca is not more easily led; the animal will usually refuse to move. To subdue a llama or alpaca, gently squeeze the ear. Also, if the camelid has been handled regularly, it will often stand still if a person puts an arm gently around the animal's neck (Woods, 2006b).

Llamas can kick with their hind legs and have serrated canine teeth; many owners cut their male llama's canine teeth to prevent severe injury to humans or other animals. When males fight with other male llamas, they try to bite the jugular vein in their opponent's neck and use their chests to wrestle each other. The rescuer must be aware the llama may use these techniques when trying to dominate people. A male llama might run straight at a person, lunging at them at the last second and trying to use their chest to knock their "opponent" out of their way. Camelids can cow kick at a 90 degree angle to the side, picking the foot up and swinging it parallel to the ground; the nails on the foot are sharp and can cause severe skin lacerations.

Berserk Male Syndrome. Berserk male syndrome is a behavior problem of variable severity and is infrequently documented in llamas. A true berserk male is improperly imprinted on people and becomes very territorial and aggressive at maturity. It will typically pace the fence line screaming and spitting at approaching people and animals, and are very dangerous if anyone enters its space. These animals will treat a person like another threatening male llama—by chest butting, knocking them down, biting and grabbing at their body, and trying to wrestle. The extreme form of this behavior problem is relatively rare and is usually only seen in males.

Berserk male syndrome llamas are often easily recognized; they are very aggressive, spitting and climbing the fence to get at the human target. The screaming sound they produce is called *orgling* and resembles a combination of a donkey's bray and an elk's bugle. If loose, these animals may have to be euthanatized by projectile weapons to protect human safety.

Birds (e.g., Turkey, Chicken, Ostrich, Emu)

Poultry. Turkeys and chickens are technically not large animals; however, they are handled like commercial large animals in large numbers in trailers. There is minimal information regarding the proper response to incidents involving these species. Poultry are raised in large commercial houses with 5,000–40,000 animals per house and are transported to slaughter processing facilities on large trucks in open wire cages, usually at night. An individual turkey can weigh from 9 to 35 lb (4–16 kg). Chickens weigh 3–5 pounds (1.4–2.3 kg) and can be challenging to catch, manipulate, and carry. Most cannot fly due to their heavy weight (bred for meat), but they can still move faster than a human.

Poultry have a tendency to flutter and make a lot of noise; this can increase the hysteria and reaction of the remaining poultry in the flock (Woods, 2006a). They may hide under objects or the overturned trailer. Poultry are extremely sensitive to heat and cold (like pigs) and can suffocate in their travel cages in overturned trucks. These species can die from stress and fear. When handled calmly, many flocks can be herded. Portable fencing is an excellent method of containing them. Individual poultry can be trapped in hand nets and returned to the flock.

Ostriches. Ostriches are normally classified as exotics and are not covered in detail within the scope of this book. An ostrich can run 70 kph (44 mph). They can be dangerous, especially males during breeding season. Their feet and legs are their primary defensive weapons. Rescuers should never stand in front of one of these birds. A quick forward thrust of their foot with its extended claw can disembowel a person, and the powerful blow of a kick can break arms and legs (Spruill, 2004). In addition, they may attack and knock down unfamiliar handlers. These birds can kick forward or backward, and the forces produced by these kicks approach that of a horse kick. Only professionals should attempt to handle these animals. Ostriches tend to panic easily but are very curious; a handler might be able to tempt them into an enclosure with grain or an object that piques the animal's curiosity (such as a bright object).

Crowding boards (e.g., plywood, backboard, or portable fencing panels), a shepherd's crook, and a hood can be used to handle these animals more safely. People who handle ostriches regularly have a shepherd's crook; they catch the animal around its neck and lead it using the crook. Professional handlers may throw a bola or lariat to trap the feet and legs of ostriches and emus—however, this requires practice and great skill.

Prolonged chases and exertion should be avoided. Capture myopathy and sudden death can occur due to hyperthermia in birds. Rescuers should avoid handling the wings to restrain or capture these animals; they are very delicate (Spruill, 2004). Portable fencing is an excellent solution to these scenarios; the animal can usually be driven into an enclosure or trailer using this equipment.

Emu. Easier to handle and more common are the ostrich's cousins, emus. These birds are good escapees and are smaller than ostriches, but they are no less intimidating. Many of these animals interact daily with people. Emus can learn to "swim;" they can walk along the bottom with their head held above the water surface like a periscope. These animals are very commonly kept as pets or alternative livestock. Some owners released their emus after the animals' livestock value crashed in the specialty egg and feather market in the 1990s.

Emus also can kick forward and backward like ostriches, but with less force. They have small spines on the back of the legs; zoo personnel recommend wearing coveralls for protection when handling these animals. If for some reason the bird must be individually handled, the rescuer should align their body perpendicular to the animal, with their hands encircling its neck and the rear end, and step sideways to encourage the animal to walk straight into the horse trailer or enclosure.

Catching emus is a challenge because they are very fast; however, they are not very intelligent. These animals are the exception to the rule that rescuers should avoid tying the legs of an animal for restraint. If it is necessary to tie the bird, its legs should be tied together as well as tied to the bird's body to reduce the risk of human injury. The bird's legs should be strapped together and underneath the bird, and the bird should be encircled with webbing, hay string, rope, or duct tape, but not tight enough to inhibit breathing.

The easiest way to handle emus, as well as commercial turkeys and chickens, is with portable containment equipment. Attempting to catch, restrain, and/or halter a bird can increase the animal's stress and the risk of human injury. Using portable fencing to drive the birds into a portable corral, then moving the corral with the birds enclosed, results in reduced stress for the birds and lower stress for the people involved.

One of the interesting and useful habits of ostriches and emus is their tendency to run along the face of obstacles such as fences. Under normal circumstances, they will usually wear a path along the fence line of their paddocks. This trait can be used to the rescuers' benefit. For example, in 2004 an emu was weaving back and forth at the fence along the interstate, so the Mississippi rescuers parked two rows of cars bumper-to-bumper to form a funnel, and parked a horse trailer at the mouth of the funnel. They then used a piece of portable fencing to drive the animal into the trailer (Figure 4.22). This method may also be successful for other animals; however, it is important to note that horses may attempt to jump the vehicles.

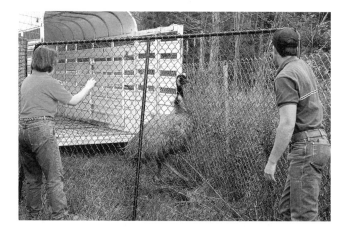

Figure 4.22 *Rescuers in Mississippi work to drive an emu into a horse trailer beside the interstate, using cars as a funnel to block escape on either side. Use of a portable gate section was an effective method of driving the animal safely. Photo courtesy Carla Huston.*

Subungulates (Elephants)

There are two species of elephants: African elephants and Asian elephants. African elephants (*Loxodonta africana*) are the larger of the two species and are most easily identified by their large ears (shaped like the continent of Africa), visible tusks on both sexes, and concave (swayed) backs. Asian elephants (*Elephas maximus*) have smaller ears, visible tusks limited to males, less wrinkled skin, one "finger" at the end of their trunk, and convex (dome-shaped) backs.

Elephants have a hearing range between 1 and 20,000 Hz. The very low frequency sounds they use for normal communication are in the "infrasound" range that is not audible to humans. Acoustic biologists have revealed that auditory communication at other frequencies reveals an entire language previously unknown to humans. Elephants have low-pitched communication that can be heard by other elephants for miles, and they are constantly communicating. One researcher played tapes of African elephants in the wild to elephants in a New Jersey zoo. Their immediate reaction was to huddle together, with their heads facing outward for protection, and listen intently to the sounds.

These animals can be extremely dangerous and should always be handled by a highly trained elephant handler. Elephants are intelligent and capable of solving problems such as walking up a ramp, and they have been observed to assist other elephants out of traps. However, elephants are the largest animals on land. The largest elephant on record was an adult male African elephant that weighed 10,886 kg (24,000 lb) and stood 3.96 m (13 ft) tall. African elephants grow larger than Asian elephants and may commonly reach 5,000 kg (11,000 lb) and 3 m (10 feet) tall at the shoulder.

Incidents involving elephants have been reported and include: elephants that get loose and rampage through a crowd of people, then the local community; injured elephants that cannot get up and need support; and elephants trapped in trailer wrecks, ravines, or holes. Unfortunately, responding officers called to perform field euthanasia of rampaging animals can expend many bullets on the animal before killing it.

Elephants may be loose when circus train cars or trailers overturn. Unfortunately, incidents involving elephants often conclude with the death of the animal; this is often necessary to prevent further human injury or death. In a 1992 incident in Palm Bay, Florida, an elephant rampaged through the circus grounds, sending six people to the hospital. Unable to get it under control, officers shot at it for 15 minutes until a man arrived with bullets large enough to finish the job. Numerous lawsuits resulted from this incident, including those filed by spectators and police involved in the shooting. Similarly, in 1998 a circus elephant in Kathmandu, Nepal, trampled her handler and ran loose in the downtown area, injuring bystanders in the confusion. Police chased the elephant to a secluded area and shot it 40 times, finally killing the animal.

In 1997 in Albuquerque, New Mexico, police investigating an apparently abandoned trailer in a hotel parking lot found nearly a dozen exotic animals, including eight llamas and three elephants. One elephant was dead, and investigators reported that the temperature inside the trailer exceeded 49°C (120°F) due to poor ventilation. Policemen were challenged with providing ventilation to the animals while waiting for an animal handler and investigators to arrive, which they did with portable fans. In 1998, a performing elephant was injured and found prostrate at an English circus wintering depot, probably after fighting with other elephants in the enclosure. Local firemen attempted to raise and support the animal using a sling, air bag, winch, and tackle. Her condition deteriorated and she died within 24 hours.

As another example, in July 2005 a bull elephant fell into a pit latrine in Embori, Africa, and had exhausted itself trying to escape. Local farmers intended to kill the animal for its meat, but the World Society for the Protection of Animals (WSPA) flew elephant experts in with webbing and ropes to sedate the animal and attempt to rescue it. Webbing was placed in a forward assist configuration (see Chapter 15) and attached to a tractor, which slowly pulled it free (Figure 4.23). Once freed, the animal returned to the forest.

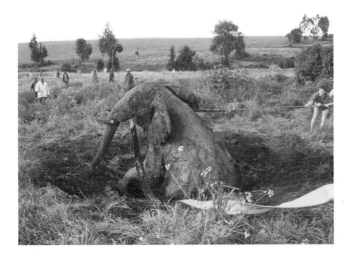

Figure 4.23 *This wild elephant fell into an outdoor open latrine in Embori, Africa. Responders flew and drove to the site to assist with webbing and vehicles. An animal this large and dangerous requires significant planning and attention to safety for responders. Courtesy of MountKenyaTrust.org.*

Large Carnivore Zoologics

Large cat species, wild dog species, and bear species are classified as carnivores. Techniques for recapture or handling of large carnivores are beyond the scope of this book. While it is possible that the manipulation techniques covered in this book may be applied to a 250 kg (550 lb) lion, rescuers should never attempt to assist any exotic large cat without assistance of a zoo veterinarian and specially trained zoo personnel. In addition, a sniper with appropriate ammunition should be on the scene to perform euthanasia of the animal if it attacks a human.

Large cats, wolves, and bears are so dangerous to humans (especially under the stress and disorientation of escape) that humane destruction of the animal may be the appropriate course of action (Wolfe, 2004). A lion commonly has 200–300 kg (440–660 lb) of weight behind its power and prowess; a large bear may weigh well over 500 kg (1,100 lb). To demonstrate how dangerous these animals can be, normal protocols within zoos mandate the availability of trained marksmen and firearms during certain procedures involving large carnivorous animals. These animals are predators; they capture and kill other animals larger than humans for food, wield offensive and defensive weapons, and are many times stronger than a human. Most are solitary ambush predators or stalk their prey. Rescue calls may involve large wild cats kept as pets, but these animals are extremely unpredictable and aggressive, particularly in stressful scenarios. The critical distance at which they will attack is very different from prey animals (Moxley, 2004).

While waiting for professional zoological help, baited traps for live capture may be employed in an attempt to recapture an exotic animal. If the incident is a trailer overturn or vehicle accident, responders should attempt to maintain the integrity of the vehicle until appropriate veterinary support and chemical capture drugs can be brought to the scene. An example of an appropriate field expedient trap is a square Dumpster baited with food with its doors and lids secured. When dealing with a large carnivore in a disaster situation, a skilled marksman should be present and prepared to shoot the animal with darts loaded with chemical capture drugs. Another marksman should be prepared to shoot to kill the carnivore if human life is threatened. Injured carnivores are extremely dangerous and prone to attack (Randles, 2004; Moxley, 2004).

In 1995 in Idaho, 15 large cats (tigers, lions, and ligers) escaped from a private game farm fenced with chicken wire. Over 50 sheriff's deputies, SWAT teams, fish and game officers, and Idaho State Police troopers hunted the escaped animals. A helicopter with a heat-sensing device was used to help search for the escaped cats. The local town was closed while all of the animals were found and shot.

Large animal escape prevention planning and response using a trained response team are features of most modern zoos. Most modern zoos feature semiannual drills and even include mock escapees in animal suits to test their response systems.

ACRONYMS USED IN CHAPTER 4

HazMat   Hazardous Materials

5 Technical Large Animal Emergency Rescue Scene Management

Dr. Rebecca Gimenez

INTRODUCTION

There is a tendency for animal incidents to become spectator events, and large numbers of untrained people may become directly involved with the rescue effort. Members of the media often focus on the "heroic rescue," but do not convey the resulting iatrogenic injuries of the animal. It is not just an animal emergency; it is also a human emergency and a human public safety incident.

Those working in technical large animal emergency rescue (TLAER) incidents must have excellent communication skills to deal with people and with other agencies; they must be able to use the incident command system (ICS) to promote effective relationships and be able to work together as a team to make sure rescuers, bystanders, and operational personnel are as safe as possible. Once human safety issues have been addressed, the safety and concerns for the animal victim can be addressed. When responding to a TLAER incident, the initial assessment may only hint at what else may become involved in the scenario (Figure 5.1).

Professional protocols for scene safety and security, approach to the rescue effort, use of the ICS, and victim care should be established for TLAER scenes. A coordinated response to a large animal emergency relies on standards of care for animals that are based on realistic situations, sensible equipment and practical training, and that consider the well-being of the animal.

INCIDENT COMMAND SYSTEM OVERVIEW

Definition of the Incident Command System

As the model tool for command, control, and coordination of a response of any size, the ICS provides a means for agencies to work toward a common goal of protecting life, property, and environment. The ICS uses business principles of management, efficiency, and effectiveness applied to emergency response (FEMA, 1998). Today it is an all-risk system that is appropriate for all fire and non-fire emergencies, including TLAER, as a method of applying leadership and organization to any emergency incident.

Brief History of the ICS

The ICS was first enacted in California in the 1970s, when the Department of Forestry recognized the need for a command management system using standardized terminology and communications, consolidated action plans, and business management principles. The ICS was established based on military principles of hierarchical command and delegation of duties to qualified individuals. The ICS divides the response effort into separate areas of responsibility, establishes an individual in charge of the response effort, determines the roles of personnel, and allows individuals to supervise three to five subordinates.

The system is flexible and can be expanded or reduced in response to the number of agencies and responders involved. For safety reasons, there should always be a minimum of two people present on any scene; the ICS will clarify which of these two is in command. Alternatively, the ICS can be expanded to incorporate many thousands of professionals and volunteers with tens or hundreds of organizations and agencies involved, as in the response to the September 11, 2001, World Trade Center terrorist attacks.

The Standardized Emergency Management System includes animal services. Veterinarians have two main directives during a disaster response: to transport and care for animals displaced by a disaster event and to return them to their rightful owner as soon as practical. The California Veterinary Medical Association (CVMA) was able to accomplish these goals during

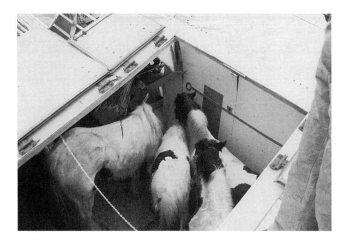

Figure 5.1 *The initial assessment of this overturned trailer full of horses will require the input of the veterinarian and the technical rescue personnel to develop an effective IAP. It is not possible to prepare for every configuration or eventuality, but an understanding of the basic considerations will allow professionals to appropriately react and adapt. The quarantine chain across the door indicates an additional challenge to the triage and transport of live animals from this scene. Courtesy of Gary McFarland.*

several California disasters by coordinating with other agencies. Other goals important to consider might include the following: animal medical care, animal shelter setup and management (logistics), recovery, protecting the public from loose animals, public and environmental health, search and rescue support, disease control, owner accessibility to animals, housing and care for animals of owners displaced for extended periods, public relations, epidemiologic surveys and consultations for zoonotic disease outbreak potential, carcass disposal, and notifying the owners of deceased animals (Nixon, 2006).

Definition of Emergency Scene

An emergency scene can be defined as a location designated by the potential need for emergency medical care or extrication methods. This location is quickly identified by emergency vehicles with flashing lights, rescue equipment, and emergency personnel. These scenes represent special hazards.

An emergency scene is under the authority of the first arriving emergency personnel, which includes emergency medical services (EMS) personnel, until the arrival of the fire or law enforcement official with authority having jurisdiction. In most jurisdictions any ambulance, police, fire, rescue, recovery, or towing vehicle authorized by the state, county, or municipality to respond to an incident is referred to as an *authorized emergency vehicle*. *Emergency services personnel* refers to fire/rescue, police/law enforcement, or EMS personnel responding to an emergency incident.

SPEAKING THE EMERGENCY LANGUAGE

An understanding of and certification in the ICS at the basic level is crucial for anyone working in the emergency management and disaster arenas. The Federal Emergency Management Agency (FEMA) Emergency Management Institute Web site for online courses includes Incident Command (basic 100 level) as well as three animal disaster courses that provide one-hour blocks of instruction for continuing education credit (Animals in Disasters, Animal Community in Disasters, and Large Animals in Disasters, all led by Dr. Sebastian Heath). These courses are prerequisites for participation on many animal rescue teams, along with other training events; it is important for people to understand the overall picture in disasters and in animal incidents.

Responders should strive to use the ICS to ensure that the scene is as safe as possible for the rescuers; once that has been accomplished, they can focus on making it safe for the animal victim. The ICS emphasizes the safest and most efficient means of dealing with any emergency by using a team approach, planning for efficient use of resources, and stressing risk assessment and safety. After performing the scene and risk assessments, the operational personnel develop an incident action plan (IAP), perform the rescue, and perform a post-rescue review (debriefing). The lessons learned on an incident can be applied to subsequent rescue scenarios.

On human incident scenes, emergency responders are familiar with each other and know each other's capabilities, weaknesses, and strengths. They all speak the same "language" in an emergency, and everyone on scene uses common terminology; this allows volunteers, agencies, and professionals to work together across boundaries and communicate effectively with all emergency response groups. Standardized training for emergency personnel establishes universal skill sets that facilitate cooperation.

In large animal incidents, there will often be responders (veterinarian, volunteer animal experts, wildlife officers, animal control officers, humane officers) participating who may be unfamiliar with ICS structure or behavior on scene; these individuals and groups can present special challenges and liabilities. The benefit of establishing relationships cannot be overstated (Figure 5.2). The ability of individuals and team members to establish effective relationships with other agencies and external organizations is critical to success. This will often include animal control, fire department, and state police personnel; it may also include wildlife/natural resources officials, the state veterinarian's office, harbor police, and emergency operations center (EOC) personnel. Knowledge of the resources and personnel assets available from other agencies is important, as is earning their trust by demonstrating that the volunteer or stranger is capable of

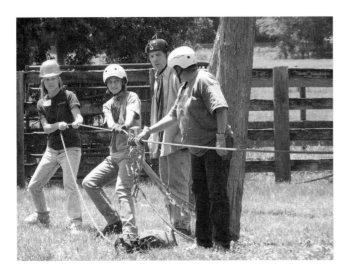

Figure 5.2 *The incident command system is a process that is best learned from hands-on experience, not just by reading a book or learning in a class. Teamwork is required to assemble a large animal emergency and disaster rescue team. Leaders should plan on realistic, hands-on training events to improve the skills of team members. Courtesy of Tori Miller.*

performing his or her assigned duties in a safe, professional, and efficient manner.

THE INCIDENT COMMAND SYSTEM IN TLAER

Large animal rescue can be exciting for the personnel involved. TLAER incident response uses concepts similar to those used in human rescue techniques, but differs in that normal team structure and function may be overridden by the human emotional response to the animal's situation. Scene protocols should not change for a large animal incident. Scene security, safety, and risk assessment will not change and may be of greater importance than in other scenarios because of the large number of bystanders that typically appear at animal rescues and the higher risk of human injury associated with these scenes. The safety of the rescuers, human victims, and bystanders should be the primary concern from the first moment the perimeter is set. A secure perimeter is paramount around the incident to protect bystanders as well as responders, the animal(s), and the scene. At incidents observed by the author, a large number of untrained bystanders will express a desire to assist the animal, despite a lack of understanding of the risks involved. However, the ICS and normal scene protocols should be employed and the team approach to disaster assistance for animals should be emphasized, focusing on the basic methods of removal of large animals from various scenarios. The simplest and lowest-risk alternatives should be used to allow safe rescues, especially in a resource-poor disaster environment.

The incident commander (IC) and safety officer (SO) should not permit anyone to enter a trailer that contains a large animal until the animal has been sedated or anesthetized, or the advice of a veterinarian has been provided, even if the cow or horse appears to be standing in the trailer. According to Jennifer Woods (2006b), "It is suicidal to get into a confined space like that with 500 kg of scared and possibly injured animal." Incidents involving large animal transport constitute confined-space rescue with obstacles. Human injuries have occurred under routine livestock loading and unloading. A veterinarian related his story of a response to a trailer overturn on an interstate highway, with six horses in the trailer and divider gates between each animal. To tranquilize each horse during the extrication process, the veterinarian crawled over each of the downed horses to get access to the next horse. Reflecting on the incident, the veterinarian admitted that the procedure was dangerous and inappropriate. If the horses had struggled violently, the veterinarian could have been crushed or kicked. In a similar situation, a mounted police officer in Louisiana crawled into an overturned two-horse trailer with the divider still in place and literally crawled over one horse, purportedly to give an injection of sedative in the animal's jugular vein. Subsequent evaluations of the rescue effort revealed that the horse's tail vein was accessible from outside the trailer, and tranquilization could have been easily accomplished without compromising the officer's safety.

The instinct of prey animals is to get up, regardless of injury. They may scramble or struggle violently, especially when stimulated by loud noises, a touch, or the movement of other animals or humans in the trailer. If the veterinarian cannot access the jugular vein, other veins (e.g., tail vein, cephalic vein, transverse facial vein, etc.) may be accessible from outside the trailer. Intramuscular injection may be the most practical approach if venous access is not possible. All options should be considered, with safety as the main objective, before a decision is made.

Professionalism on the Scene

Using the ICS sets the tone of the incident, demonstrates professionalism, and aligns with the National Incident Management System. The ICS clearly defines to whom each team member should report and for what purpose or duty. Making recommendations or providing suggestions does not place a volunteer or veterinarian in charge; this duty should be restricted to the IC. All personnel involved must accept the leader's authority, follow his or her directions, and support the decisions. Knowledge of the ICS allows everyone to work across boundaries and among all emergency response and volunteer groups at the local, regional, and national level.

A single person should never attempt to rescue a large animal without assistance. Two is the minimum number of personnel allowed to respond to an incident; one will assume the roles of IC and SO, and the other individual will assume the roles of operations and animal handler. The person performing the role of animal handler may become too focused on the rescue efforts to recognize danger; the IC/SO is responsible for monitoring the situation and preserving the handler's safety. As when suppressing a fire, the buddy system (two in and two out) exists to ensure the safety of rescue personnel. Everyone on scene must constantly work to reduce the danger, risk, and confusion, thus maximizing safety for personnel and for the animal victim.

There are very few emergencies where the responders cannot make an IAP immediately before implementing the rescue effort. Unless the animal victim is drowning or becoming a medical casualty (e.g., hyper- or hypothermic, showing clinical signs of shock, etc.), there is sufficient time for proper planning. There is rarely a reason to hurry, and it is wise to take the time necessary to plan and organize a good rescue effort. If the animal's life is in immediate danger (e.g., the animal is being swept downstream, drowning in mud or in a pool, etc.), the responders should consider options to lessen the risk by draining the pool, restraining the animal with its head supported out of the mud, etc. Otherwise, the risk assessment may need to include euthanasia as an option for resolution of the situation (see Chapter 13).

Teamwork is critical for the safety of all team members. Each member should understand his or her role in the response effort. With one experienced person in charge as the IC, a team approach provides the best chance of achieving a safe, organized, and efficient rescue effort. Proper planning, organization, training, and practice are necessary for specialty rescue scenarios such as TLAER.

Team Identification. Trained TLAER response teams and volunteers should create a hat, uniform, or T-shirt with an appropriate logo. Each team member's credentials (training, identification, etc.) should be properly documented, and individuals should have a laminated version of the credentials with them on the scene. A uniform allows other responders to easily recognize members of that group and presents a professional appearance.

Communication

People are the true communicators, not the radios and various gadgets used on the scene by human responders. Radios are not the prime communicators, they are a tool. Good communication skills allow coordination on scene and make the rescue faster, safer, and more efficient. It is easy to become focused on the rescue itself and lose sight of the importance of communication on scene. All responders need to know what is happening, when it is going to happen, and what their individual roles are in the rescue effort (see Chapter 22).

Poor communication is the primary complaint reported in post-rescue debriefings. Make sure the animal handler is well informed of the rescue plan and the handler's role. The handler should also be warned when other rescuers anticipate an event (e.g., loud sound, sudden light, etc.) to prepare for the animal's response to the stimulus.

Working with Nongovernmental Organizations

Over the last 20 years, there has been a move to actively include nongovernmental organizations, such as humane groups, in disaster planning for animals. In particular, the Humane Society of the United States has served as a model planner at the local, state, and national levels, promoting training and organization of disaster animal response teams as well as coordinating the national credentialing and resource typing of animal response teams with FEMA.

COMMON TLAER CONCERNS FROM THE ICS PERSPECTIVE

The Long-Term Response Factor Is Common

A common theme in large animal emergency rescue is a long-term response factor, indicating that the animal has often been in its predicament for an hour or more prior to its discovery by the owner or caretaker. Several more hours may elapse while the owner and friends attempt the rescue before calling a veterinarian or emergency personnel. By the time appropriately equipped personnel arrive on the scene, the animal may be exhausted or further injured by its struggles or the unsuccessful rescue attempt.

Escape Planning

Responders should remember that prey animals may respond as if the rescuers are predators. The best IAP will have a plan A (the rescue plan) and a plan B (an emergency escape route). The escape plan should include the assignment of safety buddies, identification of a clear escape route for the responders, and methods of dispersing groups of people.

Knowledge of Large Animal Behavior. Responders may become lulled into a false sense of security on the scene and be seriously injured if they erroneously assume that the animal cannot move. Trapped animals will often begin to struggle violently as soon as someone opens a door or window on the overturned trailer, touches the entrapped animal, or makes a sudden loud noise that stimulates the animal.

Operational personnel and animal handlers need to have a clear path for escape.

Emergency responders should consider a silent approach to the scene as ideal; if that is not possible, the sirens should be turned off, but the lights should be left on. Similarly, if the decision is made to cut metal (e.g., the roof of the trailer, etc.), responders should understand that many of the common rescue tools (e.g., air chisels) are very loud. The tool should be started away from the confined space, and the animal's reactions to that sound should be evaluated. With the tool still on, the responder should slowly approach the animal to allow it to become accustomed to the sound of the tool. If the animal continues to struggle excessively or panic in response to the tool, the tool should be withdrawn and should not be used. For example, during the response to an overturned horse trailer in Colorado, the responding fire department tried to use cutting tools to remove six horses. Three horses were fatally injured during their panicked attempts to escape the trailer and the sounds.

Patient Assessment

A thorough patient assessment should be performed (see Chapter 17). If a veterinarian is not available, EMS personnel on the scene should be able to perform a basic assessment. A veterinarian can also provide assistance over the phone to the EMS personnel on the scene. Local and state laws should be consulted when responders are unsure of the legal aspects of the rescue effort. Laws and regulations vary by state: In some states the EMS personnel could face penalties or charges for practicing veterinary medicine without a license. Temperature, pulse rate, respiratory rate, and other parameters have species-specific normal values of which EMS personnel may be unaware. If available, a credentialed veterinary technician can perform an assessment and communicate with the veterinarian. With appropriate and timely treatment, large animals can recover from what may initially look like severe injuries. Responders should be aware that blood on an animal involved in trauma could be that of a co-traumatized human, thus gloves are mandatory for protection from infectious diseases (e.g., human immunodeficiency virus, hepatitis, etc.).

Triage. In a field environment, especially following a disaster, those animals that have a minimal chance of survival should be triaged as "expectant," and humane euthanasia should be performed or a natural death allowed. Materials and human resources should be conserved for victims that are more likely to survive.

Prioritize the Rescue Method

The best TLAER rescue efforts prioritize the methods to be used. The responders should attempt to make the rescue as low-risk, low-tech, and most efficient as possible. Although there are situations where advanced equipment and specialty methods may be necessary, those incidents usually require more time and planning and represent increased risk to the health and safety of the rescuers and animal victim. If a piece of webbing can be used to effect a successful rescue, a helicopter is unnecessary. Increasing the complexity of the equipment or plan often increases the chance of error and injury.

Responders should implement the simplest course of action (COA) first. COA plans are assigned the letters A, B, and C, which are associated with increasing levels of technical expertise. If A COA is unsuccessful, then COA B should be attempted. COA C is enacted if A and B are unsuccessful. Fully trained team members should supervise the less-qualified members. The fire service uses a system of Awareness, Operational, and Technical levels of training in each specialty and does not attempt a Technical level rescue with personnel who are only trained to the Awareness level.

Responders should always select the technique that is associated with the least amount of danger for the animal victim(s) and the rescuer(s). Usually, the lower-technology methods are faster and/or more efficient. The speed of rescue success improves with knowledge and practice. Time invested in planning and coordination, followed by a successful rescue, is far more positive than a poorly conceived plan that requires hours to extricate the victim.

Leadership

In some TLAER incidents, the personnel on the scene may be limited to the veterinarian, a few bystanders, and the owner. A basic knowledge of ICS leadership and operational planning ideals will assist with the organization of any rescue effort. Working as a team on a large animal rescue scene is no different from working as a team to combat a structure fire. A review of videotaped large animal responses has revealed a consistent theme: Once the human victims are removed from the TLAER scene, safety protocols and the ICS are often discarded. Freelancing is extremely dangerous in any rescue scenario, and responders should take the time to call and wait for assistance.

The lack of ICS infrastructure on the scene will substantially delay the effort, regardless of the rescue type. Identification of tasks, assignment of individuals, and teamwork will suffer unless they are properly managed. In certain large emergency and disaster scenarios, the planner will need to develop maps and perform reconnaissance, especially in search and rescue operations. The IC is the focal point for contact with other agencies that may respond as well as local authorities.

Teamwork is important, and the best teams have clearly identified leaders. Subordinate members of the team follow instructions without objection or hesitation. In return, the team leader (IC) must understand the ICS, maintain control of the situation, enforce consequences for insubordination and maintain the teamwork concept, and delegate tasks to other personnel on scene. In addition, the IC must be able to communicate with all team members; potential solutions may originate from any team member who is aware that their input is valued by the IC. Knowing how to "plug in" to the ICS system is crucial, which is why potential volunteer responders should learn the ICS and leadership through hands-on, as well as classroom, training.

Prevent Conflict between Emergency Responders and Owners/Bystanders

Due to the strength of the human–animal bond, TLAER incidents tend to get out of control due to bystander and owner involvement. As an example of many aspects of the worst-case scenario, a person in Sanford, Florida, went outside to investigate a noise in the backyard and found a 20 m wide (66 ft) sinkhole, with one barn and two horses at the bottom. The owner called friends and 911, and then moved the remaining horses to a nearby pasture. The two animal victims were trapped in the approximately 10 m deep (33 ft) sink hole, which was slowly filling with water. One horse was lying down, and the other standing almost on top of it, amid an amalgamation of barn materials, trees, and other debris. By the time the police and firefighters arrived, there were over 100 people standing around the sink hole (Figure 5.3).

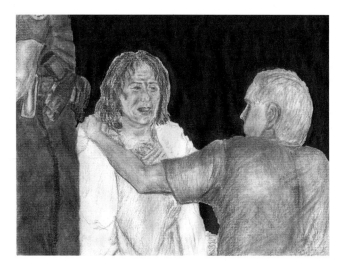

Figure 5.3 *In Sanford, Florida, a sinkhole collapsed and swallowed a barn and two horses. Although the emergency responders attempted to save the animals, the rescue effort was unsuccessful. This owner's face illustrates the horror and pain suffered by people who are very attached to their animals; to this owner, the situation is not just an animal incident, but a human incident. Responders on scene may have residual emotional reactions to incidents involving animals and children, especially those that are unsuccessful or involve trauma to the victim. Addressing the mental health needs of the owner and responders is of vital importance. Courtesy of Julie Casil.*

The immediate response of law enforcement and responders was to force the people at least 75 m (250 ft) away from potentially unstable edges of the sink hole to minimize the risk of further ground collapse. Although this decision was made with human safety in mind, the bystanders erroneously assumed that the responders were uninterested in rescuing the horses.

The potential conflict with the bystanders was resolved by communication; one person in the crowd was a retired police officer who also has horses, and he became the liaison between the crowd and the responders. A crane was readied in case the horses had to be lifted. During the planning and initial rescue efforts, the bottom-most horse drowned in the rising water. In an attempt to save the surviving horse, a lark's foot configuration of the forward assist was used. Although the lark's foot configuration and forward assist were appropriate, the webbing was attached to a very large winch. The rescuers were unaware that the horse was trapped in mud; the traction applied was unable to overcome the suction of the mud, and the horse died from severe thoracic trauma.

This scenario exemplifies many of the risks associated with TLAER efforts. First, most TLAER incidents attract a large number of bystanders that may create challenges and increase the risks of injury or death. Untrained human bystanders placed themselves at risk of injury or death due to their overwhelming desire to rescue the animals and hampered the rescue attempts by distracting the emergency personnel. Because the primary mission of the emergency personnel is to ensure human safety, additional effort was necessary to control the large crowd of bystanders. In addition, the diversion of attention and manpower to ensure human safety decreased the number of responders able to assist the animals. Inefficient planning and execution of the response plan contributed to the drowning death of one horse. Lack of knowledge of the scene (e.g., the strong anchoring forces applied by the mud) contributed to the death of the remaining animal. Constraints of the situation included the presence of an animal, darkness, the instability of the ground surrounding the sink hole, and the presence of a large crowd. Fortunately, no human injuries occurred during the rescue effort. The responders made a heroic effort that failed in the end. Since this incident, the county has formed a large animal rescue team consisting of policemen, firefighters, and experienced horse handlers. Despite the unfortunate outcome, many lessons were learned that will benefit other animals in TLAER situations.

HOW ICS WORKS ON TLAER INCIDENTS

Following the ICS approach on a TLAER scene allows volunteers and specially trained responders to understand where they plug in to the system. The IC works with several different groups.

First Responders

Police, fire, and EMS personnel—paramedics and emergency medical technicians (EMTs)—will be first responders on the scene if it occurs in a public area (e.g., on the road, at a public event, etc.). The 911 dispatch system allows rapid notification of the responders and ensures minimal dispatch time for them to respond (see Chapter 22). During the process of setting up the incident command, they will often inquire what resources are locally available (e.g., portable cattle fencing panels, trailers for animal transport, etc.). Providing the dispatch office and fire department with booklets containing phone numbers and contact information for sources of commonly needed equipment or facilities may expedite the arrival of the necessary equipment and trained personnel. This information should be previously gathered and organized and updated as necessary.

Media

Animal incidents are remarkable in their ability to attract bystanders and the media. When media photographers hear "animal rescue" over their police scanners, they mobilize quickly to the scene (Figure 5.4). Assume there will be media present at a TLAER incident. Due to the time involved in planning the response to an incident involving an animal, there is often ample time for the media to arrive.

Communication is key in determining if the media will be a help or hindrance to the rescue effort. Trained personnel can adequately communicate with the media to promote the role of ICS, emphasize the impor-

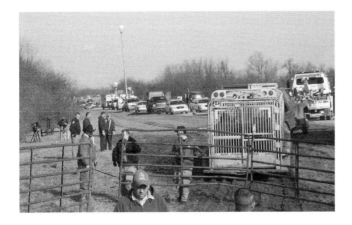

Figure 5.4 *The scene at an overturned cattle trailer on I-75 in Kentucky demonstrates the expected chaos of large animal rescue scenes on a major highway. Members of the media, bystanders, heavily congested traffic, and the transportation of a large number of animals from the scene present challenges that may hinder the rescue effort. The responders used cattle panels for containment of the animals before access was cut in the roof of the trailer to allow the live animals to escape the trailer. A rescue trailer is in place to transport animals from the scene. (Note: The overturned trailer is not visible in this photo.) Courtesy of Nathan Slovis.*

tance of proper training, and serve to educate the public about correct methods of animal rescue. However, poor or no communication with the media is more likely to result in the portrayal of the rescue as entertainment or an exaggerated dramatic event to evoke emotional responses in the viewers. Some veterinary organizations and disaster-related conferences are now offering training classes in proper communication with the media.

The media can be a hindrance to the rescue event if the coverage is associated with excessive noise or activity. For example, media helicopters create noise and wind turbulence that can induce panic in prey species. In addition, the noise generated by the helicopters can interfere with interpersonal communication on the scene; this can endanger the responders and the animal victim(s).

Public Information Officer

The pubic information officer (PIO) coordinates all media inquiries and the release of official information through the public affairs officer (PAO) at the EOC. Animal incidents present an excellent opportunity for the PIO to educate the public about the efforts to protect both life and property. Working with the media can be challenging, but by excluding them the PAO and PIO may lose control of the situation and the flow of information. On the other hand, media access to the developing scene should be controlled to ensure the safety of all involved. Media representatives may not be aware of the effects of their presence on the scene; for example, a flashbulb can induce a panic response in a trapped animal, and the animal's reaction could place the responder and the animal at risk of injury.

Media Treatment of Large Animal Rescue Incidents. The PIO should use the media to the responders' advantage in these scenarios by allowing them to take photographs and gather information about the rescue effort; these reports can be great public relations opportunities for the department, jurisdiction, or team.

An illustration of this concept occurred at a TLAER training in Massachusetts in 2005. A student that was supposed to pull the pins from a vertical lift was unable to pull hard enough to release both ends simultaneously; the front end of the sling released, but the back end remained secured to the hoist device. The demonstration animal was hanging by the rear sling for several seconds and was bucking until the other pin was pulled and the rear sling attachment was released. When released completely, the uninjured horse started grazing and appeared unconcerned by the events. Two photographers were present and obtained good-quality photographs of the entire day of training; however, despite many photographs depicting proper and efficient techniques performed that day, the photograph

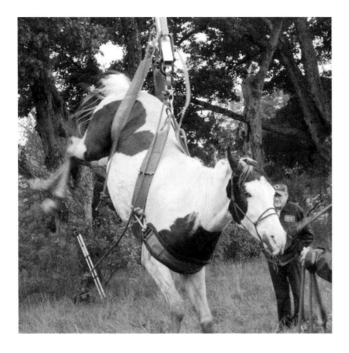

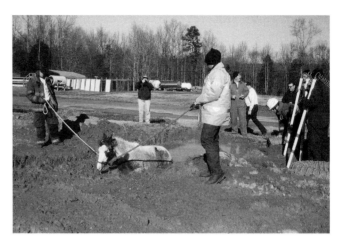

Figure 5.6   This photo shows first responders arriving on the scene and performing a preliminary scene assessment. The animal handler has attached a halter and lead ropes to the animal in the mud. Taking a few minutes to adequately plan the rescue is critical to success. Courtesy Mary Gabriel.

Figure 5.5   In this training scenario, a student failed to open the snap shackles at set down, and the unsedated demonstration horse fought the pressure on its abdomen by bucking. The PIO educated the press present about the purpose of live animal training and received excellent coverage the next day. Courtesy Claudia Sarti.

of the horse bucking in the sling was displayed on the front page of the local paper on the following day (Figure 5.5). Fortunately, the reporters had been educated during the session, and the article reflected that hands-on training and live demonstration animals are important, even when things go wrong.

Incident Commander

The person in charge at the incident is the IC, who must direct the response while maintaining the first priority: the safety of emergency responders and the public. The IC should be fully qualified to manage the response, including organizing and controlling personnel and equipment resources, maintaining accountability, developing an IAP, and coordinating activities. The IC function is assigned by rank and seniority of the first responders on the scene. It also allows transfer of the command function as other responders arrive, based on the primary authority for overall control of the incident. Furthermore, it assigns all the positions working for the IC, based on the size of the incident and number of personnel available.

Safety Officer (Operations and Public Safety)

The SO monitors and ensures the safety of all response personnel and bystanders on the scene and reports directly to the IC. Despite attention to safety protocols, responders and bystanders are injured every year. Military and civilian emergency response and rescue orga-

nizations spend millions of dollars each year to prevent or limit injuries and deaths in training and live incidents. The chaos often associated with animal incidents can compromise the safety of the rescuers and the animal victim if it interferes with good judgment and common sense. Tunnel vision and the desire to provide compassionate assistance to animals have occasionally led responders into unsafe conditions without a backup plan. Take the time to think, plan, and ensure the safety of the responders and the animal patient (J. Baker, 2005a).

In addition to the presence of the struggling or fearful animal, responders must determine if the dangerous conditions that entrapped or injured the animal are still present. Conditions such as floodwater, mud holes, sink holes, and ice may be obvious (Figure 5.6). Other situations such as electrical wires, wire fencing, chemical or biological hazardous materials (HazMat) dangers (including those used for weapons), and explosive or flammable material may be present but not readily visible. Scene assessment should include an evaluation of the animal's likely reaction to humans and how the animal's reaction may affect the situation. The scene should be evaluated to determine if there is a risk that the animal could leap forward and fall off a ledge, fall into water, fracture a limb, or sustain other severe injuries while struggling violently near wire or fencing materials. Do handlers and operational personnel have escape routes if the animal starts to struggle or falls? Is there room to let the animal move?

Human malevolence may also pose significant and unpredicted risks for responders. In war zones as well as domestic incidents, terrorists and other criminals have used injured animals to lure well-meaning responders and then detonate explosive devices or ambush the responders with gunfire when they are in range (J. Baker, 2006).

Security. Scene security is important in order to prevent equipment theft, injury to responders while focusing on the rescue effort, or possible loss of control by the owner. All motor vehicles and pedestrians must obey and not interfere with the duties of emergency personnel, and they must not block access to or exit from the emergency scene. As the IC's eyes and ears for safety and security, the SO ensures that scene security is organized, well-intentioned people are restricted from access to the animal victim(s), and bystanders do not hinder the rescue effort and are shielded from observing procedures such as euthanasia. The SO may assign an owner assistance officer to provide mental health support to the owner and/or bystanders. These scenes can be emotionally charged, increasing the level of danger for the animal and the responders.

Assess the Situation. In an emergency incident, there is often excitement, anxiety, chaos, and confusion. Rushing into a rescue attempt without proper planning can place the rescuer at risk; an animal victim is already involved, and the rescuers' goals should include preventing additional victims. Anyone responding to help an injured or entrapped animal should stop and assess the situation carefully before approaching the large animal. Taking the time to develop a plan can significantly reduce effort and injury on the part of the animal victim and the responders.

Disregard of scene assessment and safety could lead to injury or death of the intended rescuers. For this reason, other than neighborhood and on-the-farm emergencies, volunteer responders untrained in technical rescue methods and ICS should not be allowed to assist on the scene. Responders should maintain perspective on the incident: neighbors helping neighbors in the height of an acute crisis is admirable but can be dangerous.

Responders should maintain a healthy suspicion about the motivations of people affected by these incidents. During the floods associated with Hurricane Floyd (1999), an owner worried about his horses and dogs told emergency management there was a person left at home. When responders took him to check the facility, they realized he had deceived them in order to evacuate his animals. Although his concern for the animals was admirable, the use of valuable resources in the immediate time after a disaster should be reserved for human victims; the owner and his animals would have been better served by evacuation prior to the hurricane. It has been said that disasters and emergencies can bring out the best and the worst in people; people have stolen drugs or equipment from a fire apparatus or ambulance while responder's attention is diverted to performing rescues.

An incident featured in a newspaper involved a house fire where the human family members evacuated safely, then told the firefighters "Bob's still in the house!" The firefighters entered the dwelling to rescue Bob, and realized that Bob was a pet pig. The rescue effort was successful in that there were no injuries to personnel or the animal; however, the firefighters' lives were placed at great risk due to a human emotional response. People love their animals, often consider them members of the family, and may place their lives—or those of the responders—in jeopardy in order to save the animal's life.

Immediately Dangerous to Life and Health. Large animals can pose an immediate threat to life and body and can cause irreversible adverse health effects classified by the fire service as immediately dangerous to health and life. In particular, large animals can interfere with a rescuer's ability to escape unaided from the rescue environment. Large animals are prey animals with extremely fast reaction times; they react instinctively, and humans often cannot get out of the way quickly enough to escape injury. They are heavy, large, and naturally armed with powerful weapons (e.g., horns, hooves, teeth, powerful necks, etc.). Responders in large animal incidents must learn to predict what the animal might do in a worst-case scenario, and the SO must have a feel for these concerns (Figure 5.7).

The noise, yelling, lights, sirens, and other chaotic circumstances surrounding animal emergencies can heighten the panic responses of the animal victim. Animal owners and enthusiasts must rise above the idealism and emotion that make them think their animals "love" them and would never hurt them. In fact, studies have demonstrated that owners are most

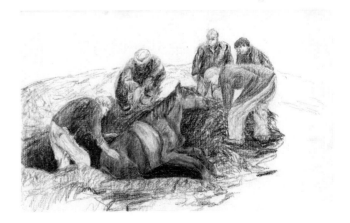

Figure 5.7 *An exhausted horse in a mud hole is exhibiting signs of shock. Responders have minimal equipment available but should be concerned about the proximity of personnel to the animal without primary restraint on the head and proper positioning to prevent being crushed if the animal reacts. Large animals typically relax and lie still until stimulated by a noise, touch, or a frightening sight. Courtesy of Julie Casil.*

commonly injured by their own animals. While animals can form apparently strong attachments to humans, they are capable of severely injuring their owners if the animal perceives the owner as a threat. For this reason, responders should avoid approaching an injured or entrapped animal without assistance. Similarly, children should be taught to recognize dangerous or suspect situations and seek help rather than attempt to rescue or assist unfamiliar animals.

Maximize Visibility. From a safety perspective, every rescuer should be concerned about being visible to others. The second most common cause of death of emergency responders is vehicular injury while on scene or when trying to direct traffic around an incident scene. The California Highway Patrol lost two officers to vehicular injuries within a six-month period in 2006 (Nixon, 2006). Make sure everyone is readily visible; reflective gear, lights, and traffic signals all help to minimize the danger of secondary accident victims. Many large animal incidents occur near roads, and responders should make sure that approaching traffic can easily see equipment and personnel (Figure 5.8). The use of signage and bright yellow or green attire with reflective tape increases visibility.

There are many examples that emphasize the importance of road safety considerations. A person was changing a tire on his horse trailer beside the road when a tractor trailer driver sideswiped the horse trailer and overturned his rig. The horses and owner were not seriously injured, but the tractor trailer driver was killed

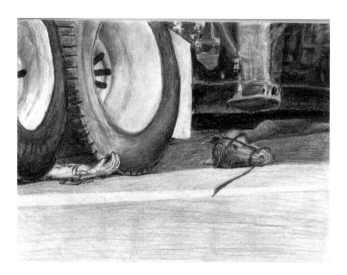

Figure 5.8 *A young person riding beside a road lost control of the animal and was unable to stop the horse; both were crushed by a tractor trailer. Preventive methods include limiting animals from roadsides without an appropriate level of rider skill. These types of incidents are possible crime scenes with human and animal fatalities or may require euthanasia of the animal. Responding to roadside incidents is associated with increased risk of responder injury from traffic. Courtesy of Julie Casil.*

when the overturned rig collided with a tree. An incident like this can happen any time and illustrates why drivers should not stop on narrow shoulders to change a tire on the vehicle or trailer—the width of the shoulder is insufficient to allow safe repair. Drivers should slowly drive the vehicle to a safer section of the road with a wider shoulder and pull off the road as far as possible. In addition to increasing the driver's safety, pulling as far off the road as possible decreases animal stress induced by the sounds and vibrations of passing high-speed traffic.

Manage the Workload. Managing the workload is the SO's job. It is easy for animal handlers and responders on scenes to overexert themselves when confronted with a large operation and few assets. To manage this, teams should require adequate rest and hydration, especially when working in extreme environmental conditions.

Logistics Personnel

Logistics personnel are responsible for providing facilities, services, and materials (including extra personnel) requested for use at the incident. Specialized equipment, such as wreckers, cranes, and fire trucks, are provided by logistics, as are specially trained personnel (e.g., trench rescue teams, etc.). Additional resources unique to large animal emergencies may include a veterinarian, portable fencing panels, livestock trailers, and carcass haulers.

Operations Personnel

Operations personnel implement the IAP by performing the hands-on activities associated with the response effort. When responding to an incident involving large animals, all responders must emphasize safety, good timing, and excellent communication. The operations section chief reports directly to the IC to request resources and updates the IC on the current situation. The operations section chief will be supervising different personnel.

Animal Handler. The animal handler should be skilled with the species involved in the incident. The handler approaches the animal, directs the containment, catches and handles the large animal. The handler must communicate well with operations personnel, and the scene should be kept as quiet as possible so that the animal can focus on the handler. If the animal is distracted by other sounds and movements, the animal handler may find it difficult to gauge the reactions of the animal. Operational personnel should give the animal handler a safe working position and an escape route.

Sufficient and safe room for the animal and human to maneuver is critical, particularly once the animal is freed from its entrapment. Most experienced handlers recommend a minimum of a 15 m (50 ft) radius around the animal. If there are apparatus, equipment, and bystanders in the way, the animal handler will have a very difficult time trying to safely handle the animal and lead it to transportation or containment. The SO should not allow emergency response vehicles to approach an animal scene as closely as they do at human scenes. A secure perimeter should be established to protect responders and bystanders from the animal victim's unpredicted or panicky responses.

Operational Personnel. Operational personnel are those who place any appliances on the animal, set up and operate extrication equipment, employ rope systems, and perform the work of the rescue. They must be sensitive to the animal handler's input and efforts to manage the animal, with emphasis on moving calmly and quietly around the animal.

Veterinarian

Veterinarians and veterinary technicians are highly trained medical personnel who should be encouraged to become involved at the community and county level in emergency response planning for animals and public health considerations. The 911 dispatcher should have a resource binder with information on the closest large animal veterinarian, preferably with ICS training and background. Knowledge of one another's capabilities is important on the scene; preferably, veterinarians willing to provide assistance in these situations should be identified and their contact information kept on record.

Veterinarians are called upon to manage animal industries (especially commercial food animal facilities), sheltering issues, foreign animal disease outbreaks, or animals affected by natural disasters (Baker, 2000). In any situation involving animals, the community will expect the veterinary professionals to provide health care as well as information and support related to the disaster. Veterinarians can assist themselves, their practices, and their communities by developing personal action plans, preparing clinic disaster plans, establishing contact with the local emergency management office, maintaining emergency equipment and supplies, conducting client education, and conducting emergency/disaster drills. The best response always starts at the local level (Baker, 2000).

Medical Expertise. It is essential to have veterinary medical assistance for most incidents involving large animals. Animals are very susceptible to stress situations, even more so than the average human victim. Large animals can develop muscle damage, hypothermia, dehydration, cardiovascular shock, and kidney failure in a short period of time. A veterinarian, veterinary technician, and/or an "animedic" (e.g., animal paramedics, Helsinborg Fire Department, Sweden) should be part of the animal rescue team.

In the United States, veterinary technicians and veterinary students are becoming increasingly interested and involved in the technical aspects of large animal rescue training. Veterinary medicine has become more specialized since the 1970s, and a small animal veterinary practitioner may not have the medications, equipment, or species-specific knowledge of animal behavior necessary on an incident scene involving large animals. Ideally, TLAER volunteers and professionals should make contact and establish working relationships with local veterinarians before the incident occurs.

Just as very few physicians have training in field rescue procedures, for veterinarians TLAER is not currently part of the curriculum in veterinary colleges in any country. It is mostly the responsibility of the fire and rescue brigades to determine which of the local large animal veterinarians are willing to become trained in technical emergency rescue and the ICS and become members of the rescue team (P. Baker, 2005). As with human incidents, a responder with expert medical knowledge but lacking basic rescue knowledge can be a liability on a large animal rescue scene; alternatively, an experienced responder without basic medical knowledge can also be a liability. In modern fire departments, firefighters are cross-trained to the EMT level or above to ensure that they have knowledge of CPR and basic first aid and are able to provide medical assistance. Cross-training in aspects of the ICS should be provided to the veterinarian and veterinary technicians who agree to cooperate in the response effort.

Veterinarian Works for Operations. The large animal veterinarian should work directly for the operations section chief and may also be requested to communicate directly with the IC. The IC is rarely a veterinarian, unless the scene receives a small, local response. In most cases, a local veterinarian who is not an integrally trained member of the rescue team will function best as an advisor to the SO and IC. The strong suggestion that the veterinarian should be working within the ICS system is based on past experiences and reports where the title of IC was essentially ceded to the veterinarian. Despite their high level of medical training, very few veterinarians are prepared to assume the IC function due to lack of ICS certification, nor have they had training in response safety, heavy rescue, or other aspects of incident scene management.

Veterinarians are equipped with euthanasia solution, sedatives, analgesics, antibiotics, anesthetics, and intravenous fluids on the scale required by large animals, and are the most qualified personnel to assess the medical condition of the large animal on the scene. They work with and treat large animals on a daily basis, and they can assist with chemical and physical animal restraint. Ideally, the veterinarian should train ahead of time with the local rescue team, obtain expertise in rescue work and ICS, and make sure they know their role within the ICS structure.

Veterinarians are accustomed to working with owners in difficult medical scenarios. The veterinarian should communicate well with the animal owner; this is especially important when the owner is requesting or insisting on a course of therapy or action that is not in the best interest of the animal victim. For example, owners often request sedation for horses that appear to be struggling inside a trailer; the owner should be made aware that a heavily sedated animal may not be able to participate in its own rescue and may jeopardize itself and/or the responders.

Getting the Veterinarian to the Scene. Veterinary access to the scene may be challenging. Many large animal veterinary practitioners operate mobile units, and the veterinarian may be far from the scene; travel time to the scene may be prolonged due to distance and traffic. In addition, the veterinarian may be detained by medical emergencies. Alternate veterinary resources should be identified and contacted. A police escort may be necessary to facilitate the veterinarian's arrival, especially for roadside incidents. Veterinarians with special interest in emergency and disaster response may seek additional expertise; in one case, a veterinarian attended the South Carolina Police Academy and became a reserve police officer in order to facilitate access to incident scenes to assist animals. Jurisdictional laws determine what options might be available.

Some local and state laws prohibit veterinarians from putting a flashing light on top of their vehicle. In most states, responders should at a minimum be certified local disaster or emergency service workers with appropriate training. Proper protocol should be followed when using flashing lights, and the driver will be held liable for any accidents caused while responding to a scene.

Special Considerations for Veterinary Support. The local 911 dispatch office should be provided with a copy of an annually updated list of veterinarians in the region with ICS and TLAER training and who have indicated their willingness to respond and assist on incident scenes (see Chapter 22).

Veterinarians are not required to respond to these types of incidents. There is little profit in rendering veterinary assistance on an incident scene, and the veterinarian often loses time and income from the effort. The veterinarian may be required to leave a paying client to assist with the emergency, interrupting service to that client for an hour or more. The day's appointments must often be rescheduled due to the time consumed by the emergency response. In addition, the veterinarian might not be paid for veterinary services provided on an incident scene.

Legal and Financial Considerations. The veterinarian should consider the legal and financial aspects of emergency response before agreeing to respond to these incidents; close attention should be paid to the Good Samaritan laws in the state in which the veterinarian is licensed. These laws are intended to protect healthcare providers and rescuers from being sued when they render aid to victims, provided that the person uses reasonable and prudent guidelines for care using the resources available at the time. Several states have promulgated Good Samaritan laws for animals, and the state animal response team and county animal response team should become involved in these legislative efforts.

In many states, a veterinarian who accepts a cup of coffee or even a dollar for his or her efforts may be held liable because he or she is offering a professional service. Veterinarians carry a liability umbrella policy on their practice, and those interested in emergency rescue might wish to consult with their insurance agent regarding increased liability umbrella coverage and other options. If the veterinarian's insurer is not willing or able to provide umbrella coverage, the state veterinary medical association may be able to assist. For example, a local response group in California was able to get additional insurance coverage through the CVMA because the veterinarians' insurers were not willing to write a separate policy for the group. Although the veterinarian's opinions are often sought during an emergency, post-incident emotional responses sometimes lead to lawsuits. Some veterinarians choose not to charge for their services on a scene; this does not always relieve a veterinarian of liability issues since they are considered the expert. Many malpractice suits against veterinarians are based on human injury during a veterinary examination; similarly, the veterinarian may be sued for injuries to bystanders who place themselves in harm's way during the rescue. Some veterinarians provide an itemized donation suggestion that lists everything they provided, suggests a fair charge by the hour for their time, and lists all expenses. (Donated work is not deductible on taxes, but donated supplies are deductible.) This book only introduces these issues, but does not make an attempt to cover the subjects of liability and legalities for veterinary care. However, from a management perspective, if veterinarians can't be covered from liability and malpractice claims, they will not be able to help on the scene. Veterinarians interested in this work might be well advised to consult with their legal and insurance advisors.

Patient Care for Animals. Professional emergency responders and veterinarians should use standardized patient protocols for large animals and be able to apply to the large animal rescue scene all the techniques required by any other type of heavy rescue (Figure 5.9).

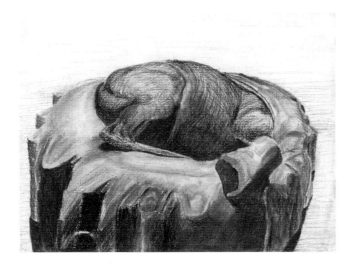

Figure 5.9 *This animal was asphyxiated when it fell or climbed into a tire feeder in the pasture. This case illustrates the complexity of heavy rescue tools necessary to cut into a large tire. Large animals are consistently capable of getting into places and equipment that would seem impossible to the average person. Courtesy of Julie Casil.*

Victim

A victim is already a victim, and an animal victim must take a lower priority than a human victim. An exception to this rule exists when the animal victim has to be removed from the situation first to allow access to the human victim (e.g., a horse and rider have fallen into a trench, and the horse's body is on top of the rider). Part of a good risk assessment is to assess whether or not the victim can be rescued without risking severe injury or fatality on the rescuers' part. It is rescue dictum that no human victim is worth the injury or death of a human rescuer, much less an animal victim. Many people have an emotionally charged reaction to animal incidents because the animal is viewed to be "innocent" (similar to children and handicapped persons). The IC must evaluate the chance of harm to the rescuers and take responsibility for these decisions. The IC should always seek the counsel of the SO.

STANDARD OPERATING GUIDELINES

General standard operating guidelines for a large animal incident should not be different from that for any other type of rescue scene that professional emergency responders would attend. The breadth of a unit's capabilities should be conveyed accurately within the community. For example, a unit trained for swiftwater rescues may not be adequately trained for confined space operations; similarly, the veterinary medical assistance teams, now redesignated as the National Veterinary Response Teams, do not perform field rescues of animals. Understanding the missions of response teams in a disaster or emergency scenario

will contribute to better utilization of specialty teams on scene.

Establish Command

Upon arrival, the SO should immediately establish bystander control and a security perimeter under the command of the IC. In large animal emergencies, establishing control can be difficult if the owner or any bystanders consider themselves experienced animal handlers; these individuals may question the authority of the responders or may disregard the IC's and SO's instructions. Communication is vital, but police enforcement of the security perimeter may be necessary.

Formulate an IAP

Formulating an IAP may be as simple as an oral discussion of the IC's intent for the rescue or as elaborate as a written plan (with attachments) for a large, multi-jurisdictional response, documenting specific responsibilities, response goals, and operational objectives. The IC ensures that all personnel and assets on scene understand the IAP and implement their roles.

Based on the dispatcher's information, the initial deployment or callout may provide a mental picture to responders, but the situation may change on scene. In addition, the scenario may change quickly based on the actions of the animals involved. Responders must remain flexible to shifting scenario challenges; alternate suggestions and courses of action should be considered. Suggestions from bystanders with large animal experience may be useful while developing the plan or implementing the rescue effort.

Perform a Risk Assessment

Risk assessment is not a form to be completed; it is a dynamic estimation of the situation and the hazards. On the scene, it is supposed to encourage responders and leaders to evaluate the options as well as what could go wrong during the response. When performing the risk assessment, the IC must consider and balance the risks versus the gains of the efforts and determine how much risk is acceptable. If the animal victim's injuries indicate that euthanasia will be necessary, it may be more prudent to euthanatize the animal (if this can be performed safely) than to extricate it and euthanize it afterward. Euthanatized animals should be removed as if they are still alive, if possible. This effort shows respect for the animal, the animal's owner, and public opinion.

Evaluate Hazards. The IC should assess the hazards present on the scene, as well as those that are associated with the rescue methods required to accomplish the objective. The IC will then decide if the rescue is worth the risk to the responders. With human victims, it is rare for the search and rescue community to make a "no" decision unless the risk to responders is extremely high (e.g., requesting a helicopter rescue during a hurricane or entering a collapsed mine).

Due to the growing popularity of challenging or extreme sports, such as base jumping, bungee jumping, extreme trail riding, and rock climbing, the subject of risk assessment has become controversial in the last 10 years in the rescue community. Risk-takers hike or ride to areas with poor access, then call 911 when they become lost or trapped. Some search and rescue organizations and county rescue teams have started to charge these individuals for their rescue services and levy fines on people who start natural disasters (such as wildfires). In large animal rescue, the practical and pragmatic aspects must take precedence when considering the amount of resources and the risks to personnel.

Establish Acceptable Risk. The IC should establish an acceptable level of risk based on the overall scenario. If the IC decides to extricate a bull from a hole, they should also determine the events or time limit that will dictate that the rescue effort be abandoned. Factors such as darkness, rising water, dangerous actions or responses by the animal victim, inability to obtain veterinary care, and inadequate TLAER training may play roles in this decision.

The "no go" decision should be made at the earliest possible time. This decision may be based on a predetermined time period, a set number of unsuccessful rescue attempts, or the occurrence of a severe injury (e.g., fractured limb) to the animal. The author has a videotape of a bull down a 25 m deep hole surrounded by rock faces; the animal is bruised but otherwise appears uninjured. If the equipment to rescue the bull is not available, or if no one is trained to perform rappelling and rope system placement, is the bull going to be rescued? (See Chapter 22.)

Implement Safety Precautions. Safety precautions vary depending on the scenario. Utilization of the ICS and trained personnel will minimize the hazards. The IC should brief everyone to make sure they know the situation and the intent.

If the chosen method is not successful, responders should try another method. Repeating the same unsuccessful method is not likely to ensure success and increases the time required to perform the rescue. In one incident involving a horse trapped in a ravine, 12 people were pulling on a rope attached to the animal's halter in an attempt to pull the horse up a 45-degree incline. The horse was not assisting in its own rescue because it was pulling and jerking backward. The responders attempted this method for two hours and were eventually successful in getting the horse up the slope to the trail. The rescue would likely have required less time and effort if webbing was placed around the horse's thorax and between its front legs and a forward assist used; in this case, the horse would have been less likely to resist assistance and would participate in its own rescue. If the rescue is not working well, responders should stop and consider other options. If one method is working poorly, improvements should be made or another method should be attempted. A suggestion in some jurisdictions has been to videotape the rescue effort. If the first attempt fails, sometimes reviewing the videotape on scene will make it immediately obvious what is going wrong, and the problem can be corrected.

Staging Area

A staging area is a place where equipment, supplies, and personnel are assembled and processed. Consider a highway construction crew installing a pipe: although many passersby observe a number of people who appear to be standing around while a few are working, this is not the case. There is a reason for this scenario: the few people working at that time must perform their tasks before the next workers can perform their jobs. Those people that are standing around are in a staging area, waiting until their skills are needed. Personnel in the staging area should be prepared, alert, and available.

On some TLAER scenes, the IC may consider using bystanders for particular jobs (e.g., making a human containment fence, pulling on rope systems, etc.). If possible, bystander assistance with minor jobs (e.g., retrieving grain or hay, getting hot water, bringing a trailer or cattle panels, etc.) will allow skilled responders more time to concentrate on their efforts. This allows the bystanders to contribute to the rescue effort in a safe manner and can also divert their attention and decrease their distractive influence. In addition, they may develop a positive image of the response effort and act as advocates for the responders. The liability is lessened when bystanders are sent for supplies and equipment compared to allowing them to contain animals or pull on a rope. The IC must balance the risk versus the benefit.

ANIMAL OWNER

In most cases the animal's owner will be on a TLAER scene. In others (e.g., loose animals, natural disasters, trailer wrecks, barn fires, etc.) the owner may be undergoing treatment by EMS personnel, been transported away from scene, or is not present. The owner and their friends may be of little value to the rescue attempt, or their emotional responses may hinder the rescue effort. The owner can provide important information, such as pre-existing medical conditions, vision problems, behavioral issues, and pregnancy, that can be significant considerations in formulating the IAP. The consulting veterinarian should listen to the owner's concerns and communicate anything significant to the IC.

Consulting with the owner might make the rescue more successful and may reduce liability concerns. Consider having one person (an owner assistance officer can be designated, or the PIO may fill this role) stay with the owner to prevent the owner from inserting himself into the rescue effort; this may require the intervention of law enforcement personnel. The owner assistance officer can explain the events as they occur and psychologically prepare the owner (and possibly the bystanders) for possible outcomes. Efforts by the PIO will reduce agitation and anxiety. When the owner and bystanders have a basic understanding of the process and why certain procedures are used, they are less likely to interfere with the rescue effort.

The PIO or team member delegated to interact with the owner should be compassionate; to many animal owners, their animals are part of their family. During an emergency, the emotional relationship the owner shares with the animals may interfere with the owner's ability to make good and rational decisions. Very few owners are able to effectively assist with the rescue. Listening to their concerns and addressing those that are valid—such as recent surgery on a specific area of the animal—will potentially help the rescue effort and also help the owner feel that he or she is contributing to the rescue in a positive manner. In cases where the owner has less emotional attachment to the animals, such as a load of beef cattle destined for slaughter, the owner may be more able to actively assist in the rescue effort.

If the animal is injured, it is common for the owner to feel guilty for directly or indirectly causing the incident (e.g., failing to address low tire pressure or perform routine trailer maintenance, waiting too long to evacuate prior to a hurricane or wildfire, etc.). This guilt may further cloud the owner's judgment in the situation. In addition, the owner's perception of the animal's pain or discomfort may be exaggerated by their emotional attachment to the animal. An example of this occurred in South Carolina, when a horse was trapped underneath a culvert. The situation was a straightforward rescue scenario that required minimal time. The animal owner's spouse was frantic and requested that the veterinarian euthanatize the animal because it was perceived that the animal was in severe distress. The spouse was removed to an area where the rescue could not be observed, and the horse was successfully extricated from the culvert with minimal injury.

Ulterior Motives. Unfortunately, there have been incidents that were intentionally caused by people as part of an insurance fraud scheme. Barn fires are the more common incidents of this type, although trailer wrecks have also been implicated. Although that scenario is considered rare, emergency responders should not hesitate to bring in law enforcement if there are questions as to the intent or cause of the incident. Rarely are animal incidents intentionally staged, but some incidents (e.g., barn fire arsons, loosed animals, etc.) are more commonly criminally motivated. Theft of large animals (particularly valuable cattle and horses) is not uncommon and should be considered when animals are missing from a property without obvious routes or evidence of escape; this will require the owner to submit a report to law enforcement. There is great expertise available in the area of stolen animal recovery, and proactive placement of microchips can aid in the recovery or identification of animals in this situation. Timely response and reporting are also critical to the effort (Metcalf, 2006).

Animal Incidents Are Human Incidents

The animal owner will often be emotionally involved and stressed when an incident involves a large companion animal (see Figure 5.3 above). The animal owner is an important component of a successful large animal rescue, not as a rescuer but as a source of information about the animal victim (e.g., temperament, age, medical conditions, etc.). When dealing with an owner who is distraught, responders should realize that it is a family emergency to that person, and the owner presents a scene safety issue to responders simply because that person may be willing to risk his or her life to save the animal. Responders should assess whether the owner is going to be an asset or a liability on scene. Owner reactions vary from incident to incident.

The American Animal Hospital Association completed a study in 1993 in which they reported that 83% of pet owners will risk their lives to save their pets. Owners have died reentering a burning house to save their pet. They have also died because they refused to leave their companion animals before, during, or after Hurricane Katrina (2005), or because they waited too long to evacuate their horses from an approaching wildfire. That scenario should not be allowed to happen; no human should die saving an animal. TLAER-trained rescue teams can be of great benefit by minimizing the risks of human injury in animal rescue scenarios.

Bystanders (Emergencies) and Self-Deployed Volunteers (Disasters)

On most incident scenes involving animals, there will be bystanders and Good Samaritans who want to assist in the rescue effort. Responders should assume that these individuals have no formal ICS training and may have inaccurate views of their own training and experience. As stated previously, professionalism and proper communication with these individuals can determine if they will help or hinder the response effort. Perceived inappropriate, callous, or cruel handling of the animal will not be tolerated by bystanders and will invariably be reported to the media and other members of the public; a successful rescue can be tainted in the public's eye by allegations of mishandling. Few volunteers possess the training (HazMat, CPR, first aid, animal handling and care, safety), up-to-date personal vaccinations (rabies, hepatitis A and C, etc.), and ICS training in order to contribute to a safe and effective response in a disaster (McBride, 2000).

If a passerby has excellent large animal experience, the IC may want to consider his or her suggestions and advice on a case-by-case basis. In general, it is not recommended that an untrained volunteer be allowed to assist on the scene.

FOLLOW-UP ON THE VICTIM

At the Scene

Once the animal is successfully extricated, its health status should be thoroughly evaluated by a veterinarian. If the animal has been trapped for an extended period of time, the rescue effort was prolonged, the animal is stressed or the environment conditions were unfavorable, the animal's health status may decline after the rescue. Large animals are physically strong and powerful, but they can be surprisingly delicate and easily stressed (see Chapter 17). In many cases, the animal has been trapped for an unknown period of time; therefore, injuries may not be obvious at the time of the incident.

A veterinarian should be on the scene to evaluate the animal as soon as possible. What looks like a tiny scratch to untrained personnel might be a punctured, potentially septic joint or tendon sheath. Wounds over the body cavities (thorax, abdomen) should be evaluated thoroughly to make sure that the body cavities have not been contaminated.

The animal(s) should be cleaned with warm water and dried with towels to facilitate the identification of any possible injuries. In some situations the animal may be too cold or medically unstable to justify soaking them with water. Mud prevents the hair from insulating the animal's body and should be removed with vigorous brushing. Chilled animals should be blanketed. Several rescuers have noted that blow dryers and confined space forced air fans work well for warming and drying animal victims, but these appliances should be used with caution because they may induce panic responses in some animals. Others have used kerosene forced-air heaters to warm and dry animals following ice and mud rescue (Gimenez, 2004a).

Cardiopulmonary shock is a primary concern during the immediate post-rescue period if there has been pressure on a body cavity (thorax, abdomen) that was suddenly and rapidly relieved; the rapid generation of negative pressure within the body cavity can lead to fluid influx into that cavity from the bloodstream.

The veterinarian should complete a thorough physical examination of the animal victim(s); he or she may prescribe pain relief or anti-inflammatory medications for suspected pain and inflammation. Fluid therapy may be required because stressed large animals quickly become dehydrated; this is exacerbated by sweating and high ambient temperatures.

If the animal was trapped in a recumbent position for a prolonged period of time, it may exhibit signs of myositis (muscle inflammation) and nerve damage due to extended pressure on the animal's "down" side.

Non-veterinary personnel should not be permitted to administer drugs to animals on the scene unless directed to do so by the veterinarian. Many horse owners maintain their own stock of anti-inflammatory and pain-relieving medications such as flunixin meglumine (Banamine) and phenylbutazone ("bute"). These medications should only be used under veterinary supervision; potentially fatal complications may develop when they are administered to dehydrated, stressed, or ill animals.

Post-incident Health Issues

It is important to remember that an animal may appear normal for several days after an incident before developing a life-threatening illness. Colic, laminitis, respiratory disease, diarrhea, and lameness are examples of diseases that may be observed during the post-incident period.

The severity of skin and muscle damage may not be immediately evident; horses that were apparently normal when rescued have begun to slough skin and muscle tissue several days after the incident. Underlying problems may develop, and the veterinarian should communicate to the owner that these animal(s) will need veterinary follow-up after the rescue. For example, a horse was trapped between a bridge and a tree. Immediately after the horse was extricated, the veterinarian on the scene began treatment with intravenous fluids, analgesics, antibiotics, and wound repair. The animal was walked slowly to a nearby stall and appeared to be improving despite severe bruising, trauma, and over six hours of entrapment and struggling. Despite immediate and appropriate treatment, the horse died nine days later. A necropsy was not performed; therefore, it was impossible to relate the death to the stress of the incident. However, this case emphasizes the importance of veterinary evaluation following a large animal incident, regardless of the apparent good health of the animal (see Chapter 17).

There are reports of successfully rescued horses, livestock, and zoologics that died from complications hours to days after a rescue, so the owner and veterinarian must monitor the animal(s) closely for changes in attitude, appetite, or general health. It is recommended that the owner record the animal's body temperature twice daily for at least one week after the rescue in case pneumonia, sepsis, laminitis, or other stress-related disease conditions develop. If there are any changes, the owner should have the animal examined by a veterinarian.

ACRONYMS USED IN CHAPTER 5

AAHA	American Animal Hospital Association
AHJ	Authority having jurisdiction
CART	County animal response team
COA	Course of action
CPR	Cardiopulmonary resuscitation
CVMA	California Veterinary Medical Association
DART	Disaster animal response teams
EMI	Emergency Management Institute
EMS	Emergency medical services
EMT	Emergency medical technician
EOC	Emergency operations center
FEMA	Federal Emergency Management Agency
HazMat	Hazardous materials
HSUS	Humane Society of the United States
IAP	Incident action plan
IC	Incident commander
ICS	Incident command system
NIMS	National Incident Management System
PA	Public affairs officer
PIO	Public information officer
SART	State animal response team
SEMS	Standardized Emergency Management System
SO	Safety officer
SOG	Standard operating guidelines
SPP	Standard patient protocol
TLAER	Technical large animal emergency rescue
VMAT	Veterinary medical assistance team

6 Understanding Large Animal Restraint in Technical Large Animal Rescue Incidents

Dr. Rebecca Gimenez

INTRODUCTION

The victims discussed in this text are not animals that a person or even many persons can easily pick up, shift, or lift. Even a young calf or foal is very strong and weighs close to 50 kg (110 lb) at birth; restraining one is more challenging than one would expect. In general, containment is a better and safer solution than capture, and responders should use commonsense restraint methods that do not rely on physical strength. Although human victims can often be carried by one or two responders, increasing the number of responders to accommodate the increased weight of the animal victim is not an acceptable plan.

A great number of veterinarians and responders would probably agree with one equine veterinarian's comment on his personal approach to dangerous large animals. According to Mike Graper (2005), "My philosophy is that "wild" (i.e., crazy, unmanageable) horses get to live and die like wild horses, and tame horses get to see veterinarians; it is up to the owner to make conditions safe for the horse and for the vet."

Although behavioral conditioning can be beneficial in many situations, it is best to expect the animal victim to be unpredictable and fearful, with minimal handling experience. A combination of physical restraint methods will probably be necessary to ensure the safety of the responders and may prevent the animal from further injuring itself.

An understanding of basic methods of physical and chemical restraint will provide technical large animal emergency rescue (TLAER) responders with options for restraining large animals while solving the difficult problem of extrication. This chapter does not attempt to detail chemical restraint dosages and capture equipment, topics which are covered adequately in other texts, but provides an introduction to the challenges that may be encountered within the context of a TLAER incident (see Appendix 4).

GAME CAPTURE OPERATIONS

Game reserves in many countries are fenced to protect the animals within their boundaries as well as the neighboring communities, crops, and livestock. The KwaZulu-Natal Nature Conservation Service's policy in South Africa is to catch animals rather than cull them. To date this service has caught more than 141,000 animals of 41 different species; most of the animals are delivered to new habitats, and revenues derived from game animal sales are used for conservation programs. Since the 1960s, techniques pioneered and developed by this program have been used in large-scale game capture operations throughout southern Africa and around the world. Many of these techniques, or modifications of them, can be applied to TLAER situations.

Passive Capture

The simplest, most economical, and least stressful method of containing large animals is to attract them to a central point with food and or water. Many cattle ranchers in the western United States use this method to capture herds of cattle with one-way trap doors into the capture site, and it is considered an excellent method for catching brumbies (wild horses) in Australia. Temporary trap paddocks can be erected at a strategic location; sites selection should be based on knowledge of animal movement, the potential for significant impact on the local environment, and accessibility by vehicle for removal of trapped animals.

Wildlife experts in Africa use a similar method for capturing hippopotamuses. Once the hippopotamuses are accustomed to the site, the construction of a capture enclosure can commence around the attractant.

However, this method is time-consuming and unsuitable for large-scale capture operations involving many animals or when time is of the essence.

A trial in Australia demonstrated that horses could be trapped effectively in both steel yards and trap paddocks. During an eight-month trial, 114 horses in 19 separate herds were captured. Researchers observed that the location and size of yards and paddocks are important to the success of the trap and to the welfare of captured horses. Wild horses could be lured into the traps using salt, lucerne hay, and molasses. Coacher or Judas horses that had been educated to artificial feeds, fences, and holding yards assisted in drawing horses into these traps (NSW, 2005). Animals should be located, gathered and moved using low stress stock-handling (LSS) techniques. In Australia, adherence to low stress stock handling techniques are required for the capture, movement, and handling of all feral horses undertaken during government capture programs (NSW, 2006).

Chemical Capture

Chemical capture methods can be used to capture all species of prey animals, but it is not a preferred method. However, unless selected animals are to be removed, the only animals routinely caught by using chemical restraint are elephants, rhinoceroses, and giraffes. Unless the responder has considerable experience in the use of this capture method, the authors recommend that the advice of a wildlife veterinarian be obtained. Public perception of animal rescue efforts has been altered by the news and entertainment media; due to dramatic portrayals and selective coverage of rescue efforts, many people believe that wild, large animals can be handled easily. In reality, large zoologic animals can be extremely dangerous. For example, zebras are wild animals that can viciously bite or kick with intent to kill, and they have only sporadically been trained, not domesticated, by very accomplished animal behaviorists and circus trainers.

The jurisdiction researching the use of chemical capture and immobilization should provide correct (and updated) training and certification for personnel, attention to safety, proper equipment, and regular practice. The ability to perform safe chemical capture can be of great benefit to local animal control offices or humane societies.

Early Techniques. Early rhinoceros capture techniques in Africa, pioneered by Dr. Ian Player and Dr. Tony Hawthorn, involved darting large doses of immobilizing drugs into the animals. The animal was then followed with vehicles and horses as the drugs took effect; once the animal exhibited signs of sedation, the rhinoceros was roped and forced into transport crates. Although effective, the technique was cumbersome and dangerous for humans and rhinos; the animal

could take up to 20 minutes to go down, traveling several kilometers in the process. In 1963 the drug M99, a powerful morphine derivative, became available. This drug took effect rapidly and could be delivered in small doses. An antidote was also available that enabled the team to walk the dazed animal to a waiting capture crate, minimizing stress compared to earlier methods. This made the process much safer for the humans and for the animals.

Another breakthrough occurred in the early 1970s with the introduction of helicopters into game capture operations, allowing officials to locate animals by air and dart them with minimal stress. In 1992, capture operations again improved when a helicopter was used to airlift rhinoceroses for the first time where management policies prohibited the use of vehicles. With modern technology, rhinoceros mortalities during moving operations or in the bomas (named for heavily fortified livestock enclosures in Africa) have declined to less than 1%. Modifications of these helicopter sling load methods can be used in TLAER-related scenarios. Similarly, helicopter platform net gun, herding/mustering, and darting operations are commonly used for capturing wild burros and horses in the United States (see Chapter 18).

Dangers to the Animals. Chemical capture methods in large animals are associated with the highest rates of compromised animals and the highest number of fatalities due to capture myopathy (CM) and accidental death or injury. For these reasons it is rarely considered appropriate for use in TLAER scenarios. If used, the process must involve veterinary oversight to prevent injury or death to personnel or animals. The using of guns or darts to shoot a sedative into the shoulder or hip of a large mammal requires knowledge of the proper dosage and adequate logistical support to track a darted mammal until the sedative takes effect. For example, using ground techniques, 23 (9 male, 14 female) wild horses (*Equus caballus*) in the Great Basin Desert were immobilized with succinylcholine chloride. Induction and recovery times were rapid, and most animals were returned to their original bands within 10 minutes. Dosages ranged from 0.66 to 0.77 mg/kg body weight. Neither abortions nor changes in herd membership or status were observed; however, concerted efforts for up to 24 hours were needed to return some animals to original bands, and three non-drug-related mortalities (13%) occurred. For reference, the frequency of death loss experienced with traditional capture methods of feral animals is 2%–4% (Berger et al., 1983).

Darting and Chemical Capture. Darting equipment is most often owned by animal control and veterinarians and is used in limited situations, often as a last resort.

Due to media coverage of chemical captures, the general public often believes that a darted animal will immediately collapse. However, the real-life situation varies greatly from these dramatic portrayals. An experienced wildlife veterinarian estimated that the shortest time period from dart placement to recumbency was approximately 42 seconds (Amass, 1999). Horses are capable of covering 10–16.5 m (33–54 1/2 ft) per second at a gallop; in 42 seconds, the horse has traveled 420–693 m (approximately 1,400–2,300 ft).

Hazards, such as ditches, holes, trees, trenches, water, and equipment, can present severe risks of injury to the sedated and fleeing animal. Location, habitat, and the time required for sedation should be considered in order to avoid injury or drowning of sedated mammals. When animals are scared and running, the alarm reaction is driving them beyond their flight distance. They may fall or run into obstacles because they do not have control. The animal may break a leg or its neck when it falls, necessitating euthanasia, or exhaust itself to the point of severe muscle damage (CM).

When considering darting an animal, the owner should be made to understand the risks associated with the procedure. Because the intended subject is often moving, perfect aim and dart placement is not often possible. Potentially fatal complications can occur if darts pierce body cavities, joints, tendon sheaths, or other structures. Anxious animals often require higher or additional doses, further increasing the risk of serious injury or death.

Personnel Safety. Some of the drugs used for these procedures by professionals can be fatal to humans (e.g., carfentanyl, M-99, etc.), even in very small doses. If the sharpshooter accidentally hits a person, or if a dart explodes in the shooter's face during loading, the results are often deadly. Some of these drugs do not have antidotes.

Sedation tends to be so commonplace for large animals that most people assume it is safe for the animal and that once the animal is sedated, it cannot injure anyone. Although the animal's fear responses are diminished by sedation/tranquilization, it is still capable of inducing human injury. In addition, there is a human tendency to underestimate the potential for a sedated animal to kick, strike, or bite with speed and accuracy.

Typical sedation posture of the horse includes a head position below the level of the heart (llamas and cattle will most often lay down), drooping and relaxed lips, and decreased ear movement (Figure 6.1). They may also drool, and their eyes may appear unfocused. Some animals may appear very sedate, but unexpectedly awaken to kick or bite.

Sedation or tranquilization is not a substitute for proper training. For example, when the author first started training animals for TLAER she could not

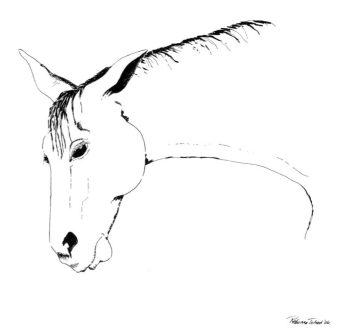

Figure 6.1 *A sedated animal typically looks sleepy, with a lowered head, relaxed ears, droopy eyelids and lips, and a distant expression. Courtesy of Becky Tolson.*

imagine that a horse would submit to the demonstrations in slings and under heavy equipment without low levels of sedation. Even with low doses, she was kicked and bitten several times by the horses in training events. Since she began training the horses to do the demonstrations without being sedated, no one has been kicked or bitten.

Correct Drug and Dosage. Only a veterinarian should evaluate an animal and administer drugs on scene. The use of chemical restraint drugs in the correct dosage is a primary reason why veterinarians are called to the scene of a large animal incident. This chapter will not attempt to cover this subject, but instead suggests that the interested responder talk to a local large animal practitioner.

Veterinarians are encouraged to consult with specialists when asked to participate in unique scenarios involving exotic wildlife species. For example, a veterinarian attempted to use published doses for chemical restraint to restrain a zebra and remove an oral growth. The attempt was unsuccessful, despite an extremely high cumulative dose. Following consultation with a zoo veterinarian, a new drug combination was used successfully to immobilize and treat the zebra.

Wild animals do not respond to chemical restraint in the same manner as domesticated species; they may require significantly higher or lower doses to produce the same effect. It is also important to note that recovery from sedation in a wild animal may not be as smooth as that observed in a domestic herbivore. The fight-or-flight response often causes the animal to make premature attempts to rise or attempt to flee before it has regained sufficient strength and coordination.

Correct Equipment. The dart used for most large animals has a large, barbed needle; the barb anchors the needle in the animal's hide to allow drug delivery without dislodging the needle from the skin. The veterinarian must surgically excise the dart after the animal is immobilized to minimize trauma; manual removal of the dart is not recommended. On close examination of the darted area, one will observe a dark circle (approximately 7.6 cm, or 3 in., in diameter) centered around the needle puncture site. There must be sufficient power in the firing charge to enable the dart to penetrate the hide, but the deceleration trauma will cause a hematoma, which may develop into an abscess. Darting is not often performed on privately owned horses. In addition, horses that develop abscesses at the darting site require daily treatment; this can be difficult to achieve if the horse cannot be readily caught. Darting is a legitimate tool in the response kit, but needs to be considered a last-resort solution.

Sedated prey mammals should be closely monitored and should not be released until they recover normal locomotor capabilities as determined by a veterinarian. Exceptions to this rule include large, dangerous species that pose a risk of injury or death to the responder. Such species (e.g., elephant, large carnivores, etc.) should be placed in secure sites where they will not be subject to physical harm or extremes of temperature and can be monitored from a safe distance.

Types of Equipment Available. There are many items available for chemical capture and immobilization, including dart guns, blow guns, rifles, CO_2 pistols, and different types and sizes of darts. The equipment is expensive and sold as specialty items. In some situations (e.g., zoos, exotic animal facilities, animal control) dart guns are required components of the emergency response toolkit. For example, at one major U.S. zoo, a silverback gorilla escaped its zoo enclosure twice in the middle of the night. The zoo's response team, well equipped with physical restraint and chemical capture equipment and trained in TLAER procedures, were able to recapture the animal both times with a dart. The backup plan, or "plan B," in their standard operating protocol is a marksman with a lethal bullet. For large, dangerous animals (especially large exotics and primates), lethal force must be included in the backup plan in case the animal charges a person or threatens public safety (see Chapter 13).

The most useful equipment for emergency responders on large animal scenes is the bang or jab stick used to sedate or anesthetize animals that are trapped out of reach of veterinary or response personnel. Despite the name, it is not intended to be banged or jabbed into

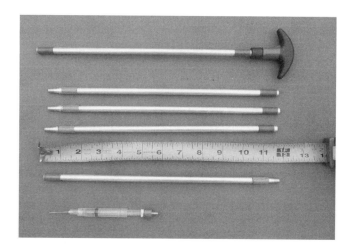

Figure 6.2 *An improvised jab stick, constructed from a 3 cc Luer-Lok® syringe, a hypodermic needle, and a shotgun cleaning kit.*

the animal; forceful application will prevent the drug from being effectively injected and will certainly startle the animal. Instead, a smooth, forward-pushing motion into a large muscle mass is preferred. A simple do-it-yourself version can be made with a 3 cc syringe with a Luer-Lok® hub, a hypodermic needle, and a shotgun cleaning kit. The syringe plunger is placed on the end of the assembled cleaning kit and pushed into the syringe barrel (Figure 6.2). This method allows intramuscular injection from a safer distance and is well suited for use on animals in overturned horse trailers, trapped in wells, etc.

Mass Capture Using the Oelofse Method

This method was devised in the Hluhluwe-Umfolozi Park (South Africa) by Jan Oelofse in the late 1960s while employed by the KwaZulu-Natal Nature Conservation Service. To use this technique, a large funnel-shaped site (approx 300 m, or 984 ft) is constructed using opaque plastic suspended by cables. At the widest open end, a plastic curtain is used, which is then closed once the desired animals are inside the site. The animals are herded down to the narrowest end using a series of curtains to gradually reduce the size of the holding area. The final crush has a loading ramp where transport vehicles are in position to receive the animals. This commonly used method is effective for catching herds of exotic animals such as water buffalo and zebra in Africa and for wild horses in America.

Modifications of this method used for emergency rescues would include portable fencing or corral panels to form a funnel, to enclose a small group of animals, or to drive them toward safe containment. A human chain is effective in some cases; this may present an increased risk of human injury if the animals panic or if humans penetrate too far inside the animal's flight distance and action zones, inciting a flight response from the animal. Other suggestions that have been successfully used on scenes are police caution tape, videocassette tape pulled from the cassette, or white one-quarter-inch electric fencing tape (with or without electrical charge) tied and strung between trees or obstacles to form a containment area.

Drive Net Capture

Probably the oldest method used in mass game capture, this method is still used today in Africa for catching animals such as deer in dense bush. Approximately 100 m (330 ft) of rope netting is woven through the bush, and animals are driven into the nets by a line of beaters (literally, people beating the bushes to create noise). There must be sufficient personnel in the vicinity of the nets to restrain and tranquilize the animals. There are minimal applications for this method in TLAER.

Drop Net Capture

In this method, a cargo net is suspended on a line strung between two trees or posts over a specific place the target animal is likely to enter. The trigger is baited with a favorite food of the quarry and is triggered by the animal when the bait is touched. It can also be triggered by a hidden operator pulling a string from some distance away or by radio. In African wildlife capture, unattended cargo net capture tools can be fitted with transmitters that signal triggering to a receiver up to 62 km (38 miles) away.

Net Gun Capture

A cannon net gun can be set to cover a specific area. In one study, a remotely fired net gun was used at a waterhole for capturing wild goats and urial (a breed of wild sheep) in an area where helicopters could not be used. Twenty-six goats and eight urial were caught, with a capture effort of 12.5 person-hours per goat and 59.5 person hours per urial. Up to four animals were caught at once, and multiple captures accounted for 74% of all captures for both species. The researchers noted that a remotely fired net gun should be effective for capturing other species at waterholes or other sites where the animals' presence could be predicted (Edge, 1989).

Because animals caught with a suspended drop net capture tool or cannon net gun have not been frightened by pursuit or the presence of humans, their stress is minimal. Once entangled in the net, the animal ceases to struggle, rolls into a comfortable position, and can relax before humans appear. These versatile tools are low-cost, humane, and very portable. The drop net capture method features a guaranteed capture because the animal must be in the center of the net to trigger the capture tool and may represent an excellent method to capture shy or loose animals in TLAER incidents.

A Comment on Live Capture

Scientists seeking to capture, mark, and release mammals for research purposes have a special responsibility to both the integrity of their research and the animals they handle to ensure their capture methods are humane and animals are released in the best possible condition. The primary methods used for live capture include trapping and netting. These techniques are designed to keep captive animals alive, uninjured, well provisioned, and in comfortable conditions while awaiting subsequent processing and release. Emergency responders can learn much from these methods.

Great care should be exercised while transporting newly captured feral animals. When necessary, injection with long- and short-acting tranquillizers may be used prior to transportation, but only in consultation with a veterinarian.

Corral traps are designed to enable herding of large mammals along fences or runways into a corral. This technique is commonly used by wildlife personnel in research or management procedures involving large ungulates and kangaroos. As with cannon nets, another technique of choice in the wildlife profession, care should be taken to avoid injury to captured mammals. When corral traps or nets are used, all animals captured must be attended to as quickly as possible to prevent panic or injury.

CAPTURE MYOPATHY

If an animal is chased or runs too far, sometimes their muscles become so exhausted that the tissue begins to break down, which may result in a commonly fatal syndrome called CM (capture myopathy). (See Chapter 20.) Especially when chased beyond the point of recovery, many animals can literally be run to death. Cardiomyopathy is a similar condition in which an animal develops spasms and may literally drop dead from the stress. This is a significant risk in some species, but capture stress can be a major problem associated with the capture of all large prey animals. Contrary to popular belief, domesticated and wild prey animals are not necessarily physically fit; responders should strive to avoid overexertion of the animals during capture operations. Chasing should be avoided, and containment and capture should be conducted in a slow manner using LSS handling methods and avoiding extremes of environmental conditions (see Chapter 4).

In the 1980s, four different capture methods were evaluated for evidence of stress or CM in hematologic, biochemical, and physiological parameters in 634 bighorn sheep (*Ovis canadensis*). Animals were captured by four techniques: drop net (*n* = 158), drive net (*n* = 249), chemical immobilization (*n* = 90), and the net gun (*n* = 137). Post-capture biological parameters were compared according to four different outcomes: normal, stressed or compromised, CM mortality, and accidental mortality. Differences were reported between outcome groups relative to certain physical parameters, including temperature and respiratory rate. Laboratory values compared among groups included creatinine phosphokinase (CPK), lactic dehydrogenase (LDH), serum glutamic oxaloacetic transaminase (SGOT), blood urea nitrogen (BUN), glucose, white blood cell (WBC) count, and plasma pH. The goal of the study was to find methods that could identify animals that are more likely to develop CM and require treatment prior to release.

Of the fatalities observed, 5% (2 of 40) had been captured by the net gun, and fewer than 4% (1 of 27) by drive net. Two animals that died within a month of release in the follow-up group also had been caught with the net gun. The single surviving CM case had been captured by the net gun (Kock et al., 1987a).

In the same study, the physiological parameters (temperature, pulse, and respiration), selected biochemical parameters (cortisol, CPK, SGOT, LDH, alkaline phosphatase, potassium, sodium, chloride, creatinine, BUN, selenium, glucose, total protein, plasma pH, and plasma carbon dioxide levels) and selected hematological parameters (packed cell volume, hemoglobin, red blood cell count, and WBC count) were compared among bighorn sheep captured by the four methods.

Biological parameters affected by stress, including temperature, respiration, cortisol, CPK, SGOT, potassium, glucose, and WBCs revealed significant differences among capture methods. Some blood parameter differences, including temperature, respiration, cortisol, glucose, and WBCs, could be explained partially by the distribution of age and sex within capture method groups. Drop net and net gun methods of capture appeared to produce the least amount of alteration to biological parameters related to capture stress and capture mortality. The drive net was similar to the former methods, while chemical immobilization caused the greatest alterations in the physiological, biochemical, and hematological parameters (Kock et al., 1987c).

The net gun was found to have considerable advantages over the use of ground nets and chemical immobilization methods for capturing bighorn sheep. The use of the net gun resulted in the lowest proportion of compromised sheep (11%, or 15/137), no CM mortality, and a 2% (2/137) accidental mortality. The use of drop nets resulted in 15% compromised sheep (24/158), a CM mortality rate of 2% (3/158), and an accidental mortality rate of 1% (2/158) (Kock et al., 1987b).

A similar proportion of sheep were compromised with the drive nets (16%, 39/249), which also had the highest CM mortality rate at 3% (7/249) and an acci-

dental mortality rate of less than 1% (2/249). Chemical immobilization resulted in the most compromised sheep at 19% (17/90), a CM mortality rate of 2% (2/90), and the most accidental deaths at 6% (5/90). Drop nets and drive nets were comparable when combining total mortality with rates for compromised bighorn sheep, 18% and 19%, respectively (29/158 and 48/249). Chemical immobilization had the highest combined measure of risk at 27% (24/90) and net gun the lowest at 12% (17/137) (Kock et al., 1987b).

CHEMICAL RESTRAINT IN TLAER

Veterinarians have access to a number of very effective sedatives, particularly for horses. Some of these pharmaceuticals are found in the barns and trailers of animal owners. Nonveterinary personnel should not be allowed to administer these medications to animals without veterinary supervision. Each drug poses the risk of side effects for each species, and the veterinarian is trained to be aware of these risks, consider the risk/benefit of these effects, and be prepared to treat complications as they occur. Furthermore, a number of pharmaceuticals acting on the central nervous system are also controlled substances. What may be an effective dose for a horse may not be effective when administered to a zebra or a cow. If the owner has already administered medications to the animal, they should inform the veterinarian immediately upon his or her arrival.

Sedation is unnecessary and not recommended for some animals. If the animal is geriatric, exhibiting clinical signs of shock, or standing in water, sedation should be avoided unless the veterinarian on the scene determines that it is absolutely necessary. Sedated animals lower their heads. If the animal is standing in water, the handler will need to support the animal's head and neck to prevent it from drowning—they can drown in depths in which humans can stand (Figure 6.3).

There will be TLAER situations where no human can or should get in the same space with the animal to employ physical restraint (e.g., inside an overturned trailer, down in a well, etc.). The responders should evaluate the possible use of chemical restraint for these scenarios in consultation with a veterinarian.

There can be severe risk of injury if the animal prematurely awakens from the sedation. It may resume struggling or make violent attempts to escape, placing the animal handler in peril. Veterinarians and their staff are trained to evaluate the animal's level of sedation and can provide additional sedative when necessary. Unexpected behavior during sedation can occur and illustrates the importance of using live animals in training. Responders should never assume that a sedated horse cannot react and kick with great force and accuracy.

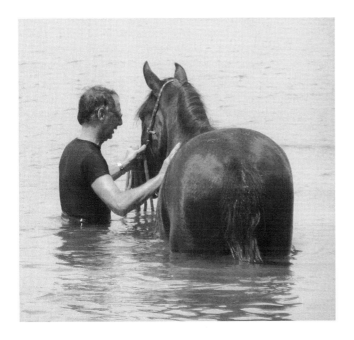

Figure 6.3 *A horse trapped in water should be carefully evaluated before sedation is considered, because the sedated horse could drown if its head drops below the water level. Here the animal is haltered for primary restraint, and the handler is staying in a safe position. Responders should consider using an inner tube to provide floatation for the horse's head. Courtesy of Rebecca Gimenez.*

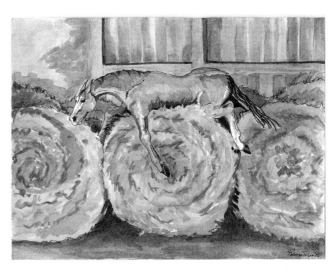

Figure 6.4 *A horse that climbed on top of a hay bale attempting to reach better-quality hay appears to be an easy rescue. However, when approached, the animal may struggle and represent a challenge to the animal handler to halter and restrain while responders remove bales to free the animal. Alternatively, using the front legs as anchor points is risky unless the horse is very cooperative. Courtesy of Becky Tolson.*

Recovery from Sedation or Anesthesia

Once the animal has been extricated, it should be allowed to rest until it rises on its own. If the animal has been sedated or anesthetized, it should be maintained in as relaxed and quiet an environment as possible until it is awake and strong enough to get up on its own. Large animals can be injured when waking up from sedation; if they attempt to stand before they can support themselves, they can fracture their neck or a limb. When the animal is ready to rise, the handler should give the animal sufficient freedom to move its head and neck to be able to find balance as it rises.

PHYSICAL RESTRAINT

Initially, the best restraint method may be to avoid approaching the animal until experienced personnel arrive on the scene. If the animal is to be approached, responders should select a simple physical restraint method until the veterinarian arrives and can provide advice on further restraint methods.

Simple Methods

Simple methods should be used to allow the animal(s) to remain calm. A prey animal can often be calmed by allowing it to eat; responders should provide forage in the form of grass, hay, or alfalfa. If a herd of cattle is loose, allowing them to graze until an adequate number of personnel are on the scene facilitates herding them toward containment and safety. In addition, responders should encourage all personnel (including bystanders) on the scene to talk in low tones and remain as quiet as possible.

Halter and Lead Rope

A halter is important for guidance and restraint of the animal victim, but it is never intended to be used as an anchor point during a rescue. An animal, like a human, should never be pulled by its head and neck because serious injury could result.

Rescuers should not negate the ability of the animal to use its head and neck. Jerking on the animal's head will cause injury, and steady pressure may induce the animal to fight the pressure. Smaller species may be coerced to move when enough pulling power is applied, but large animals have leverage, height, and weight advantages over responders. If the responders are positioned above the animal, gravity provides an additional advantage to the animal.

ANCHOR POINTS IN RESCUE

Unacceptable Anchor Points

Rescuers should apply standards of rescue that maximize the medical chances of the victim's survival and that will minimize injury. With the exception of a victim in dorsal recumbency, applying rescue equipment to the most fragile parts of a large animal (i.e., the lower legs, head, and neck) should be avoided (Figure 6.4).

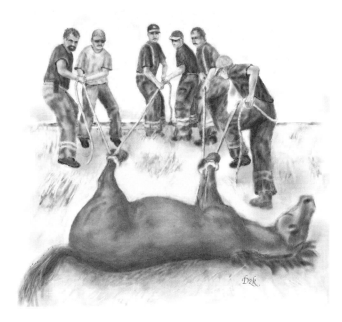

Figure 6.5 *Responders attempt to drag a sedated horse out of a ditch using the lower legs. Although the pastern may appear to be a readily available and functional handle, placing ropes can be dangerous to personnel. Pulling a horse by the pasterns may cause severe trauma to the animal. If lower legs must be used, add padding to protect the limbs. Courtesy of Michael Dzurak.*

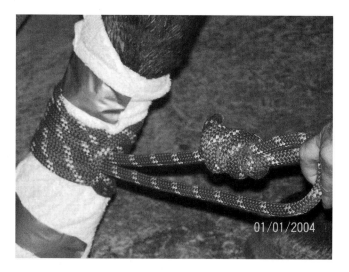

Figure 6.6 *When the torso cannot be used as a safe anchor point for a rescue, applying a Prusik loop to the leg over padding is an effective field expedient. Multiple loops will further spread the pressure across the limb surface, minimizing injury. Courtesy of Rebecca Gimenez.*

The Lower Limbs. Although the anatomy of the lower limb appears suitable for anchoring ropes (especially the pastern), a cow or horse's lower limb is not a handle. A reflex reaction, called the withdrawal response, produces strong contraction of the limbs in response to strong tension; thus, the animal will reflexively fight the restraints. Placing ropes or webbing on the lower limbs requires close proximity to the animal's limbs; this can be very dangerous, especially in recumbent animals. If the lower limbs must be used, rescuers should ensure sufficient protection and increase the contact area of the rope or webbing with the skin, while supporting the head and neck (Figure 6.5).

Horse skin is approximately the same thickness as human skin. On the lower limbs, the absence of muscle or fat increases the risk of injury to the animal's soft tissues (including ligaments, tendons, blood vessels, and nerves). The animal's hair may obscure visible lesions from kicks, rope burns, bumps, bruises, etc.; however, the lack of a visible skin wound does not preclude a deeper injury.

When the animal is trapped in dorsal recumbency (the animal is on its back), the lower legs are often the only anchor points available for rescue. In this case, padded webbing should be used to maximize the surface area of the rescue material in contact with the skin (see Chapter 15). In the absence of webbing, wrapping a Prusik hitch around the lower limb over padding

from a shirt or towel is a field-expedient method of using rope that allows increased surface area and protection to the leg (Figure 6.6).

Degloving injuries are avulsions of skin and a variable amount of soft tissues. These injuries frequently occur when an animal's hoof or foot becomes entrapped by sharp objects (e.g., wire fencing, hard plastic, metal, etc.). The animal's struggles to free the limb against the sharp edges shears the skin and tissues of the lower limb away from the bone; this effort can literally rip the skin and deeper tissues off of the lower limb.

The Head and Neck. The head and neck of large animals are not appropriate anchor points. There are documented cases of animals suffering neurological injury from pressure placed on the head and neck in rescue scenarios. The opposition reflex will cause the animal to fight the well-intentioned restraint and pressure. Using a rope (e.g., lasso or noose) to pull the animal by the neck or for rescue purposes is an unprofessional approach to TLAER (Figure 6.7). The author has documented numerous incidents where the animal survived a incident, only to be strangulated by well-intentioned but unknowledgeable rescuers. For example, a cattle owner applied a power winch cable in a cinch configuration around the neck of a cow stuck in mud. Before the winch could be stopped, the animal was decapitated by the cable.

The ears of donkeys and pigs are not suitable anchor points. Ears are composed of cartilage and skin and can be permanently damaged by excessive pressure, tension, or twisting.

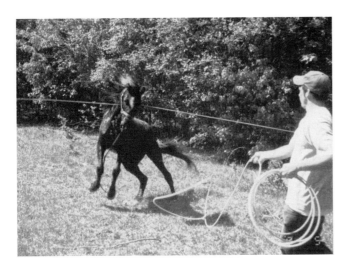

Figure 6.7 *A mustang is roped by numerous cowboys and fights the pressure around its neck. This is not an acceptable method of restraint in TLAER and may contribute to injuries. Courtesy of Tomas Gimenez.*

Rescue Anchor Points on a Large Animal

Regardless of the incident environment, freeing a large animal means that it needs to be moved up, down, forward, backward, or to the side. With the exception of an animal in dorsal recumbency, moving a large animal in any of these directions can be safely accomplished by attaching webbing around either the chest or posterior abdomen/pelvis, or both portions of the torso (see Chapters 15 and 16).

POSITION AND TIMING

Contrary to instincts, the safest place responders can be is well out of the animal's way or in close contact with the animal at its shoulder. Unless proximity to the animal is necessary, rescuers should remain out of range of the animal's teeth and limbs. As stated in Chapter 4, the energy delivered by a striking or kicking limb is increased as momentum and muscle contraction force the limb away from the body; responders in close proximity to the animal are less likely to be injured because of the lower forces at that distance. The conscientious use of handles, canes, and other physical extensions of the responders' arms (Figure 6.8) should be employed to minimize the risk of getting kicked while placing an appliance, especially with animals below ground level and those demonstrating fearful behavior (Figure 6.9). (See Chapter 15.)

Reaction Time

As previously stated, the reaction times of prey species are faster than human reaction times. Studies in horses revealed that the response to noxious stimuli differed between the forelimbs and hind limbs. In response to electrode stimulation, forelimb responses (e.g., lifting

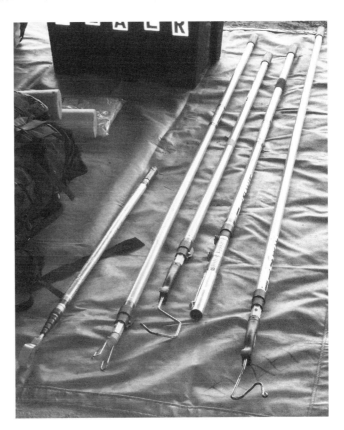

Figure 6.8 *Basic safety equipment that serves as an extension of the arm can allow personnel to place equipment from a safe distance, particularly on recumbent animals. Left to right: A long piece of 10 cm (4 in.) webbing can be thrown or unrolled; an aluminum golf ball retriever can extend up to 7 m (23 ft) to pick up pilot lines under trailers; painter's poles as the platform for three different interchangeable tips (push pole, S-hook, and carabineer hold-open); a boat hook has various uses to push or pull objects and webbing; a simple aluminum cane with a rubber handle makes an excellent leg or webbing handler while the operator can remain at a distance. Courtesy of Axel Gimenez.*

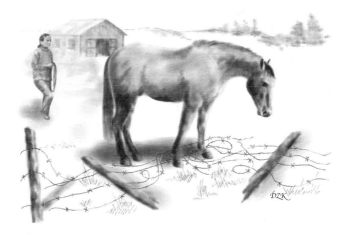

Figure 6.9 *A horse trapped in a barbed wire fence is a dangerous scenario for the animal handler who is approaching to assist and restrain the animal. While the handler is attempting to halter the animal and help it, the animal may move and further entangle and injure itself. Caution should be used when cutting barbed wire because the wire may recoil when tension is released. Courtesy of Michael Dzurak.*

the limb) were significantly faster than hind limb responses. The strength of the stimulus required to elicit a response from a hind limb was more than twice the strength to elicit a response from a forelimb, but the behavioral reaction to hind limb stimulation was significantly stronger (Spadavecchia et al., 2003). Humans working with prey species, particularly fearful prey species, should be cognizant of the rapid reaction times and pronounced behavioral reactions. The hind limbs of prey species have evolved to provide powerful propulsion during flight efforts; this powerful musculature also imparts extremely powerful force to kicks.

Many researchers have confirmed that the reaction to sound is faster than the reaction to light; mean auditory reaction times range from 140 to 160 milliseconds and visual reaction times range from 180 to 200 milliseconds (Galton, 1899; Woodworth and Schlosberg, 1954; von Fieandt et al., 1956; Welford, 1980; Brebner and Welford, 1980). The difference in these times may be due to the time required for the stimulus to reach the brain from the sensory organ; an auditory stimulus requires 8–10 milliseconds to reach the brain (Kemp, 1973), but a visual stimulus requires 20–40 milliseconds (Marshall et al., 1943). Reaction time to touch is intermediate, at 155 milliseconds (Robinson, 1934). Once a sound stimulus has been transmitted, the brain still must process the stimulus, determine an appropriate reaction, and command the muscles to respond. The conduction speed of signals in the brain is approximately 100 m per second, and decreases to approximately 70 m per second in the peripheral nervous system (to the limbs). Assuming an average height of 1.8 m (approximately 6 ft), 0.026 seconds elapse as the brain transmits the signal to the feet.

Several studies have determined that the time for human motor preparation (e.g., tensing muscles) and motor response (in this case, pressing the spacebar on a keyboard) was the same in all three types (auditory, touch, visual) of reaction time tests, implying that the differences in reaction time were due to processing time (Miller and Low, 2001). Differences in reaction time between these types of stimuli persist whether the subject is asked to make a simple response or a complex response (Sanders, 1998). Most of these studies were conducted on athletes and subjects that were trained to react to the stimuli.

A scared running horse can cover approximately 16.5 m (54 ft) in one second, and their stride length ranges from 3 to 9 m (10–30 ft). The prey animal's reaction time is approximately half of a human's 180–200 millisecond reaction time, emphasizing that a human is not likely to be able to move rapidly enough to escape injury from a surging horse. A healthy horse can rise from lateral recumbency (flat on its side) to a standing position in less than one second, often

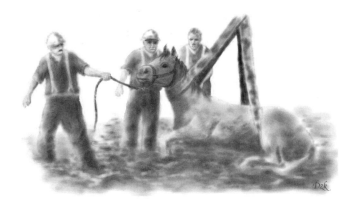

Figure 6.10   *A horse being assisted to its feet using improper modifications of the simple web sling. Placing the webbing under the neck for a vertical lift can cause injury to the neck structures and pulling on the head at the same time is counterproductive because it does not permit the animal to balance itself. Courtesy of Michael Dzurak.*

before the handler has realized the animal is attempting to stand.

Assisting Animals

Large animals use their heads and necks to maintain their balance; these structures constitute 10% of the animal's total body weight. Freedom of head and neck movement is an essential component of forward movement. An animal that is healthy should not be prevented from using its head and neck to climb a steep bank or hill or to rise from a recumbent position. A halter and lead rope are important to help maintain control of a horse and to prevent it from leaving the scene of an incident, but should not be used as rescue anchor points (Figure 6.10). Horses and cattle do not stand or walk well on asphalt or flat, slick surfaces, nor do they negotiate stairs and ramps well. A simple solution includes placing rugs across the slick surface (e.g., trailer sidewalls, etc.) or floors. Llamas can negotiate difficult or slick terrain more adequately than cattle and horses because of the pads on their feet.

CONDITIONING AND PREVENTION FOR LARGE ANIMAL OWNERS

Low-stress handling methods and desensitization of large prey species reduce the risks of injury to humans and animals and can have a positive effect on production and performance. For example, a cattle farm in Clifton, Tennessee, features a program of LSS handling methods for their 30-plus cow and calf operation. The program includes regular movement of the herd through the chute and head gate system without subjecting the cows to procedures. This desensitizes the animals to physical restraint and confinement, regular handling of young stock by personnel, low-stress weaning procedures, and early acclimatization to encourage the herd to come when called (for grain, range cubes, or movement to fresh pasture). This farmer's young cattle are in high demand at sale time, and all heifers are purchased directly from the farm by local operations (Dzurak, 2006).

Animals that are accustomed to being caught, safely led, and loaded in a trailer (e.g., in darkness, wind, heavy rain, etc.) will be more likely to survive because they can be efficiently evacuated. Desensitized animals are less likely to exhibit a panic response to frightening situations. In addition, a calm and quiet approach by rescuers reduces the risk of a panic response. For example, one of the author's horses became entrapped by 40 m (132 ft) of rolled up wire in a strange pasture. Walking into the pasture, the owner saw the horse standing quietly and uninjured, with both front legs wrapped in woven wire fence. The owner was able to call for help to cut the wire from the animal's limbs and back her calmly out of the wire.

These scenarios demonstrate the benefits of desensitization. When a horse (which had been imprinted and desensitized) rolled over and became cast with his legs through a fence, a friend discovered the animal. Recumbent animals may exhibit a panic response when approached by a perceived predator (such as an unfamiliar human); using a calm, quiet approach, the person was able to approach the horse, avoid its panic response, and restrain it until assistance could arrive. Once the horse was free from its entrapment, it rose uninjured and ran off.

METHODS OF PHYSICAL RESTRAINT

As a general rule, responders should use the minimal amount of restraint needed for that situation and that individual animal. Proper physical restraint should be the first method employed, and chemical restraint should be used only when necessary. A twitch or Scotch hobble is not necessary for every horse encountered on TLAER scenes. If the animal is recumbent and exhausted, there may be no need for physical or chemical restraint. If an animal is sedated, it is less likely to be able to participate in its own rescue. Unsedated animals are better able to respond with physical effort when asked; if the animal is cooperating with the handler, it should be rewarded by relaxing the pressure.

The next rule is to use the maximum amount of restraint that is needed for rescuers to remain safe when working with an aggressive or unpredictable animal. When working with large animals, responders should understand the industry standards for handling livestock and horses: 10 cm (4 in.) steel tubing and 2.5 cm

(1 in.) steel panels between the animal and all personnel. When handling exotic animals, increased protection for the humans is required. Adult buffalo and zebras routinely destroy conventional livestock facilities (Dennis, 2003). Although these standards provide adequate protection for responders and are desirable, they are often not practical or available on a rescue scene. Available safety equipment and field-expedient obstacles should be used.

Halter and Lead Rope
In horses and show cattle that allow themselves to be caught, the simplest and best form of physical restraint is a good quality halter and lead rope. Although no human can safely hold onto a truly terrified prey animal, a halter and long lead rope provide the best physical restraint possible to keep the handler and animal connected.

Secondary Containment
To prevent animals from leaving the scene after they have been rescued, responders should consider containment around the scene with portable fencing, cattle panels, or fladry (see Chapter 8).

Shoulder Twitch
The shoulder twitch is a favorite for horse owners because it is simple, easily learned, and can be performed from a safe position near the shoulder. This technique is not recommended for use on any other large animal—cattle skin is too thick for this technique, and grasping the skin of llamas, sheep, or goats in this way will injure them.

To achieve this twitch, one should grasp a piece of shoulder skin with the fingers along the line of the shoulder, a very obvious area of the horse. Grasp a 10–15 cm (4–6 in.) square section of skin and roll it slightly over the knuckles. This is an acupressure point and will distract the horse. The technique allows flexibility; the handler can increase pressure by rolling the skin around the knuckles, or release pressure (by partially unrolling the skin) to reward the animal when it is cooperating.

Young Animal Restraint
Young prey species are often underestimated. Despite their smaller stature, young animals are capable of inducing severe injury. In addition, young animals that have not been handled may panic in response to restraint attempts. Although some young animals may be wearing halters, they are not broken to the lead and will fight pressure on the halter. These animals are most efficiently restrained with a firm "hug,"

with one arm around the animal's chest and the other around its buttocks or gently grasping and lifting the tail at a 90-degree angle. Excessive pressure on the tail or head may induce a form of cataplexy, where the foal collapses in the handler's arms; as soon as pressure is relieved, the animal will often struggle.

This restraint technique is more difficult in larger foals and calves due to the strength of their struggles. Therefore, it should not be considered a long-term restraint option.

Contralateral Limb Lift

Distracting a horse by forcing it to concentrate on balance can also be effective in certain situations. The contralateral limb lift technique is often used by veterinarians and is performed by picking up and holding a front leg off the ground. Obviously, this technique is risky on an aggressive, panicking, biting, or kicking animal because it places the handler in close proximity to the limbs. It is also possible to use a hobble strap to hold up the front leg. This technique is based on methods used in Australia to teach an aggressive horse to yield to the trainer; the horse reportedly realizes that the person has the power to prevent the animal from taking flight; this is a rather nonaggressive way for the human to assume the alpha leader position. Hobble straps should only be used by advanced animal handlers. Responders should be aware that lifting a mule's or donkey's front leg will not prevent it from kicking with a hind limb.

Recumbent Animal Restraint

It is sometimes easier and safer to force foals and calves to lie down and then use a person's body weight to restrain the animal. Recumbent prey animals are still extremely strong, and their instinctive drive to rise and stand can increase the strength of their struggles. On the other hand, some animals relax completely once they realize that they are overpowered. However, stimulation with pressure or loud noises will often cause the animal to rise (or attempt to do so).

There is a theory that a person can keep a recumbent horse down by placing a knee on the muscle of the animal's neck (without obstructing the trachea and carotid artery or jugular vein) and tilting the animal's nose upward by grasping the cheek piece or nose piece of the halter (Figure 6.11). Reality has shown that a seven-month-old, 250 kg (550 lb) horse is capable of throwing two firefighters off and rising to a standing position in less than one second. When attempting to restrain recumbent animals, handlers should protect their face so they are not hit in the head by flailing limbs or the thrashing of the animal's head.

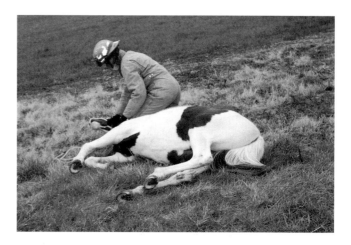

Figure 6.11 *Personnel can encourage recumbent horses to remain recumbent by kneeling and placing body weight on the neck and tipping the horse's nose upward using the halter. The animal handler must be aware of the potential danger posed by the struggling hind limbs. Courtesy of Axel Gimenez.*

Twitches

The upper lip twitch is the most commonly used means of physical restraint of horses (Figure 6.12). There are several types of twitch available, including rope twitches, chain twitches, and humane twitches (with several variations). Twitches can be dangerous when used by an inexperienced animal handler; if the animal suddenly pulls away and the twitch handle is pulled from the handler's grip, the swinging free end of the twitch can induce severe injury before the other end dislodges from the horse's upper lip. Fatalities have occurred when handlers—or bystanders—were struck in the head by a loose twitch. A twitch with a 1.5 m (5 ft) handle increases the chance that the handler will be able to maintain a grip on the device.

Twitches are effective when appropriately used. These devices apply pressure on an acupressure point, inducing the release of endorphins that induce a euphoria-like state of relaxation. Some horses have learned to anticipate the application of the twitch and are adept at avoiding placement on the upper lip. A small population of horses violently resist the application of a twitch and may strike, rear, or bite.

The pressure on a lip twitch cannot be released to reward good behavior. This device should be applied for a limited time period (10–15 minutes) because it can act as a tourniquet. Once the upper lip has become numb from decreased blood flow, the acupressure and sedation effect of the twitch ceases.

The Stablizer acts on similar principles and is available in several sizes to accommodate a variety of head sizes. This device applies pressure on the gums above the teeth and below the upper lip simultaneously with pressure on the poll area directly behind the animal's ears. The authors have used this device on numerous

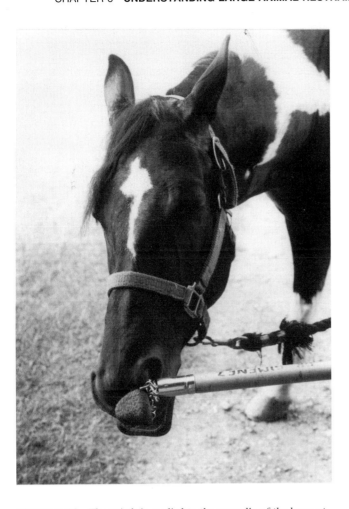

Figure 6.12 *The twitch is applied to the upper lip of the horse at an acupressure point; this causes an animal to relax and accept some procedures that may be slightly uncomfortable. Only experienced animal handlers should use this method and for limited time periods, because the effect will be lost when the lip becomes numb from congestion of blood flow. Courtesy of Tomas Gimenez.*

occasions in training and live rescue scenarios and consider it to be an underused physical restraint tool that responders should consider a suitable alternative to standard twitches or chains.

Lip, Nose, and Chin Chains

Lip, mouth, and under- or over-the-nose halter chains are other devices that are commonly used in the horse industry but should be avoided by inexperienced handlers. The lip chain consists of a piece of small-gauge chain passing underneath the horse's top lip at the gum line and from one side of the halter to the other. The over-the-nose chain passes from one side of the halter over the nose and attaches to the other side of the halter. The under-the-nose, or chin chain, passes from one side of the halter underneath the horse's jaw and fastens on the opposite side of the halter. A mouth chain passes from one side through the horse's mouth (where a bit would be located) and fastens on the opposite side.

When improperly applied, these methods can be inhumane. A gentle tug on the chain is usually all that is required; jerking or sharply pulling on the chain is painful for the horse and may cause the animal to back up, rear, strike, or paw. If the horse reacts violently to the pressure, it may rear up, lose its balance, fall over backward, and sustain severe (and possibly fatal) injuries. Similarly, these methods should be used with caution in areas with low ceilings; if the horse rears in response to pressure, it can sustain a severe cranial injury if its skull impacts a low beam, ceiling, or low-hanging object.

Ear Twist

Twisting a prey species' ears is not an acceptable means of physical restraint. The technique is often very effective in temporarily immobilizing the animal, but it is considered inhumane by most owners and professionals because it is very painful for the animal. It is possible to damage or break the cartilage in the ears of pigs, cows, or horses. Historically, some handlers would bite the animal's ear with their teeth; this can be very dangerous for the handler and is very painful for the animal.

Nose Tongs

Nose tongs have been used for many years by the cattle industry to restrain the head while the animal is caught in a head gate or squeeze chute. They act by placing pressure on very sensitive areas inside both nostrils. The use of this device is not encouraged or recommended in TLAER scenarios.

Scotch Hobble

The Scotch hobble is a commonly used method of physical restraint, particularly for the castration of large male animals; use of these hobbles allows access to the testicles with reduced risk of being kicked by the rear legs. It is an advanced form of restraint that should only be used by animal handlers with significant experience. A rope loop is tied around the animal's lower neck and another loop to the pastern of one of the rear legs (on the recumbent animal, the "up" limb).

Barrel Hitch

In cattle and other ruminants, a barrel hitch of rope, starting with a loop around the neck and hitched around the animal's abdomen at the level of the sternum and the hips, provides a method for recumbent restraint. When the free end is pulled, the pressure placed on the animal's back and abdomen will induce it to lie down and remain recumbent until the pressure is released. TLAER instructors have used this method to allow students to manipulate webbing onto recumbent demonstration animals without using sedation or other physical restraint on the animals (Figure 6.13).

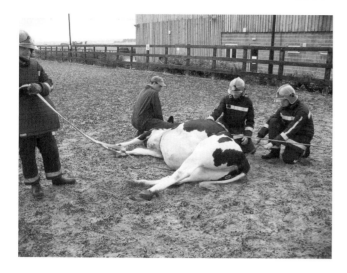

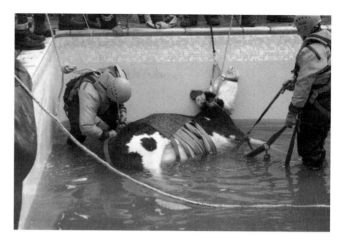

Figure 6.13 A demonstration dairy cow is laid down using the barrel hitch method to allow students in the United Kingdom to practice the emplacement of webbing in the Hampshire slip configuration. As long as tension is maintained on the free end of the rope, the animal will stay down. Courtesy of Paul Baker.

Figure 6.14 A beef cow that fell into a suburban pool is anesthetized by a veterinarian and readied for vertical lift. The level of the water in the pool was lowered by the responding fire department to prevent the animal from drowning, and the head is supported by responders. Courtesy of Paul Baker.

COMBINING PHYSICAL AND CHEMICAL RESTRAINT

Neither physical nor chemical restraint will completely stop an animal from injuring itself or humans. Some species and individual animals metabolize drugs at different rates from others; similarly, a drug that is effective in one species may have absolutely no effect on another. Responders should remember that the industry standard includes steel chutes, panels, and stocks to handle large animals. If responders are not separated from a large animal by an inch or more of solid steel, they are risking their life unless there is an adequate safety plan in place. Animal handling experience does not completely protect handlers from injury; humans are injured or killed every year while performing routine procedures on animals. All person-

nel involved in a TLAER situation should remain vigilant at all times. The induction of general anesthesia by a veterinarian may be necessary in some cases to ensure the safety of responding personnel as well as the animal (Figure 6.14).

ACRONYMS USED IN CHAPTER 6

BUN   Blood urea nitrogen
CM   Capture myopathy
CPK   Creatinine phosphokinase
LDH   Lactic dehydrogenase
LSS   Low stress stock [handling]
SGOT   Serum glutamic oxaloacetic transaminase
TLAER Technical large animal emergency rescue
WBC   White blood cell

7 Water and Unstable Ground Rescues

Dr. Rebecca Gimenez

INTRODUCTION

Swiftwater, floodwater, ice, and mud rescue environments are extremely dangerous and represent some of the most hazardous and unknown conditions rescuers will encounter. The addition of large animal victim(s) with their inherent danger and unpredictability makes large animal incidents of this type more hazardous and demands a high level of training, appropriate equipment, prioritization, and preparation on a local basis (Figure 7.1). Measures that could prevent many of these tragedies include fencing off pond or river access, riders staying on the trail, and crossing only at safe fording areas.

Any large animal emergency or disaster scenario that involves water hazards should be considered the most difficult and potentially dangerous scenario. Paradoxically, these may also be the most urgent of all rescue scenarios due to the threat of drowning, incoming tides, water current, hypothermia, or asphyxiation by the pressure of mud. Many water scenarios (floodwaters, ice, mud, quiet ponds, or swiftwater) contain unexpected and unique hazards for both trained and untrained rescuers.

WATER RESCUE PHILOSOPHY

The building blocks of any successful rescue include training, practice, experience, and good judgment (Ray, 1999). The types of rescue considered for these environments should be prioritized and a "go" or "no go" decision made based on the risk assessment, personnel and equipment available, the existing conditions, the physical health and behavior of the animal victim, and the difficulty in operation of the equipment and of the necessary techniques required to rescue the animal. The procedures in this chapter should not be attempted by personnel without certified training in water (swiftwater and floodwater) rescue, and/or surface ice rescue. Certified personnel should update their certifications regularly.

The Current State of Training

Human rescue training is available in swiftwater or floodwater rescue and safety as well as surface ice rescue. These courses teach the student to be aware of the unexpected; reinforce options for self-rescue; and present victim rescue strategies at the awareness, operational, and technical levels. An operational and technical swiftwater or surface ice rescue course (e.g., Sierra Rescue, Rescue Three International) allows students to practice methods for rescuing human victims; unfortunately, most of these methods are not applicable to large animals.

A technical animal rescue course (with emphasis on small animal concerns) involving swiftwater, low-angle rappel, and floodwater aspects has been offered as a three-day course through Code 3 Associates, Rescue Three International, and the American Humane Association since the 1990s. In 2005, these organizations began to offer large animal rescue training as an optional fourth day of the course.

Animal victims of emergencies and disasters are rarely considered or discussed in mainstream training books, standard operating procedure, or materials used as references or instructional manuals by the fire service and other emergency responders. Prioritization of rescue methods is never more important than when ice, swiftwater, and floodwaters are involved in the scenario. Improved techniques and awareness of challenges and dangers inherent with water rescue are required for responder teams to practice and enact (Figure 7.2).

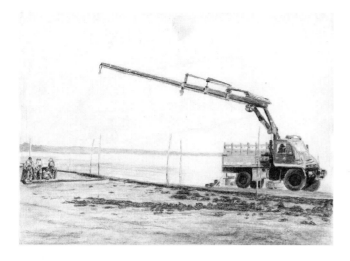

Figure 7.1 *The use of an extendable crane and plywood on the surface of tidal mud to reach the animal is demonstrated in this rescue scenario. The injection of air or water next to the extremities using a mud lance is simultaneous with the vertical lift or horizontal haul and negates the suction effect of the mud. These incidents are hazardous, and an appropriate response requires proper training and equipment. Courtesy of Julie Casil.*

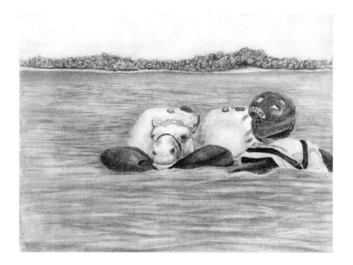

Figure 7.2 *Maintaining a large animal's head above the water surface is critical in water rescue scenarios. Flotation devices must provide good flotation to the animal's head and neck. In field testing, any device that allowed a sling under the animal to support its weight between air logs or hoses and provided flotation under the head was effective. Courtesy of Julie Casil.*

Water and unstable ground scenarios affect large numbers of animals and livestock, demonstrated by Hurricane Katrina in 2005. Floods can kill large numbers of livestock (90,000 beef cattle in 1997 in the Midwest; 1,200 dairy cattle in Oregon in 1996; more than 3,000 dairy cattle in Washington in 1991; Heath, 1999). Forty of the 100 counties in North Carolina were affected by flooding from Hurricane Floyd in 1999, with a total estimate of $13 million in livestock losses (Hudson

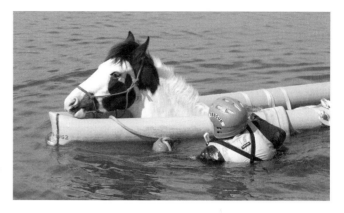

Figure 7.3 *Once the animal has been brought to a water depth where it can stand, the animal handler should restrain the animal while operational personnel remove the floatation device and other equipment. In this training scenario in Kentucky, the handler is bringing the animal toward shore. Courtesy of Axel Gimenez.*

et al., 2001). Although the total number of livestock deaths "represented a small percentage . . . when compared with North Carolina's total livestock population" (NCDA&CS, 1999), there were numerous valuable livestock and companion animals lost in these disasters.

Attitudes

Flooding is the single most frequent and widespread disaster and emergency situation both in the United States and abroad, and it can account for high numbers of human and animal losses. Flooding can occur anywhere; this is often overlooked by humans who do not live near bodies of water. There are numerous videos and pictures from flood and swiftwater rescue attempts over the last 25 years, many of which have served as examples of improperly executed and inadequately planned rescue methods. For example, four people in a bass boat entering the Mississippi River during its flood phase in 1993 to save a drowning animal is a reminder of the need for training and awareness and of the difficulty of handling large animals when water environments are encountered (Figure 7.3).

General information about flooding deaths from the Centre for Research on the Epidemiology of Disasters (CRED) database is available. The Office of U.S. Foreign Disaster Assistance/CRED International Disaster Database contains essential core data on the occurrence and effects of over 12,800 mass disasters in the world from 1900 to the present.

Due to media coverage of Hurricane Katrina and similar disaster events, many people tend to erroneously think that a major hurricane or long-term heavy rain is necessary to cause local flooding. Flash flooding is a common event in desert areas such as the southwestern United States; rainstorms miles away drain quickly across the flat ground to flood channels and can cause unexpected downstream flooding on an apparently sunny day. A beaver dam or poorly constructed human dam can burst and flood everything downstream. These types of flash floods can cause destruction of permanent structures and fencing and will frequently displace large animals.

Farmers in the Amazon Basin of South America experience flooding of their homes and pastures for three to six months of the year. They have learned to mitigate the damage and prevent livestock loss during the wet season by placing their cattle on large rafts of trees strapped together, delivering forage to their animals daily. This demonstrates the value of preparedness and mitigation.

WHERE ANGELS (SHOULD) FEAR TO TREAD

Trained firefighters and emergency personnel have drowned in swiftwater, ice, and floodwater environments. In 2005, the total number of U.S. on-duty firefighter fatalities was 106, including 2 deaths from drowning (1.88%). This reflects the 1.7% trend demonstrated by the 19 on-duty firefighter deaths that occurred between 1990 and 2005 due to drowning in water rescue operations (floodwater, swiftwater, and SCUBA dive operations) (FEMA, 2007). Although the UK firefighting community lost 1 on-duty member to drowning between 1999 and 2002, 13 others nearly drowned during this period (Health and Safety Executive, 2003).

Even in developed countries, drowning is among the top four causes of accidental human death. Approximately 500,000 people drown each year worldwide; many of these deaths are in undeveloped countries and result from natural disasters. A startling number of fire and police personnel worldwide are nonswimmers or weak swimmers (Advanced Rescue Technology, 2004). According to the Centers for Disease Control, more lives are lost in the United States each year to drowning than to fire. In 2002, 2,670 people were killed in fires (not including firefighters), compared to 3,281 accidental drownings and an additional 519 boating accident-related drownings reported by the U.S. Coast Guard (Rigg, 2005).

A study of 2,213 flood fatalities in Australia that occurred between 1788 and 1996 (Coates, 1999) discusses the causes of death and indicates the hazards associated with the rescue process: of the total deaths, 6.1% occurred while being rescued, 1.4% of deaths were rescue personnel, and 3.4% of the fatalities were volunteer rescuers. The disparity between the numbers of professional versus volunteer rescuers killed is directly related to training; a higher death rate was observed in untrained individuals. Interestingly, the study also showed that 8.3% of the fatalities occurred when victims attempted to retrieve stock or property (Coates, 1999).

Flash flood-related fatalities in the United States have been well documented (Jonkman, 2003). Annually, 23%–43% of people in the United States killed in flash flooding is due to persons being swept into the water (French et al., 1983; Mooney, 1983). Fatalities due to rescue efforts were reported to be 2%–3% (Mooney, 1983; French et al., 1983). The U.S. National Weather Service data sheets on 571 flash flood fatalities for the period 1995–2000 show similar patterns with respect to causes of death (Jonkman, 2003).

Five of 52 (10%) human deaths after Hurricane Floyd (1999) were rescue workers. The leading cause of death after the disaster was drowning, and 24 (67%) deaths involved occupants of motor vehicles trapped in floodwaters. Seven deaths occurred during transport by boat; flotation devices were not worn by any of the decedents (MMWR, 2000).

There is very little data available on the number of horse and livestock owners who drown working with livestock or riding animals (Figure 7.4). One study from Oklahoma covering the period 1988–1994 found that 5% of riding fatalities were due to drowning (eight total) while on horseback (Shariat, 1996). Of these four occurred in a pond (chasing a bull, breaking a horse, or moving cattle), one in a river, and one in a flooded pasture. Two were linked to the horse wearing a tie-down so that it could not lift its head; both the horse and the human died. Four of the riders who drowned were nonswimmers; in two cases flooding was a contributory factor (Kola, 1996). A North Carolina study reported two riding-associated drowning fatalities in a 10-year period (MMWR, 1990).

As an example of the danger, in one Oklahoma incident a 29-year-old man and family members were riding horses in rising floodwater, herding cattle to

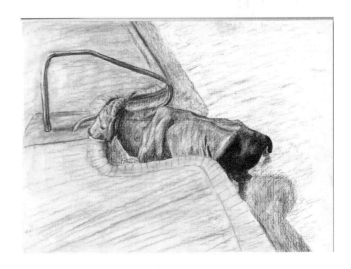

Figure 7.4 *A cow in a suburban backyard pool is a water-related rescue scenario that represents danger to well-meaning bystanders. Without assistance, most animals cannot climb the steps and may exhaust themselves swimming or struggling in deep water. Courtesy of Julie Casil.*

higher ground. The man's horse was standing in what appeared to be shallow water in a flooded pasture. The horse stepped into a drop-off and fell, throwing the rider from the saddle and into the rising water. The man was last seen swimming toward a grove of trees; he went under and never resurfaced. His body was found three hours later in 2 m (7 ft) of water. The horse survived.

Prevention for Riders

Mounted police officers and search and rescue mounted posse members should know how to swim before going into water of any depth; only 2 inches of water is sufficient to cover the mouth or nose and lead to drowning. Riders should be aware of proper use of tack and equipment around water (e.g., remove tie-downs). Mounted riders should avoid muddy bogs or dangerous terrain; if the horse is wary about entering the mud, there is probably a good reason for the concern. Horses should not be ridden in heavy rains or flood conditions in areas scattered with ditches, ravines, and rolling terrain because dangerous drop-offs may be obscured by seemingly shallow water (Shariat, 1996). Warnings given to motorists caught during flash flood conditions should apply to horseback riders. Crossing a road with an unknown depth of water flowing over its surface should be avoided. An inexperienced rider or nonswimmer should never attempt swimming a horse while mounted as the rider is commonly separated from the horse in these situations (MMWR, 1990).

Have a Policy

In water, ice, and mud rescue the solutions are not easy. Binoculars should be used to perform the risk assessment without committing personnel into the rescue environment (Fire Service Guides, 1998). Responders should develop a unit policy including criteria to determine if it is a "go" or "no go" situation for each scenario (e.g., flood, swiftwater, ice, mud, beach). If the unit policy includes rescue attempts, the unit must procure the proper equipment, schedule regular training, and ensure that fit and trained personnel are available. Or, the unit should set up a memorandum of understanding with another unit that can provide this equipment and personnel. The time and monetary investments in the correct equipment, training, regular recertifications, and practice scenarios can be significant.

THE "SIZE-UP"

The safety officer (SO) and incident commander (IC) will do a sizing up to evaluate the risk and determine whether the appropriate equipment, personnel, and training are available. Factors to be considered include the availability of water transport (e.g., boats, barges, etc.), experienced personnel (including boat captains),

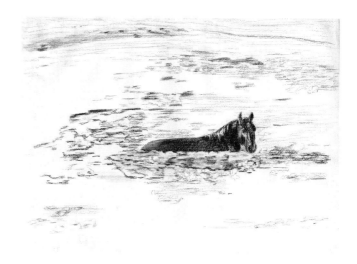

Figure 7.5 *A large animal victim trapped in ice quickly becomes hypothermic and unable to assist itself. Without appropriate surface ice rescue training, PPE, and strict attention to scene safety, responders should not go out on the surface of the ice. Shorebound responders can break a path through the ice to the victim with heavy objects or chainsaws. Courtesy of Julie Casil.*

personal protective equipment (PPE), proper attention to personal safety in watercraft, and a backup plan if the boat propeller becomes inoperable due to damage from unseen hazards (Figure 7.5).

A cow standing in 1 m (3.3 ft) of slowly moving floodwater may appear to be in less danger than one that is 10 m (33 feet) away on the other side of a 60 cm (2 ft) deep, swiftly flowing creek water; however, both can be similarly dangerous. The animal could be trapped and immobilized by unseen debris such as fencing, barbed wire, mud, a vehicle, a hole, or a tree branch. The animal may have been trapped for a prolonged period of time in cold water. The water may be contaminated by toxic chemicals and untreated sewage. By the time disaster animal rescuers get to a flood zone, it might be as much as 72 hours after the initial callout and disaster onset; animals will often be exhausted and dehydrated and may have immersion injuries. Alternatively, if the animal has not been trapped for a long period, it may be struggling and more difficult to handle. In swiftwater scenarios, neither animals nor rescuers may be able to walk across even a shallow creek without losing their footing and being swept downstream.

A major theme of this book is to provide understanding of the risks involved in handling large animals. In these water scenarios, there are two dangers: the victim and the water/ice/mud. Approach and position become crucial. When in the water with the animal, the tendency for responders is to focus on the rescue technique and placement of equipment, to the detriment of personal safety. When approached by boats, floating hoses, or a person in a personal flotation device

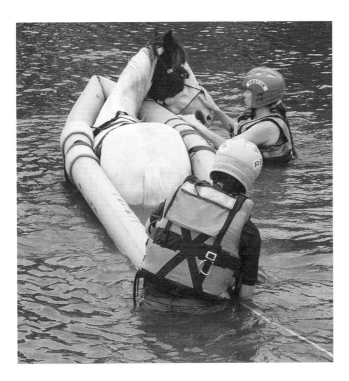

Figure 7.6 In this demonstration of a large animal flotation device made from inflated supply hose, one operations person is also acting as the animal handler while the second pinches the two ends of the fire hose together with webbing. Webbing (10 cm, or 4 in., wide) is slung under the animal to support it, and 2.5-cm (1-in.) webbing is tied over the top of the animal to prevent it from jumping out of the device. The animal should be gradually approached and allowed to become accustomed to the equipment. Courtesy of Rebecca Gimenez.

(PFD), most animals react with concern and/or fear; it is advised that rescuers approach the animals from the front in a very slow manner to allow them to become accustomed to their presence (Figure 7.6)

For example, in a 1922 incident a horse was found standing on a low head dam in less than 1 m (3.28 ft) of water. The horse was blind, and the lone responder in the rowboat did not appear to have any obvious source of assistance or safety equipment. The result of the rescue effort is unknown, but even with modern rescue equipment and techniques this can be a very difficult scenario to resolve. Low head dams are structures typically built to back up water into a reservoir (including some swimming holes). The wall-like structures pool water as it flows over the dam's crest and drops to a lower level. The dropping water creates a dangerous hydraulic "keeper" recirculation that causes a backwash effect; the backwash carries debris or victims back toward the face of the dam, where the water washing over its crest washes them toward a point downstream called a *boil line*. The boil line continually circulates water from below the surface toward the face of the dam. Victims caught in the boil can become trapped in the rapidly circulating water

and drown. In certain states low head dams are outlawed or being destroyed because of the dangers associated with them.

Public Health Concerns

Trapped animals will often be dehydrated despite being surrounded by floodwater because materials dissolved in the water make it unpotable (undrinkable). Chemicals such as pesticides, solvents, fertilizers, paint, and other materials often contaminate floodwater. Contamination can also originate from flooded septic systems and public wastewater treatment facilities, carcasses, and flooded cemeteries (Baker, 2000).

Major public health issues such as this may prevent responders from being able to assist humans and animals because of concerns for rescuer safety and availability of appropriate PPE (Murphy, 2006). The hazards of contaminated floodwater were demonstrated during Hurricane Katrina (2005), when floodwater resulted in widespread dermatological (skin) injuries in both humans and animals (T. Gimenez, 2005).

Better Use of Resources

Responders should develop a water rescue policy for animals in the local jurisdiction that addresses both swiftwater and floodwater scenarios. The policy will inform the decision for "go" or "no go." This policy will require a constant risk assessment cycle to determine if there is sufficient training, PPE, personnel, and equipment to attempt animal rescues in emergencies. Consider that in complex disasters human rescues will be ongoing and will probably require a significant percentage of the available resources. Many areas do not have sufficient resources to perform human and animal rescue. They rely on trained and equipped certified volunteer groups for animal rescues in disasters, with the understanding that quick response from those volunteers may not be possible during local emergencies.

The best use of boat resources might be to take veterinarians to the scene to perform triage and minor treatment, providing hay and fresh water to stranded animals, and obtaining a GPS grid coordinate so that the animals can be located and transported when the water recedes. A thorough preassessment of needs, resources, and locations of animals should be coordinated through the emergency operations center. Initial assessment personnel in helicopters who will screen the disaster area may provide much information to field rescuers.

Attempting to approach and restrain frightened and stranded animals may force the animals into deeper water, increasing the animals' risk of injury or death. If the floodwaters are not actively rising, the animal(s) can often be safely supported in their location until the waters recede.

During the aftermath of Hurricane Katrina in September 2005, a National Guard Boeing CH-47 Chinook

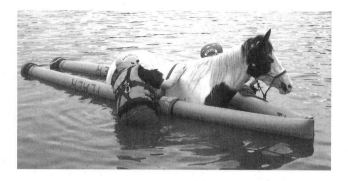

Figure 7.7 *The inflated supply hose floatation device is attached to a demonstration animal in approximately 1 m of water by firefighter/rescue students practicing this technique using locally available equipment. Courtesy of Rebecca Gimenez.*

helicopter crew attempted to salvage a cattle barge for the purpose of moving 100 cattle trapped on an island. The crew had previously dropped bales of hay to the trapped animals to provide them with food until they could be safely rescued. Unfortunately, the vessel was not recovered before the crew was ordered to fly out of the path of the approaching Hurricane Rita. The animals survived by swimming to high land (National Guard Bureau, 2005).

This policy will require a constant risk assessment cycle to determine if there is sufficient training, PPE, personnel, and locally available equipment to attempt animal rescues in emergencies and disasters (Figure 7.7).

Healthy animals will usually be found stranded on higher ground—they can all swim short distances if necessary. Animals that appear to be standing in the middle of floodwater are either on the highest ground (e.g., barn roof, ridge top, etc.) in the immediate area or are trapped in wire fencing or other materials. Swimming is a very physically demanding activity that few animals can sustain for more than a few hundred meters at a time.

Structural and Ground Collapse

It is not uncommon for sheds and barns to lose their structural integrity and collapse when the sand foundation of the poles is washed away by floodwater. Rescuers should be cautious about entering structures affected by flooding because the buildings' structural integrity may be weak and collapse may be imminent.

Karst landscapes form when water dissolves limestone-type rocks and are most common in Kentucky and Florida. Sinkholes and caves are seen on the surface, but these structures represent a complicated balance between erosion and the water table in these areas. It is not uncommon for cattle and horses in their own pastures to fall into a hole that literally opens beneath them in these geologically active areas. The SO on the scene should evaluate the risk versus benefit of sending

rescuers into flooded, potentially collapsing structures or unstable ground such as large sinkholes in karst topography (Cobb and Currens, 2001).

Types of Flooding

Coastal floods (storm surges) occur along ocean coasts and big lakes. Wind pushes the waves, leading to high water levels and flooding of the coastal areas, especially if the surge occurs simultaneously with a high tide.

River floods occur when rivers or creeks flood outside their normal boundaries. This may occur due to dikes or dams being breached by high precipitation levels upstream, melting snow, or blockage.

Flash floods occur after high-intensity local rainfall. A rapid rise in water levels and severe rainfall in the flooding location occurs often in deserts and mountainous areas. The U.S. National Weather Service has defined flash floods as those that follow within a few hours of heavy or excessive rain, a dam or levee failure, or a sudden release of water impounded by an ice dam.

Drainage floods occur when high precipitation levels overwhelm normal public or natural drainage systems.

Water can be moving (swiftwater), still (static), or tidal (waves and incoming tides). It can be found at the lowest point of almost any terrain feature, in sinkholes, ditches, and manmade obstacles, and it is often combined with mud.

BARGE AND BOAT RESCUES

Since the 15th century, large animals have been moved on and off ships and barges by using canvas slings; however, this is a time- and equipment-intensive method. The safest, lowest risk, and most recommended method for rescue of large animals from stillwater and floodwater scenarios is the use of a heavy-duty barge with a ramp that can drop and allow the animals to walk onto the barge. Military landing craft or barges that bring riprap and rock to shorelines of lakes and rivers are perfect for this job, and the metal ramps can be covered with rubber mats or plywood to provide footing for the animals. This type of specialty resource is something that needs to be incorporated into disaster preparation plans; local responders should identify these resources before they are needed.

After a hurricane in 2001, the Louisiana State University veterinarians were asked to assist with sedating 12 horses that needed to be moved approximately 4 km (2.5 miles) across fairly shallow water (1–2 m, or 3.3–6.6 ft) to a levee from which they could be evacuated by vehicles. The horses were 300–400 kg (660–880 lbs) each and appeared to have little experience with handling and restraint by humans. There was a cattle chute on a patch of ground above water level, totaling approximately 1 1/2 acres of dry ground; part of this area was being used by a Coast Guard helicopter that was lifting two horses. The chute was located 50 m (55 yd) from a road where the barge was able to moor.

The barge was essentially a flat-topped structure 40 cm (15.7 in.) above the water surface with no sides, approximately 2 m (6.6 ft) × 4 m (13 ft), with a 25-horse power motor. In the cattle chute, the horses were sedated heavily with intravenous detomidine hydrochloride. The horses were restrained on the edge of the road adjacent to the barge and were then anesthetized with ketamine hydrochloride.

When each horse became recumbent, a group of people lifted the animal onto the barge and slid each across the barge to accommodate 3–4 recumbent animals per trip. Jugular catheters were inserted, and triple-drip anesthesia (intravenous administration of a mixture of xylazine hydrochloride, ketamine hydrochloride, and guaiafenesin) was administered to maintain anesthesia for the barge ride of approximately 20 minutes. At the levee the animals were pulled off the barge onto the bank in a manner similar to that used to load them. The horses were allowed to recover on the levee then led into stock trailers for transport. Responders moved 10 horses on the barges in the time the helicopter lift team moved 2 animals.

A veterinarian on the scene remarked that if a walk-on/walk-off barge could be designed like a horse trailer (with slots for the horses to enter), they could be tied, sedated, and moved standing (Hubert, 2006). Furthermore, if anesthesia is necessary for injured animals or animals that require excessive restraint, padding the surface of the barge and providing shade to protect the animals from heat and direct sunlight would be of benefit. Said Hubert (2006), "Sides on the barge would have prevented our greatest fear—that if an animal struggled, it would fall over the side and into the water."

Although a barge specifically made for transporting cattle or large animals is ideal, especially if it can be moored close to the bank or high ground, in most communities that equipment is rare. Traditional barges may have inappropriate footing; hooved mammals cannot easily walk up a steep ramp or keep their footing on a slick surface such as plywood (Figure 7.8). If using equipment barges, sisal or rubber mats or rugs should be placed to provide traction on ramps or slick surfaces.

If leading animals by boat, the tail and long mane hairs of horses should be tied up so that they do not float out and become caught in the blades of the motor while moving; the authors documented two cases where this occurred and caused severe injury to the animals. Providing flotation for the head of the animal, such as an inflated inner tube tied under the halter, works well to keep the animal's chin and nostrils above water.

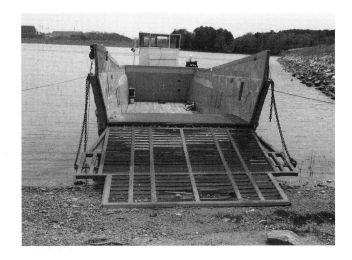

Figure 7.8 *An equipment barge such as this may be used to load and transport large animals. Heavy rubber mats or plywood should be used to cover the open metal ramps to the deck, and animals may need to be sedated to prevent their attempts to jump out of the transport while under way. Courtesy of Tomas Gimenez.*

When possible, the animal should be walked in shallow, slowly moving water. Fractious and nervous animals may attempt to jump into the boat or pull away from it; they should be tied to the side of the boat to prevent this, not held by a person who could be pulled into the water by the animal. Small craft may be capsized by a large animal; for this reason, an appropriately sized craft should be used.

Leading haltered animals through deep water is very difficult because animals can swim faster than humans and may end up pulling the human by the lead rope. In addition, they are very difficult to guide. Positioning one person with a lead rope on each side of the haltered animal allows better control and gives the animal sufficient room to move. The water should not be any deeper than 1 m (3.3 ft) when using this method with halter-broken horses. However, impromptu rescues of horses from flooding barns will commonly feature one person leading each horse from stalls to safety; catching, haltering, and leading animals out of a barn in rapidly rising water poses extreme danger for personnel and the animals. Concerns about the structural integrity of the barn must also be taken into account (Figure 7.9).

Based on evaluation of videotaped attempts to employ these methods with varying degrees of success, responders should attempt to drive animals that cannot be haltered. Animals should not be lassoed and towed behind boats, as they may be asphyxiated by the lasso. Roping the horns of cattle and towing them with a boat will tend to force the animals' nostrils into the water as their heads are pulled forward by the horns and thus cannot be recommended. Barges lacking sides or railings are not appropriate for conveying

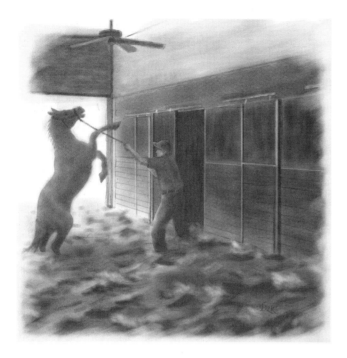

Figure 7.9 *This scenario from Greenville, South Carolina, illustrates the importance of disaster planning for flooding scenarios. Just catching, haltering, and leading animals under these conditions is difficult and dangerous, there needs to be an evacuation plan and more than just one person should be present. Courtesy of Michael Dzurak.*

animals unless they are anesthetized. Placing a conscious, standing large animal in a rescue boat is very dangerous due to the animal's unpredictability; the standing animal is tall enough to raise the center of gravity of the boat and may capsize it (Ray, 1999) if the animal panics and struggles. Small foals and calves may be sedated or anesthetized and trussed (legs tied together) in a boat for transport. Smaller craft may be adequate for transporting goats and sheep, but they must be contained or sedated so they don't jump off the craft. For small animals swimming in the water, the craft can be brought up next to the animal and webbing slung under it to lift and roll it into the craft.

Field-expedient solutions proposed have included using a Zodiac-type inflatable boat with the floor cut out to form a floating sling. In June 2006, the Animal Rescue League of Boston successfully extricated a pony from a flooded barn with this method. In general, any device that slings the animal between floating pieces works very well, preventing the animal from climbing up on it or from rolling out of it. Another proposed method is to float a pontoon boat with an empty center over the animal and lift the animal in a sling in the center to stabilize it for transport; however, it is suspected that this type of vessel would perform poorly in fast-moving water.

PRIORITIZING THE RESCUE

As with all animal rescue situations, human safety is the first priority. Proper planning and attention to safety avoids the necessity of rescuing the rescuers. Water is so dangerous that despite every effort to be safe and prepared, human fatalities—including those of trained and experienced rescuers—occur every year.

Sending a rescuer with a halter and lead rope to catch a beef cow trapped on an island of high ground surrounded by floodwater is generally a poor use of resources. A better plan would involve providing hay and fresh water to the animal until responders are able to return to contain and transport the animal. On the other hand, the trapped animal might be a show cow that is accustomed to human handling and is trained to lead. Each animal is an individual. If the water continues to rise, options include containment, barge transport, or euthanasia.

Prioritize the Rescue Method—ReThRoG-H

Large animal water rescue methods have been adapted from human and small animal water rescue training (Ray, 1999). Water rescues of conscious humans are often facilitated by the human's ability to understand verbal instructions such as "come here" or "swim that way," as well as the ability to grasp a floating object or thrown rope. The acronym ReThRoG-H summarizes the order of methods used in human and small animal rescue: reach, throw, row, go, and helicopter. However, these methods must be adapted and may not be applicable to large animal water rescue scenarios.

Reach. In human and small animal rescue, a water rescue is most simply and safely attempted from the safety of the bank by reaching out with a pole for the victim to grasp (humans) or is used to catch a part of the small animal (collar) (Ray, 1999). This method cannot be applied safely to most large animal water rescue scenarios; even if a person is able to catch the halter of a swimming animal with a pole or cane, the animal's weight and momentum would likely pull the rescuer into the water.

There are very few scenarios in which this technique would be effective with large animals. If attempted, the rescuers on the bank need to be in appropriate swiftwater PPE so that if they are accidentally pulled into the water they can save themselves. Large animals respond to flooding by seeking high ground. They do not grasp or climb onto floating objects and may be frightened by any such objects that approach them.

Throw. Throwing a floating object to a human or small animal victim may be successful, but it is very difficult to assist a large animal with this method. Some might consider trying to lasso the swimming animal; roping is very difficult if not regularly practiced. In addition, access to the head and neck is often limited because large animals tend to swim with only their nostrils above the water's surface. It may be possible to rope horned cattle, but the roper may be pulled into the water by the animal. This method may be successful if the rescuer anchors the free end of the rope to a strong anchor point on the bank and allows the force of the water to push the animal toward the bank.

The throwing method is easily complicated by obstacles and may lead to the animal or rescuer becoming tangled in the rope and drowning. If the animal's limb(s) become entangled (e.g., in ropes, webbing, etc.), it may panic and may drown itself during the struggle. There are very few water scenarios where throwing would be effective for large animal rescue.

Rescuers should never be allowed to tie themselves to anything in water, particularly to any part of a large animal. Care should be taken to ensure ropes do not become coiled around people or body parts to prevent dragging and injury.

Row. The rowing method requires the rescuer(s) to enter the rescue environment (water) with the victim in either a boat or watercraft, or enter the water from the bank, and is associated with higher risk of injury (Ray, 1999). The technique requires proper planning, PPE, appropriate training and equipment, and appropriate watercraft. Swimming animals are extremely difficult to handle or direct. In cases where animals are standing in shallower water, they might be approached or driven with a boat to direct their movements; haltered and tied to a boat; driven onto a barge (safest and best method); pulled to the bank to be lifted, sedated, onto a barge; or pulled behind a boat using a halter and flotation device to keep the head above water and a forward assist to anchor the body as the animal swims. All of these methods are difficult and dangerous, requiring training and practice in the use of this equipment. Another suggested method to control the movement of a swimming animal involves the use of inflated fire hoses on the water surface to form a funnel to direct the animal to high ground.

Go. Swimming rescue can be performed in human rescue situations, but it is not without inherent risk. Do not allow anyone to jump into the water to save an animal (or for that matter, a human) without a plan, preparation, and backup. This method should never be attempted with swimming large animals; they are difficult to steer or control in water, they markedly outweigh their rescuers, and their moving limbs can easily injure a human.

If the animals are standing in shallow water (1 m, or 3.3 ft, or less), the animal handler may enter the water to attach webbing for a horizontal drag or vertical lift (Figure 7.10), attempt flotation with a modified

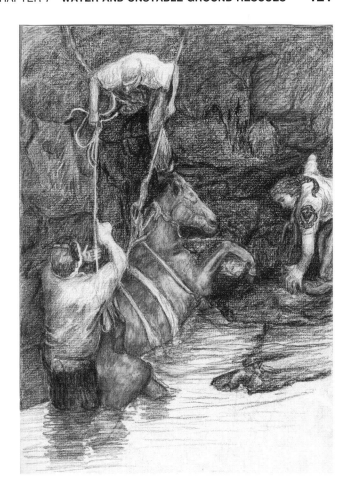

Figure 7.10 *An exhausted horse is brought up next to the steep bank that it had unsuccessfully spent hours trying to climb to escape the river. Local responders applied webbing around the body of the animal in a modification of the sideways drag. This response demonstrates the challenges of removing a large animal that cannot assist itself. Courtesy of Julie Casil.*

equine flotation device, or apply an Anderson Sling in preparation for helicopter sling load. These are high-risk options requiring experienced handlers and training and practice in the use of this equipment in water.

Helicopter. Helicopter rescue should be the choice of last resort in most situations, but it is effective for specific scenarios (see Chapter 18).

WATER-RELATED MEDICAL CONCERNS

Hypothermia is a significant contributor to the cascade of events that is observed in stressed animals in cold conditions (see Chapter 20). Even the relatively warm water (25°C, 77° F) found in the canals in Florida will cause a decrease in the animal's body temperature; rescued animals have been reported to have body temperature losses of 1–3°C (2–5° F) when rescued after two to six hours in the water (Kastner, 2005).

In nonmoving cold water the animal can be expected to lose body temperature 25 times faster than in air; if the water is moving, the convection current will remove heat from the body of the animal 250 times faster (Ray, 1999). A short time spent in cold water environments can cause immersion hypothermia and make the animal unable to assist in its own rescue (Park, 2006).

Dermatological conditions of the skin contracted by standing in floodwater for several days have been described and include both fungal and bacterial infections. Significant numbers of these cases were reported in both large and small animals after large hurricanes and may occur with or without hazardous materials in the floodwater. Animals that stand in water for two to five days will usually have severe bacterial and fungal infections. A 2000 study from North Carolina State University College of Veterinary Medicine (CVM) indicated the most effective treatment for these conditions was to hose the affected skin with cold water at low pressure twice a day and apply tincture of green soap spray and let it dry (drying in the sun is even better). If the injury is touched, rubbed, scrubbed, or bandaged, it may deglove and expose bone, joint surfaces, tendons, ligaments, or tendon sheaths (with potentially fatal consequences). Following the CVM's treatment regime, the wounds were healing and regrowing hair three weeks later (Vivrette et al., 2001).

Fire ants (*Solenopsis invicta*) are significant hazards in the southern United States. When their mound is flooded, fire ants join together to form a raft of living ants that floats downstream until it encounters a tree, an animal victim, or a human rescuer, and they climb on to dry safety. These ants grip onto the animal's (or human's) skin and inject an alkaloid venom called piperidine; the venom is extremely irritating, and produces a burning sensation (hence the name *fire ant*). The sites form blisters that may last for several days. There is not much prevention for this other than a good dry suit, but it can be a serious health hazard for rescuers and victims. An animal assaulted by 60,000 fire ants will be frantic from the pain and will endanger itself and everyone else in the vicinity. Some rescue personnel are allergic to multiple stings by these insects, and life-threatening anaphylactic reactions have been reported.

SPECIAL CONSIDERATIONS

Sports Events

Three day eventing, marathon carriage driving, and other equine sports accidents at water obstacles on or off the course can involve significant numbers of bystanders, terrified and thrashing equids, harnesses and heavy carriages on top of humans and horses, and severely injured humans in varying depths of water (Figure 7.11). The first action recommended is to cut the harness or bridles, freeing the animals to swim

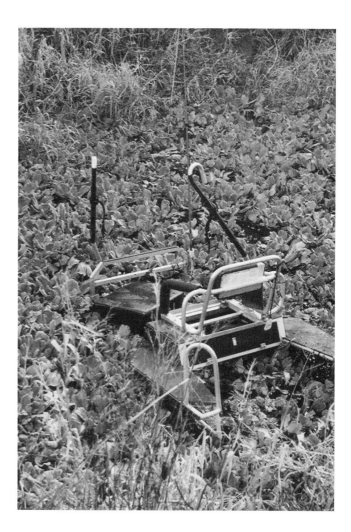

Figure 7.11 *When this carriage with two horses veered off a driving competition course and landed in a Wellington, Florida, canal, quick-thinking owners and bystanders cut the harnesses off the animals to release them. The animals swam out of the canal and were contained by bystanders. Courtesy of Jeff Galloway.*

away from the wreck; responders can then effectively and safely deal with the human victim(s) (Galloway, 2006).

Although the water may appear shallow and still, these scenarios are very dangerous. While they may not appear to require the same level of preparation as floodwater scenarios, they may still involve many humans standing in the water (often trying to hold the horse's head above water) with an excited, injured, and struggling equid. The paramedics on call at these events (for human injuries) should be aware of safety zones around large animals while they work to save the rider/driver who may be trapped underneath the horse(s) or in the harness.

Canalized Watercourses

Flood channels, temporary water diversion devices, canals, and other canalized watercourses represent significant swiftwater hazards to rescuers. These types of concrete channels are present in many communities; they are commonly used to channel water through downtown areas or steep and desert terrains. If a large animal falls into one of these canals, it cannot easily escape. These canals should be fenced to prevent animals and children from gaining access.

In certain parts of the world, these canals are designed to handle flash-flood water; it does not have to be raining locally for water to be passing through the canals. Flumes are concrete channels designed for flood control. Flume rescues will often require vertical lift techniques because the sides of the channel, even if dry and only 1 m (3 ft) deep, are too high and steep to allow a large animal to jump out or over. Water released through these channels often moves extremely fast. The responders' first call should be to the public works department to divert the flow of the water while personnel and the victim are in the flume. In dry channels with standing animals, the simplest method would be to dump a truckload of dirt in the channel to make a ramp to walk the animal out (Gilman, 2003).

The Norco Animal Control and Fire Department in California have responded to several scenarios where an animal became cast in this type of channel and could not get its feet positioned underneath itself to rise. The animals were sedated, and rescuers pushed the Rescue Glide under its body. Webbing was placed in a forward assist with lark's foot pattern and a backward drag configuration, and rescuers slid the entire animal up and over the lip of the channel on the Rescue Glide.

The markedly steep sides of most manmade canals prevent animals from climbing out and often aggravate rescue attempts. In some areas (south Florida) the sides of the canal are made of coral rock; this substance is extremely rough and lacerates the legs and body of any animal (or human) attempting to walk through it. Further complications may include reptiles (e.g., snakes, alligators) and insects (e.g., fire ants, black flies, mosquitoes) in the water with the rescuers and victim. Reptiles should be driven away or relocated by knowledgeable responders; alligators over 2 m (6 ft) in length can be extremely aggressive and dangerous to both victims and responders.

Pools

Large animals that have fallen into swimming pools present one of the most common large animal dispatch calls for fire department assistance in the United States and abroad (Figure 7.12). Owners commonly allow their animals to graze in the yard, or loose animals may wander through the neighborhood. Local fire departments are capable of draining a pool quickly, providing enough time for rescuers to design an extrication plan.

Strategies for removing an animal from a pool may include driving the animal up the steps. Placing forward assist webbing will help by guiding the animal

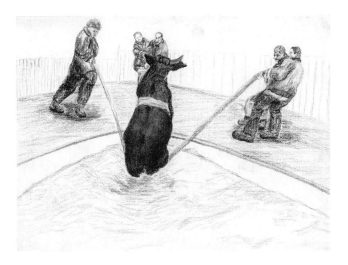

Figure 7.12 *Cattle and other livestock commonly land in pools if allowed to run loose and are often difficult to restrain because they are not used to being haltered. In this case, animal control and firefighters use a forward assist to encourage the animal to climb the steps of the pool. An inflated fire hose can be strung across the pool to limit movement to one area of the pool and effectively confine the animal. Courtesy of Julie Casil.*

and supplementing its forward motion. Other tested methods include webbing placed around the hindquarters of the animal or vertical lift.

Special challenges include the animal landing on a pool cover that may support its weight temporarily while attached, but ensnare its legs and cause it to drown if the cover is cut at the edges. Other pool covers are extremely lightweight and will trap only the legs and drown the animal rapidly; these must be quickly cut loose from the animal.

When asking an animal to walk up a steep bank or steps, personnel should allow the animal sufficient room to navigate the ramp or steps; a guiding rope on the halter and a forward assist around the chest are also recommended. Driving the animal from behind is more effective than pulling on its head and allows the animal to provide muscle power for its own rescue.

Exotic or Endangered Large Animal Wildlife

As an example of possibly the ultimate large animal water rescue, in 1997 an endangered loggerhead sea turtle weighing approximately 294 kg (650 lb) was caught by its flipper in a buoy chain in the Charleston, South Carolina, area. The Charleston Rescue Squad, very proactive in TLAER training and practice, responded, along with several other agencies (U.S. Coast Guard, emergency medical service [EMS], South Carolina Department of Natural Resources, public safety, and sheriff's departments).

Five divers entered the water with the massive animal to cut the chain with underwater cutting equipment; this effort required nearly three hours to cut a link in the weighted chain, free the turtle, and reattach the chain with a shackle. Divers were not able to maneuver the large sea animal, approximately the size of a small car, or move the chain, which was attached to a 453 kg (1,000 lb) counterweight. The risks were numerous: the animal thrashed at the sight of the divers and support personnel in boats. There was a small risk that a rescuer could be bitten by the beak of the frightened animal and a more significant risk of a rescuer being crushed between the large animal and the buoy. The Coast Guard allowed the divers to cut a link in the chain with a large, hydraulic bolt cutter; once the animal was freed, the chain was reattached with a shackle (Jones, 2002).

SEDATION PROTOCOLS

Sedatives and tranquilizers are available, but not necessary in every case. In water, ice, and unstable ground situations or where cardiovascular shock is a concern, chemical sedation should not be used without veterinary recommendation and supervision. Most sedatives cause the animal's head to droop closer to the ground (or water). It might be necessary to delegate a rescuer to hold the animal's head above the water so it can breathe; to accomplish this, the rescuer would be in a potentially dangerous position directly in front of the animal. Sedated animals can still kick, strike, and bite. Rescuers should remain vigilant and maintain safe distances and positions.

PROPER PERSONAL PROTECTIVE EQUIPMENT FOR RESCUERS

Responders should dress appropriately for the situation. Firefighters in turnouts or bunker gear have drowned on several occasions, and it is the opinion of the author that drown-proofing training in a static pool does not accurately represent operational conditions. All personnel within 3 m (9.8 ft) of the hazard (water, ice, or mud) must wear appropriate gear, equipment, or PPE for water rescue, not bunker gear (Ray, 1999). Recommendations include the following:

- Water rescue helmet: These helmets have holes to allow water around the head; in contrast, the bill of a standard fire helmet will often hold the rescuer's head below the water level. The Styrofoam insulation of these helmets decreases their weight and provides flotation and protection from objects.
- PFD: PFDs designed for whitewater or swiftwater use (U.S. Coast Guard Type III or V) should be used and should be outfitted with a knife, whistle, and reflective material.
- Dry/wet suit: Dry and wet suits provide thermal protection and protection. When water contaminated with hazardous materials (HazMat) is present or suspected, a dry suit is recommended.

- Shoes: Rescuers should wear hard sole neoprene booties to protect their feet from debris, rocks, sharp objects, and other unseen hazards.
- Gloves: Gloves should be worn to protect rescuers' hands from unseen hazards, sharp objects, rope burns, lacerations, and scratches.
- Goggles: Based on the incident, goggles may be worn to prevent HazMat-contaminated water from being splashed into their eyes.

WATER BEHAVIOR

Water in any form (swiftwater, floodwater, wave, or static) can be extremely dangerous. The behavior of water is beyond the scope of this book, and appropriate recommended resources are found on-line. When the speed of water doubles, the force it exerts on an object or victim is quadrupled. As previously stated, no one (rescuers or bystanders) should be positioned downstream of the victim or tied to anything (e.g., the animal or an object) while in water. Floodwaters are often contaminated with HazMat, and the victims' and rescuers' lives may be at risk. Over 90% of the training in swiftwater rescue is composed of teaching prospective rescuers how to rescue themselves (Ray, 2006).

COMMERCIAL FOOD ANIMALS

Based on flooding incidents over the last decade and information gained from the leadership of the North Carolina State Animal Response Team (SART) and North Carolina Department of Agriculture and Consumer Services (NCDA&CS), there is no reason that commercial animals should be exposed to floods except under catastrophic conditions. Zoning restrictions, building codes, and regulated uses of 100- and 500-year flood zones should restrict commercial animal facilities from areas appropriate for crops or pasture. This is an example of the concept of mitigation to limit the severity of damage sustained from a disaster.

Hurricane Floyd caused unprecedented flooding across most of eastern North Carolina in 1999, adversely affecting pets and livestock. Livestock losses included 2,107,857 poultry, 1,180 cattle, 28,000 hogs, and 752,970 turkeys. To minimize public health threats, state and federal officials incinerated the dead animals. The estimated livestock damage was over $13 million. Agricultural facilities and farm structures, many of which were not insured against flood losses, were damaged. The total damage to farm structures was estimated to be $256,341,000 (NCDA&CS, 1999). Much of the floodwater was tainted with raw sewage, pesticides, agricultural waste, petroleum products, and dead farm animals.

Commercial livestock drowned in floodwaters. Animals were also lost or injured as the result of starvation, dehydration, heatstroke, and falls through or

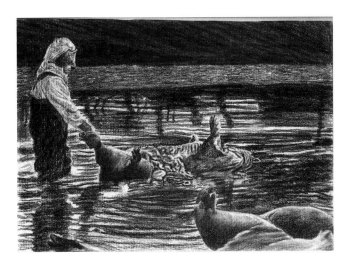

Figure 7.13 *After Hurricane Floyd, thousands of pigs were drowned and floated downstream in North Carolina. Days later, this is the scene that disaster workers faced. This scenario presents significant risk to public health. Courtesy of Julie Casil.*

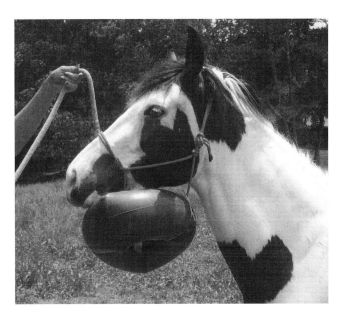

Figure 7.14 *When animals are trapped in mud, water, or ice and need support for the head and neck while waiting for rescue, an inner tube may be tied under the halter to allow the head to maintain buoyancy. Courtesy of Helen Keulemans.*

from barn roofs. Other animals were lost when they wandered away from facilities with damaged structures and fencing.

Despite the efforts of rescuers, food animals salvaged from the floodwaters cannot be allowed to enter the human food supply without appropriate withdrawal times; appropriate withdrawal times may not be known for these situations. Public health and food safety issues **must** be considered when food animals are involved in disaster situations (Figure 7.13).

Following Hurricane Floyd, the state of North Carolina and the Federal Emergency Management Agency (FEMA) have been purchasing property in flood-prone areas to prevent commercial development and to reduce the risk of loss or damage of life and property. As of 2002, 1,888 units of land had been approved by FEMA for purchase at a cost of $135.3 million. Another 2,534 units, at a cost of $136.1 million, were under review (NCDA&CS, 1999).

INDIVIDUAL ANIMAL FLOTATION RESCUE FROM WATER

The ideal solution for rescuing individual animals in floodwater environments has not yet been developed. As of this publication, research and development of safe and effective methods is ongoing. After Hurricane Floyd (1999), members of National Veterinary Response Team, formerly Veterinary Medical Assistance Team-3, and the North Carolina State Veterinarian's Office spent two days attempting to rescue a herd of over 300 cows stranded on the only high ground for miles as the water continued to rise. Several of the smaller animals were able to be sedated and lifted into a boat for transport. Several methods were attempted to float the

remaining animals out of the flood zone, with no success. Helicopter rescue was not an option for these animals.

The abdomens and torsos of large animals float relatively well because of the gas present within their digestive systems; however, their heads and necks are very heavy and difficult to keep above the water line. Inflated fire hoses or pool flotation devices have been used. Although they provide flotation, these objects are unstable and often ineffective. Any flotation device for large animals must maintain the animal's head above water (Figure 7.14). Swimming large animals expend significant amounts of energy attempting to keep their nostrils above water.

The dangerous consideration with any animal flotation device is that a rescuer must enter the water with the animal, inside its action zone. The risks associated with sedating an animal in the water may be justified in some situations; if performed, flotation for the head (e.g., inflated inner tubes) should always be available.

Animals that have been struggling in water for a prolonged period of time may be sufficiently exhausted that they may stand quietly to be harnessed into a large animal flotation device (LAFD). Early research and development efforts included placing flotation underneath the animal to lift the entire animal out of the water, but the animals struggled excessively in response to these devices and often rolled out of them.

The authors devised a LAFD using high-flotation air logs, using a sling to hang the animal between the flotation logs (Figure 7.15). This device is similar to a vertical lift sling method and allows freedom of

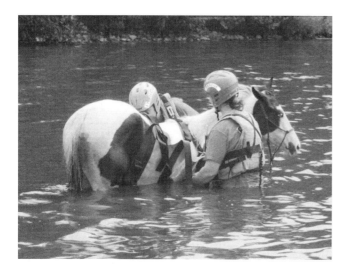

Figure 7.15 *Responders attach the belly portion of a sling for a flotation device underneath an animal trapped in a floodwater scenario far from dry land. One operational person is also acting as the animal handler. Courtesy of Nathan Slovis.*

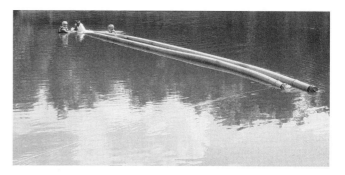

Figure 7.16 *In the initial development phases of the inflated supply hose flotation device, a 23-m (76-ft) length of supply hose was used. Although it worked well, it was difficult for responders to manipulate in the water due to its length. A shorter section is recommended for this purpose. Courtesy of Nathan Slovis.*

movement of the animal's limbs for swimming or walking. Animals used in 24 live demonstrations of this equipment by the author over a four-year period (2002–2006) adapted to the device quickly; after a short struggle, the animals relaxed into the sling and rested their noses on the head flotation device. Attaching an inner tube under the halter or allowing the animal's head to rest on the prow of the inflated fire hose provides sufficient buoyancy to keep the animal's nostrils above water.

Experimentation during these demonstrations has revealed that a horse in this type of flotation device can be successfully pulled with a fireboat or an inflatable raft powered by human effort (Park, 2006). An easy pace should be maintained while pulling the animal so that wakes (waves created by the motion of the boat) are smooth and do not push water into the animal's nostrils; this is especially important if the animal is sedated.

INFLATED SUPPLY HOSE LARGE ANIMAL FLOATATION DEVICE

Firemen from the Lexington, Kentucky, Fire Department attending TLAER training in 2005 asked if an air-inflated supply fire hose could be used to float/rescue a large animal standing in floodwater. Collaboration of the firefighters and the author resulted in the successful development of an inflated supply hose LAFD. The device consists of a 12 m (40 ft) section of supply hose, inflated approximately 50% with air, with Storz™ caps on each end to provide watertight seals. It was folded so that it partially encircled the animal, with a modified surcingle/sling tied to the animal in the water to hold the hose in place (Figure 7.16).

The biggest problem with the initial method was that the supply hose was too long, buoyant, and hard to control by the rescuers. To address this problem, the authors purchased a specialty 6.1 m (20 ft) section of 10.16 cm (4 in.) supply hose. Surcingle-type flat fire hose webbing, a western girth, or wide strapping is tied underneath the abdomen and over the back of the horse to keep it confined in the LAFD (Figure 7.17).

The convenience of this method is that the "prow" (or front) of the device is underneath the animal's head, allowing it to rest its head on the hose and maintain its nostrils above water level.

Inflated fire hoses can also be used as flotation support for responders on ice and in water rescues. A partially inflated 30 m (98 ft) length of hose can also be used as a floating device to reach a drowning person while responders remain safely out of the water.

Requirements for Employment of Large Animal Flotation Device

All equipment except the halter and lead rope for the horse should remain inside the boat or raft until they are used. The animal handlers will request pieces of equipment to be handed to them by the boat personnel as they are needed. As stated previously, responders should be trained and certified in water rescue techniques.

Equipment. Certain equipment is necessary for animal rescue using a LAFD.

- Belly support webbing 1 m long, made of fire hose or 10.16 cm (4 in.) wide webbing with loops on each end (two each)
- Strap webbing 2.5 cm (1 in.) wide and 3–4 m long (two each)
- Supply fire hose 5–6 m (15–20 ft) long fitted with a Storz cap on each end and inflated slightly more than

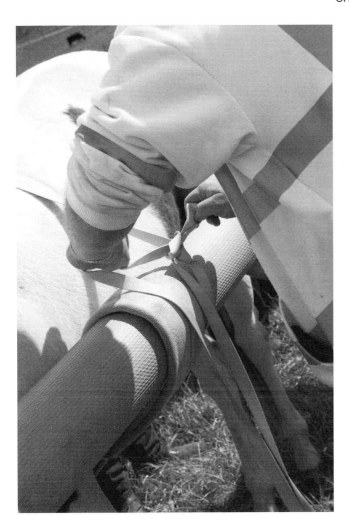

Figure 7.17 *The belly webbing goes under the animal, behind the front legs and in front of the back legs. Additional webbing should be tied over the animal to hold the flotation device in place when the animal moves in the water. Courtesy of Axel Gimenez.*

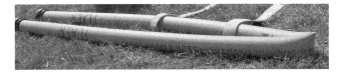

Figure 7.18 *The inflated supply hose flotation device consists of an air-inflated supply hose and webbing for slinging under the animal's body. Operational personnel and handlers must be strong swimmers and use water safety equipment. Courtesy of Axel Gimenez.*

Personnel. As in all rescue scenarios, an IC is necessary to direct the efforts. A SO, whether an individual assigned the task or the IC assuming the duty, is vital in water rescue situations. Ideally, one team member should assume the role of SO on land and another serve as SO on the rescue boat. Other necessary personnel include the following:

- Boat personnel: One person should be dedicated to operating the rescue boat, while other operational personnel coordinate with the animal handlers to provide the equipment and monitor the animal as it is towed. Boat personnel should remain in the boat and should **not** enter the water unless there is an emergency with the animal or personnel. All personnel must wear PFDs.
- Animal handler: One handler should hold the animal's halter/lead rope for restraint and possibly support the head of the animal while it is sedated; this person must wear complete water rescue gear and rescue PFDs. It is imperative that this person be a competent swimmer.
- Operational personnel: One person should be positioned on each side of the horse to attach the equipment; one may also serve as the animal handler. These individuals must wear complete water rescue gear and rescue PFDs. They must also be competent swimmers.

Procedure for Employing Large Animal Flotation Device. Proper deployment of the LAFD can be performed in approximately 10 minutes by appropriately trained personnel using equipment as described above. The procedure is as follows:

1. The animal handler arrives by boat, enters the water, and approaches the stranded animal (the water should be no more than approximately 1 m, or 3 ft, deep). The halter is placed and a long lead rope is attached. Animal handlers should ensure that they remain out of reach of the animals' legs to avoid being pulled under if the animal should begin to swim or struggle. If the animal is not halter broken, this is a serious complication that may require darting or termination of the effort. *Note:* Many animals need to be slightly sedated to prevent

halfway with air (one each). (See Figure 7.18.) Alternatively, two air logs (engineered for at least 181 kg, 400 lb, lift can be used to float the animal, but are not appropriate for lifting it out of the water).

- Breast collar or western cinch to prevent the animal from swimming out of the modified LAFD (one each)
- Kernmantle ropes with carabiners and Prusik hitches of various sizes (assortment)
- Various sizes of inflated inner tubes
- Halter and lead rope appropriate for the species and size of the animal (one each)
- Complete water rescue gear (e.g., PFD, helmet, foot protection) for the animal handler and operational personnel who will be in or near water; minimum of one PFD for each person in the boat or raft
- Air bottle with adaptor and manifold, or air can (one each)
- Air-fill lines (two each)
- Polypropylene towrope (one each)

struggling; the head may need to be supported by another rescuer while the animal is being fitted with the LAFD. An inner tube tied under the chin on the halter works well.

2. Two additional operational personnel are brought by boat to the animal's location. *Note:* To avoid or reduce the risk of a panic response by the animal, the boat should approach slowly and remain as far from the animal as practical. All responders should use soft, soothing voices. The boat pilot should be vigilant and keep the engine propeller away from people, the animal victim, and the rescue equipment. The horse's tail should be tied up so that stray hair does not get caught on equipment or submerged hazards.

3. Operational personnel enter the water near the animal with the folded fire hose floating on top of the water. The folded end of the hose should be placed at the animal's head. The hose should be slowly floated around the animal and not lifted over the animal's head. Placement of the bend of the hose directly in front of the animal allows it to place its chin on the hose. *Note:* The hose is very difficult to manipulate in the water unless it is maintained in a folded configuration. Shorter lengths of 4.57–6.1 m (15–20 ft) are easier to handle.

4. Two pieces of body support webbing or short pieces of looped fire hose 10.16 cm (4 in.) wide and 1 m (3.3 ft) long is passed under the animal's chest and abdomen directly behind the front legs and directly in front of the hind legs.

5. The body supports are tied with webbing to create straps underneath and over the top of the animal's body, allowing the straps and body support webbing to lay behind the shoulder/withers and in front of the back legs at the flank. *Note:* The flank (the area in front of the hind legs) is where the bucking strap is placed on rodeo horses and bulls. Animals may initially resent pressure in this area; therefore, the webbing should be placed and tightened gently from a safe distance.

6. The body support straps are firmly attached to the body support webbing and around the animal to prevent slipping and to ensure that the sling remains attached to the body as the animal swims or struggles. *Note:* Personnel should ensure that there are no hanging loops of webbing or ropes that could become entangled in the animal's limbs or entrap a rescuer.

7. A breast collar can be attached to both sides of the hose using a friction wrap of webbing, and it should be placed directly in front of the chest. This equipment prevents the horse from slipping forward out of the modified LAFD.

8. Two Prusik loops are hitched around the supply hose as attachment points for the boat towrope. *Note:* If using an air log flotation system, the (deflated) logs should be snapped to the four snaps on each side of the animal's belly support. Boat personnel connect the air lines to the air source (e.g., breathing air, tank, etc.)

and pass the free end of both air lines to operational personnel, who connect the air lines to each of the air logs. The air logs are then inflated individually or simultaneously. Alternatively, the preinflated logs can be floated to the animal and attached to the four snaps on the belly support sling. A carabiner/Prusik combination is used to connect the ends of the air logs. The Prusik loop in front must be placed over the animal's neck to prevent entanglement of the forelegs. The carabiner-rope-Prusik combination allows the air logs to be adjusted for height and pulls them close to the animal's body. Loops and ropes should be secured so that they do not hang where they can become entangled. If additional flotation is necessary, boat personnel can inflate an inner tube with the can of air or the air lines and hand it to an animal handler. The inner tube should be placed under the chin of the animal for additional flotation in deeper water.

9. The animal handler leads the animal into deeper water. As the water depth increases and the animal's body sinks, it will begin to hang in the webbing and relax with its chin on the "prow" of the LAFD (Figure 7.19). Operational personnel may have to drive the animal forward into deeper water by waving their arms. *Note:* Once the animal's feet are off supporting ground, most animals will attempt to swim unless sedated. If the animal begins to struggle against the restraint, it should be allowed to swim around the handler in circles until it tires; swimming requires physical exertion and the animal will soon tire and become more cooperative. Once correctly in the LAFD, the animal will relax and hang in the sling system; the animal's struggles usually last 30 seconds or less.

10. A floating polypropylene (not nylon) towrope is connected to carabiners, which are connected with

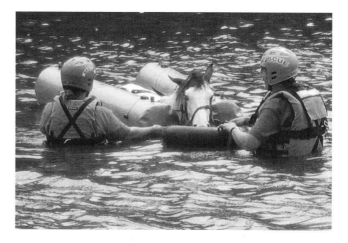

Figure 7.19 *In a training scenario at Eastern Kentucky University, a student animal handler demonstrates the large animal flotation device (LAFD) in 5 m (16 ft) of slack water. The horse is able to relax into the sling and comfortably rest its head on the "prow" of the device. Courtesy of Axel Gimenez.*

Prusik loops onto the capped ends of the supply hose. The animal is pulled slowly in a backward direction (the rear end of the animal is pulled in the direction of dry ground); this prevents wake water from entering the horse's nostrils. In addition, animal victims may be more cooperative when they cannot see the boat pulling them.

11. The animal handler and operational personnel return to the boat and make themselves available if there are complications or problems.

12. Once close to shallow water the animal handler(s) reenter the water, disconnect the LAFD from the towrope and lead the animal toward the shore. Once the animal's feet touch the ground, the animal may struggle and fight to escape the water. Removing the flotation device is performed in reverse of its employment and can be completed while the animal is still in shallow water or out of the water. *Note:* Handlers should be aware that the animal may buck and rear when its feet touch the ground. It is often difficult for handlers to attain leverage on the animal's head to direct it, especially when the animal is opposing the effort; it is more difficult if the rescuer's feet are unable to reach the bottom. Using a long lead rope allows a responder on the bank to catch the animal and remove the LAFD as it emerges from the water.

MUD AND UNSTABLE SURFACE RESCUES

Mud provides another dangerous aspect to consider in large animal rescue. Mud falls into the definition of "unstable ground," which includes mud, ice, soft sand, gravel, sludge, in both inland and coastal areas (Lane, 2004). Mud exerts a powerful suction effect on the victim, and removing any animal over 10 kg (22 lb) can be challenging (Figure 7.20). This suction effect can be overcome with the injection of air or water into the mud around the victim. Using a mud lance to inject the air or water around the legs and under the animal's abdomen simultaneously with the vertical lift or horizontal drag effort has demonstrated great efficacy in numerous live rescues and demonstrations with live animal victims trapped in mud.

Placing a cofferdam (a temporary structure to keep an area dry while surrounded by water) around the animal victim is difficult, equipment- and skill-intensive, time consuming, and potentially dangerous. This technique has been associated with poor results in human rescues. A cofferdam for a large animal rescue would have to be larger than for a human and subject to higher water pressures, increasing the risk of failure.

Mud rescue challenges are similar to water but may be more insidious. During the rescue attempt, a rescuer may suddenly realize she/he is as entrapped as the animal victim. If this occurs, the animal rescue must be interrupted while the human rescuer is extricated.

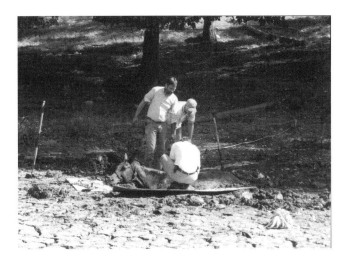

Figure 7.20 *This horse became stuck in a pond bed during a drought. The owner had attempted to dig the animal out for over two hours before calling emergency responders; unfortunately, his efforts only worsened the animal's entrapment. Only four people were on scene for this rescue. Courtesy of Rebecca Gimenez.*

Quicksand

Quicksand is a type of running soil formed when regular sand, silt, mud, or gravel contacts a flowing water source, usually an underground stream or spring. Under normal conditions tiny grains of sand have intergranular pressure and friction sufficient to support the weight of something walking on top of it. When flowing water or upward hydrostatic pressure causes water to move between the particles of sand, it acts as a lubricant to reduce the friction and cohesion and forms a suspension. Large animals have a great weight supported on a relatively small surface area (their feet or hooves). Human feet have larger surface areas, and humans are less likely than animals to fall through the surface crust.

This type of soil is rarely more than 1 m (3 ft) deep. The largest threats are starvation, exposure, or the inability of the animal to defend itself from predators. It is difficult to visually identify quicksand before walking into it because leaves and sticks, or a crust of dried sand, can cover and hide the liquefied material until something steps on it and falls through. Quicksand can form underwater, snaring animals as they cross rivers or walk along the shore of oceans or lakes. Because quicksand can develop as water from underground springs percolates upward into the sand, the condition is best stabilized by removing or diverting the water; this may not be possible in field situations.

Because quicksand is more dense than water, an animal will actually float (if it relaxes) more easily than in pure water. Pulling on a mired animal creates suction that is stronger than the animals' muscles; technically, this is a partial vacuum because air or water is unable to fill the void left by the object or extremity. Digging in quicksand is often ineffective and traps the animal deeper in the material as it flows to refill the holes. Animals that struggle will drown rapidly in quicksand, especially if the head has no floatation or support.

Quicksand Can Be a Deathtrap. In 1964, two college students were hiking in the swampland south of Florida's Lake Okeechobee. The lead hiker was walking along the sandy bank of a small stream when his feet suddenly disappeared into the sand. He was quickly chest deep in thick sand. His fellow hiker extended a tree branch, but the entrapped hiker was unable to free his hands to grab the limb and sank deeper into the sand until he had completely disappeared.

Not only do people vanish into mud and quicksand, but vehicles and animals have also disappeared without a trace. Quicksand is a fascinating phenomenon of nature that requires cautious respect. Tidal flats are particularly dangerous. In September of 1988, a woman became mired in the mud flats near Turnagain, Alaska, when she attempted to push a trailer out of the mud. Her husband worked for two hours and managed to free one of her legs. Emergency rescue was called, and a team worked to free the woman, but was unable to extricate her before the tide came in and she drowned.

The extrication of human victims is best achieved by having someone pull with a rope while the victim swims out with extremely slow, deliberate motions. For obvious reasons, this is not an option for animal victims. There are reports of human victims swimming 4 m (13 ft) in an eight-hour period to escape without assistance by moving their bodies very slowly into a horizontal position, floating face up. Leveraging against an object, such as a large walking stick, can ease the task.

Quicksand rescues require significant planning and commonsense. In 2001, three deer in a South Carolina state park became mired in "pluff mud" (local name for quicksand) 30 m (98 ft) from the bank. The Charleston Rescue Squad and the Department of Natural Resources wildlife officers were dispatched but refused to enter the mud for safety reasons. The responders waited for the tide to rise and approached the animals on the surface of the water in an airboat. They sedated the animals, injected air to extract them from the mud, strapped them to a human rescue basket, transported them to dry land, and released them. The rescue was efficiently planned and executed without human or animal injury.

Mud

Deep mud at rest is similar to quicksand but may be more difficult to escape because it possesses a more solid structure and creates a stronger partial vacuum as an object or extremity is removed. It is easy for a relaxed

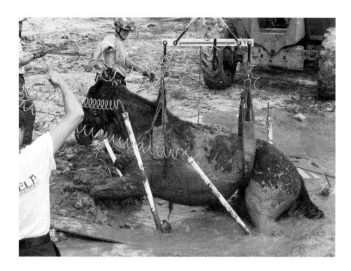

Figure 7.21 *This horse is being extricated using a vertical lift from the mud while responders force air under each extremity as it rises through the mud. Courtesy of Tori Miller.*

animal to float on top of the mud, but struggling and attempts to dig the animal out may cause it to sink further into the mud. The viscosity (resistance to flow) of the mud is related to the type of soil suspended in the water (e.g., clay, sand, organic humus, etc.). Mud can vary widely in consistency. Rescuing an animal trapped in mud 3 m (9 ft) from hard ground can be as challenging as rescuing one 40 ms (130 ft) away (Figure 7.21). Digging is the most common method initially attempted, but is ineffective in softer mud because the mud quickly refills the hole. If the mud is sufficiently dry or sandy, digging attempts may have limited success. Rescuers should not enter the mud with the animal due to the significant risk of injury and human entrapment (altering an animal rescue attempt into an animal and human rescue attempt).

In a 2002 case in Ohio, a horse was mired in mud that appeared to be dry on the surface. The rider asked a backhoe excavator on the scene to remove the mud from around one side of the horse. An analysis of this incident would indicate that extreme caution is necessary because of the high risk of accidental injury to the horse when heavy equipment is used. This was a simple approach and allowed the horse to roll onto it's back– away from the entrapping mud– and rise to its feet by itself. One limitation to the use of heavy equipment is the need for the equipment to be rapidly withdrawn when the animal is struggling. In addition, the noise and vibration generated by heavy equipment often induce a panic response from the animal victim. As in all rescue situations, a good quality halter and lead rope are essential.

Mudslide, Debris Flow, Lahar

Mudslides and mudflows can range in consistency from muddy water to a coarse, pasty substance resembling wet concrete. A lahar is a mudflow consisting of volcanic debris and water; these flows possess high energy and speed and can cover several dozen meters per second for long distances.

Mudslides and volcanic debris flows pose a threefold hazard; they have the ability to crush, bury, and dislocate. The force exerted by flowing mud and the debris it may carry can crush structures, people, and animals. Mud can flow around and over objects to entrap them or bury them entirely. For humans and animals this may result in death due to asphyxiation or hypothermia. The flows can also carry structures or victims for large distances.

FIND A BETTER ANCHOR POINT

Pulling on the victim's head is ineffective and dangerous. However, this method has often been employed by inexperienced rescuers because the head and part of the neck were the only parts of the animal's body that were readily accessible. A veterinary practitioner reported putting a horse down after struggling to remove it by pulling on the head and attempting to dig the mud from around it's body in a dried pond bottom for over six hours (Stafford, 2006). There are documented cases of farmers using power winches and vehicles to pull cattle out of muddy ponds; because the rope or chain was anchored around the animal's head or neck, the animal was asphyxiated or decapitated by the effort. Nerve damage and facial or skull injuries can occur if the halter is used as the sole anchor point to extricate an animal from the mud. Halters should be used for restraint and guidance, not as anchors.

Increase Surface Area to Stay on Top of the Mud

Mud that entraps animals can sometimes be walked on by humans simply because the ratio of the surface area of a human's feet to their body weight is much larger than that of a prey animal. Rescuers need to increase their surface area-to-weight ratio to safely approach the victim and prevent becoming trapped in the mud themselves. This is accomplished by spreading weight distribution over a larger surface area. Effective means of increasing weight distribution include using an inflatable ice rescue path or plywood sheeting (Figure 7.22). An inflated inner tube should be placed under the chin of the animal for supplemental flotation; this method is extremely effective in scenarios where the animal is exhausted and may not be able to keep its nostrils above the mud.

The Partial Vacuum Effect

A less dangerous approach uses air or water injection to fill the space and negate the partial vacuum effect as the victim's extremity is pulled out of the mud. Mud can exert a strong suction or vacuum effect, often

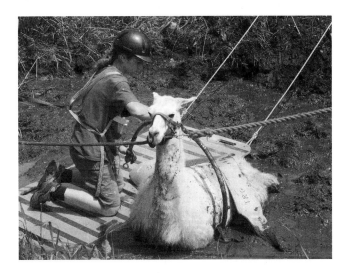

Figure 7.22 *A plywood board with antiskid tape and ropes to allow positioning is placed next to a trapped llama to allow an operational person to approach and work safely. This responder is employing the Nikopoulos needle around the belly of the animal to feed a pilot line, followed by webbing, underneath the animal's abdomen and thorax in configuration for a vertical lift. Courtesy of Claudia Sarti.*

making it many times harder to overcome the partial vacuum of the mud than to overcome the weight of the victim. The partial vacuum effect of mud on the body and long extremities of animals and humans can exert more force than the gravitational forces (weight) exerted on the victim. The joints and muscles may become severely damaged if excessive force is used to lift the victim without negating the vacuum effect of the mud. The use of winches should be avoided in both human and animal rescue. Manual, rope, or mechanical rope systems are recommended because they allow greater control of the pulling effort.

The injection of air or water into the mud to negate the suction or vacuum effect has been used for years to extricate heavy equipment from the mud. In 2000 Allen Schwartz of Days End Farm Horse Rescue in Lisbon, Maryland, applied this technique to large animal rescue in the United States for the first time. The method has evolved to using injected air or water to negate the mud's vacuum effect on the animal's body before vertical lift techniques are employed. In the United Kingdom, rescuers have used the mud or sand lance for many years for the same purpose.

Vertical Lift Is Not Always Necessary

Many times the animal will be stuck too far from stable ground and not accessible with vehicles, cranes, or all-terrain forklifts. If the animal can be turned onto its side, the increased body surface area contact will usually keep its body on top of the mud and allow it to be dragged by the hindquarters or front torso (using the Hampshire slip, forward assist, backward drag, or Santa

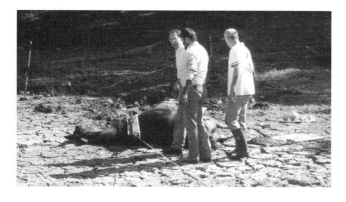

Figure 7.23 *A Santa Barbara sling was attached around the animal's body at the level of the withers, and a horizontal haul apparatus was used to shift the animal onto its side and pull it to firm ground. A tarp, plywood sheeting, or Rescue Glide underneath the animal is recommended to minimize skin trauma, and often makes the use of a winch unnecessary. Courtesy of Rebecca Gimenez.*

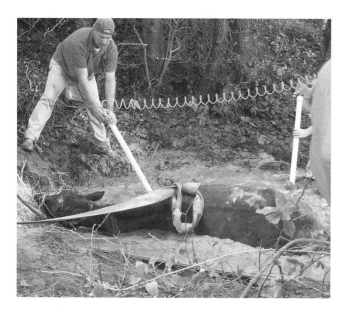

Figure 7.24 *An operational responder injects air with a PVC air injector into the mud trapping the legs of a horse while other personnel pull on the webbing around the horse in a modified Santa Barbara sling configuration. Notice the animal has been rolled onto one side to increase the surface area on top of the mud and facilitate access to the extremities. Courtesy of Tori Miller.*

Barbara sling methods) to solid ground (Figure 7.23 and Figure 7.24). (See Chapter 15.) The animals will often lie quietly as they are pulled and begin struggling when the pressure is released. Rescuers should be prepared for the animal to rise when it reaches solid footing and the pressure is released.

Inexperienced or less knowledgeable responders may position themselves behind an animal stuck in mud to push on its hindquarters, or they may position themselves too close to the animal's body without a safety buddy and safety line. The physical effort exerted

by a struggling animal can severely injure a rescuer if a thrashing body part is suddenly or unexpectedly extricated and contacts the rescuer with extreme force. The placement of webbing around the hindquarters can be used in conjunction with the forward assist, but it is not as effective when used as the sole method of forward pull.

Vertical Lift

If the animal is near stable ground, a web sling vertical lift method with a crane or mechanical rope system can be employed with simultaneous use of injected air or water to break the suction of the mud. If the animal is entrapped near a steep bank or solid footing, an A-frame or tripod may be used to lift the animal and swing it to the bank.

If a helicopter lift is considered, wide webbing and consideration of surface area contact on the body are particularly important. The Anderson Sling is the only recommended sling for helicopter sling loading of a live animal; this sling is very difficult to properly place on an animal trapped in mud. (See Chapter 18.) The World Society for the Protection of Animals reported the attempts made by inexperienced helicopter crews to rescue cattle trapped in mud and volcanic lava flows in 2005. The crews did not break the mud's suction on the animals before using the helicopter to lift the animals; unfortunately, the animals were literally cut in half as the cable tightened around their bodies. Negating the suction and vacuum of the mud is critical for mud rescues regardless of the lifting method employed.

Requirements for Employment of Mud Rescue

Equipment. Certain equipment is needed for a mud rescue of an animal victim.

- Sheet(s) of plywood or any flat board (including an EMS backboard) can be used to direct animals into a chute, block animals from a path, or support a human's weight on mud. Animals should not be allowed to walk on the boards. Modifications to these boards to increase safety and efficiency include adding tread to one side of the board to improve the footing, painting the board a bright color to protect the wood from rotting and make it easier to clean, cutting holes to facilitate grasping and carrying, and adding rope lines to facilitate moving the board on the surface of the mud.
- Fire hose of any length and size appropriate is a necessity. It can be inflated with air to serve as a flotation device for rescuers or to create a floating obstacle to drive swimming animals in the intended direction.

- A compressed air source (e.g., breathing air bottle, compressor, tank or vehicle source) with a 30 psi minimum inflation pressure is necessary for air injection to negate the suction/vacuum effect of the mud.
- A Nikopolous needle (a 2 m, or 6 ft, piece of 4 cm, or 1.5 in., electrical conduit bent into a C shape with a metal loop at far end or modified with a garden hose attachment at one end) facilitates the placement of webbing or rescue cord. (See Chapter 15.) The Nikopoulos needle is threaded through the mud around the animal; a hose attachment on the needle allows water to flow out from the opening at the front of the needle, facilitating its passage through the mud. The webbing or rescue cord is then attached to the front end, and the needle is withdrawn by threading it back around the animal in reverse of its original path. This results in webbing placement in the path created by the needle. The needle facilitates the proper placement of webbing despite submersion of the body's ideal anchor points and allows rescuers to avoid using the head and neck to extricate an animal victim.
- A sand or mud lance (4 ft, or 1.2 m long, 1 in. or 2.5 cm, stainless pipe with T handle with attachments for air or water injection) allows injection of compressed air or water into the mud to break the suction/vacuum effect on the animal's extremities.
- A Santa Barbara sling (modified heavy duty leather or nylon web surcingle heavy duty buckle and D rings around the entire surcingle) allows sideways dragging of the animal along the surface of mud or ice. *Note:* This sling is not appropriate for vertical lift.
- A section of 6.1 cm (2.5 in.) wide webbing 10 m (33 ft) long is necessary for backward drag, Hampshire slip sideways drag, or forward assist.
- Simple vertical lift equipment (see Chapter 16).
- Schwartz air injectors (15 1/2 in. [1.3 cm] PVC pipe 5 ft [1.5 m] long with slant-cut ends, end caps, and air connectors) can be used if a mud or sand lance is not available. Ideally, one air injector per limb is recommended.
- A Hampshire strop guide (2 m [6.6 ft] long, 8 cm [3.1 in.] wide stainless cold-rolled steel with slight natural bend) allows webbing or rescue cord to be pushed under the animal and threaded to the other side to establish an anchor point other than the head, neck, or legs.
- An air manifold with valves, air line, and accessories for air connectors are used to provide air pressure through the mud or sand lance or Schwartz air injectors.
- A water hose and water source are necessary for use with the Nickopolous needle; low water pressure is appropriate.
- Small-diameter rescue cord is used to attach sections of webbing to the Nikopoulos needle or strop guide

to facilitate proper placement of the webbing around the animal victim's body.
- Appropriate mechanical rescue rope systems are necessary for providing the pulling forces for extrication (see Chapter 14).
- An Ice Path (inflatable rescue path, or IRP) 5 m (16.5 ft) long allows rescue personnel to walk across the surface of the water or mud. If not available, plywood boards (as described above) can be used.

Personnel. Personnel needed for a mud rescue are the following:

- IC
- Animal handler
- Operational personnel (two to four persons)
- Designated SO

Procedure for Conducting Mud Rescue (Small or Large Animal). With planning and appropriate equipment (as described above), a team of five trained personnel can extricate most animals from mud in ten minutes.

1. All personnel should approach the animal by standing on plywood sheets or an Ice Path. All rescuers should have individual taglines to a safety buddy on safe ground or to the inflatable Ice Path.

2. The Animal handler should approach the animal and place a halter on the animal's head for guidance and physical restraint only. Sedation should be cautiously considered on an individual basis because struggling will often worsen the animal's entrapment; however, sedating a hypothermic, stressed, or medically compromised animal can increase the risk of suffocation, injury, or death. An inflated inner tube can be used to keep the animal's nostrils above the water or mud. The inner tube can be tied under the halter to maintain it in place.

3. For animals trapped deeply in mud, the Nikopolous needle can be used to thread a small-diameter rescue cord under the animal at the level of the withers (behind the foreleg). A section of webbing can be attached to the end of this small cord and pulled around and underneath the animal by reversing the path of the Nikopoulos needle (Figure 7.25). Digging should be avoided, as it will destabilize the surface of the mud.

If the animal is trapped near the surface of the mud, a Hampshire strop guide can be threaded underneath the animal. Rescue cord or webbing is attached to the free end of the guide, and the guide is pulled in reverse to thread the rescue cord or webbing under the animal's body behind the forelimbs or in front of the hind limbs.

One piece of 9 m (30 ft) webbing can be used to perform a forward assist or backward drag, a Santa Barbara surcingle, or the Hampshire slip method (Figure 7.26). Duplicate pieces of 1 m (3 ft) webbing should be

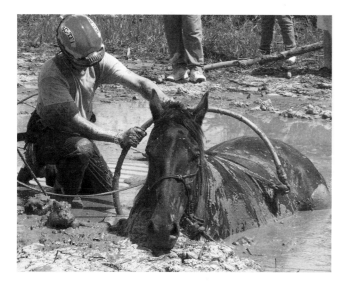

Figure 7.25 *The Nikopoulos needle is pushed down and around the animal in the mud to force a pilot line around the animal's body. Webbing can then be attached to the pilot line and placed around the animal's abdomen and thorax in preparation for a horizontal pull or vertical lift of the animal in concert with air or water injection methods. Courtesy of Tori Miller.*

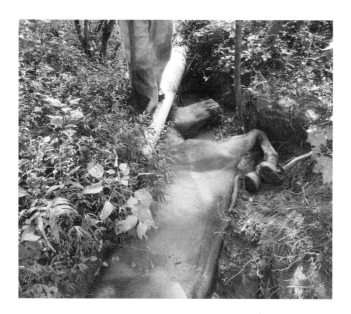

Figure 7.26 *This horse is stuck under a culvert. An appropriate and rapid rescue method would be a forward assist appliance using webbing in a lark's foot (choke) configuration around the chest. Courtesy of Tori Miller.*

used for simple vertical lift with a Becker sling or the UC Davis-Large Animal Lift (see Chapter 16).

4. The webbing is attached as appropriate for the slip, drag, or lift methods.

5. A mud lance or PVC pipe assembly is preloaded with air or water and inserted into the mud next to each leg of the animal (without injuring the animal). Air or water is forced into the mud to break the suction/

partial vacuum effect while rescuers exert forces necessary to lift, pull, or drag the animal out of the mud. This is repeated as necessary. *Note:* Rolling the animal so that it is in lateral recumbency (on its side) increases the body surface area in contact with the mud and facilitates dragging the animal across the surface. Placing the animal's body onto an Ice Path, Rescue Glide, heavy duty tarp, or sheet of plywood may facilitate the effort. Rope systems may be anchored to the plywood or Rescue Glide; however, many animals must be pulled by their bodies with webbing around the body as the anchor, but not the head and neck or legs.

Mechanical rope systems or human power may be considered for pulling on the load (victim). Most animals will relax and lie quietly when pressure is applied across their body; however, they may begin to struggle as soon as the pressure is relieved. A quick release or an emergency knife should be readily available to cut the ropes if necessary. A halter and lead rope should be placed on the animal for control and restraint when the animal reaches solid ground.

Specialty Equipment for Unstable Ground Rescue

Ice Path or Inflatable Rescue Path. The IRP is a component of the animal rescue equipment inventory of the UK fire brigades. The Hampshire and Kent Fire and Rescue Services have led the effort in developing technologies for animal mud rescue. With hundreds of miles of coastline and inland waterways in the United Kingdom, this is an extremely common response scenario for their jurisdictions.

This device allows firefighters to access areas of unstable ground such as mud or ice, but is not suitable for swiftwater rescue. It can also be used as a floating raft platform on water. It can support up to 500 kg (1,100 lb) by displacing and spreading the weight over a larger surface area. It is a 5 m (16 1/2 ft) long, 1.5 m (5 ft) wide, reinforced rubber platform deployed with air from a standard cylinder. Multiple IRPs can be leapfrogged to reach a victim far from stable ground. A rigid, inflatable boat can be used to deliver the IRP to the rescue scene away from shore (P. Baker, 2006).

The IRP has two sides: one with a tread surface to provide stable, nonslip footing for personnel, and another with a slick surface. Personnel can walk on the treaded surface of an IRP placed over still water (less than 1 m [3 ft] deep), ice, or mud. The slick side of the IRP is useful for pulling a "packaged" (restrained) animal up a bank or over the surface of mud or other obstacles (e.g., roots, boulders, etc.) to reduce the friction and facilitate the pulling effort (Green, 2005). Lubricant may be added on top of the IRP to further facilitate the effort.

Mats for Traversing Unstable Ground. Heavy-duty epoxy Mo-Mat panels (15 m [50 ft] lengths) have been used since the 1940s by Department of Defense forces in the United States and by drilling and mining operations worldwide to traverse beachheads and unstable ground. If soft conditions are encountered, the panels can be used in leapfrog fashion to reach the rescue site with vehicles. Unfortunately, these systems require heavy equipment for placement and are no longer manufactured.

To solve the problem of moving vehicles over soft soils the U.S. Army Corps of Engineers' Engineer Research and Development Center (ERDC) developed new materials and matting systems for rapid construction of roadways. The ERDC investigated the use of a combination of geosynthetics, mat systems, and strong soil layers to surface roadways in civil engineering applications (ERDC, 2006; Santoni and Tingle., 2002).

Mud Lance (Sand Lance). This equipment is a one-piece stainless steel lance 1.2 m (4 ft) long with connections for air or water. This equipment is also ideal for forcing water into overheated hay bales to prevent combustion. Compressed air is most commonly used to loosen dry materials, and water is used for wet materials. Employment of this device is simple: the hose is connected from the cylinder regulator outlet to the quick-connect inlet coupling on the mud lance, and the lance is inserted into the mud.

For safe operation, the operator should wear a wet/dry suit as appropriate, gloves, and safety goggles. The victim's eyes should be protected if mud and debris is a concern. The operator should not bend the lance. The mud lance is retracted and reinserted in the mud surrounding an extremity. Care should be taken when inserting the lance to avoid direct contact with the animal victim's limbs. The mud lance is manufactured using heavy-gauge stainless steel and should be periodically tested with normal supply media (8 bar compressed air and 8 bar for water) to ensure its integrity. A homemade lance constructed of stainless steel by a local welder at the request of the authors has been extremely effective.

ICE RESCUE

Ice rescue of a large animal is a particularly challenging scenario because it involves a rescue environment that is extremely dangerous (water), a potentially dangerous and unpredictable victim, and extremely cold conditions. The correct equipment, surface suits, and training are required for the preparation and attempt of these rescues. If the proper gear and training are not available, ice rescue should not be attempted (Hendrick and Zaferes, 1999). Binoculars can be used to perform the risk assessment before committing personnel to the rescue environment (Fire Service Guides, 1998).

Current State of Technology for Large Animal Ice Rescue

Roping or lassoing a large animal and pulling it from the ice trap by its head or neck is not a professional or recommended approach to large animal ice rescue. As previously mentioned, animals can be injured or asphyxiated by pressure from the rope. In addition, this method often pulls the animal through the ice like the prow of a ship; instead, pulling the animal across the surface of the ice provides less resistance.

Ice rescue of large animals does not require equipment beyond that required for human surface ice rescue. Simple rescues can be performed with basic equipment and adequately trained and prepared personnel. In 2004, the Wilmington, Ohio, rescue squad and fire department were called to assist with four Belgian draft horses that had become trapped by ice. Two of the animals drowned prior to the department's arrival, but they were able to perform an effective rescue of the remaining two animals. Chain saws were used to cut a path to the animals (10 m [33 ft] from the bank), and the ice was removed from the cut path. Willow trees were encased in the ice for a 3 m (10 ft) distance, and underwater cutting saws were necessary to remove the trees and enable the rescue. The animals were exhausted and cold, but able to swim to the bank. The animals were led to a nearby barn and warmed with kerosene jet heaters and blankets and were provided immediate veterinary treatment. Several similar rescues using this method have reported excellent results but may require a sense of urgency due to the risk of the victim drowning.

Equine Emergency Response Unit of Kansas City, Missouri, was dispatched to a farm where a horse had walked out onto a frozen pond attempting to find water, falling through the ice 2 m (6 1/2 ft) from shore. A sledge hammer and pry bar were used to break a path in the ice to the horse. With encouragement, the horse exited the water and ice under its own power (Thompson, 2006).

In a similar incident in West Virginia, a horse drinking from a creek slipped into the ice and became recumbent and exhausted. Rescuers applied a web sling to make a vertical lift. Difficulties were initially encountered when the wrecker could not be placed close enough to the bank to allow the boom to reach the sling. This was mitigated by digging the bank back to stable soil and filling the holes. The animal sustained severe lacerations on its legs from thrashing on the sharp edges of the ice. Once rescued to dry ground, a veterinarian was on scene to treat the hypothermic and injured animal.

Vertical Lifts from Small Ice or Mud Holes

A small ice hole is a challenge because the animal must be lifted vertically to allow its pelvis (hips) and hind legs to clear the surface and prevent injury. If a wider

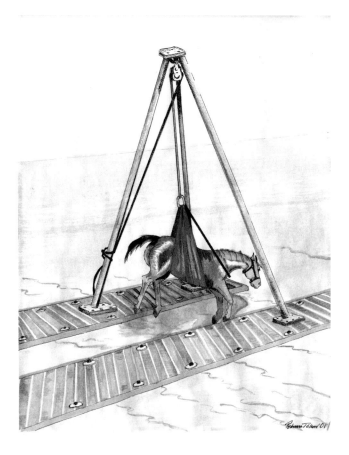

Figure 7.27 A horse in tidal mud in the United Kingdom is being lifted using a tripod stabilized on unstable ground by use of inflatable rescue paths (IRPs) and simple vertical lift techniques. The IRP in the center will slide under the lifted animal, the animal will be set down on top of it, and the IRP with the animal's body weight on it will be pulled to shore. *Courtesy of Becky Tolson.*

opening can be made, there will be more room available to maneuver the victim. Heavy lift equipment, tripods, and A-frames (see Chapter 16) are not appropriate or safe when used directly on top of ice surfaces; the heavy weight of these pieces of equipment is distributed on the small surface area of the devices' legs and will pierce and fall through the ice surface. In certain situations (depending upon the animal victim's weight and the thickness of the mud or ice), an IRP can be employed to provide a stable surface and distribute the device's weight over a larger area. Three IRPs should be used: two are placed on either side of the animal to support the legs of the tripod lifting frame (two legs of the tripod are placed on one path) (Figure 7.27). When the animal is lifted clear from the hole, a third IRP is slid into place underneath the animal to seal the hole opening and avoid dropping the animal back into the hole in the event the equipment fails. The sedated animal is then lowered on to the third IRP path and moved to safety by dragging the rescue path with the animal on top of it. This procedure is the same for mud as it is for ice.

In this situation, with nothing else available, a forward assist web sling in a lark's foot (choke) configuration can be used. The webbing is passed around the chest at the level of the sternum and withers and passed between the front legs to the lifting equipment for an overhead lift (see Chapter 15). If overhead lift equipment is not available, webbing can be placed around the chest (and possibly the abdomen) in a lark's foot configuration, and the animal can be rolled onto its side (perhaps on a tarp or Rescue Glide) and manually pulled using a Hampshire slip or forward assist method.

It may be necessary to sedate the animal to prevent it from attempting to stand on the ice when it has been extricated from the hole. Flotation support for the animal's head while it is in the water can be provided using an inner tube tied under the halter or inflated fire hose or PFD placed underneath the animal's head.

Other successful ice rescues of large animals have included breaking the ice from the shore out to the animal with a heavy object (tire, concrete block, chunk of metal) tied to a rope and thrown repeatedly to make a small trail. This prevents the rescuers from getting onto the ice themselves.

ACRONYMS USED IN CHAPTER 7

ART	Advanced Rescue Technology
CRED	Centre for Research on the Epidemiology of Disasters
CVM	College of Veterinary Medicine
EMS	Emergency Medical Services
ERDC	Engineer Research and Development Center
FEMA	Federal Emergency Management Agency
HazMat	Hazardous Materials
IC	Incident Commander
IRP	Inflatable Rescue Paths
LAFD	Large Animal Flotation Device
PFD	Personal Flotation Device
PPE	Personal Protective Equipment
PVC	Polyvinylchloride
ReThRoG-H	Reach, throw, row, go, and helicopter
SO	Safety Officer
WSPA	World Society for the Protection of Animals

WEB SITE RESOURCES

www.rescue3.com
www.code3associates.org/tar.html
www.cred.be
www.ncfloodmaps.com/pubdocs/historicdata.htm
www.UNMUSEUM.org
http://www.tenspider.net/security-hazards/lahar-mud-quicksand.html
www.wsfb.co.uk/equipment/irp.htm
http://www.hosetechnologies.co.uk/11-Lance.pdf

8 Loose Large Animals

Dr. Rebecca Gimenez

INTRODUCTION

Unfortunately, loose large animals are an extremely common scenario worldwide, contributing to significant injuries and deaths of people in vehicles that hit them. Animals may also attack people. Loose animals can injure themselves easily, cause destruction of property and equipment, and disrupt community function and safety. Injured animals and intact males of most large animal species can be aggressive and dangerous, while even tame ones can accidentally injure well-meaning rescuers as a result of their fear and flight responses (Figure 8.1).

Prevention includes educating residents of a community to maintain safe fencing and to avoid releasing animals from a trailer without first establishing proper containment. On local and state levels, prevention of loose animals would include support of animal control officers and humane society efforts to increase the quality of fencing as well as laws that would mandate stiff consequences for owners of loose animals, especially repeat offenders.

A vehicle doesn't have to impact a large animal very hard or fast to throw the animal over the hood of the vehicle and into the windshield; the center of gravity of a large animal is higher than most car bumpers, and they are lifted by the impact of the bumper and grill and the momentum of the vehicle. When impacted, the animal's body rolls over into the vehicle and can injure or kill the occupants. This situation most commonly involves deer, moose, cattle, and horses.

In typical wrecks, pigs, goats, or cattle may be thrown onto the roadway when a livestock hauler overturns or is split open by an obstacle; alternately, they may fall out due to an unlatched or damaged door or ramp. In general, these animals will graze in the median or on the side of the roadway unless chased or frightened. It is more difficult to effectively drive or contain excited or frightened prey animals. Previously described methods of driving and containment, based on knowledge of these species' behaviors (see Chapter 4), are more effective and efficient.

LOOSE ANIMALS CAN BE DEADLY

A study released in 2004 by the Centers for Disease Control and Prevention estimated 247,000 major incidents between animals and vehicles per year on U.S. roadways, contributing to over 26,000 injuries (more than 10%) and 200 human deaths. This study estimated that 9 out of 10 animal-related wrecks involved moose and deer, but other animal species represented included cattle, horses, squirrels, bears, dogs, raccoons, and alligators. In 2006 a loose donkey on a Texas interstate caused a fatal collision between two tractor trailers when one driver swerved to avoid the animal. The animal continued to run loose for three hours until animal control officers lassoed it and transported it away from the scene.

It can be difficult for vehicle drivers to see prey animals from an adequate distance because the hair of prey animals diffracts incoming light; as the headlight beams from an approaching vehicle reaches the animal, its hairs bend the light and decrease the animal's visibility in the incident light beam from the headlights. This characteristic evolved as a protective mechanism to decrease detection by predators. Most large animals cannot be seen in the road in the dark until the driver is approximately 50m (165ft) from the animal (Gimenez, 2006c). At highway speeds a driver cannot see the animal in time to react, much less stop or avoid hitting it. Even in daylight, animals beside the roadway can be very difficult to see from the road. The unpredictable behavior of many prey species can increase the

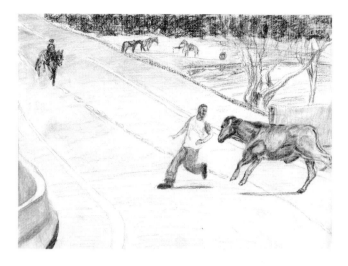

Figure 8.1 *Responders should not tease or chase livestock, especially when the animal is loose. The assistance of a professional cowboy with a lariat to catch and hold (not drag) the animal while waiting for transportation assets is suggested. Courtesy of Julie Casil.*

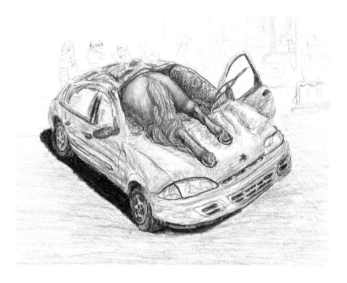

Figure 8.2 *Loose large animals cause severe injuries and death of drivers globally. The hair shaft of the animal's fur refracts an incident light beam from headlights, making it almost impossible to see the animal until the driver is too close to stop. Education of animal owners, increased standards for fencing, and a system of fines for repeat offenders could decrease the incidence of these tragedies. Courtesy of Julie Casil.*

risk of impact and injury. The natural colors of prey animals tend to be dark and earth-toned; from an evolutionary standpoint, bright colors and patterns increase the risk of predation (Figure 8.2).

According to a 2001 study, there were 3,192 accidents in Texas that involved an animal impacted by a vehicle. Out of a total of 323,958 incidents, there were 1,601 human injuries and 12 human fatalities. In most cases, the accident causes severe injury or is fatal for the animal.

LEGAL ASPECTS OF LOOSE ANIMALS

All U.S. states and many other countries have applicable livestock laws concerning the relationships between animal ownership, property, vehicle operation, and the animals themselves. These laws tend to be complex and should be investigated by responders in their jurisdiction. Even the legal definition of a "fence" can vary; for example, California law 17121 defines a "lawful fence" as follows:

> A lawful fence is any fence which is good, strong, substantial, and sufficient to prevent the ingress and egress of livestock. No wire fence is a good and substantial fence within the meaning of this article unless it has three tightly stretched barbed wires securely fastened to posts of reasonable strength, firmly set in the ground not more than one rod apart, one of which wires shall be at least four feet above the surface of the ground. Any kind of wire or other fence of height, strength and capacity equal to or greater than the wire fence herein described is a good and substantial fence within the meaning of this article. The term "lawful fence" includes cattle guards of such width, depth, rail spacing, and construction as will effectively turn livestock.

State and local laws may base their definitions of acceptable fencing as that which contains one's own livestock or that excludes other livestock. Most states require owners to make a reasonable effort to maintain fences to keep livestock off public roadways. The laws often provide for liability if a motor vehicle or train strikes an animal, but whether the liability lies with the owner of the animal or the operator of the vehicle may differ between jurisdictions.

The language of most U.S. state laws concerning the operation of vehicles near livestock is similar to California law 21759:

> The driver of any vehicle approaching any horse drawn vehicle, any ridden animal, or any livestock shall exercise proper control of his vehicle and shall reduce speed or stop as may appear necessary or as may be signaled or otherwise requested by any person driving, riding or in charge of the animal or livestock in order to avoid frightening and to safeguard the animal or livestock and to insure the safety of any person driving or riding the animal or in charge of the livestock.

However, for animals that are not under the direct control and charge of a person, the owner may be subject to liability if the animal is struck, similar to California 16902: regarding permitting livestock on a highway, "A person that owns or controls the possession of any livestock shall not willfully or negligently permit any of the livestock to stray upon, or remain unaccompanied by a person in charge or control of the livestock upon, a public highway . . ."

In some U.S. counties, there are still free-range grazing laws; these may alter the legal implications of a collision with an animal (Nixon, 2006). For example, also in California 16902, regarding presumptions or inferences in actions for motor vehicle collisions with animals: "In any civil action which is brought by the owner, driver, or occupant of a motor vehicle, or by their personal representatives or assignees, or by the owner of livestock, for damages which are caused by collision between any motor vehicle and any domestic animal on a highway, there is no presumption or inference that the collision was due to negligence on behalf of the owner or the person in possession of the animal." In other words, the owners may not be held liable for injury or damage when free-ranging animals are involved.

The disposition of livestock captured by someone other than the owner (animal control, humane society, private persons) as strays, and the capturers' responsibilities for returning the animals or keeping them, vary widely between states. Brand laws in most states address the registration of brands for identifying livestock and horses, written bills of sales, and a system of inspection of livestock sold at auction or moved inter- or intrastate. Much of this portion of the law is directly aimed at preventing the theft of livestock and horses, which is still a common crime across the country.

DEVELOP A PLAN TO RECOVER THE ANIMAL(S)

Responders should encourage all humans on scene to remain calm and work to develop a strategy to recover the animal(s). Teamwork with bystanders and rescuers combined with close attention to prey animal herding behaviors will provide safe tactics to confront the dangerous scenario of a loose animal on the road, on the trail, or at livestock events. Options for containing the animals include driving them into a pasture, cutting the fence on the interstate, or driving them into a backyard or more confined area. "Catching" a prey animal is rarely the correct strategy to employ. Instead, a professional should use concepts based on animals' motivations, such as food enticement, containment, and use of Judas animals. While it may seem an impossible task, good preparation and effective employment of a strategy will increase the chances of success.

Use Prey Animal Motivations to Your Advantage

Food and herd membership are strong motivations for large animals. Some animals will recognize and be attracted to the sound of shaking grain in a bag or

bucket or the sight and smell of hay thrown on the grass. A loose animal will tend to go toward familiar surroundings (e.g., trailhead, pasture, trailer, barn, etc.) and may be more easily driven toward these areas. Many loose animal rescue scenarios involve animals that are far from home and in unfamiliar surroundings. When searching for loose animals, responders should first check livestock facilities close to the scene; animals will be attracted to local livestock.

In group scenarios, catching one animal (preferably the dominant animal of the group) often allows the handler to lead the others, because the animals' herd instincts keep them together. Handlers should avoid approaching animals that give off negative body language and instead catch one that appears interested in treats or human contact. For example, trained responders were driving on Highway 89 in Utah when they observed two horses grazing beside the road outside of a barbed wire fence. The rescuer approached the horses with an emergency halter and treats in hand (Figure 8.3) and used proper body language and knowledge of horse behavior. By approaching the horse exhibiting positive body language and offering it a treat, the animal was safely and efficiently caught and restrained. Both horses were then led to safety inside a nearby fence.

Professional responders should encourage the use of behavioral cues as opposed to force to control large animals, and they should avoid capture deadlines (see Chapter 4). Loose animals do not respond to force in the same manner as confined animals. Instructors in livestock handling courses encourage owners and professional handlers to learn to use proper body language, the flight zones of the animal, their herding instincts,

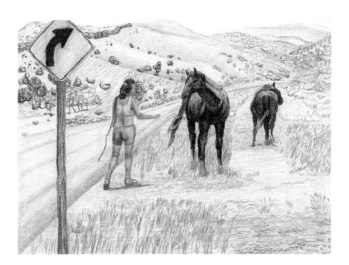

Figure 8.3 *Appropriate body language, voice, and treats encourage loose animals to allow the animal handler to approach them in these scenarios. The body language of the closest horse shows its interest in the treat as it allows the handler to enter its action zone. Courtesy of Julie Casil.*

and animals' stress responses to the benefit of the handlers on live scenes (Woods, 2005).

Behavior is much easier to use to the rescuer's advantage; although using animal behavior is simple, it is a learned skill like anything else in the specialty rescue field. For example, if there is another animal trapped (e.g., in a septic tank, mud, or overturned trailer), it is often advisable to keep a Judas animal standing calmly within the line of sight of the trapped animal during the extrication process. If the trapped animal can see another of its own species, it will be calmer during the rescue.

Fear Reaction

In the wild, predators tend to attack the prey animal's back or the hind legs; from there they grip, bite, and claw to disable their prey. As previously described (see Chapter 4), prey species often cannot see objects or animals (including humans) approaching from the rear; the animal's fight or flight response may be evoked before the animal realizes that the perceived predator is not a threat. In addition, some large animals may have had negative experiences with humans in the past that will impact their response to approaching rescuers.

On a rescue scene, the animal is usually in an unfamiliar setting and will predictably react with fear. Using a Judas animal to catch animals of the same species is a good idea but will not work with a different species of animal. For example many horses are fearful of sheep, pigs, goats, or llamas. Camelids are inherently curious and will aggressively approach and inspect another animal of any species; this may incite a fearful response by a horse unfamiliar with these species and increase the risks of injury or loss of the handler's control over the animal.

Behavior Dictates Animal Reactions

Prey animals are easily frightened and their herd mentality can cause one excitable loose animal to excite other animals; multiple animals running loose generates a dangerous scenario, especially on roadways. There are many examples of one loose, excited animal at a show or event causing other animals to break loose of their ties or handlers and stampede through the showground. The danger increases with the number of animals and if equipment (e.g., carriages, saddles, gates, or boards pulled from the wall, etc.) is being dragged. If a horse is hindered by the reins or a tipped saddle, or is dragging an object it pulled loose (e.g., limb, carriage pieces, fence post), it may panic and seriously injure itself or others. Its fear might make it injure any person that gets close to it. Responders should use caution when approaching an animal that is visibly shaking with fear. It is often advisable to first try to cut away the offending object with a sharp knife before attempting to catch the animal. Sometimes asking the animal to back up under control will allow the handler to maintain control better than leading the animal forward.

An animal is relaxed enough to be approached when it stops or turns, stands still, and looks at the handler with both eyes. Instead of approaching the animal, the handlers should back up slightly and call the animal by name or talk in low, soothing tones. If the animal moves toward the handler, the handler should keep backing away to encourage the loose animal to continue approaching him or her. Offering a treat, forage, or a piece of candy is often helpful in these situations. If the animal is nervously pacing back and forth or in circles around the handler, the handler should stay relaxed and allow the animal to keep moving its feet and approach as it feels more comfortable; eventually, it will turn to look at the handler with both eyes.

Herding Instinct

The instinct to stay with the herd is genetically hardwired into the behavior of prey animals; they are often fearful when alone. Human ancestors in Europe and North America used this tendency to hunt auroch (an extinct species of cattle), deer, and horses by driving entire herds of these animals off cliffs to their deaths for slaughter. Horses have been known to return to a burning barn to rejoin their herd mates, only to perish in the fire. The herd bond can be used to the rescuers' benefit to keep a group of animals together and move them as a group.

When others of the same species are not available, prey species may seek and maintain the company of other species; modern examples of this are horses that are paired with chicken, goat, pig, or kitten companions. Many horsemanship instructors recommend that horse owners establish themselves as their horse's companion in place of other animals.

Once one animal is caught and haltered, it can serve as the "magnet animal" to lead the other loose animals toward safe containment: this animal is called the Judas animal. If one animal of the group cannot be caught, the animal handler should consider using a Judas animal of the same species to attract the loose animals to the original enclosure or site of release. The Judas animal can be led slowly away from the other animals to see if they will follow it off the roadway and into a yard, pasture, or other form of containment. If the Judas can be kept standing calmly and eating forage or grain, the other animals will be attracted to the forage and relaxed by the calmness and presence of the Judas animal.

In a 2004 example, a bystander was driving down the interstate in South Carolina with horses on a trailer and saw animal control officers attempting to slow traffic and catch a loose horse running on the road. The driver pulled off the road onto the emergency lane and opened the windows to let her horses safely stick their heads out of the trailer. Almost immediately they whinnied at the other horse, which came to the trailer and allowed itself to be caught.

The use of a Judas animal is one of the best ways to catch a loose animal and is an excellent example of using the animal's instinctive behaviors to the rescuers' benefit. The maternal instinct is even stronger than the herding instinct; nursing offspring will instinctively follow their dams. The maternal instinct can also be used to bring an adult female animal to a specific place if her offspring can be safely caught and restrained in the safe area. Calves have been placed in the back of vehicles and driven slowly to containment as the cow followed the vehicle, and mares have willingly loaded onto trailers where their foals are restrained.

The Bureau of Land Management (BLM) is often contacted to capture mustangs that have escaped their owners when attempts by the local animal control or humane society have been unsuccessful. This is a common occurrence across the United States; the freeze brand identification on the animal's neck identifies these horses as wild mustangs. Considered a living part of the historical heritage of the Old West, mustangs are subject to special regulations regarding their handling and treatment. The mustangs, often purchased at auctions by well-intended people, still possess wild behaviors that can make them dangerous to uneducated or unprepared owners. The BLM employs cowboys to catch escaped wild horses. These employees consistently find the use of Judas horses to be one of the best methods for recapturing these animals, and their ideas can be applied to rescue efforts (Smythe, 2006).

In 2000, a recently purchased wild mustang stallion bolted off the horse trailer, jumped the fence, and continued running, still dragging its lead rope. The stallion was found 20 km (over 12 miles) away in a junk yard in Greenville, South Carolina. The local animal control office called the BLM to collect the horse. The BLM employee showed up on the scene with a Judas horse and trailer. The cowboy hid under the neck and chest of his horse and backed it toward the approaching mustang. When the dangling lead rope was within reach, the cowboy tied it to his horse's saddle and led his horse onto a stock trailer. The mustang followed the horse onto the trailer and was successfully recaptured with minimal stress.

ON-ROAD RESCUES

If a loose animal crosses roads, responders should take precautions to flag and warn drivers that there is a loose animal along the road; this will help prevent secondary incidents such as a vehicle impacting the animal. It may be necessary to cut a fence or enlist bystanders to make a human chain to close escape routes and form a containment area. Any time the large animal gets near or on a road, there is significant danger. People

have been seriously injured or killed chasing animals near active traffic lanes. The animal will not perceive the road as being a danger zone and may unpredictably dart into traffic.

Responders can be hit by an approaching driver if the animal jumps or runs in front of the vehicle; drivers swerve wildly to avoid hitting animals or unexpected obstacles and can roll their vehicle, hit a tree, or responders. Road safety is the priority on these scenes to keep rescuers, the animal(s), and drivers safe. Flares, signals, and reflective clothing and gear increase visibility (even during daylight hours) and warn drivers of the danger.

Use of Herding Dogs

The question may arise whether or not trained herding dogs should be used on the scene to round up loose cattle and other livestock. Unfortunately, in most areas there are very few well-trained and practiced dog/owner teams that can be employed. Untrained dogs or personnel can hinder the effort by increasing the loose animals' panic level and scattering the group.

Well-trained herding dogs have been used in numerous scenarios in several countries, and they are an excellent and effective method of driving and containing large animals (excluding horses). Cattle- and sheep-herding dogs can quickly round up and drive livestock into containment more efficiently and with less distress than cowboys on horseback or people using portable fencing. Local response organizations should identify if these dogs are available in the area and make prior arrangements for their services as needed.

PREVENTION FOR LARGE ANIMAL OWNERS

There are some practical ways for owners to protect their animals.

- Make sure all trail horses or other large animals are under physical control at all times (haltered with a good-quality lead rope), especially when ponying (leading from another horse) and packing. Use strong overhead tie lines in campgrounds and at rest stops.
- Ensure quality fencing at facilities and check for downed fencing after all storms. Consider using double-barrier fencing for young stock and intact males. Goats and sheep are particularly well known for escaping.
- Teach horses to be willingly tied, led, or ponied and accustomed to trail conditions. Invest time desensitizing horses to strange objects, noises, and events.
- Teach horses to come to people and readily be caught and loaded on a horse trailer, regardless of the conditions (e.g., dark, cold, windy, raining, changing barometric pressure, etc.).

- Use permanent internal and external identification methods on all animals (brand, microchip, identification tag on halter or bridle) to increase the likelihood that your animal will be returned to you when found.
- Riders should wear a fanny pack stocked with a minimum of a cell phone (with global positioning satellite capability), local map, 4–7 m (13–23 ft) of cord to use as an emergency rope halter, and nonperishable treats.
- In backcountry situations where grazing is allowed, use hobbles on stock to limit their movement. Bells can also be used to facilitate locating stock that have wandered despite the hobbles.

Special Focus—Catching a Loose Horse

At some point in their horse-related activities, most riders have been on a runaway horse or had one pull away from them on the ground. The animal does not have to be actually running to be a runaway; a runaway animal is no longer under a person's control or influence. If a horse runs away with a rider aboard, the worst thing that can be done is to chase the horse. If not chased, most horses will return to the herd. The accompanying riders should stop and form a small group to encourage the horse to return to the herd. One person can dismount from his or her horse and lead it, following the loose horse slowly. If the runaway horse stops or turns toward the group, the group should stop and let it come to the horses. One person should dismount and try calling the horse's name and shaking something in his or her hand as though it were grain or a treat. If the horse is maintaining a 10–30 m (33–100 ft) flight distance, it helps to approach the horse leading a quiet horse. Those approaching the animal should use a soothing voice, avoid looking the loose horse directly in the eye, advance toward the horse's shoulder, and groom its neck with their hand to comfort it. An emergency rope halter or belt may be used to restrain the horse temporarily.

If there are other riders on horseback, they should dismount to prevent further excitement and possible runaways. The group of riders should walk their horses in the opposite direction from the loose horse. If the runaway horse does not return within three to five minutes, the riders should call the ranger station and/or 911 for assistance.

If a horse gets loose close to a road or heavily populated area, the rider should immediately call 911 and report the incident and location. Communication with the responders should include the exact location of the loose animal or the exact location it was last seen. The caller should request that responders avoid using flashing lights and sirens when responding to a loose animal incident.

When Animals Get Truly Lost

Sometimes an animal will be sufficiently distracted, injured, or close enough to familiar territory that it leaves the group. Walking other horses in the opposite direction may cause the loose horse to return to the group. Horses should never be chased with other horses; chasing them increases the risk of injury and risk that the horse will be frightened by the approaching animal. Riders should move slowly down the trail in the direction the horse went, and dismount and walk toward the horse. When close, the loose horse may come to the horse being led and allow itself to be caught.

If the animal gets truly lost, their tracks should be followed to where the animal goes off the trail. This point should be marked on the ground and the map. Standard search procedures should be used to avoid searchers from becoming lost. Horses tend to stay on a trail and travel uphill. They instinctively prefer open areas with grass or forage where they feel safer because they can see approaching predators. Horses and pack llamas are less likely to go downhill or into deep woods or brush, unless it is the only source of water. Cattle, on the other hand, tend to browse in deep brush.

Using established search procedures, back-up riders and people on foot should be assigned to track the animal. They should search the trails and obvious areas first; it is rare for a horse to move cross-country unless there are wide open areas of desert, pastures, or fields. Cattle and llamas will usually find the best grazing or browsing available. Local saddle clubs, mounted search and rescue, or mounted police organizations should be contacted for assistance in finding the animal(s), while using appropriate search procedures.

APPROACHING A LOOSE ANIMAL

All prey animals share a herd mentality; if one herd member exhibits fear or panic, the remaining animals will be on guard and more excitable. If one animal is injured or cannot move very fast, the herd will not wait or slow down for that animal; elephants are an exception to this rule. Use of the correct approach toward the animal(s) is crucial to catching them. (See Chapter 4.)

Predators, including humans, tend to focus on the object of their interest and move toward it in a direct line. In contrast, prey animals are indirect thinkers that use approach and retreat methods to reach their destination. As a result of these differences, the predatory, direct approach is often unsuccessful in catching a prey animal. Eye pressure (resulting from direct eye contact with the animals) and incorrect body placement or language will cause the herd to move or scatter (Figure 8.4).

Reacting to Aggression

Responders should make themselves appear as intimidating as possible if an animal becomes aggressive and

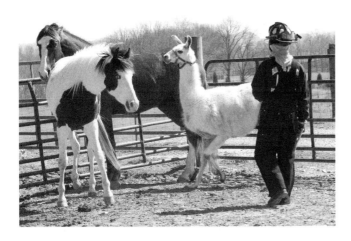

Figure 8.4 *A firefighter approaches animals that have been contained inside portable fencing and an existing fence obstacle. Exerting too much pressure on the animals with this type of aggressive body posture will cause the animals to resist capture. Courtesy of Axel Gimenez.*

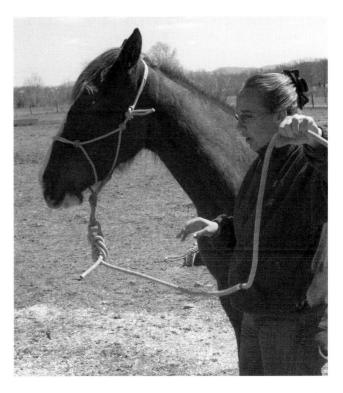

Figure 8.5 *The use of an emergency rope halter allows the animal handler to use one section of rope to fit the head of any size animal or species of large animal. A figure eight on a loop on the end of a 7 m (23 ft) rope is slipped around the animal's neck, and a loop of the free end of the rope is pushed through the bight and over the animal's nose. The free end becomes the lead rope. Courtesy of Axel Gimenez.*

attacks; however, this is not recommended with aggressive stallions, bulls, boars, all elephants, male camelids, male large birds, and all large female animals with nursing offspring. Those animals are deadly, and appropriate physical protection for the rescuers are required. For less dangerous animals, raising the hands to wave or clap and raising the voice pitch are often effective. Eye contact is threatening to a prey species, but it is recommended that responders avoid physical contact and step behind an obstacle to prevent injury. Fearful or enraged animals can inflict severe injury or death. Experienced animal handlers are essential in these circumstances.

Herding by Driving or Leading

If it is obvious which animals in the herd are the alpha (lead) animals, attempts should be made to catch or confine these animals first. The rest of the herd (especially horses and llamas) may follow those animals. Loose animals should be allowed time to realize that they are isolated; once they realize this, they will follow the herd. Prey animals' strong bond to the herd can be used to the rescuers' advantage to keep a herd of prey animals together to lead or drive them to safety.

THE EMERGENCY ROPE HALTER

A 7 m (23 ft) piece of 9 to 15 mm (5/16 to 9/16 in.) nylon braid boating cord can easily be packed into saddlebags, a pack, or kept in a vehicle for use as an emergency rope halter and sturdy lead rope. This halter will fit any size prey animal's head (Figure 8.5). *Note:* These directions are intended for haltering an animal that is accustomed to being haltered (e.g., horses or show livestock); animals that are wild, not adapted to

humans, or aggressive should be contained in a confined area until an experienced animal handler or a transport resource arrives. Attempting to halter wild animals is difficult, dangerous, and may cause the animal to injure itself in its attempts to escape.

It is possible to use a 2–3 m (6–9 ft) stick or pole to gently place this type of halter on a wild or uncooperative horse in a confined area, with much patience by an experienced animal handler. Animals that are not accustomed to halters and are not broke to lead cannot be expected to understand the concepts of pressure and release upon which halters are based. Experienced animal handlers should carefully evaluate the risks associated with haltering these animals.

1. Tie a figure eight on a loop in one end of the rope and hold the rest of the rope looped softly in the left hand. This knot has a special purpose; later, a short length of rope will be fed through the open loop in the knot to complete the halter.

2. Approach the animal from its left at the shoulder, groom it with the knotted end of the rope, and using the right hand, slip it over the neck at the shoulder. Treats are recommended to entice the animal to approach. Unless the animal is trapped in mud or exhausted, handlers will not be able to halter a wild or

unbroken animal. These animals should be contained in a small area until help and transport arrive. Handlers should always keep their face out of the way to prevent getting struck by the animal's head if it moves to avoid the rope.

3. Catch the figure eight knot under the neck and gather it to make a loop around the neck. This does not provide adequate control, but the animal has yielded to the handler's efforts. Gloves are recommended to prevent rope burn if the horse reacts and pulls away. If the animal starts to pull away, it should not be chased; the handler should step away and attempt to pull the animal's head and neck softly toward the handler's body. The handler should continue talking in low tones and rubbing the animal to keep it calm.

4. Gently slide the rope loop that has been placed around the neck closer to the poll (behind the ears), talking softly to keep the animal relaxed. Handlers should not touch the animal's ears or try to pet its face; these actions can cause anxiety for some animals.

5. Feed a .5 m (1 3/75 ft) loop of excess rope through the bight (loop) of the knot under the animal's chin. This loop will become the nose piece when pushed gently up over the animal's nose. Avoid touching the hairs of the lips and nostrils as the loop is lifted over the nose.

6. Fit the emergency halter around the nose and poll by pulling on the rope end, and use the extra length of rope as a lead rope. The animal handler must maintain the tightness of this halter, as it is an inherently loose knot (Figure 8.6). *Note:* Do not attempt to tie any animal with this (or any other) halter. The emergency rope halter loop will loosen and slip off the animal's nose and head if not maintained by tension on the rope. A standard halter should be placed on the animal as soon as possible (Figure 8.7).

Tying Animals on the Scene

Animals that have been caught on a rescue scene should not be tied. It is rare for cattle or exotic species to be accustomed to wearing halters, and it is unlikely that they will accept being led or tied. Most animals that can be haltered and led will not tolerate standing tied near traffic, crowds of humans, generators, lights, or emergency equipment. When startled, animals will fight the restraint and may break free again. If the animal has been tied to an object that is not well anchored (e.g., tree limb, fence post, cattle panel, etc.), the object will break or pull loose and be dragged by the animal; this will increase the animal's fear and risk of injury.

Animals should not be roped around the neck to catch them, and they absolutely should not be tied if roped. In 2000 a cow jumped out of a trailer on a South Carolina interstate highway. The cow survived the fall, but was asphyxiated when it was lassoed and tied to a guardrail. The tie rings on the sides of horse trailers are

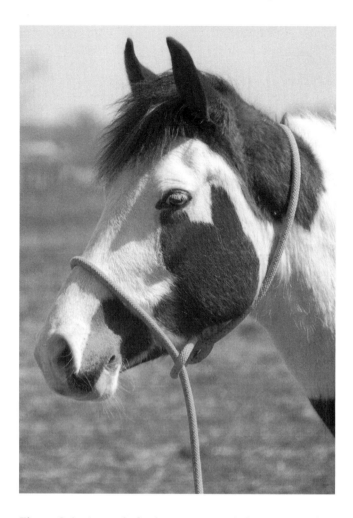

Figure 8.6 *A properly fitted emergency rope halter. Courtesy of Al Filice.*

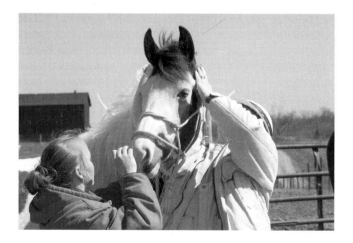

Figure 8.7 *The handler has successfully haltered the animal using an emergency rope halter and is adding a rope halter over the top for proper control. A second handler is offering a treat to distract the animal. Courtesy of Axel Gimenez.*

easily pulled free or broken by an animal fighting restraint and should not be used in a rescue environment. Many young animals, especially horses, are not accustomed to being tied and might fracture their necks fighting the restraint. If the restraint is made of good-quality, unbreakable rope, the animal can asphyxiate, fall, and fracture its pelvis, or otherwise injure itself.

A handler should remain with the animal to prevent it from getting loose again. In addition to restraint with a halter and lead rope, the animal should be confined inside a portable corral or other field-expedient secondary containment. A very effective way of keeping a restrained animal calm is to offer it good-quality hay until transport arrives.

Darting Loose Animals

Chemical restraint using a dart for delivery of appropriate drugs should rarely be used for capturing loose large animals because the animal's health and safety should be carefully considered (see Chapter 6). Personnel using these methods must have correct equipment, veterinary oversight, and certification in the use of these drugs and equipment (Figure 8.8).

Field Euthanasia in Exigent Circumstances

Loose animals that seriously threaten humans due to their aggression, fear reactions, or by threatening motorists in high-speed traffic areas may have to be euthanatized by projectile weapon; however, a good evaluation of the situation is recommended. In one example, a loose bull was found grazing in a soccer field in Seneca, South Carolina. Due to a concern for public safety, local law enforcement officials shot the animal before considering other options, such as closing the gates to the public field. The public outcry in response

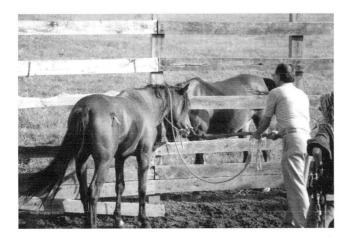

Figure 8.8 *A darted young stallion is cautiously approached in secondary confinement by a responder using a 2 m (7 ft) stick to thread an emergency rope halter over the animal's head. The dart causes a significant hematoma in the hide of the animal when it hits, and often must be surgically excised. Courtesy of Rebecca Gimenez.*

to this animal's death was enormous, since it was a trained circus animal and tame. If possible, a method of confining or driving animals to safety should be used before lethal force is employed. In another incident, a truckload of 19 bison overturned and several escaped; the insurance company was contacted and requested that the animals be shot before they could cause a secondary motor vehicle accident. (See Chapter 13.) In these types of circumstances, the decision for lethal force may be warranted.

BASIC HANDLING SKILLS

Animal handlers should practice the following basic large animal handling skills.

Leading the Animal

The person with the most large animal handling experience should be designated the animal handler. A response scene is not an appropriate place to learn to catch, halter, and lead animals. These are skills that must be practiced, just as rope rescue skills are practiced by emergency responders. Potential animal handlers should be encouraged to work with a local farm to practice their handling skills on a regular basis.

Very few large animals other than horses and camelids are accustomed to being led, unless they are used for show purposes. In general, livestock should be held in containment instead of individually led. Animals trapped in mud or similar circumstances should be haltered so that once freed, they cannot escape, and secondary containment should be made available.

Equipment Recommendations. For better leverage and safety, the animal handler should attach a long lead rope to the halter. Good quality 2.5 cm (1 in.) yacht braid or cotton is recommended. A lead rope at least 5 m (16.4 ft) long is recommended, so that the animal can be allowed to jump and run in a circle while the handler maintains a safe distance. The lead ropes found in most tack stores are approximately 3 m (10 ft) long and are too short for rescue use. When leading the animal, the animal handler should wear gloves to improve the grip and protect his or her hands.

Body Position. The animal handler should attempt to stand at the shoulder on the animal's left side, out of range of the front and hind hooves. In contrast to what is taught to most show handlers, 1 m (3 ft) of free rope is recommended between the animal's halter and the handler's right hand. Tighter restraint may be resented by some animals. In addition, this length allows the handler extra time to respond to the horse's movements (Figure 8.9). Handlers should avoid holding the halter because they can be injured or dragged if their fingers become entrapped in the halter rings or buckles

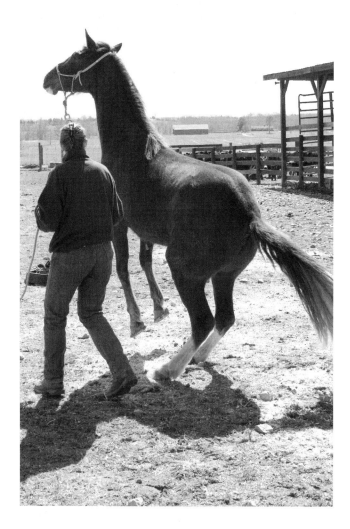

Figure 8.9 *The animal handler should always maintain a safe distance (approximately 1 m, or 3 ft) between the animal and themselves for safety in case the animal rears or bolts in panic. This greater distance gives the animal handler leverage and the animal room to relax. Courtesy of Axel Gimenez.*

(Parelli, 2006). Most importantly, the handler will have no leverage, and the animal will be able to get away more easily.

When leading an animal, the handler should walk at a confident pace that is comfortable for the animal. The animal should be encouraged to walk at the handler's shoulder: allowing the animal to walk ahead of the handler increases the risk of being kicked, whereas animals that walk behind the owner may pull away, lunge forward, strike, rear, or bite. If the animal refuses to walk forward, the handler can encourage it to do so by pulling at a 45-degree angle to the side; pulling the animal slightly off balance will encourage it to step forward. Another operational person can encourage the animal forward by gentle clucking from a safe distance behind it. Responders should not be allowed to use a vehicle or ropes around the rear end to push or pull

the animal forward; a forward assist is more effective if additional impulsion is necessary. (See Chapter 15.)

When the Animal Becomes Scared. If the animal is scared by an object or moving obstacle, the handler should attempt to stand between the animal and the intimidating source. If the handler is on the opposite side, he or she is more likely to be crushed or trampled by an animal attempting to escape the source of its fear. Shaking the lead rope forcefully may divert the animal's attention and may prevent the person from being trampled. Equipment, vehicle noises, and crowds of people might scare the animal. The handler should be given plenty of room to lead the animal and avoid narrow spaces that the animal may rush through in its attempt to escape.

If the animal tries to jerk loose or run away, the animal handler should attempt to limit the animal's progress in a straight line by pulling its head to one side and driving its hindquarters in the opposite direction (Lyons, 1992). This is most easily accomplished when the animal handler steps backward and pulls the lead rope in that direction, turning the animal's head toward him or her. If an animal is allowed to get its head 180 degrees away from the animal handler, the animal will have a leverage advantage, and the handler might not be able to stop the animal from running away.

When releasing the animal into a paddock, pasture, or trailer, the animal handler should stand toward the front of the animal, release the halter buckles or tie, then quickly step backward away from the animal. Excited horses will often whirl around quickly, kick, and run away. Children and adults have been severely injured or killed when this happened and they were unable to react quickly enough to escape injury (Park, 2004).

Driving a Herd

Many large animals (e.g., cattle, llamas, alpacas, emus, pigs, etc.) and some horses are not accustomed to individual handling and haltering, so they should instead be handled as a herd or in small groups. If the group of animals can be kept calm and moved slowly, it will be relatively easy to move them into containment. Containment may include cutting the fence on the interstate to move them out of the lanes of traffic, into a portable corral, or into a tennis court or other fenced area. If the herd scatters, the animals will become more excited and increase their speed of movement.

Moving a Herd. Do not allow people to shout, clap their hands, or make loud sounds to move animals. For most prey species, the presence of a human will encourage them to move 180 degrees away from the human; this tendency can facilitate animal movement by correctly positioning personnel to slowly drive the animal in the desired direction. The calmer the animals can be kept, the easier it will be to keep them together and move them into a safe containment area. Some animals will follow a person with flakes of alfalfa hay walking toward containment.

In some areas of the United States, it is common for local cowboys to be called to round up cattle escaped from overturned cattle trailers. These scenarios can be disastrous; the cattle may scatter in many directions unless the cowboys can keep the animals together and calm. In others, the use of a mounted posse has been effective, as has the use of trained herding dogs.

Using Portable Fencing. Personnel moving a herd of animals using portable fencing should be encouraged to look at the ground and use their peripheral vision to watch the animals' movement. As previously stated, eye pressure (i.e., direct eye contact) is often sufficient to move many prey animals and may discourage them from entering the containment area.

By keeping their movements fluid and calm, people become less threatening to the animals when containing them inside portable fencing. All personnel should be encouraged to use as little noise as possible and minimize talking to low tones. Most livestock accept containment and as long as the humans stay on the outside of the fence, the animals will remain relaxed (Figure 8.10).

Portable Fencing Alternatives. There are several variations of portable fencing that can be used to drive, contain, or move large animals

- When containing animals that don't represent an obvious threat to human life, forming a human chain (a line of people holding hands) to encircle loose animals or using humans to make a funnel to drive the animals into or out of an area can be successful. As recommended when driving animals, all personnel should move slowly and make minimal noise while looking at the animals out of their peripheral vision.

- Using a line of people holding a movable barrier (e.g., film from a videocassette tape, police tape, electric fencing tape, etc.) can be helpful. Alternately, this type of "fencing" can be tied between trees and obstacles to help funnel animals into a particular area or to ward them away from others such as obstacles, cliffs, or holes.

- Using 1.5 m (5 ft) tall steel cattle panels or another portable barrier (such as wooden pallets tied together) is effective for containment but may be difficult to move quickly. These are viable options to use on scenes where animals need to be released from confinement in an overturned trailer and reloaded onto another trailer. The containment should be assembled before the animals are released from the trailer.

- The author recommends 1.5 m (5 ft) tall mesh plastic fencing with polyvinylchloride (PVC) supports attached to the fencing approximately every 3 m (10 ft; Figure 8.11). Unrolled snow fencing, bolts of fabric, or similar materials will also work with varying degrees of success based on their pliability and ability to be supported by humans. The supports make convenient handles. If an animal tries to challenge or bluff the fence, it can be shaken in a way that will sufficiently discourage the animal from continuing its challenge.

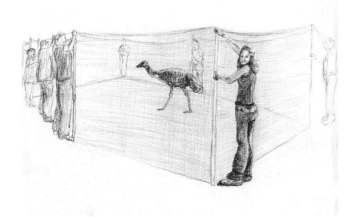

Figure 8.10 *Use of plastic fencing to contain and drive large animals represents a lightweight, inexpensive, and highly portable method of maintaining safety for animals and the humans assisting them. Here, a portable fence is used to move a captured emu to a transport trailer for delivery to animal control facilities. Courtesy of Julie Casil.*

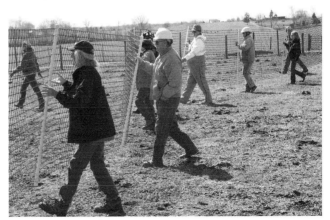

Figure 8.11 *Responders practice using portable plastic fencing supported by PVC handles to contain loose animals during a training scenario. The smooth coordination of people at both ends of the fence is crucial to maintaining the shape of the fence and avoiding obstacles. Courtesy of Axel Gimenez.*

Support the Portable Fence. Personnel should use the natural features (e.g., cliff, river, hedges) and obstacles (e.g., an existing line of fencing or the side of a building) of the terrain to support the portable corral. Maximize the size of the containment area and try to maintain rounded corners; animals that run into a square corner are more likely to jump the barrier instead of turning to follow it.

The biggest challenge associated with this type of containment is coordinating all personnel to move in a slow, calm, and nonthreatening manner to enclose the animals using any existing barrier (e.g., fencing, terrain, etc.) to assist with containment. There should be an operations person directing the movement of the humans (with or without fencing) to enclose the animals. When possible, the containment area should be set up ahead of time and the animals should be driven slowly into it.

Portable fencing can be used to drive animals into a stock trailer or other transportation and is easier and safer than trying to push and pull an unwilling animal into a trailer (Figure 8.12). The fencing can be configured as a funnel to push animals into a trailer, as a block to prevent them from going into obstacles or over cliffs, or as temporary confinement.

Trailer Loading

Loading prey animals into a trailer can be difficult without proper equipment and an understanding of prey animal behavior. If at all possible, experienced animal handlers should be available to provide guidance and advice when loading large animals. This skill requires significant practice in various situations (e.g., darkness, inclement weather, etc.).

For groups of animals and livestock, a stock trailer provides adequate space for animals to load. Cattle panels can be used to close the gap and crowd the animals into the trailer. Instead of shouting and chasing the animals into the trailer, responders should allow the animals a few seconds to investigate the trailer and load calmly. This approach will minimize injuries to the animals and responders. Once loaded, the animals should be separated using cut gates or dividers as appropriate.

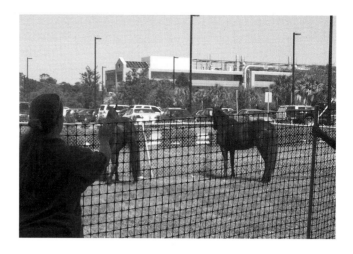

Figure 8.12 *Loose horses in an urban area represent a significant hazard. Using portable fencing and existing obstacles (in this case a fence) to contain them is a safe way of reducing the threat of secondary incidents or entrapment by the animals. Courtesy of Tori Miller.*

For camelids, goats, ratites, pigs, and sheep, the trailer should be enclosed to prevent the animals from jumping out and to shield them from environmental conditions (e.g., heat, cold, sunlight). Camelids usually lie down in transit, but camels have been reported to jump out of trailers. Goats and sheep are capable jumpers.

For horses, a stock trailer is often preferred because many horses will load more easily into the open space of the stock trailer than a traditional straight- or slant-load trailer. Some horses do not load readily into any type of trailer, while others willingly load regardless of trailer type. There is abundant educational information on loading horses into trailers available to interested personnel.

ACRONYMS USED IN CHAPTER 8

BLM   Bureau of Land Management
GPS   Global positioning satellite
PVC   Polyvinylchloride

9 Trailer Incidents

Dr. Tomas Gimenez and Dr. Rebecca Gimenez

INTRODUCTION

Emergencies involving large animals trapped in an overturned (Figure 9.1) or wrecked trailer are far too common but have allowed on-site research and development of new techniques to decrease stress and iatrogenic injuries while extracting large animals from these predicaments. *Trailer incident* in this chapter refers to trailers ranging in size from the common bumper-pull two-horse trailer to a commercial hauling van pulled by a semi-tractor with 9–16 horses. Certain aspects of commercial livestock hauler overturns have specialty training and response concerns; the reader is encouraged to review the standard operating protocol (SOP) for response to those special incidents (see Chapter 21).

The value of prevention by performing regular maintenance on the trailer cannot be overstated. A mismatch in vehicle towing capacity versus trailer and load size is known to contribute to the majority of horse trailer incidents. These prevention strategies are mentioned here for awareness purposes but are well covered in other texts. Unusual incidents such as trailers hit by trains, lifted on top of barns or in trees during tornados, or a car impacted in the horse compartment are rarely preventable and represent true accidents.

Usually, responders arrive on the scene and find several well-meaning civilians getting in the trailer and trying to drag the animals out using ropes around the animals' legs and necks. The driver/animal owner may be injured and need medical attention; however, this person may resist medical treatment until he or she is assured that the animals are safe. In some cases, the trailer may be precariously positioned near a ravine or bridge abutment. Traffic is stopped in both directions, and a crowd rapidly gathers.

An incident action plan (IAP) should be generated based on many criteria. It is important to consider all of the options for removing the animals before resorting to cutting tools; if there is a safe method for leading, lifting, dragging, or rolling the animals out of the trailer, it is preferable to the use of cutting tools. There may be a time-sensitive concern for the medical condition of the animals. Other factors include the estimated time of arrival of the veterinarian called to the scene and the environmental, incident scene, and vehicle hazards on the scene. The extrication strategy may involve removing the horse from the trailer or cutting the trailer from around the horse. This chapter focuses on the response options to these types of emergencies.

Despite the apparent need for a rapid response, very few on-road emergency responses must be conducted in a great hurry. Although law enforcement, bystanders, the owner, and the media may be pressuring responders to hasten the rescue, a trailer wreck must be approached similar to any other extrication scene. Using the incident command system (ICS), responders should establish scene management and control mechanisms for traffic and devise an action plan (see Chapter 5).

Trailers are available in a wide variety of configurations and are generally built to be extremely strong. As long as the animal victim stays within the confines of the trailer, the chances are good that the animal will not only survive, but experience only minor injuries in an incident. Even incidents of rollovers or crushed trailers have reported minor injuries to animals that remained within them.

There are many options available to rescue teams responding to a crushed or overturned trailer; several represent updated technologies or methodologies borrowed from heavy rope rescue techniques. These techniques have been tested in multiple training scenarios using real trailers of different sizes and weights, as well as in actual rescue scenarios (Fox, 2006). The

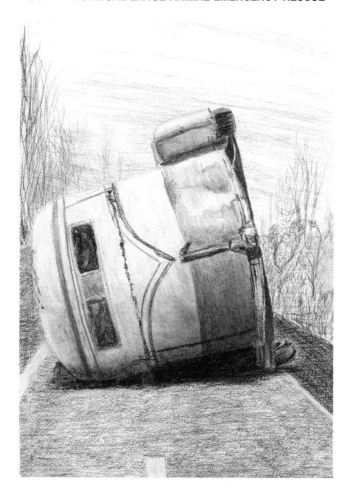

Figure 9.1 *There is no uniform approach to a rescue scene with an overturned trailer. Responders should consider the orientation of the animals inside, the resources available, and the on-scene conditions before selecting a safe method of releasing the animals, extricating the animals, or righting the trailer. Courtesy of Julie Casil.*

equipment specific to each of these technologies is affordable and easy to collect into a rescue equipment cache for a veterinary practice, veterinary school, or regional equine response unit.

The use of these techniques requires specific patient care protocols, SOPs, and a rescue team trained in the employment of the equipment. Trailer incidents involving animals are highly emotional settings and may involve numerous bystanders, the owner, and emergency responders. According to Kandee Haertel (2000), "The horse inside the trailer is the valuable commodity, not the trailer. Trailers are expensive, but the horse should be your primary consideration. Are you handling a multimillion dollar breeding stallion or someone's very special friend? It is in the best interest of the rescuer to consider each horse as absolutely irreplaceable." (Professionals in emergency equine care should be educated in the latest technology and equipment available to them for use in everyday as well as emergency situations.)

INCIDENT PREVENTION

The most common causes of trailer incidents are a mismatch between trailer and towing vehicle; lack of proper preventive maintenance, lack of knowledge regarding how to drive a vehicle towing a loaded horse trailer or how to properly hitch a trailer, and poor craftsmanship/quality control on the part of the trailer manufacturer. There are excellent texts and resources available that cover the important topics of trailer maintenance, towing vehicle selection, trailer-loading training of the horse, trailer driving strategies, and general trailer safety that are outside the scope of this book.

There should be a minimum of two axles on livestock and horse trailers so that if a tire fails, the other wheel and tire will support the trailer while the driver exits traffic lanes. One-axle horse or livestock trailers are unsafe for transporting animals and should not be purchased for this purpose. One roadside assistance provider recommends that owners carry two spare tires for their horse trailers due to the prevalence of multiple tire blowouts (Cole, 2005).

Drivers should not allow animals to stick their heads out of the trailer windows during transport; this increases the risk that the animal's head or entire body will be ejected from the trailer in an accident. There are two documented cases of a close-passing vehicle decapitating horses that were allowed to hang their heads out of the trailer windows. Other deaths have occurred when the free end of a lead rope was hanging or blown out of the open window and wrapped around the trailer axle, causing the horse to be decapitated or suffer a broken neck.

BASIC TRAILER CONSTRUCTION

There are over 100 different horse/livestock trailer manufacturers represented in the equine/livestock industry. No two trailers are exactly the same; fortunately, most use similar construction methods, design configurations, and basic materials. There is no such thing as a "typical" horse trailer—configurations include single horse in-line, straight-load for multiple horses, slant-load for multiple horses, and stock trailers. In-line trailers position the horses parallel to the direction of motion, whereas slant-load trailers position them on a 30- to 40-degree diagonal. Stock trailers are commonly open, with one or more partitions that can swing to form square compartments within the open trailer.

Most horse trailers in the United States are hitched by a fifth wheel/gooseneck or bumper-pull (tag-along) method; in the United Kingdom, the bumper-pull hitch is most common due to tow vehicle size restrictions. Trailers may have recreational vehicle-like (RV-like) living quarters with full kitchens, bedrooms, and bathrooms. Some have slide-out portions for added space in the living quarters that makes the trailer essentially an RV with a compartment for horses in the back.

Most trailers have a tack room for equipment and saddles; it can be located in the front or back of the trailer. Some trailers may convey a carriage (up to 750 kg, or 1,650 lb) in a compartment near the horses that may have to be removed to gain access to the animals. Many people haul multiple species of animals on the same trailer (e.g., horses and cattle, horses and dogs, goats and cattle, zoo animals, llamas and alpacas).

COMMON TRAILER CONFIGURATIONS

Commercial or Private Shippers

Some owners never personally transport their animals; they ship their horses in commercial or private horse vans or lorries. Transport capacity in these lorries or trailers may range from 2 to 14 horses. The horses are usually positioned in-line and head-to-head (facing each other) within the horse compartment, and 3 horses across. Other options are slant-load or rear-facing configurations. The partitions are removable to make compartments for mares and foals, extra large or special horse loads, etc. There is no access to the horse compartment from the cab of most commercial semi-tractor trailers. The horses are loaded via a ramp that slides from the frame underneath the horses; wooden slides are lifted and attached to keep the horses centered on the ramp as they load or unload. Most horses are held in place with chains from the partitions or sides of the trailer to their halters, and the horse compartment will often feature numerous obstacles (including human attendants).

Bumper-pull Trailer

Bumper-pull trailers are available in in-line (or straight load) and slant-load configurations. Some have doors and ramps on the front of the trailer as well as the back, and others may be configured so that the animals ride with their rump toward the towing vehicle (i.e., facing backward). Many animals find it less stressful to have their heads positioned toward the back of the trailer (Creiger, 2005). If there is a ramp, it may or may not be part of the door that allows access to the horse compartment. If the ramp does not form a wall of the compartment, it must usually be lowered or opened to give access to the doors, which are then opened to allow access to the horse compartment. Some of the older steel trailers have exposed springs (similar to those on garage doors) that can cause serious injury in an accident, and they should be of concern to responders. The post between the back doors of two-door trailers is for attachment of the doors and may be removed safely without compromising the structural integrity of the trailer.

Gooseneck Trailer

Most modern gooseneck trailers are slant-loading trailers; the horses are loaded from the right side of the trailer's rear and positioned facing the left diagonal. The left rear door often secures the tack compartment (for saddle and equipment storage). If one of these trailers is turned on its side in a wreck, the tack compartment becomes a 1 m (3 ft) obstacle for the animals to either jump over or crawl under. It is unlikely that a horse will crawl underneath the compartment, and jumping it can result in severe injury to the horse's head, neck, or limbs. Llamas, goats, and some cattle may get on their "knees" to crawl out of a trailer; they must be contained to prevent them from getting loose.

Tack compartments in modern trailers may have retractable pins that allow the tack compartment walls to be removed, but often these are welded or rusted in place and hard to remove if the trailer's frame or walls have been damaged. The post between the back doors of the trailer is for attachment of the doors and may be removed safely without affecting the structural integrity of the trailer.

Hitch Concerns. Gooseneck trailers are towed with pickup trucks or semi-tractors; the gooseneck hitch attaches to a ball hitch that is placed on the floor of the truck bed over the rear axle. Bumper-pull trailers anchor on a hitch ball below the rear bumper of the tow vehicle. These trailers have been towed by cars, trucks, and sport utility vehicles (SUVs). A major difference between the gooseneck trailer (common in the United States) and the bumper-pull trailer is that much of the weight of the gooseneck trailer is on the hitch over the rear axle of the towing vehicle. Bumper-pull trailers place less weight on the tongue and hitch, and the amount of weight exerted on the hitch can change significantly as the animals shift or the vehicle moves.

Large pickup trucks are optimal for pulling gooseneck trailers. Short-bed pickup trucks restrict the maneuverability of the truck/trailer combination and are therefore not suitable for pulling gooseneck trailers. Large SUVs are the most appropriate vehicles for towing bumper-pull trailers. Trailer purchasers often ask which of these hitch types is safer: if a well-made trailer is hitched correctly, maintained, loaded properly, and driven defensively, both types are very safe (Figure 9.2).

A mismatch between trailer weight and vehicle weight is the root of many trailering incidents. SUVs are top-heavy (i.e., they have a higher center of gravity). In addition, these vehicles tend to have "softer" springs to create a smoother ride for human passengers; however, these springs can contribute to vehicle sway and increase the difficulty of maintaining control of the vehicle. All tires should be inflated to the tire

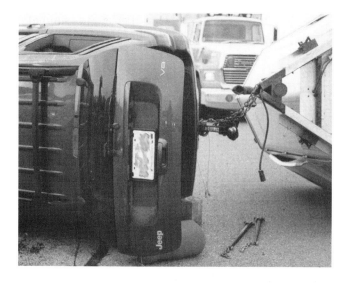

Figure 9.2   *One of the most common contributors to trailer accidents is failure to correctly connect the trailer to the hitch on the towing vehicle. Note that the mount with ball is in the receiver, the coupler collar is closed, and the safety chains are attached to the towing vehicle. Sway bars are unnecessary if using a towing vehicle appropriate for the horse trailer and with correct weight distribution. Courtesy Jennifer Woods.*

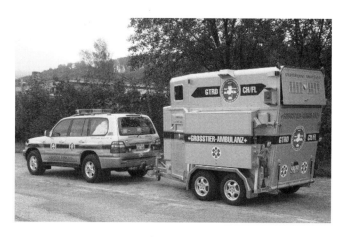

Figure 9.3   *This trailer shows the type of lightweight trailer commonly used in the European Community. Lightweight trailers minimize the tow weight and allow a smaller vehicle to be used but must be carefully evaluated for safe braking capabilities with the weight of animals in the trailer. Courtesy GTRO CH/FL.*

manufacturer's recommendation, not to the lower pressures recommended to provide a smoother ride. Combined with a bumper-pull trailer, these concerns increase the risk that the rig will sway, jackknife, or flip over. Trailers are not aerodynamically designed; a strong crosswind over 56 kph (35 mph) can overturn a trailer and provides another reason for owners to evacuate early before high-wind event disasters (e.g., hurricanes).

A small truck or car towing a large trailer occupied by horses is not appropriate. Towing a live animal that may shift its weight around is significantly different from towing a boat or camping trailer. The shifting weight of animal(s) in the trailer can make the trailer sway and should be prevented with proper loading procedures. If the towing vehicle is unable to control the sway of the trailer, it may cause a wreck. Bumper-pull trailers are more prone to sway due to the location of the hitch behind the vehicle instead of centered over the rear axle. Most gooseneck trailers are longer than bumper pulls and are less likely to sway because the trailer becomes an integral part of the towing vehicle–trailer combination. Also, it should be noted that swaying of the trailer (resulting from vehicle mismatch, improper loading, or hitching) can initiate a harmonic effect that will cause the trailer to continue to sway with increasing severity. The only way to stop a swaying trailer is to slow the vehicle as quickly and safely as possible without slamming on the brakes (which could cause it to jackknife).

TOWING A TRAILER

The European Community requires that a vehicle used to tow a trailer exceed the weight of the trailer loaded with horses. This regulation automatically limits a lightweight two-horse bumper-pull trailer to being towed by the largest four-wheel vehicle available (Figure 9.3). European trailer manufacturers have worked to make their trailers as light as possible, constructing them of fiberglass and composites, to allow large horses to be towed with lighter vehicles. Very light trailers may be unsafe at higher speeds and when passing large trucks on major highways. These lightweight trailers are tall, wide, and well engineered. In some cases they are so lightweight the owner does not have to back the truck to hitch the trailer; instead, he or she can grab the handle on the unloaded trailer and pull it to the truck hitch.

A horse trailer in the United Kingdom is rated according to its maximum authorized mass, which is the maximum weight of the trailer plus what it is carrying (e.g., horses, tack, etc.). To legally tow a trailer in the United Kingdom, a driver must pass a large goods vehicle test in addition to the regular driver's license (category entitlement B + E or greater). The large goods test requires drivers to demonstrate their ability to perform an off-road reverse maneuver, controlled stop, coupling and uncoupling, making left and right turns, and driving on the open road.

In the United States, drivers can tow a horse trailer with almost any type of vehicle. Most states have few or no requirements or regulations pertaining to horse trailers, and there are minimal federal regulations for driving tow vehicles with trailers. Some states do not require the registration or annual inspections of horse trailers.

Articles in popular horse magazines often emphasize the size of the engine, but few address the braking capacity or load range for the towing vehicle. The horsepower and torque of the engine of the towing vehicle provide power and pulling control, but the engine is less important than the braking power and weight of the towing vehicle. It is more important that the vehicle can stop the trailer. The brakes on the trailer are made to complement, not replace the brakes on the towing vehicle. Hydraulic and electrical brakes on the trailer should be regularly inspected to ensure they are functioning in accordance with the manufacturer's specifications.

The price of the trailer does not appear to directly relate to the quality of the manufactured product. Trailer manufacturers are poorly regulated, except through Department of Transportation regulations for weight, tires, and height/width. Surveys of the undercarriages and construction quality of a wide variety of horse trailers by researchers (Cole, 2006; Gimenez, 2006a) have revealed serious concerns within the livestock/horse trailer industry regarding the following points:

- Poor quality tires, incorrect tire rating (usually well underrated), or tire size for trailer mass and tire inflation level
- Poor overall design, protection/insulation, and installation of wiring for brakes and electrical system
- Poor quality control (engineering, design, manufacture, and installation) and poor quality of flooring materials, axles, cross-members, and sheet metal edging
- Only the minimum required lighting and reflective materials to make the trailer readily visible on the road and in the dark

Mitigation Efforts

Owners and Drivers. Some horse clubs and other livestock organizations offer trailer safety rodeo days for local owners and staff. These educational events should be designed to help people learn to safely hitch and tow their trailer and understand the challenges for an animal being hauled (Cole, 2006). Recently offered events such as this have featured each driver navigating their personally owned trailer through stations as follows:

- Qualified personnel (professional trailer repair technicians) evaluate each trailer for safety and make recommendations to the owner regarding the floors, brakes, tires, wheels, hitches, electrical system, and wiring.
- Owners experience riding in the back of a horse trailer under good and poor driving conditions (e.g., speed, rough terrain, driver errors, braking) with their arms tied behind their backs (to simulate being on four hooves with no arms to stabilize themselves)
- A qualified judge evaluates the owner unhitching and rehitching the trailer to the towing vehicle
- A qualified judge evaluates and times the driver negotiating a simple obstacle course (e.g., forward motion, emergency stop, obstacles, tight turns, backing up through cones, and parking)

Feedback is then provided to the owners on their trailers' safety and their driving skills, which can assist them in understanding their personal responsibilities to their animals and other drivers.

Emergency Response Volunteers. As stated previously, responders should obtain training in the handling of horses and livestock. A basic skill set should include safe haltering and leading and encouraging animals to move into an enclosure (e.g., cattle panels, portable fencing, tennis court, etc.) for their safety. These skills should also be regularly practiced. A trailer wreck should not be the first time personnel have handled a horse. There should be a standard IAP incorporated into the department's planning guidance for responding to these incidents. (See Chapters 5 and 21.)

COMMON CAUSES OF INCIDENTS

Homemade Trailers

Homemade trailers can be found on the road. The primary safety concern with these trailers is that the trailer hitch may have been built at home by simply welding steel to the truck's frame. The attachment point between the trailer hitch and the towing vehicle's frame is the point of highest stress between the trailer and towing vehicle, similar to the junction between the end of a bridge and the road. It is because of this point of highest stress that commercial hitches and receivers have some degree of flexibility built into them to avoid stress fractures. A conventional welding point may not provide the necessary flexibility and can cause catastrophic failures. Welding points of concern are connections of the axles to the frame of the trailer and the neck of the trailer (from the hitch to where it attaches to the frame of the trailer).

Other homemade conveyances for large animals may include covered or uncovered cages set into the back of pickup trucks and modified horse compartments on the back of a van, truck, or RV frame (Figure 9.4). The primary concerns with these vehicles are the location of the vehicle's center of gravity with the weight of a large animal in the back and how that affects the vehicle in poor driving conditions.

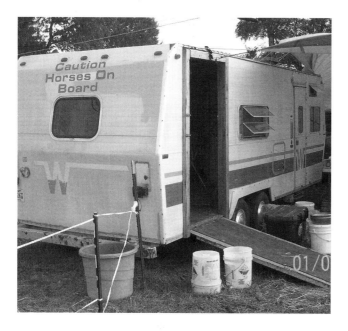

Figure 9.4 *The types of conveyance used to transport large animals varies from SUVs and custom trailers to homemade or retrofitted vehicles such as this. Most of these vehicles do not indicate what type(s) of animals might be inside the compartment. Courtesy of Tori Miller.*

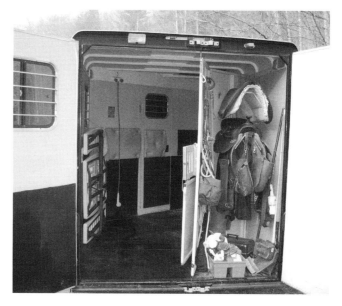

Figure 9.5 *The rear of this trailer shows a reversed configuration from the standard, with the tack compartment on the right and dividers turning the animals to stand with their heads to the right and away from the center of the road. This allows animals to be unloaded through the escape door at the front and away from the traffic In an emergency situation. Courtesy of Tomas Gimenez.*

Incorrectly Hitched Trailer

Failure to correctly hitch the trailer to the towing vehicle is a common cause of trailer accidents. Most common faults include the following:

- Incorrect hitch ball size for coupler
- Failure to lock the coupler
- Failure to lock receiver in hitch
- Failure to connect electrical system, brakes, and/or safety switch to towing vehicle
- Failure to tighten nut on hitch ball

The driver towing a trailer should never assume that somebody else (e.g., family member, etc.) correctly hitched the trailer. It is ultimately the driver's responsibility to make sure that the trailer is properly hitched before loading any animals and getting on the road. At least one roadside assistance provider that specializes in horse trailer owners provides a trailer hitching safety publication for owners (Cole, 2006).

A correctly hitched trailer will remain hitched, even in catastrophic conditions. For example, a train hit a trailer crossing the tracks in Georgia, and despite the impact, the gooseneck was still hitched to the truck after the accident. Unfortunately, the horse was ejected through a window and died, but the photographic documentation shows that the structural integrity of these trailers is excellent. In another collision, between a sand truck and a three-horse trailer in Loxahatchee, Florida, the trucks and trailer rolled and flipped numerous times in an incident that killed all of the drivers

and passengers in the vehicles, as well as the horses in the trailer. Although the nose of the trailer pushed the frame and hitch of the truck forward over 1 m (3 ft), it was still attached.

Load Plan

In two-horse, in-line (straight load) bumper-pull trailers, a single horse should always be loaded on the left side of the trailer so that the horse's weight will help maintain the trailer toward the center, or crown, of the road. If the driver is hauling something heavier than the horse in the other stall, the heaviest object or horse should be loaded on the left (e.g., motorcycles, heavy furniture, etc.). It is preferable for the gates and dividers of the trailer to be locked in place at all times; any imbalance can cause accidents if an animal paws, shifts, or falls in the compartment and causes the trailer to sway. The animal should have sufficient headroom to be able to move its head to maintain balance while in transport. Unsecured objects in the trailer compartment with the animals can be dangerous if they shift or slide into or underneath the animals; in addition, they can be obstacles to extrication in a wreck.

In most slant-load trailers, the animals are loaded through the right rear door and face to the left of the trailer at a 30- to 45-degree angle diagonal. However, there are trailers that do not fit this configuration (Figure 9.5). Animals should be loaded over the axles where possible; if hauling a minimum number of horses versus a full trailer, owners should consult trailer manufacturer's recommendations before loading the trailer.

Animals may be ejected from the trailer during a collision or overturn, while others may remain in the trailer. It is generally safer for an animal to remain inside a trailer until appropriate egress can be coordinated. Ejected animals are often injured by going through the window, door, or roof of the trailer, or landing on the road surface at velocity. As with human victims, ejected animal victims have a poor chance of survival.

HUMAN PASSENGERS IN TRAILERS

Allowing a person to ride in the trailer with animals, either healthy or sick and injured, especially in the animal compartment, is dangerous. Some drivers allow their children or pets to remain in the living quarters of the trailer while on the road; this is similarly dangerous. Wireless camera systems provide readily available and economical solutions for visually monitoring horses during transport.

Remember that human victims take priority over animal victims in a rescue scenario. The trailer should be thoroughly searched for human victims in the living quarters area (including the gooseneck area of the trailer).

Some commercial transports hire animal caretakers to ride in the horse compartment during transport; there may be as many as eight human victims in an overturned semi-trailer fully loaded with horses. Commercial interstate haulers may be partitioned in multiple configurations and contain up to 16 large animals; these types of transport may have more humans than horses in the trailer, and there may be attendants, veterinarians, or grooms in the trailer. Excellent information on the humane aspects of handling, transportation guidelines, legalities of traveling with animals, and shipment restrictions can be found through the Animal Transportation Association (www.aata.org).

Keep People Out of the Trailer

It is very dangerous to allow anyone (e.g., veterinarian, firefighter, bystander, or owner) to enter a trailer (including one that is not overturned) with a frightened and possibly injured animal. There are common situations where animals become entrapped in nonmoving trailers; they may jump over a divider; scramble, fall down, and become pinned under the divider or another animal; or unsuccessfully attempt to jump out of the trailer through the escape door. These animals are often frantic and scrambling. No one should be permitted to enter the trailer until the animal is sedated.

For example, in 2000 a horse being hauled on an interstate highway through Ohio attempted to jump through the right escape door of the trailer during transport. The owner stopped immediately, next to the guard rail. When emergency personnel responded, they stopped traffic and pulled the trailer away from the guard rail to get access to the animal. The front half of the animal's body was outside the door and its rear end was hung on the chest-bar. After the animal was sedated, the chest-bar was cut from the left compartment of the trailer by a responder, and the animal was moved out the door onto the ground. An analysis of this incident would suggest that the driver should have driven to the end of the guard rail, providing more room for the extrication. Waiting for the veterinarian was a safe decision on the part of the responders.

OBSTACLES TO EXTRICATION

In the effort to keep their animals safely within the confines of their trailer and make them comfortable, owners may have a wide variety of equipment and gear in the travel compartment of the trailer with the animals. All of these objects may become entangling obstacles to the animals and responders trying to assist.

Trailer Ties

Most horses will be in divided stanchions or stalls during trailer transport. Many are tied by their lead ropes or trailer ties or straps attached to their halters and tied to a ring above the trailer window or anchored to the support pole. In contrast, cattle are rarely tied in trailers and rarely loaded into single stalls. Most horses are haltered when inside a trailer, but very few other large animals will be wearing halters.

Tie straps are made of 2.5 cm (1 in.) nylon with a standard snap on one end and a "panic" snap on the other. If there is a load on the strap, it is impossible to undo the standard snap; in these situations, the panic snap is designed to be opened by manually moving a sliding cover that allows the clasp to spring loose.

In a slant-load trailer that has rolled on its right side, the animals will be hanging from what has become the topmost (roof) portion of the trailer. If the trailer rolls onto its left side, the animal's heads will be tied to what has become the bottommost (floor) portion of the trailer. Animals can be asphyxiated by the tie or rope and halter; it may need to be cut using a serrated knife or by releasing the panic snap. Without entering the trailer, rescuers can use a long pole to attach a carabiner to the animal's halter (Figure 9.6), then safely cut the nylon tie strap with a seat belt cutter or good-quality serrated knife on a pole (Figure 9.7). This allows the handler to have a primary method of restraint on the animal when it emerges from the trailer.

The most dangerous tie straps for rescuers and animal victims are bungee-type tie straps. The horse may be hanging from the strap or pulling back in a desperate attempt to flee. The horse is effectively loading energy (storing energy) in the bungee tie that will be released when the tie is cut. Once a loaded

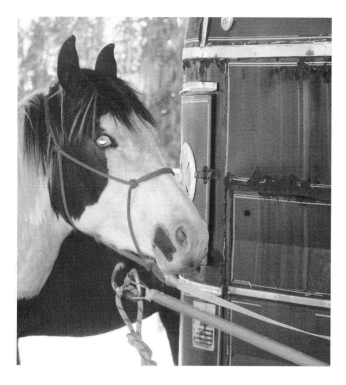

Figure 9.6 In this demonstration, a long pole with a carabiner in an open holder is extended 4 m into a simulated trailer to allow responders to attach a lead line to the demonstration "trapped horse" being held by a trailer tie. This minimizes the chance of injury to rescuers by keeping them out of the trailer compartment. Courtesy of Tori Miller.

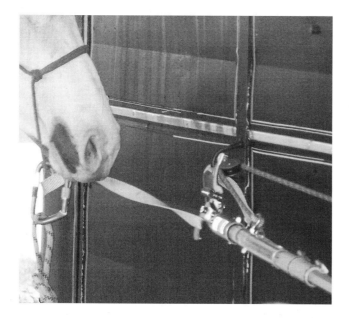

Figure 9.7 A pole cutter on an extra-long painter's pole allows responders to cut the trailer tie from a simulated trapped animal from over 4 m away. Always check to see if the horse is tied to the trailer before extrication begins. Whether the horse is to walk out on its own or is going to be dragged out of the trailer, always attach a long line to the halter prior to cutting the tie strap. These procedures should be performed from the outside of the trailer with the aid of extension poles. Courtesy of Axel Gimenez.

bungee-type tie is cut, it will whip around inside the trailer and can cause eye or facial injuries to the animal victim and/or rescuer. There are documented cases of humans and horses sustaining severe injuries from these types of ties and two cases of loaded, tied horses able to completely exit a trailer while still attached to the fully loaded bungee tie (Blackburn, 2004).

The metal hardware is often the weakest link in the tie strap, but it is not often sufficiently weak to break under extreme loading conditions. The tie strap must be strong enough to keep the animal from turning around or biting its neighbor while in the trailer, but it does not need to be strong enough to hang the weight of a horse from it. Use of a breakaway halter with a leather poll or breakable tie strap (with baling twine as the weakest link) in the trailer will prevent animals from breaking their necks or hanging from the trailer in an accident. A tie strap that will break under a significant load and free the animal during an incident is commercially available. The advantage of some types of these straps is that it will remain attached to the halter and can be used as a lead rope.

Dividers

A simple trailer accident where the brakes are applied suddenly may cause horses to lose their footing and fall under the center or front divider. They may be minimally injured but unable to stand because there is not enough room to rise. Removing the center divider by pulling (or cutting) the pins may allow the animals to stand. Animals should be untied because they need their heads and necks to balance themselves. Horses usually need to get their legs out in front of their bodies and propel with their hindquarters to rise. In contrast, cattle rise rump first, kneeling on their front end and stepping up. They can rise to a standing position in a smaller space than a horse.

TRAIN VERSUS TRAILER

In a retrospective study of more than 200 incidents involving horse trailers, researchers noticed an overrepresentation of incidents involving gooseneck horse trailers caught on railroad crossings (Gimenez and Gimenez, 2006b). Almost all of these incidents resulted in the loss of human and/or equine life. Drivers of vehicles pulling trailers should heed the low-clearance caution signs at the railroad track crossing. All gooseneck and bumper-pull trailers are low clearance, having only a few inches of clearance from the road. Drivers should consider alternative routes that do not cross low-clearance railroad tracks. If the driver is unable to avoid crossing railroad tracks, they should proceed cautiously, especially when the tracks are higher than the road grade.

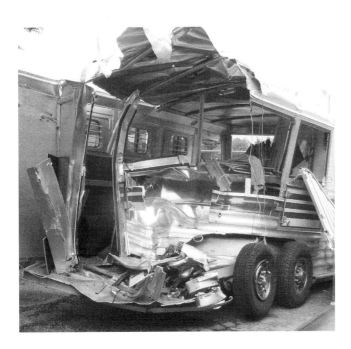

Figure 9.8 *This trailer was hit in the center by a train and split in half. This photo reveals the interior of the trailer where one horse was standing upon impact. Prevention by education of drivers and appropriate signage at high-center railroad crossings will prevent these tragedies. Courtesy of Tomas Gimenez.*

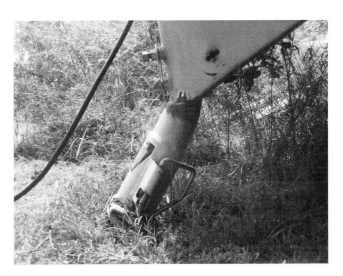

Figure 9.9 *Although this towing combination was in a collision with a train, the gooseneck hitch is bent but remains attached to the ball, which was ripped from the bed of the truck. This illustrates that a safely hitched trailer will normally remain hitched unless involved in a catastrophic wreck. Courtesy of Tomas Gimenez.*

For example, a driver in Blacksburg, South Carolina, attempted to tow a loaded gooseneck trailer across a marked railroad crossing and became stuck on the raised tracks. A train was approaching and unable to stop. Unfortunately, only two of the three horses in the trailer were able to be removed before impact; death was considered instantaneous for the remaining animal, and the trailer was literally cut in two (Figure 9.8). The gooseneck remained hitched to the ball of the hitch, but the hitch plate was ripped from the truck bed (Figure 9.9). An analysis of this incident would suggest that educational prevention efforts to trailer drivers about the dangers of railroad crossings would be in order, and it has been since provided to the industry (Cole, 2006).

If a horse trailer becomes lodged on a railroad crossing, the driver or responders should call 911 immediately, whether or not a train may be near. Emergency dispatch agencies can contact railroad companies and alert them of the situation. Additionally, all humans and animals should be evacuated from the tow vehicle and trailer. Evacuating the animals from the trailer serves two purposes: it removes the animals from harm's way, but it will also reduce the weight in the trailer. This may sufficiently raise the trailer and allow it to dislodge from the tracks and complete the crossing safely, or back up off the tracks. The animals should be taken as far from the railroad track as possible to prevent a panic response if a train approaches or passes.

Most railroad crossings and some road crossings or turnouts are built up, making them slightly higher than the surrounding roadway. Drivers should cautiously evaluate these locations before attempting to turn into or cross them. When the truck tires pass over the high point and approach the lower roadway grade, the rear tires of the trailer may still be on the low roadway grade on the initial side of the crossing; this can cause the front of the gooseneck trailer to "bottom out" on the high point of the roadway. While bumper-pull trailers are less susceptible to this problem, it is important to raise the jack stand to a level that will provide sufficient clearance in these situations.

WHAT IS IN THE TRAILER?

Responders should never assume they know what is in the horse trailer: llamas, cattle, pigs, furniture, immigrants, farm vehicles, motorcycles, mattresses, dogs, gas tanks, and unidentified hazardous items may be in the compartment with the horses or alone. For example, a veterinary technician reported driving three 4.2–4.8 m (14–16 ft) long Siamese crocodiles in a horse trailer from Ocala to St. Augustine, Florida. Exotic circus animals are moved daily across the country, often in unmarked trailers (Witte, 2005).

Miniature horses, llamas, and other specialty livestock may be transported in alternative vehicles, not horse trailers. This might include standard cars, vans, or custom conversion type vehicles (Figure 9.10). In a motor vehicle accident, the animals will be in the

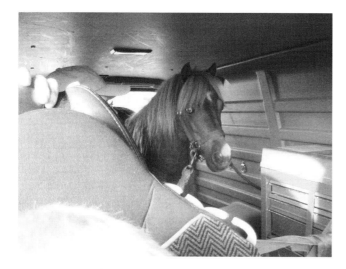

Figure 9.10 *Many different and unexpected transportation methods are used for large animals; in this case, the pony is being transported in an electrician's van with human passengers. A child is in a booster seat, a passenger is seated in the back of the van with the pony, and another is driving. In a motor vehicle accident, this animal will provide another concern to responders attempting to assist the human victims. In addition, the animal is not separated from the human passengers and may cause human injury in an accident. Courtesy of Tomas Gimenez.*

compartment with the human victims and must take second priority for rescue.

SPECIAL HAZARDS

Potential fire hazards exist in most horse trailers. Electrical connections to the trailer should be removed or cut. Propane cylinders should be mounted under the gooseneck on the outside of the trailer behind the towing vehicle, but they may be found anywhere inside the trailer or mounted on the nose of the hitch. Extra hay may be stored in the feed manger, wood shavings may be spread on the floor where the animals stand, and many trailers have wooden floors covered with rubber mats. Some trailers have wooden walls or rubber-lined walls that increase the amount of combustible materials.

It is very common for trailers with human living quarters (factory or homemade) to have one or more propane tanks. The only legal and safe location for such tanks is on the trailer tongue in bumper-pull trailers or under the gooseneck portion or the trailer in gooseneck trailers. This also means that in a front-end collision the trailer's propane tanks will be one of the first structures to hit the back of the tow vehicle. Trailers with propane tanks may have an ignited pilot light in the stove and/or refrigerator inside the trailer. Responders should also be aware of the possibility of

propane, gasoline, or kerosene tanks in illegal locations inside the trailer.

There may be hazardous materials in the trailer, such as gasoline for an onboard generator or flammable fluids used for horse care (e.g., alcohol, fly repellants, cleaners, hoof polish, etc.). If the emergency breakaway battery is damaged, battery acid may be released. People who camp with their horses will often have lighter fluid, charcoal, and firewood onboard, as well as a variety of human and equine grooming and cleaning products that may be hazardous (particularly if mixed).

The heavy-duty springs on the rear ramp and door of some trailers can be dangerous both to responders and to animals. Use extreme caution when removing these. Many ramps have lifting assistance systems such as hydraulic arms or tightened springs at the base of the ramp that may be dangerous when compromised in an incident.

Doors and divider gates may or may not be attached correctly with lynch pins to maintain their position and may fall onto responders if not stabilized.

PLANNING A TRIP

Regardless of the scenario and planned trip duration, owners and drivers of trailers should be prepared to provide initial assistance on scene in event of a trailer accident until professional emergency responders arrive. Resources and equipment recommendations would include the following at the minimum:

- Flashlight (do not shine this into trailer, as it may panic the animals).
- Cell phone (charged) with emergency contact(s) for people who can help with the horses.
- Flares or warning triangles.
- Reflective gear for human personnel.
- Fire extinguisher (large).
- Extra halters and long lead ropes or emergency rope halters.
- Equine and human first aid kit.
- Tire-changing equipment.
- Two spare tires for trailer.
- Stabling guide or similar resource for stabling out of town.
- Membership in a roadside assistance service specializing in helping people towing horse trailers. (Some of the largest vehicle roadside assistance organizations do not provide roadside assistance to tow vehicles with horse trailers, or for vehicles with dual wheels.)
- Emergency information for emergency responders (Figure 9.11) posted in the trailer and truck in case the driver/owner is injured and cannot make decisions for the animals.

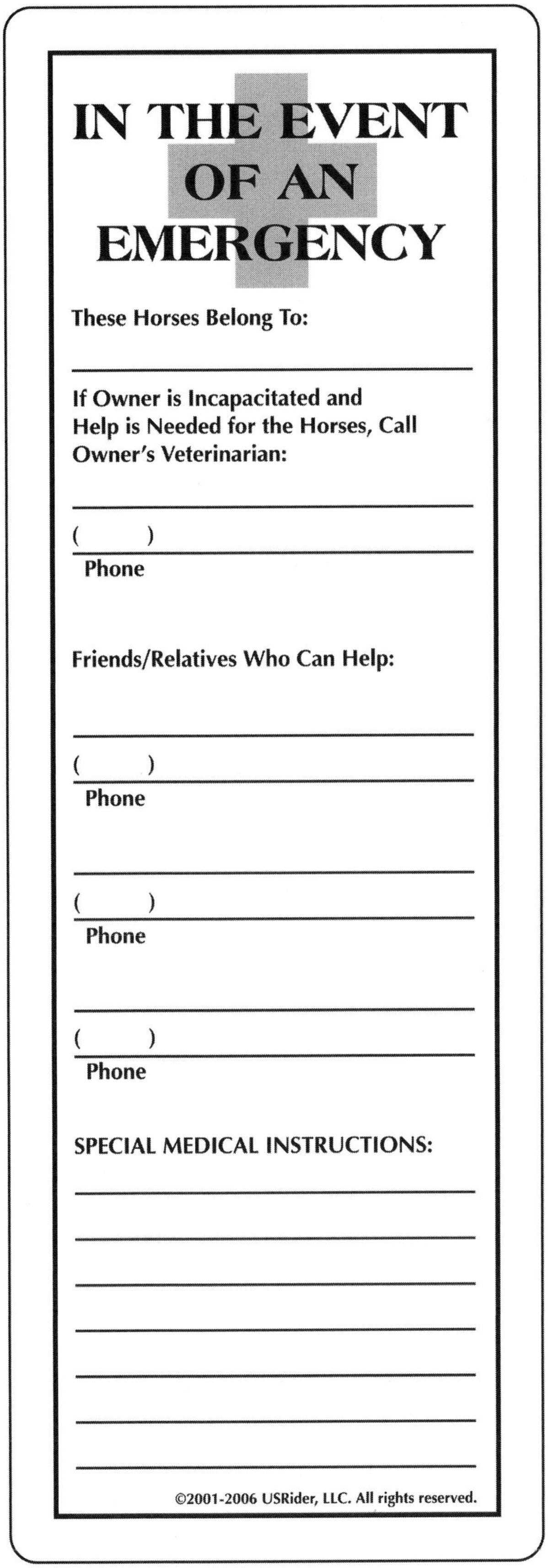

IN THE EVENT OF AN EMERGENCY

These Horses Belong To:

_____

If Owner is Incapacitated and Help is Needed for the Horses, Call Owner's Veterinarian:

_____
_____
(   )
Phone

Friends/Relatives Who Can Help:

_____
(   )
Phone

_____
(   )
Phone

_____
(   )
Phone

SPECIAL MEDICAL INSTRUCTIONS:

_____
_____
_____
_____
_____
_____
_____

- A folder containing the equine infectious anemia test (Coggins test) certificate, health certificates, insurance information, etc., with stickers placed on the trailer alerting emergency responders to the emergency information in the book (Figure 9.12).
- An "at the next exit" book with information regarding veterinarians, hospitals, tire and vehicle repair shops near the planned travel route. These books are usually available at truck stops.

RESPONDING TO THE INCIDENT—INSTRUCTIONS FOR THE DRIVER

Drivers should take certain actions after an accident or other incident.

- Call 911 immediately.
- Stay out of traffic lanes and set out warning triangles and flares.
- If there is a person in the trailer, he or she should be evaluated first. Injured humans are first priority in an accident.
- Perform an overall assessment by checking on the animals through a window or opening. Do not allow anyone to enter the trailer or open doors and windows.
- If trailer is still upright, chock the wheels with available means or, if possible, move it away from traffic lanes.

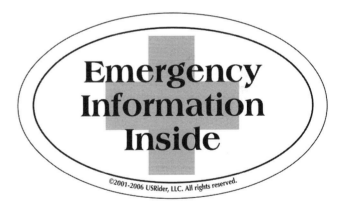

Figure 9.12 _This sticker serves to notify emergency responders that valuable emergency contact information related to the animals in the vehicle is within the vehicle or trailer. Owners and shippers should consider using this kind of notification to alert emergency responders. Courtesy Mark Cole. Used by permission._

Figure 9.11 _This emergency contact form is an example of documentation that may be in the vehicle or trailer. Many owners will have health and contact information on a sticker like this or in a folder or book in the trailer or vehicle. Emergency responders should look for this information from the owner if available. Courtesy of Mark Cole. Used by permission._

- Assess the health of the horse(s) through the window (e.g., watch nostril flare, assess general attitude, etc.).
- Keep animals cool with water spray or fans if the ambient temperature is high.
- Give hay or forage to animals to keep them calm until assistance arrives.
- If animals are loose on roadway, contain them (see Chapter 8) or have a person catch them with a halter and lead rope. Do not tie animals once caught.
- Do not let horses out of the trailer without halters and lead ropes in place to allow proper restraint. Similarly, livestock should remain on the trailer until assistance arrives and containment is established.
- Remove tack and obstacles to make a clear path to the horses for rescuers.

ANIMALS THAT HAVE FALLEN THROUGH THE TRAILER FLOOR

From the standpoint of pain, suffering, and prognosis, trailer incidents involving floor collapse are the worst possible type of incident. These incidents can be prevented by proper attention to maintenance. The presence of urine and manure initiates an oxidizing process that can corrode aluminum floors, rust the steel and metallic components of the floor, or rot wooden floors. Frame components are also subject to these effects. The damage can result in broken springs, severed U bolts and lost nuts from the bolts that hold the axle on the trailer frame. Rubber mats should be removed and the floor and frame integrity checked regularly (on an annual basis or more frequently). Rumber (rubber–lumber) is a relatively new flooring material that minimizes the corrosion problem to the floor.

Inattention to the condition of the trailer floor can be fatal. For example, the owner of a horse in Pendleton, South Carolina, borrowed a neighbor's trailer to transport the horse to a veterinary clinic. While driving through a dangerous S-curve on a steep slope, the trailer began to shake, and the driver heard a noise. The driver found a safe place to pull over 300 m (1,000 ft) further. The horse's legs had fallen through the rotten wooden flooring, and were trapped between the axle and the frame. The trailer frame had to be cut with a torch to remove the horse, which was destroyed based on the severity of its injuries (Figure 9.13).

Drivers transporting animals should pull over and stop immediately at the closest safe location on the roadside if they hear anything unusual, turn on the hazard lights, and check animals. If a horse has fallen through the trailer floor, call 911 and a veterinarian immediately. If the animal is struggling, applying a blindfold may sufficiently calm the animal (if it can be applied safely). Chemical restraint is often indicated;

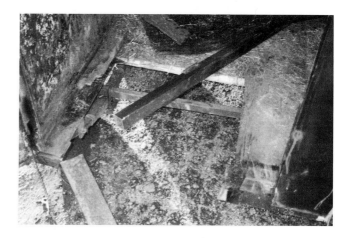

Figure 9.13 *A draft-type horse fell through the rotten floor of this trailer and was dragged approximately 300 m (1,000 ft) to a parking lot before the driver could stop in a safe zone. Here, responders cut the channel and boards to free the horse's rear legs. Due to the severity of the injuries, the animal was euthanized shortly after extrication. Courtesy of Tomas Gimenez.*

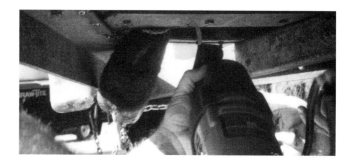

Figure 9.14 *A motorist noticed blood dripping from this trailer and stopped the driver, who tried to tie the leg of the cow up (note the rope on the limb) and drive home. The concerned motorist called 911; responders used a reciprocating saw to provide enough room to lift the leg out of the hole, and patched the trailer floor. Courtesy of Tomas Gimenez.*

those that have veterinary drugs and verbal approval by the attending veterinarian to sedate should give the correct dosage for weight and consider using a pole syringe to more safely administer the drug. In most cases, life-threatening injuries occur rapidly; many cases require humane euthanasia.

Numerous incidents where animals have fallen through the trailer floor involve flooring that is not secured in place or trailer-manufacturing processes that fail to provide appropriate support to the flooring (Figure 9.14). A horse being transported in 2004 fell between the loose boards in the trailer as the driver pulled into the gravel driveway at the veterinary facility. Despite a short drag event, immediate treatment and long-term care, the severity of the lower limb injuries eventually required euthanasia.

Related to these scenarios is the animal that falls out the back of a trailer during transport, especially those that are tied in the trailer. The author has documented four of these incidents within a two-year period. In one case in Arizona, the unsecured trailer rear doors allowed the tied animal to step out the back of the trailer, and it was dragged several hundred meters before the driver could stop the vehicle. The abrasion and friction burn injuries were severe and involved almost two square meters (22 square feet) of skin being removed by the asphalt. The animal was rehabilitated successfully.

TRAILER INCIDENT RESPONSE EQUIPMENT

Exhaustive detail on the types of rescue and extrication tools and their use is not within the scope of this book; however, some highlights for each are provided here.

Standard Rescue Equipment
- Stabilizing struts.
- Cribbing (various sizes of lumber).
- Airbags with air source.
- Tarps.
- General hand tools.
- Rope rescue systems and ancillary equipment.
- Cutting equipment (air chisel, K-12 saw, hydraulic cutters and spreaders). *Note:* The simplest, most common and most useful cutting equipment is a powerful (28 V) cordless reciprocating saw with demolition blades.

Specialized Rescue Equipment
- Rope halters or emergency rope halters (see Chapter 8).
- Two sections of webbing (10 cm × 10.7 m; 4 in. × 3 ft) with a loop on each end (long, wide tow straps are very suitable).
- Portable fencing/cattle panels (see Chapter 21).
- Obstetrical lubricant or liquid clothing detergent.
- Extension poles with the following attachments:
  Open carabiner holder (for attaching a long lead line to the halter).
  Professional pruning hook/blade (for cutting tie straps).
  Hook (for passing webbing over/under animal).

The most suitable extension poles are high quality (hexagonal) roller paint poles from large hardware stores or professional paint suppliers. Consumer-grade roller paint poles are not acceptable because they will bend when extended. Alternatively, a pike pole from the fire engine can be used, but it is heavier than the

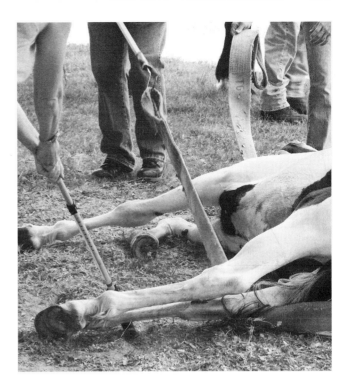

Figure 9.15 *A variety of equipment can be used as extensions of the human arm, including human walking canes, boat hooks, painter pole extensions, tree trimmers, and golf ball retrievers. Aluminum equipment is lightweight and allows the passage of lines or equipment without having to enter the compartment with the animal(s). Courtesy of Tori Miller.*

roller paint pole and may not be long enough in some cases.
- Leg cane (for lifting/moving horse's legs) (Figure 9.15).
- Rescue Glide with accessories.

Cutting into the Trailer

There may be a need to use cutting tools to remove jammed metal obstacles inside the trailer (e.g., door hinges, divider gate hinges, back door post, etc.). Cutting the trailer should be avoided if possible; there are many better options for removing the animals safely. If holes are to be made in the trailer, they must be large to allow safe egress for a large animal. The cut opening should be a minimum of 1.9 m × 1 m (6 ft × 3.5 ft), with all cut edges protected by tarps or foam pool noodles. It is better to remove the entire roof, floor, or side wall of the trailer. If making a hole, responders should attempt to cut the metal like a door (i.e., cut the top, one side, and a bottom) and pry the metal back on the uncut side.

The metal should not be pried during the cutting process; the animals may attempt to bolt through the hole when they see light and can seriously injure rescuers as well as themselves (Fox and Fox, 2000).

The veterinarian can help rescuers weigh the decision to use fast-cutting tools that are likely to generate stress in the animals (e.g., from noise, sparks, or vibration) over a short period versus slower tools that will take longer to get the job done but induce less stress. Some cutting tools are very noisy and cause vibration. The hollow trailer will act like an echo chamber, amplifying every noise. The noise and vibration can panic the animals inside the trailer, and sedation is recommended when these cutting methods are used. The cuts should be planned for efficiency and minimal cutting time. Once a cut has been started, it should be finished even if the animals struggle.

Cutting Tools. Cutting tools include the following.

- Air chisel: This tool is very loud, very effective and rapid, but it generates vibration and can panic the animal victims inside the trailer. If possible, the animals should be sedated using a bang or jab stick prior to use of this tool. The animal's eyes should be covered to protect them from sparks and debris. Ear plugs can be made from cotton, socks, or feminine hygiene products, but may be impossible to apply without risk of injury.
- Light power generation: Lighting from rescue vehicles is necessary, but it must be located a safe distance from the trailer in order to permit safe animal exit and movement into a safe enclosure or alternate transportation (another trailer).
- Hydraulic-powered rescue equipment: This equipment is more quiet and slow compared to air chisels. The power unit and hydraulic pump should be placed as far away as possible to reduce noise.
- Rescue rotary saws: These cutting tools are loud, very effective and fast, and produce minimal vibration.
- Hand rescue tools: Saws, hammers, and axes will all cause noise and vibration. These require a longer time to get the job done and probably are too slow to be considered viable options unless they are the only equipment available.

Note: When using cutting equipment, always assign a person to assess how the animals in the trailer are reacting to the tool noise and vibration. The tool should be turned on at a distance from the trailer and the animal's reactions assessed as the tool is brought closer to the trailer. Turning the tool on and off repeatedly will cause more stress than leaving it running continuously for the time it is needed. It is important to note that an overturned trailer will look very different from a trailer in normal configuration (Figure 9.16).

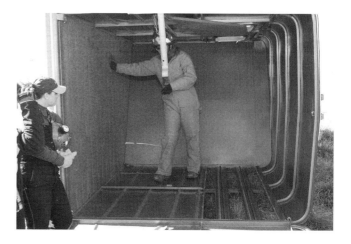

Figure 9.16 *The view of a person in an overturned demonstration trailer gives students a better idea of what to expect from these scenarios. It also demonstrates that creating a wide opening in the rear by removing all gates and dividers, blocking the floor, and allowing the animals to self-extricate may be a better solution than returning the overturned trailer to its wheels. Courtesy of Axel Gimenez.*

STANDARD OPERATING GUIDELINES FOR TRAILER INCIDENTS

The following standard operating guidelines (SOGs) are intended for emergency responders on technical large animal emergency rescue (TLAER) trailer incident scenes.

- Establish ICS procedures (see Chapter 5).
- Pay attention to scene safety (e.g., power lines, gas lines, etc.).
- Pay attention to personnel safety (e.g., reflective personal protective equipment [PPE], etc.).
- Do not allow vehicles to approach or park within 7.6 m (25 ft) of the egress path of the animals because the animals may emerge rapidly from the trailer.
- Do not allow anyone (e.g., rescuer, veterinarian, owner, etc.) to enter the trailer. All assessment and extrication procedures should be performed from outside the trailer. It is not justified to allow any human inside a transport containing one or more unpredictable and stressed large animals. Sedating and/or anesthetizing the animals may be necessary.
- Check for human victims in the trailer/van.
- Request emergency medical services (EMS) on site.
- Assign a photographer to document the scene and rescue effort for insurance, court, litigation, crime scene, or liability issues.
- Use standard SOP for traffic control (law enforcement). Large fire equipment can be used to block traffic; personnel should not be allowed to block traffic.
- Responders should minimize noise and use a silent approach. The sirens should be silenced, but the strobe lights should be operated for safety reasons.

- A large animal veterinarian should be contacted and escorted to the site. The veterinarian must be prepared to perform triage and possibly euthanize animals on site. The veterinarian should have basic knowledge of the ICS and be willing to work under the incident commander (IC) as a team member.
- Request animal transport to haul rescued animals away from scene.
- If possible, identify local, experienced horse handlers who are willing to assist on the scene. A knowledgeable handler will facilitate the rescue effort. If this person is not familiar with the ICS system, a brief introduction to the ICS will be necessary.
- Request panels or portable fencing for containment if needed.
- Consider moving the entire trailer to provide egress room before trying to extricate.
- Request wrecker(s) if needed.
- Determine the number and type of animals in the trailer.
- The IC should assign one person to accompany and interact with the driver/owner; this person is also responsible for preventing the driver/owner from interfering with the rescue operation.
- Responders should ask the driver/owner if the animals have received any medication before the emergency personnel arrive at the scene.
- Assess possible injuries and medical conditions from outside the trailer.
- Assess the position of horses/animals in trailer.
- If sedation is indicated to facilitate extrication, it should be administered from outside the trailer with the aid of a jab stick syringe extension or a syringe attached to a pike pole.
- Providing fresh grass or hay to the animals will often calm them.
- Dead animals should be covered with a dark-colored king-sized bedsheet to minimize attention and reduce the visibility of blood stains.
- In a trailer overturned on its side, the windows may become holes on the ground. If the trailer is upside down and the horse is down on one side, it may kick through the windows. Responders should attempt to block the windows with plywood or a backboard when possible.

Do **not**:

- allow vehicles and people in close proximity to the animal egress or handling area.
- forget that the effects of sedation can wear off at any time.
- use ropes around the head, neck, or legs if any better option exists (see Chapter 6).
- use winches to extricate animals; instead, use rope systems or human power on ropes.

- shine a flashlight into trailer suddenly, or take pictures using a flash, as it may panic the animals.
- drag animals out of the trailer and directly over abrasive surfaces such as asphalt, sand, or gravel; a tarp, plywood board, or plastic sheet should be placed underneath the animal.

ANIMAL PATIENT CARE IN TRAILER INCIDENTS

Large animals generate a considerable amount of heat under normal relaxed conditions in a pasture environment. A metal trailer sitting on asphalt quickly becomes a sauna as the animals generate heat in addition to the heat radiating from the road surface. It is important to avoid overheating the animals inside a trailer during an incident. An unattended animal in a hot trailer will quickly overheat and can suffer from dehydration, hyperthermia, hypovolemia, shock, and kidney failure. Due to their large muscle mass, pigs and draft type horses (e.g., Clydesdales, Percherons, Belgians, etc.) are less able to dissipate body heat than cattle or light horse breeds. If a transport incident occurs in a warm environment, it is essential to begin cooling the animals as soon as possible upon arrival at the scene. One or two team members should be assigned to spray a mist of water on the animals as needed from outside the transport. Hosing the outside of the trailer can also have a cooling effect (see Chapter 20).

If animals must remain in a trailer for a period of time, they should be monitored for signs of overheating or heat exhaustion and offered water. Providing adequate ventilation can assist in keeping the animals cool. Extreme cold is less likely to negatively affect animals unless they have been sweating.

Veterinarians should not be allowed to enter the trailer with the trapped animals to perform triage. The veterinarian should be able to perform a preliminary assessment based on the scenario, the reaction of the animals to stimuli, and observation of the animals through natural openings in the trailer.

EXTRICATION OPTIONS

Upon arriving at the scene of a trailer incident, responders must determine which option(s) they will use to free the animal victims in a safe and efficient manner. Trailers may land in unusual positions when they stop rolling or moving: upside down on the roof, on the side, even on the back doors. There is no uniform SOP for these incidents, but thinking of the trailer as an object that can be manipulated to slide the victims out may make it easier to conceptualize extrication and extraction. A combination of methods may be necessary, and the strengths and weaknesses of each are discussed below.

Perform the Assessment First

The assessment of the animals should be performed from the outside of the trailer looking through the natural openings (e.g., windows, floor slats, etc.) and may require that a team member climb on top of the trailer after it has been chocked for stability (Figure 9.17). Personnel should not be allowed to open doors or windows, even if they appear too small for an animal to pass through them. Panicked animals may attempt to jump or run through the opening when they see light entering the compartment. A team member should assess the position of the animals and the presence of obstacles (e.g., structural components of the trailer, equipment, etc.) (Figure 9.18). Even in severe rollovers, the animals may be able to stand up and be literally walked out of the trailer. In other cases, a trailer that did not overturn may contain animals that are down on their side due to hard braking and loss of balance and footing.

Stabilize the Trailer

Most trailers will need to be stabilized before attempting the actual extrication. In the case of bumper-pull or gooseneck trailers, the rescue operation will be easier if the towing vehicle is not attached to the trailer. The trailer should be unhitched or cut away from the towing vehicle after placing cribbing and/or rope systems under or on the trailer to prevent it from rocking or rolling over further. Cribbing, rescue struts, and other hydraulic systems are available through the local fire-rescue department. Details on the use of heavy specialty rescue equipment are beyond the scope of this book.

In addition to its final orientation, the overturned trailer may be in a ditch or ravine, stuck in trees, stuck in mud or water, or leaning on top of another vehicle containing human victims. It may be easier to bring the entire trailer back up to the road surface using a winch, and stabilize it in a safe area, instead of attempting extrication on unstable surfaces or on a slope. The safety officer and IC should seek the advice of the veterinarian on the scene to determine the safest compromise for the animals and the rescuers in stabilizing and orienting the trailer (Figure 9.19).

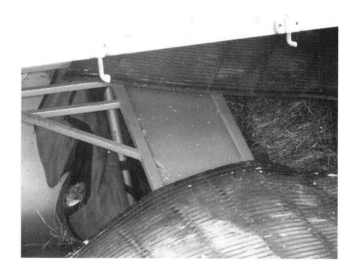

Figure 9.18 *The view inside an overturned horse trailer is a chaotic mixture of rubber mats, hay bags, tack and equipment, divider/gates, and animals. Moving any of the obstacles may stimulate violent reactions on the part of the animals trapped in the trailer. Courtesy of Tori Miller.*

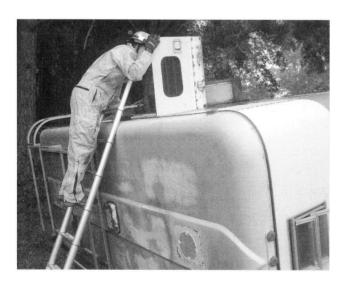

Figure 9.17 *A good assessment of what is actually in the overturned trailer should be completed once the vehicle is stabilized. Here, a firefighter uses a ladder to get up on the trailer and observe the orientation of the animals while placing webbing and round slings on the trailer for stabilization purposes. Courtesy of Al Filice.*

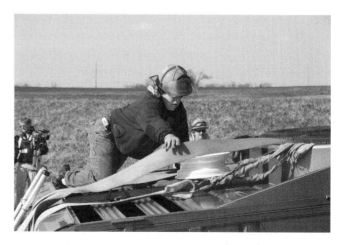

Figure 9.19 *During a TLAER training event, students learn to react to an overturned horse trailer scenario that includes media, bystanders, a hysterical horse owner, and plastic horse mannequins inside the trailer. Using the methods in this chapter, the demonstration trailer sustained no damage other than broken clearance lights. Courtesy of Axel Gimenez.*

Livestock liners, potbelly livestock trailers, and large horse vans are so large that it may not be necessary or possible to separate the trailer from the tractor, since most extrication procedures will take place through the back or roof of the trailer. Stabilization of the trailer is critical before attempting to access the animal compartment. (See Chapter 21.)

Containment and Restraint

Responders should set up a method of primary restraint (halter and lead rope) and secondary containment (e.g., panels, plastic portable fence, etc.) before allowing animals to exit the trailer. Livestock should be permitted to leave the trailer on their own without allowing a person to enter the trailer (see Chapter 21). A load of pigs or cattle released from an overturned liner will not be individually haltered for containment, but horses should not be unloaded from a trailer without a halter and long lead rope to prevent them getting loose once extricated. The use of containment and restraint should be planned and assembled before any access is attempted into the trailer (Figure 9.20).

The doors of the trailer should not be opened until the handler has control of the animal (i.e., a lead rope and halter have been placed) or an appropriate containment system (e.g., cattle panels) has been assembled for whatever species is in the trailer compartment. A lead rope 4.6–6.7 m (15–22 ft) long is recommended to provide leverage to the animal handler working with the animal. Most cattle are not accustomed to halters and leading, unless they are show cattle. If animals are not wearing halters, responders should assume they are not halter trained. It is preferred not to unload animals on the side of the road except in extreme cases (e.g., fire in truck/trailer, horses being removed from wrecked trailer, etc.). If the animals must be removed, traffic must be stopped to allow better control of the animal(s)

and to minimize the risk of secondary incidents (e.g., loose animals and/or responders impacted by moving vehicles). There are many cases where animals were extricated from trailers, only to get loose and cause a secondary wreck or injure themselves while running away. Always have a backup plan of containment with portable fencing (see Chapter 8).

Alternate Transport

Responders should make an early assessment of whether or not alternate transportation for the animal(s) will be necessary. Many trailers, even overturned ones, are roadworthy after set back on their wheels. If the trailer and/or towing vehicle are not roadworthy, alternate transport should be coordinated early in the response to minimize waiting time. Overturned liners with livestock will always require alternate transportation; for this reason, several professional slaughter companies have SOPs for the dispatch of a rescue trailer and trained response teams for these animals.

Orientation of the Animals

After an incident, animals may be in any number of orientations within the trailer; the greater the number of animal passengers, the more complicated the extrication planning. If all the animals are standing up, they can often be led from the trailer. It is more common that one or more animals will be down and underneath other animals; the standing animals will need to be released first to give the others room to stand if they are able to do so. If an animal can walk out of the trailer on its own without having to be manipulated, it is always safer for the rescuers and the animal victims (see Chapter 15).

Block the Windows

An animal is often down in a trailer because it cannot establish secure footing on the slick surfaces or its legs are caught in or through the trailer windows. Using rubber mats, plywood boards, or an EMS backboard to shove into the trailer to block the windows may allow the animals to find secure footing and stand inside the trailer.

Walk the Animals Out

On many emergency scenes with trailers, the simple approach of removing obstacles around the animals (e.g., doors, dividers, ramps, hay racks, tack room, and equipment, etc.) may be all that is needed for the animals to stand and walk out of the trailer through the normal openings. It is preferable that no humans be allowed to enter the trailer; a long lead rope can be attached to the animal's halter and trailer ties can be cut using serrated knives or cutting devices attached to extension poles.

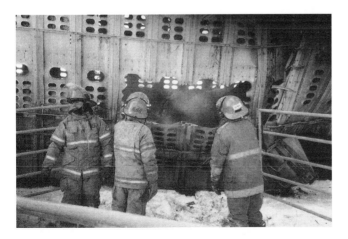

Figure 9.20 *Firefighters respond to an overturned cattle trailer by setting up primary containment before cutting into the roof or sides to release the animals. Courtesy of Jennifer Woods.*

Righting the Trailer

The method of righting the trailer discussed here involves bringing the trailer to an upright or stable position before extrication. The most stable position might not be on the wheels: it may be on the trailer roof. The technique has been expanded and is based on the work of the human emergency rescue professions. It requires the use of rope systems, air bags, web anchoring, and other basic technical equipment owned by most fire departments.

This approach is indicated only when the position of the animals has not changed significantly in relation to the trailer or where access to the animals is impossible without performing this method of rescue. However, it is very rare that this method would be selected. An example of this approach might include an overturned slant-load gooseneck trailer on its side, with horses still within the partitions, that can be easily rolled back over onto the wheels with minimal obstacles (Figures 9.21–25).

Cutting the Trailer

Cutting tools are often needed to remove jammed metal obstacles blocking the animals inside the trailer (e.g., door hinges, divider gate hinges, back door post, etc.). There are a variety of tools available to responders, including a reciprocating saw that features low noise production and adequate cutting speed. (See also the cutting tools section earlier in this chapter.) However, cutting into the sheet metal and ribs of a trailer should be the last resort in a wreck of any type. The noise will increase the stress level of the animals, and, in most cases, there are better options to use to get the animals out of the transport. This is not true of all liner wrecks and overturns (see Chapter 21).

If cutting an access opening into a trailer, it should be cut like a door, not a ramp. Animals will be reluctant

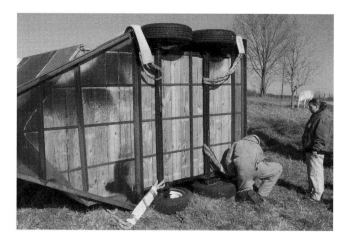

Figure 9.22 *Righting a trailer is usually a last-resort method; however, manipulation of a trailer to allow stabilization, access, and efficient extrication is very common. Large slings are emplaced, using the axles as attachment points to cradle the trailer as it is righted, to allow control of the descent. Bracing the trailer before approaching the animals inside is crucial. Courtesy of Tori Miller.*

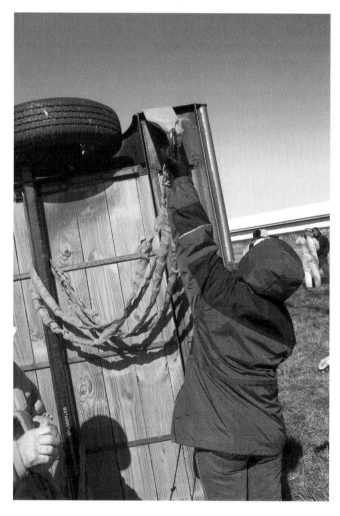

Figure 9.23 *Round slings or fire hose webbing can be emplaced around the axles of an overturned trailer to provide an anchor point that will not destroy the rope. The round sling should be passed around the outside of the wheel well, not between the axles, to distribute the force and increase control. Courtesy of Axel Gimenez.*

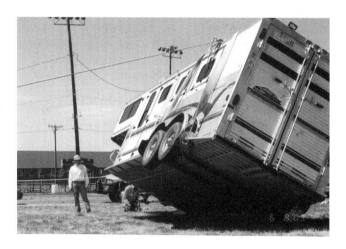

Figure 9.21 *Righting an overturned trailer is not a common response on scene, but manipulating and stabilizing trailers is a common scenario. Courtesy of Tomas Gimenez.*

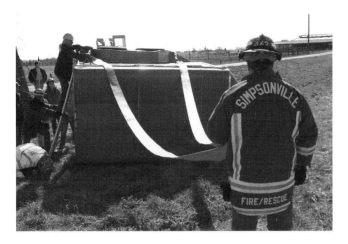

Figure 9.24 *Webbing in a "V" configuration is attached to the round sling, allowing the trailer to be supported as though cradled. In this way, the lifting and lowering sides provide control of the righting procedure. Courtesy of Axel Gimenez.*

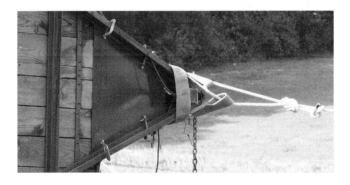

Figure 9.25 *The moving anchors at the nose of an overturned trailer may make use of short pieces of webbing or fire hose with sewn loops at each end wrapped around the hitch mechanism as anchor points to attach the ropes. Human power can be utilized on this moving anchor system to provide control of the nose during the righting procedure. Courtesy of Tori Miller.*

to walk over a ramp-type opening because it will usually be slippery due to the type of material (e.g., metal) and the presence of manure, urine, and possibly blood; additionally, the ramp may not feel solid when the animal steps onto it. When making cuts, the metal should not be pried back until the entire hole is finished being cut to prevent the animal inside from attempting to push its body through a hole that is not sufficiently large for it to pass. All jagged edges should be covered; ideal materials for this purpose are pool noodles available in large retail or toy stores.

Backward Drag Method

The backward drag method is ideal for removing an animal in an overturned trailer when the responders only have access to the rear end of the animal, and it can be emplaced without a human getting in the trailer (see Chapter 15). Where possible, tarps or other protec-

tive materials should be used to cover the metal and surfaces (including asphalt or concrete) over which the animal will be pulled.

PUTTING IT ALL TOGETHER

Every incident is different; trailer incidents, like auto wrecks, require various extrication strategies. There is no specific procedure for every incident, and responders will have to make a decision and create an IAP based on accumulated rescue knowledge, animal-handling knowledge, and experience. Trailer incidents are common and involve special aspects that are not usually part of other TLAER responses—especially the dangers associated with the road and traffic. The considerations for extricating horses from a wrecked trailer include the structural integrity, location, and position of the trailer; the position and health status of the animals inside the trailer; accessibility to the animals without having a team member entering the animal compartment; obstacles that interfere with access and egress; the possibility of removal through existing openings (i.e., doors or ramps); existing authorization for field euthanasia of severely injured animals; and the availability of an equine ambulance or alternate transportation.

Options for extrication include the following:

1. Allowing the animals to exit through existing openings (i.e., doors or ramps).
2. Creating openings and leading the animals from the trailer.
3. Repositioning and righting the trailer to a better position for removal and extrication of the horses (see Figures 9.21–9.25).

HUMAN VICTIMS

Trailer wrecks are one of the few TLAER incidents that commonly feature human victims who may be more concerned for their animals than for their own safety and injuries. When possible, obtain the name and phone numbers of their veterinarian and other contacts regarding the animals' care before the human victims are transported to the hospital. Responders should remain aware that animals are routinely transported long distances, and animals involved in an incident may be far from their homes; this is especially important when incidents occur on interstate highways or near large livestock and horse show facilities. It is important to determine if the animals are insured and their approximate value; this will assist the veterinarian on the scene when treatment or euthanasia decisions must be made.

The team member designated to interact with the owner should demonstrate compassion. The owners' animals may be very important to them, and they may be overwhelmed by the knowledge that something they did contributed to or caused the wreck or accident. The emotional value of an animal may far exceed its actual financial value. Mental health personnel may be required to assist the animal owner during the incident and response effort, particularly if the rescue effort is unsuccessful or the animals are critically injured.

TRAILER RIGHTING SOG

Although this option is one of the most rarely indicated TLAER methods, below are the exact methods to use for simple trailer stabilization or in scenarios where the trailer must be manipulated to make extrication more efficient. The procedure described below was originally developed by Captain John Fox from the Felton Fire District in California and slightly modified by the authors.

- The decision to bring the trailer back to an upright position should be based on the location and orientation of the horses relative to the position of the trailer.
- Stabilize the trailer.
- Separate the trailer from the towing vehicle.
- Following consultation with a large animal veterinarian on the scene, sedate the horses from outside the trailer using a jab stick or use the animal's tail vein (if accessible).
- Assign at least one person to monitor the horse's movement and/or behavior and report to the veterinarian.
- Keep animals cool (e.g., fan or mist, if necessary).
- If the trailer is on a slope, such as the road shoulder, it should be dragged carefully with a winch to a flat area or accessible area.
- Attach wrecker round slings or similar material around each axle but against the wheel sides, with both ends of each round sling passing around the outside of the wheel wells and not between the axles (see Figures 9.22 and 9.23).
- Connect each end of the top of the round slings to each end loop of a nylon web (4 in. wide, 50 ft long; 10 cm wide, 15 m long) with large carabiners. Lay the webbing (now forming a "V" shape) over the trailer.
- Attach the "V" end of the webbing to a heavy-duty friction system (brake tube) connected to a secure anchor.
- Create a space of 10–15 cm (4–6 in.) under the trailer with either a fulcrum or an airbag and cribbing.
- Using an extension pole with a hook, guide the end loops of a second section of webbing (4 in. × 50 ft, or 10 cm × 15 m) under the trailer until the loops meet the round slings located on the bottom end of the axles.
- Connect each webbing loop to the corresponding round sling with large gate carabiners (see Figure 9.24).
- Drape the webbing around and over the trailer toward the axle side.
- Connect the center of the webbing to either an appropriate rope mechanical advantage system or to a winch.
- Deflate the top tires so that when they land, they will not roll (but do not slash the tires).
- Attach two lines, at a 120-degree angle to each other, to the hitch portion of the trailer. These two lines will be manned with two or three people as moving anchors on each line to help prevent the trailer from pivoting during the righting procedure (see Figure 9.25).
- On a bumper-pull trailer, the trailer jack should be fully raised to prevent damage to the jack.
- If the trailer is on a slippery surface such as wet grass, asphalt, ice, or an oil spill, add a static line from the lower end of each axle under the trailer to the secure anchor with the friction system. These lines will keep the trailer from dragging during the righting procedure. These lines are normally not necessary on sand or dry grass.
- The person coordinating this operation should stand facing the trailer hitch with an unobstructed view of all systems and personnel involved.
- Commence righting the trailer in a continuous and slow manner without jerking movements; the animals may struggle or thrash.
- As soon as the trailer passes its balance point, stop the lifting movement and allow the friction system to deposit the trailer very gently on its wheels.
- Stabilize the trailer, including the tongue in a bumper-pull trailer, place wheel chocks, and proceed to unload the animals.

ACRONYMS USED IN CHAPTER 9

EMS	Emergency medical services
IAP	Incident action plan
IC	Incident commander
ICS	Incident Command System
RV	Recreational vehicle
SOG	Standard operating guidelines
SOP	Standard operating protocol
SUV	Sport utility vehicle
TLAER	Technical large animal emergency rescue

10 Barn and Wildfires

Lt. (Ret.) Jeff Galloway and Dr. Rebecca Gimenez

INTRODUCTION

Barn fires, wildland fires, and transport or trailer fires can have a devastating impact on animals and their owners. Each year, hundreds of animals die in often-preventable barn fires (Figure 10.1). In most cases the owners thought their barns were not at risk of fire. Wildfires, which consume hundreds to thousands of acres annually in most countries, threaten scattered communities. Horses and livestock in these communities must be evacuated or sheltered in place. Although rare, transportation fires (e.g., truck, trailer, or van) are significant events and present extreme challenges. Responders to any of these fire scenarios should include equine veterinary practitioners to provide medical triage, treatment, and possible euthanasia.

Volunteer fire departments are most commonly the first responders dispatched to the scene of a fire. Most barn fires burn rapidly, allowing a window of only three to five minutes to save animal lives; for this reason, bystanders and owners will most often be the rescuers. Wildfires affect broad areas, and owners and producers in risk areas should have animal evacuation plans.

Prevention is the key. Mitigation can be defined as actions taken by owners to reduce or permanently eliminate the long-term risk to life and property. Preventive actions can significantly reduce potential losses of life (human and animal) and property. It should be noted that equine and livestock veterinary practices and show facilities are also vulnerable to all the aforementioned fire scenarios. Veterinary practices may be at higher risk due to the presence of flammable (e.g., alcohol, laboratory chemicals, cleaning agents, etc.) and combustible or explosive (e.g., oxygen, anesthetic gases) agents.

Veterinary professionals are viewed as experts in preventive horse health care. Basic barn fire preven-

tion, risk assessment, and recommendations for improvements around facilities can be incorporated into the annual farm health survey. In addition, facility owners should be encouraged to request a courtesy inspection from their local fire department.

DATA REPORTING FOR BARN FIRES

In accordance with the Federal Fire Prevention and Control Act of 1974 (P.L. 93–498), the National Fire Data Center of the United States Fire Association (USFA) gathers and analyzes information on the magnitude, characteristics, and trends of fires across the United States. The National Fire Incident Reporting System (NFIRS) uses fire-reporting data to more accurately assess and combat fire problems at a national level. The data gathered by the NFIRS includes barn fires; however, livestock structure fires are subclassified as cattle, poultry, swine, or "other livestock" facilities. The other livestock facilities may include horse or hay barns. Therefore, accurate statistics with regard to horse barn fires are not available. Additionally, insurance companies do not have a centralized reporting agency for compiling such data.

A search of the veterinary and lay literature revealed information regarding assessment, treatment, and prognosis of burn injuries in horses and animals but minimal information regarding fire research or incidence reporting on barn fires. Collecting the actual number of these events is impossible at this time because there is no nationalized or centralized reporting system that specifically addresses horse barn fires. It is for this reason that much of the available knowledge of horse barn fires (both prevention and response) has been the result of anecdotal (e.g., information from firefighters, owners, and veterinarians) and media reports.

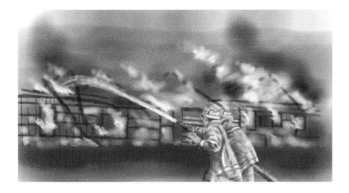

Figure 10.1 *Most barns are constructed of combustible building materials and contain many combustible materials. Animals may have only three to five minutes to be released from stalls once a fire starts before the entire structure is engulfed in smoke and flames. Courtesy of Michael Dzurak.*

This informal collection of data on barn fires has revealed that a significant number of fire events occur in winter. This finding is consistent with the results of formalized surveys conducted by fire science researchers (Loveman and Bernard, 2005). Fire investigation experts estimate that 80%–85% of horse barn fires are accidental, caused by human error (e.g., smoking cigarettes, welding near combustible materials, etc.) or electrical malfunctions. Most electrical fires occur in winter and are associated with heating buckets, water troughs, or living and office spaces. Unfortunately, without detailed NFIRS reports for the specific fires, cause and other details cannot be determined from a data review. Although media reporters provide coverage of the fire and short-term effects, they rarely have access to or receive details on the fire that may be important to disaster prevention and recovery concerns or to veterinary epidemiologists.

There are a few formal sources of available data on horse barn fires. The Fire Protection Engineering Division of the Union Carbide Chemicals Company conducted studies in the 1970s on race track stables for the New York Racing Commission. The California Thoroughbred Breeders Association and Horsemen's Benevolent and Protective Association issued a report on a study of race track stable fires.

The National Fire Protection Association (NFPA) published "Occupancy Fire Record (FR 63–2)," which describes fires in race track barns and stables. Over 90% of investigated fires in this report occurred at race tracks. This was likely because of media coverage and the requirement for investigation before insurance claims for property damage were reimbursed.

A 20-year database of horse barn fires in the state of Kentucky was compiled by members of the Lexington Fire Department, librarians, newspapers, and lay equine publications. To determine the significance of horse barn fires in Kentucky, efforts were undertaken in 1999 to uncover the primary causes of such fires (Dwyer, 1999). Twenty-eight news reports regarding horse barn fires were examined. Fires caused the deaths of 267 horses at the following locations: 23 privately owned farms, one racetrack, one racehorse training facility, one public riding stable, and one veterinary clinic barn. One report did not classify the structure type involved in the fire.

The number of horse deaths per fire in the Kentucky survey ranged from 1 to 38. In five fires, no horses were killed due to successful evacuation or the absence of animals in the structure at the time of the fire. One fire caused the death of one person. Fires occurred between the hours of 6:00 p.m. and 6:00 a.m. on 14 occasions. Seven fires occurred during daytime hours. Six reports did not state the time (Dwyer, 1999).

In an analysis of seven major horse barn fires reported by the Associated Press media from October, 2005, to February, 2006, the following statistics speak to the futility of delayed response:

- Epona Farm, Illinois—33 died, 1 rescued
- Fair Hill, Maryland—24 died, 4 rescued
- Little Full Cry Farm, Virginia—10 died, 0 rescued
- Eureka Downs, Kansas—43 died, 1 rescued
- Lutts, Tennessee—9 died, 6 rescued
- Miami County, Ohio—10 died, 2 rescued
- Norwich, Vermont—0 died, 14 rescued
- Kingsley, New Brunswick, Canada—0 died, 16 rescued

The Kingsley and Norwich fires stand out because both barns had personnel on the scene when the fires began and the horses were removed from the structure. The Norwich facility was under construction at the time of the fire. Every structure in the above incidents was considered a complete loss.

Even small barn fires require deployment of large firefighting resources. For example, in the early morning hours in February 2006, a fire began in a four-stall barn in Colorado. By the time a passerby saw the fire, called 911, and alerted the owners, the barn was fully engulfed in flames. A mare and her newborn foal were killed in the fire. Firefighters from two departments responded with a total of seven trucks and 13 personnel. They were at the scene for two hours and thirty-seven minutes, extinguishing the fire and performing overhaul and salvage. The damage was listed by the departments as extreme and quickly traced to a heat lamp used for the newborn foal.

Development of a reliable and comprehensive database as part of NFIRS would increase the ease of tracking horse barn fire incidents and provide more accurate information to the equine and insurance industries as well as to firefighters.

Economic Losses

The economic losses of horse barn fires can be devastating, with the loss of horses (with actual and sentimental value) and the cost of the structure. Other losses include tack, vehicles, equipment, and feed. Most structures are considered a total loss. In the Kentucky study, 14 reports mention the estimated value of the horse(s) and/or property lost; the total loss was estimated at ≤$5.6 million (Dwyer, 1999).

In the barn fire at the Woodbine Race Track (Toronto, Canada) in August 2002, damage to the buildings was estimated at over $1.5 million and the value of the lost horses in excess of $5 million. In the Eureka Downs, Kansas (February 2006), and the Fair Hill, Maryland (November 2005), fires, initial estimates of property damage and value of lost horses ranged from $1 million to $1.9 million. A fire that is not suppressed in the first minutes rarely fails to involve the entire structure.

Horse barn fires resulted in an estimated $124.6 million in direct damage to property in the United States between 1999 and 2000. These estimates were based on 5,800 barn structure fires (other livestock buildings included). Thirty-four people were injured and one person died in these fires (Loveman and Bernard, 2005).

Arson

Arson refers to the willful and malicious setting of fire to a structure. It may be performed as an act of revenge or malicious intent, to obscure a crime, or as insurance fraud. It is not a common cause of barn fires, but should be considered a possible cause when insured horses are lost in a barn fire. Arson (or situations that are highly suspected to be arson, but cannot be proven) represents approximately 15% of barn fires (Dwyer, 1999). People who commit arson are primarily motivated by profit or anger, with a very low percentage being true pyromaniacs. Random acts of arson are more common than insurance fraud. In the Eureka Downs, Kansas, racetrack stable fire in February 2006, arson detection dogs were brought in as part of the department's routine investigation. Arson was considered a possible cause because many of the 43 horses lost were insured. The actual cause of that fire is still under investigation at this time.

When a horse barn (or any other structure) burns, the incident commander on scene makes a determination of whether a cause is readily apparent or if further investigation is needed. If an in-depth study of the incident is required, an investigative unit is called to the scene. The actual cause of the fire may be determined within hours. However, with complex suspected arson cases, it may take days to weeks to reach a determination, and state fire marshal investigators may become involved. If the property is insured, the insurance company's investigator contacts the fire department and inspects the scene within 48 hours of the fire. After the fire investigation is completed, the fire department files a report with the NFIRS.

The most publicized and prosecuted recent barn fire arson case was in 2001. A firework maliciously thrown onto the roof of a barn ignited a fire that resulted in the deaths of 19 horses at a public boarding facility in Michigan. The firework started a fire that spread so rapidly that the night watchman on duty could save only five horses before the barn was engulfed in flames. Following a jury trial, the defendant was convicted of 19 counts of willfully and maliciously torturing or killing animals (MCL 750.50b(2)). The trial court sentenced him to three years of probation, with the first year to be served in the county jail (State of Michigan, 2004).

In 2005 four teenage girls allegedly trespassed onto a North Carolina family farm while the owners were away on vacation. They allegedly sprayed hair spray in a horse's tail, and set it on fire to watch the mare run in panic. In this case the mare was outside in a paddock, but if this event had transpired inside a barn, or if the horse had run into a structure, it could have caused a much worse incident to occur. The mare survived after tail amputation and nursing care (Hamilton, 2006).

BASIC FIRE BEHAVIOR

Responders in the TLAER area should understand the process of ignition and the basics of fire behavior so that they may assist with prevention of these incidents. A fire requires three ingredients to burn: an ignition source (e.g., spark or intense heat), a fuel source (combustible material), and oxygen. Based on the availability of oxygen, the arrangement of the combustibles, and type of fuel, the fuel source begins to smolder. Fire can smolder for hours, producing low levels of heat and smoke that may not be detected by humans or by commercial detectors. Although smoldering fires (e.g., hay fires, manure fires) are more easily brought under control, they are also the most difficult type to detect and to extinguish. Opening a smoldering bale of hay may cause ignition; it should be hosed down thoroughly, and using a mud lance to inject water into the bale has been suggested.

In a study of 28 barn fires in Kentucky, causes included electrical fire (four), suspected or confirmed arson (three), lightning strike (two), light fixture malfunction (one), electrical heater malfunction (one), overheated electrical cord attached to a fan (one), heat lamp igniting hay (one), malfunctioning lawn tractor stored in the barn (one), cigarette dropped by farm worker (one), and sparks from a welder (one). In 12 fires, the cause was not disclosed (Dwyer, 1999).

Straw bedding reaches a burning temperature of 148°C (300° F) in one to five minutes, during which time it will burn an area 3.05 m (10 ft) in diameter. It develops as much heat and burns at the same rate as gasoline. Living beings usually cannot survive more than a short exposure to 66°C (151° F). The searing heat quickly destroys the delicate tissues of the respiratory tract. Injury to the tissues can occur within one minute; for this reason, humans and animals must be rescued from a burning stall within 30 to 60 seconds. If the damage to the lungs is so severe that it impairs air exchange, the victim will suffocate. Within three minutes of exposure, the victim is dead (Zajackowski and Wheeler, 2002).

Tests in a 3.66 m ×3.66 m (12 ft ×12 ft) stall using two bales of fresh straw showed that in one minute a fast, clean-burning fire creates air temperatures reaching 190°C (374° F) for a height of 4.57 m (15 ft) above the floor. Similar tests using slow-burning straw did not develop noticeable quantities of smoke, and the temperature 4.57 m (15 ft) above the floor reached 66°C (151° F) during the first one and one-half minutes. As the fire continued to burn, dense smoke developed. At three and one-half minutes after ignition, the temperature reached 121°C (250° F) (Zajackowski and Wheeler, 2002).

When flames appear, more heat is being produced. The fire begins to rapidly expand. At this point it may be too late to save any living animals or humans in the structure. Flames move quickly unless design features of the facility slow their progress. After flame eruption, temperatures may exceed 982°C (1,800° F) within minutes at ceiling level (Zajackowski and Wheeler, 2002). Temperatures approach the flash point within three to five minutes; the flash point is the temperature at which all combustibles within that space of super-heated air will ignite. In livestock barns this space is usually the loft area above the ceiling of the first floor and below the roof. Unfortunately, in most barns this space is commonly used for storage of bedding, hay, and other combustibles. This all but guarantees loss of the building contents and any animals housed within it. It is not uncommon for a fire department to return to the scene of the initial fire hours or days later to extinguish smoldering pockets, especially in hay or straw.

An animal should be able to survive a fire less than 1 foot in diameter and/or at temperatures less than 66°C (150° F) if it is rescued within the first 30 seconds. After 30 seconds, it will suffer fatal internal injuries from smoke and heat inhalation. Horses in adjoining stalls may have five to eight minutes to be rescued, depending upon stall construction, ventilation, and separation (Zajackowski and Wheeler, 2002). All 24 horses in the Fair Hill, Maryland, fire (2005) were determined by the deputy state fire marshal to have died of smoke inhalation. Personnel on the scene reported that there were no sounds from the animals when they arrived at the fire, even though the barn was not yet fully engulfed (McKee, 2005).

In addition to the damage caused by inhaled smoke and heat, toxins released during the process of burning also induce severe tissue damage when inhaled. Carbon monoxide and carbon dioxide are common by-products of fires. When inhaled, these gases block the absorption of oxygen by the hemoglobin molecules in the red blood cells, causing asphyxiation through anoxia; although the blood continues to circulate, it does not carry a sufficient level of oxygen necessary to sustain tissue function and life. Flames do not necessarily need to be visible for this to occur (Zajackowski and Wheeler, 2002). Additionally, animals removed from burning buildings have appeared stable for several days, but rapidly destabilize and die from severe pneumonia and lung damage. Some animals rescued from barn fires may need to be euthanized on the scene or at a later time based on the extent of their internal or external injuries (Dwyer, 2006).

Horse Behavior in Barn Fires

Contrary to popular movie portrayals, horses allowed to run out of burning barns do not often run to safety. As prey species, horses are instinctively inclined to remain with the herd and seek safety. A horse that is allowed to run out of a burning barn will often run back into the barn, where its herd and its safe stall are located. Alternatively, the loose horses may run in panic down the road, causing secondary incidents if they are hit by vehicles (including vehicles responding to the fire). Although extra time is required, all horses should be haltered and led from a burning structure.

Smoke induces a panic response by the horse. The sights and sounds of frightened humans, sirens, and crackling flames compound the animal's panic. Once a horse is removed from the burning barn, it can be turned loose in a secure corral, pasture, round pen, or arena that is far from the burning structure. Ideally, a safe containment area is designated in the prepared fire evacuation plan. Trailers may be an option to contain rescued horses if they can be safely and efficiently loaded. It is preferable to have individual handlers hold the horses in a safe area. Animals should be tied as a last resort only. If a horse must be tied, the loose end of the lead rope should be tied above the highest level of the animal's head. There should be enough slack in the rope to allow the horse to lower its head to be level with its withers.

Two behaviors demonstrated by horses in stalls during barn fires are climbing the stall walls in an attempt to escape or standing silently in a corner of the stall as if waiting to die. The horse that climbs the stall walls is more likely to die because it is exposed to more dense smoke as it raises its head. In addition, the severe trauma sustained while attempting to climb the walls or climb out of the stall windows can be fatal. Generally, younger horses and stallions will try to climb the stall walls. Older horses will give up and stand in the corner of their stall, without attempting to escape. An individual horse's behavior in a smoke or fire situation cannot readily be predicted and may be the opposite of what is expected (Galloway, 2006).

An animal does not voluntarily breathe smoke; it will seek a window or other area to find the best-quality air. Recent practical demonstrations during firefighter training included using simulated smoke and practicing evacuation of horses in a fire drill situation. In these scenarios, every horse went to the stall window to get air. If air was not available at the window, the animal lowered its head to breathe at ground level.

Rescuing a horse from a stall in a fire situation is dangerous because of the damaging fire and smoke, the possibility of structure collapse, and the unpredictability of the animal. When the stall door is opened, the animal may rush over top of the handler or may be cowering at the back of the stall. Placing a halter and lead rope on the animal's head and leading it to safe containment must be done efficiently and performed with one horse at a time. This skill requires practice.

FIRE CODES AND ENFORCEMENT

National Fire Code (NFC) documents in the United States define assembly occupancies as those "used for a gathering of 50 or more persons for deliberation, worship, entertainment, eating, drinking, amusement, awaiting transportation, or similar uses," or "as a special amusement building, regardless of occupant load." They define business occupancies as those "used for account and record-keeping or the transaction of business other than mercantile." The majority of equine facilities satisfy both of these definitions and are classified as mixed occupancy structures. Once a facility meets the requirements for mixed occupancy, it must also meet the most restrictive fire- and life safety requirements for those occupancies. This distinction can lead to an enforcement dilemma (Hawthorne and Manley, 2004).

Local county governments, code enforcement commissions, and fire marshals are in the process of developing fire protection codes for barn facilities that house horses and/or other species, including codes for on-site water supply, electrical inspection, and life safety code enforcement (McKee, 2005).

NFPA 150

After a series of disastrous race track fires in 1976, the NFPA established a committee to make recommendations to the equine industry for occupancy requirements, construction, and fire protection. In 1979, the first edition of "NFPA 150 Standards on Fire Safety in Racetrack Stables" was published and accepted as an American national standard (NFPA, 2000). In 2004, the NFPA 150 Technical Committee asked the Standards Council to authorize the expansion of "NFPA 150—Racetrack Stables" to include life and fire safety requirements for humans and animals in all types of animal

housing facilities. The request was based on the National Fire Codes (NFC) classification of buildings that house animals as "storage occupancies;" this designation places barns in the same category as warehouses. The expansion was approved, and the NFPA 150 became the Technical Committee on Animal Housing Facilities to reflect the new focus (Hawthorne and Manley, 2004). It should be noted that this committee does not include a veterinarian or horse industry representative.

Three of NFPA's major documents ("NFPA 1—Uniform Fire Code," "NFPA 101—Life Safety Code," and "NFPA 5000—Building Construction and Safety Code") classify any type of animal housing facility as a "storage occupancy," defined as an "occupancy used primarily for the storage or sheltering of goods, merchandise, products, vehicles, or animals." It is typically characterized by the presence of few people, usually limited to owners and employees. If members of the public enter the building, the building can no longer be considered a storage occupancy. Depending upon the number of people, it may qualify as a mixed occupancy between storage and assembly, or storage and business.

For example, a $1,394\,m^2$ ($15,000\,ft^2$) barn of 30 stalls operated as a private horse breeding facility, would be classified as storage occupancy. The only people allowed inside the barn would be the barn's owner and employees. The same home and barn operated as a boarding facility for horses would be considered a mixed business and storage occupancy to those interpreting the definition (Hawthorne and Manley, 2004).

The structure classifications are currently determined by the local authority having jurisdiction (AHJ) and results in inconsistent treatment of such facilities across jurisdictions. To provide better guidance to AHJs, expansion of NFPA 150 will address all types of occupancy and develop provisions specific to animal-housing facilities. The Technical Committee plans to divide NFPA 150 into three major sections: (1) administrative requirements; (2) general requirements (e.g., occupancy classification, construction, fire protection, and means of egress requirements for all buildings housing animals); and (3) specific requirements for different types of facilities. Specific requirements include public access to the building in new construction and existing structures. Existing structures will be required to provide a minimum acceptable standard of life and fire safety for humans and animals (NFPA, 2000).

FIRE PLAN

Facility fire prevention starts with developing a written defensive fire plan. Copies of the plan should be posted in readily visible and accessible areas (e.g., at the front entrance gate, with neighbors, and with the local fire department). A mailbox or dry storage container can be used to store the plan; the container should be clearly labeled with the words *fire plan* in red letters on a white background.

The defensive fire plan should include the following:

- Layout of the barn with prevailing winds
- Number of horse stalls
- Fire department water supply at the barn and within 300 m (1,000 ft)
- Electric supply shut-off switch or breaker
- Hay storage location(s)
- Hazardous materials location(s)
- Emergency contact phone numbers, including veterinarians
- Emergency equine transport phone numbers
- Location of emergency paddocks

The best way to ensure a facility is prepared is to request a courtesy fire safety inspection of the facility. The inspectors will evaluate fire extinguishers (unexpired, readily accessible, easily visible, and functional), electrical wiring and conduits, code regulations for living spaces within the barn, smoke/carbon monoxide/heat detectors, storage of hay and other flammables, access and egress to the barn aisles, property and driveway access, water sources (e.g., fire hydrant, ponds for drafting, etc.). Barn and facility personnel should be familiar with the proper use of a fire extinguisher. An additional benefit to safety inspection is the familiarity with the facility that is gained by the firefighters; basic knowledge of the facility location, population, layout, specific or unique hazards, preliminary contacts, and location of water sources can increase the efficiency of a response.

Practical Considerations

Facility owners should ensure the barn or facility address is accurate in the local 911 database. A readily visible, reflective sign with 15 cm (6 in.) lettering prominently placed at the property's entrance will aid responders in locating the facility, especially in the dark. Adequate outside lighting, street lights, or motion-sensor lights will also aid responders.

Facility Access. Gaining access to properties through entrance gates is a prevalent problem for fire departments; an average, 20-ton fire truck requires a minimum opening and driveway of 3.66 m (12 ft) wide. Narrow gates, overhanging tree branches, and low power and telephone lines have hindered fire department access to facilities. For example, in Palm Beach County, Florida, a fire truck attempting to enter a narrow gate to respond to a barn fire sustained over ≤$1,000 damage to the truck because the facility entrance was less than 2.7 m (9 ft) wide. In another incident, a four-stall barn caught fire. The owner observed smoke and called 911 in the first moments of ignition. The fire department responded within three minutes, but it was unable to pass through the entrance gate or down the winding driveway to the barn. None of the horses were saved.

Padlocks, large cables, or heavy chains on the main entrance gate will hinder timely fire department access. During a response, the fire truck cannot drive over or through the locked gate or fence to get access to the property and facility. If the entrance gate has an installed numeric keypad, an emergency access device (e.g., Knox-Box) should also be installed to allow fire department access. A large fire truck requires a wide turning radius on solid ground. When possible, a fire lane should be established at the barn entrance and designated a no parking zone. Designated parking areas should be located well away from the structures to minimize the chances of vehicle gasoline ignition.

Include a local fire department representative, as well as all boarders, when designing a plan for public and private facilities. All personnel should be familiarized with the location of the written defensive fire plan (see next section). Prominently placed, reflective signage should identify emergency paddocks and pastures.

Disaster preparedness plans for wildfires, flooding, tornadoes, and hurricanes should also be devised. An evacuation plan should include an emergency destination location for all livestock, as well as a designated method of transport. It is unwise to wait until the disaster happens to make a plan. Once the plan is in place, review a safety checklist and practice regular disaster drills every six months.

Inside the Barn. When all considerations from the front entrance to the barn have been addressed, it is time to look inside the barn and continue developing fire safety precautions. This process begins with an understanding of the causes of horse deaths inside a barn during a barn fire. Animals generally die from smoke inhalation or the effects of radiant heat, not from direct fire contact. Most horses are dead within minutes of the fire's ignition, depending on the amount of smoke inside the barn, ventilation inside the barn, the construction of the barn and the prevailing winds.

The average stall is 3 m × 3 m (10 ft × 10 ft) to 3.66 m × 3.66 m (12 ft × 12 ft) in size. Burning hay and bedding (e.g., shavings or straw) reaches a temperature of 148°C (298° F) in one to five minutes. Animals must be removed in 30 seconds, before they suffer fatal burns or smoke inhalation. Horses in adjoining stalls have five to eight minutes to be rescued, depending on stall construction, ventilation, and proximity to the fire.

Layout within Facilities

Examine animal placement in stalls as it relates to the prevailing winds, the direction from which the wind strikes the barn most of the year. The stronger the prevailing winds, the faster the smoke will be pushed toward the far end of the barn. For example, in Florida an east to southeast wind prevails on the east coast, and a west to southwest wind prevails on the west coast. In mountainous regions, a downdraft blows off the mountains during the day. A method to determine the prevailing wind is to stand with the wind at your back and note the direction it blows through the barn. Use a compass to determine the prevailing wind at the barn.

Begin the layout of the horse stalls within the following guidelines: young, energetic horses; stallions; the most valued horses; or the most reactive horses should be placed at the stalls closest to the exit upwind (i.e., on the side of the barn where the wind enters the barn) from the prevailing winds. This will allow rescuers to remove these horses more quickly from smoke and get them to the safety of emergency paddocks. Other horses should be placed in the center of the barn or toward the end of the barn where the smoke will accumulate due to the prevailing wind. Remember that the layout of the animals' stalls not only depends on prevailing winds through the barn, but also on which horses will be rescued first in case of any disaster or emergency.

Professional evacuation and response training is available to horse facilities and emergency responders. Volunteers should learn to effectively use a fire extinguisher (Figure 10.2). A simple smoke drill inside the barn will determine how any horse should react, but it should be noted that they may not react the same in an extreme emergency. Only a professional barn training company, trained firefighter, or local fire department should perform smoke drills inside the barn; these drills use a theatrical smoke machine to generate

smoke that is nontoxic and will not harm horses. The placement of windsocks or a flagpole near the barn and horse paddocks allows responders to easily determine the prevailing wind direction, which will have an impact on the response strategy.

An analysis of these incidents reveals that it is sometimes possible to access animals that otherwise cannot be safely extricated through the center aisle. Firefighters recommend removing the outside wall below the window, possibly with a chainsaw or axe. The horse must be haltered to prevent it from running loose, and portable containment options can be considered. If the facility design allows, responders should consider driving the animals out of the barn down a chute or funnel to a paddock or pasture.

At the Fair Hill, Maryland, fire in 2005, the 4 surviving horses (of 28 horses in the barn) were rescued through outside-facing stable doors by responders and veterinary technicians that arrived on the scene. Access doors to the barn aisle are standard design in horse facilities, but an additional door leading from each stall to the outside (and, if possible, directly into a paddock) improves safety and the possibility of rescue during a barn fire (Figure 10.3).

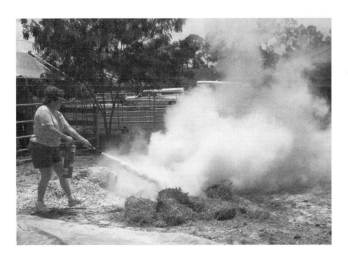

Figure 10.2 *Using a 2.2 kilogram (5 lb) ABC extinguisher to put out a small fire in hay provides practice in the proper use of an extinguisher in an emergency, but only allows 9.2 seconds of extinguishing time. Fire extinguishers are often insufficient to allow extinguishing of anything but smoldering fires in barns. Courtesy of Jeff Galloway.*

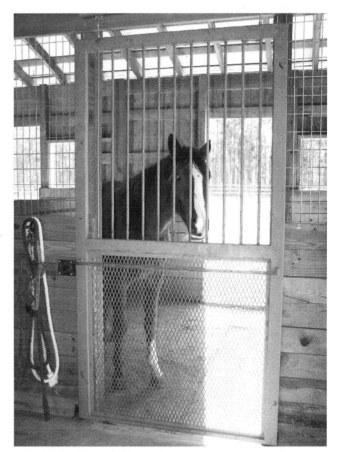

Figure 10.3 *The safest compromise for efficiency, comfort, and safety is provided by stalls with openings to the inside hallway as well as an outside paddock. Courtesy of Tori Miller.*

EVACUATION PLAN

As previously stated, advice should be sought from the local fire department when establishing fire plans. A fire evacuation plan is not effective unless practiced. It is recommended that facility owners practice a drill once every three months. Public facilities and boarding barns should practice a fire drill and review the evacuation plan once a month. This ensures that new boarders, employees, and students will be well prepared.

The fire evacuation plan should include an alternate location to house animals in an emergency. This area must be identified with *emergency paddock* signs readily visible to first responders. The emergency paddock should be far enough away from the barn that radiant heat will not cause burns to the animals or melt the fence, but should not be so far away that personnel are unable to return quickly to the barn to rescue other horses. In the apparent chaos of an emergency, personnel will not know where to put the animals unless an emergency paddock is clearly identified.

If the facility on fire does not have any pastures, a paddock, round pen, horse trailer, or neighbor's farm may be designated an emergency paddock. Practicing the evacuation plan allows personnel to detect and address its weaknesses.

Anatomy of a Barn

The most common horse barn layout has stall doors opening onto an interior hallway. This is designed for human convenience, so that the employees or owner can efficiently feed, water, and clean stalls. Numerous references promote this as an efficient barn design, but few note the benefits of stall accessibility from the outside. Modern barns, including private facilities, are commonly built on a grand scale, ranging from 25 to 100 m (83–328 ft) from end to end. Many of these barns are configured with one long aisle and no side escape routes; this feature decreases the chances of rescuing horses in a barn fire.

Most fires start within 1 m (3 ft) of ground level (e.g., dropped cigarette butt in stall bedding or insulation, sparking electrical fire at the outlet in the wall, etc.), and flames climb quickly into the roof spaces through insulation or other combustible materials. The intense heat and sparks are trapped under the caplike (usually metal) roof. As the heat increases, the combustibles begin to burn. Once the roof joists or rafters begin to burn (and eventually fail), the entire roof collapses into the interior hallway. This represents the greatest hazard to responders trying to remove animals.

Barn Construction Considerations

Materials. Barns are constructed from a variety of materials, including wood, concrete, fiberglass, and composite materials. Despite the use of modern fire retardant materials, any structure can burn.

Even concrete buildings can burn—the wooden rafters and trusses supporting the roof are combustible, as are the bedding on the floor of the stalls, forage, rubber mats, and the wooden doors on the stalls. Concrete actually contributes to increased heat once a fire starts, because it contains the heat within the walls.

Modern building methods often use light-weight wood construction as opposed to traditional post-and-beam construction. Desirable barn designs incorporate roomy, open facilities, with wider clear-span and open arenas, and barn aisles 5–7 m (16 ft, 6 in. to 23 ft) wide. This kind of construction uses gusset (or truss) plates. Gusset plates are metal plates that hold the truss joists together by friction between numerous 10 mm (.50 in.) spikes on the gusset plate and the wood. Using this construction feature, the creation of a 40 m (132 ft) clear span arena is possible. Gusset plate trusses are strong under normal conditions, and less wood and fewer nails are required to support the barn roof. This makes construction costs cheaper, and more clear span can be made available. This method of construction has been adopted widely throughout the United States.

However, since metal absorbs and conducts heat from fires more rapidly than wood, the heat rising in a burning barn is absorbed by the gusset plates and rapidly transfers to the adjoining wood. The hot metal singes the combustible wood, and eventually falls out. If the wood is not fully cured, water remains inside the wood cells. The heat from the fire turns the water into steam, and the steam pressure literally blows the gusset plates out of their position in the wood. When that occurs, the entire truss fails and forces the surrounding trusses to bear more of the loading weight of the roof. Eventually, those trusses also fail and collapse into the interior hall.

Location. Emergency response times are longer in rural areas due to longer travel distances for firefighting vehicles. Additionally, fires may burn longer before being noticed in rural areas due to lower population densities. Firefighters will seldom choose an offensive approach for agricultural facilities, instead attempting defense of nearby structures. As stated previously, wide entrance gates and driveways (minimum of 3.66 m, or 12 ft) facilitate fire equipment access.

Design. Many stables are designed to optimize convenience and comfort for the animals and humans. Fire prevention considerations might not be foremost in the building designer's mind. For existing barns, the owner should consider comprehensive fire suppression and prevention methods.

Any structure can burn, and few barns have after-hours security. This fact can lead to a delayed response or, in one reported case, the discovery of a burned-out structure the following morning. Most stables are long and narrow and may contain 4–60 stalls. Many have

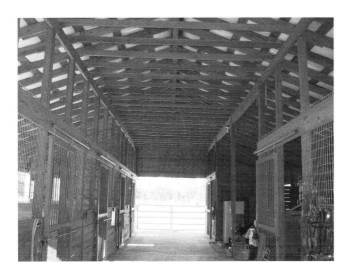

Figure 10.4 *A well-designed barn. The use of stall doors facing the inside and outside is shown here, with post-and-beam construction, easy-open sliding stall doors, excellent ventilation, and clear aisles. Barn design should ensure that defensive fire suppression and safety factors are taken into account. Courtesy of Tori Miller.*

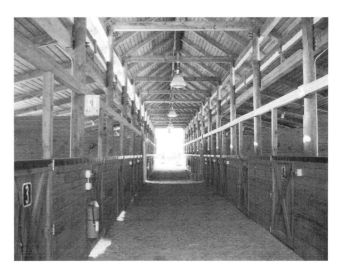

Figure 10.5 *This public overnight horse facility at South Mountain State Park, North Carolina, demonstrates a prevention stance and attention to detail with post-and-beam construction, excellent ventilation, conduit-covered electrical wiring, fire extinguishers, multiple access points, wide aisles, and a siren alarm system. Courtesy of Tomas Gimenez.*

stalls featuring Dutch doors; these doors are sectioned in the center to allow the door to be completely closed or the lower half only closed and the top half left open for ventilation. Few have rear stall doors connecting stalls with direct access to an exterior paddock or pasture. Horse barns designed with front and rear stall doors provide two exits in case of fire (Figure 10.4).

New facility construction should be designed to limit the spread of fire and maintain structural integrity as long as possible and along fire escape routes for a specific period of time (Figure 10.5). Reducing the chance of detection or alarm failure is important as well. Common methods include (1) an inspection, testing, and maintenance program for the system; (2) active monitoring; (3) design redundancy; and (4) using the simplest system that can provide appropriate coverage.

Barns should be designed so that there is a doorway leading directly outside within 30 m (100 ft) of travel distance from all portions of the building. It should be possible to exit from any point in the building in at least two directions. Dead ends longer than 12 m (40 ft) are not permitted by national code. Travel distance may be increased to 46 m (152 ft) when the barn is constructed of masonry or masonry-veneer and protected by an automatic sprinkler system (NFPA, 2000).

Firewalls, which are completely sealed and provide one hour of fire protection, are required for human living spaces. Firewalls coupled with smoke detectors, heat detectors, and carbon monoxide detectors (depending on the jurisdiction) give the best protection, although there is no substitute for common sense.

Fire curtains compartmentalize the open space in the roof trusses and slow the transfer of superheated air

and smoke through the loft space. Fire curtains are highly recommended and will prevent the truss area from becoming a tunnel for the travel of heat and flames (Zajackowski and Wheeler, 2002). Another effective form of compartmentalization is the construction of multiple smaller buildings, as seen at racetracks and large show facilities, instead of one large building.

Good ventilation is important for the health of animals kept in stalls and increases their chances of survival in a fire. Airborne particulates (e.g., dust, fine particles) will trigger most commercially available smoke detectors. For this reason, common smoke detectors may not be appropriate for most barns but should be used in all living areas. Other options may be available—ask the fire department in your area.

The NFPA recommends roof vents as an effective method for removing noxious gases, superheated air, and unburned gases. Common options include continuous open slot ridge venting; louvered or heat-activated vent monitors; or vents designed to melt, collapse, or spring open at preset temperatures (usually 100°C, or 212° F).

Management. A no smoking policy should be implemented and strictly enforced. This policy should prohibit smoking inside the barn and for a designated radius around the barn; the role of smoldering cigarettes in barn fires should not be underestimated or overlooked. In one incident, an arson investigator reported that a nesting bird picked up a burning cigarette butt and brought it in the barn. Brush, overgrown grass, and weeds should be removed within a 15 m (50 ft) radius around the barn.

Frost-free water hydrants with long hoses should be installed and fire extinguishers placed along the aisleways. Alternative water sources (e.g., pond, cistern, or swimming pool), hydrants, or standpipes should be marked and unobstructed for fire department access.

Use Fire-Retardant Materials

While it is impossible to make a livestock building completely fireproof, owners of such facilities can reduce the risk of fires by incorporating safety practices, prevention strategies, and management focus. Barn design should attempt to increase the amount of time (minutes) that it takes a fire to reach flash point. This can be accomplished by modifying building materials and contents, compartmentalizing with fire resistant barriers, and adjusting ceiling height or room volume (Zajackowski and Wheeler, 2002).

A true noncombustible building material would be a material of which no part will ignite and burn when subjected to fire. Builders and owners should look for building materials that are as noncombustible as possible. Masonry, heavy timber, and fire-retardant treated wood should be considered for all livestock building construction.

The flame-spread rating of construction materials is an estimate of how long it would take for flames to traverse the surface of the material as compared to the standard concrete block (0 rating) and dry red oak (100 rating). Fire-retardant lumber decreases flame spread by 75% to achieve a rating of 25, and it is effective for many years. The material develops a carbon char on the exposed surface that will not continue to burn, maintaining the structural integrity of the wood (Zajackowski and Wheeler, 2002).

A low smoke-development rating indicates that the material produces less smoke as it burns, resulting in increased visibility, less noxious gas liberation, and fewer sparks to propagate the spread of fire.

Fire ratings indicate how long a material may block the progression of a fire: higher-rated materials will slow the progression of the fire. Interestingly, this is the most complicated rating system. Metal siding has a low (good) flame-spread rating, but, because it is a good conductor of heat, it has a poor fire rating. Combustibles touching fire-heated metal can ignite. The bottom line is that as long as there is hay, horse shavings, and bedding inside the barn, the barn will have the potential to burn.

Electrical Service. Faulty electrical wiring and connections are leading causes of barn fires according to data compiled by the NFPA. Because it is impossible to render any facility entirely fireproof, preventive measures and mitigation techniques are critical.

- Ensure that electrical service boxes should be in a dry, dust-free location and mounted on fire-resistant materials.
- Install a main shutoff switch near the entrance and/ or exit so first responders can quickly turn off the power to the barn (without turning off power to the house, property lighting, pumps, etc).
- Modify the electrical system to maintain power to the water pumps when the building's power is interrupted. External lights with alternate power sources are also recommended for safety.
- Make sure the electrical service to the barn is "heavy duty" and the fuses are the correct rating for the electrical demand.
- Ensure that lighting fixtures should be Underwriters Laboratories listed (Margentino and Malinowski, 2004).
- Protect electrical wires with conduit to prevent rodent damage that could spark an electrical fire. Metal or polyvinyl chloride conduits should be used for every inch of wiring between every junction box. The use of plastic covered wires is not advised.
- Install lightning protection systems (i.e., lightning rods). They should be installed by a professional and correctly grounded to allow proper dissemination of the energy of a lightning bolt via a heavy-duty conducting cable to the ground.
- Minimize the need for extension cords. Install a sufficient number of electrical outlets for all appliances (e.g., clippers, heaters, fans, microwaves, etc.). If an extension cord must be used, it should be a heavy duty (low-gauge rating) cord.
- Evaluate the wiring for all appliances and light fixtures in the barn for worn or frayed cords or cracked cord insulation. This includes the wiring for electric heaters for water buckets, tanks, etc.
- Ensure that light fixtures should be free of dust, cobwebs, chaff, dead insects, or other combustible materials.
- Clean dust and dirt from electrical appliances such as fans and heaters.
- Keep heaters or heat lamps clear of combustibles, away from high traffic areas, and out of reach of livestock and children.
- Disconnect coffee pots, radios, heaters, fans, portable heaters, and other electrical appliances when not in use.
- Supervise use of any type of heater at all times. When not in use, heaters should be unplugged. *Note:* Regarding tank heaters, in one incident a water heater unit contacted the side of a 1,135 l (300 gal) plastic water tank in which it was installed. It caught fire, burning the plastic down to the level of the water. Animals can be electrocuted by these products. Superior tank heaters fit through a drain at the bottom of the water container, making it harder for an animal to access it. In very cold climates, floating

water heater styles are necessary to keep ice from forming.

- Do not use nails as hangers for electric cords.
- Cage all electric light fixtures, especially those above horses, to prevent damage or shorts.
- Make sure animals have no access to any electrical outlet, wiring, or appliance.

FIRE PROTECTION STRATEGIES

Early warning systems should permit notification of the fire service and occupant/owner and allow escape and timely removal of animals from the facility. Detection must lead to fire department notification (e.g., alarm, call to dispatch, bells) for an appropriate emergency response to occur. Reliable fire detection systems notify the owners, 911 dispatch, and/or the nearest firefighting organization by way of an automatic alarm. Many systems also feature an outside noisemaker that can be heard by nearby neighbors.

Prevention involves separating all ignition sources from fuel sources and minimizing the fuel sources that are present. Storing hay and bedding in a separate building, keeping the barn clean (including cobweb removal), and enforcing a strict no smoking policy are examples of effective tactics.

SPRINKLER SYSTEMS

A sprinkler system is an excellent investment to prevent a total loss from fire, and it is the best method of fire suppression. Sprinkler systems have allowed the rapid control and extinguishing of approximately 93% of fires when present (NFPA, 2000).

Sprinkler heads are individually activated by heat, delivering approximately 95 l (25 gal) of water per minute onto the source. Sprinkler system and fire suppression methods have been proven to extinguish or slow the progression of barn fires. Water pressure is a crucial factor in ideal functioning of this system; the system may require a separate water tank and pump to maintain sufficient water pressure. Obviously, this increases the cost associated with the system.

Wet pipe systems (pipes constantly charged with water) are cheaper and require less maintenance. Dry pipe systems must be employed where the climate drops below freezing: pressurized air or compressed nitrogen fills the lines until the sprinkler head is activated by fusible links. The pressurized air is released, priming the water into the pipes and dousing the fire. Obviously, this system is more complicated, and thus more expensive, than the wet pipe system.

A current technology used in Europe and in maritime functions may be used in the future: water mist systems. In this system, stored water is highly pressur-

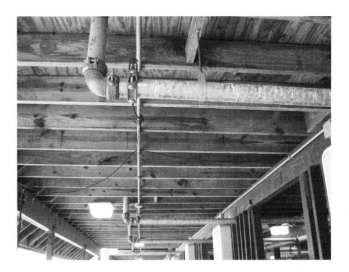

Figure 10.6 *This mounted police barn at the Kentucky Horse Park was retrofitted with a sprinkler system after an incandescent lightbulb ignited a smoldering hay loft fire that was successfully extinguished. Smoke damage to the building was significant. The sprinkler system features fusible links and a pipe with a diameter of 15 cm (6 in.) that provides water at sufficient pressure to quickly extinguish a fire. Courtesy of Tomas Gimenez.*

ized to produce fine water droplets using up to 25% less water. The system is more expensive than the previously described systems, but uses less water. Insurance companies do not currently rate premiums based on this system, but in the future it is hoped that technology advances will make it cost-effective for livestock facilities.

Automated sprinkler systems should be installed and maintained. Although the initial cost of such a system can be high, many insurance companies will reduce premiums by as much as 50%. These systems allow longer response times and reduce the risk of animal and human death. Additionally, a sprinkler system is a depreciable expense. Over time, the barn owner will save money, especially if the animals within the facility are considered valuable (Figure 10.6).

Early Warning Devices

A rule of thumb used in the firefighting profession is that fires involving combustible materials (e.g., wood, straw, hay, shavings, etc.) double in size every minute. Therefore, in 10 minutes, a small fire will increase in size over 4,000 times. This emphasizes the need for fire prevention and prompt action when faced with actual incidents (Bukowski et al., 2002).

A professional alarm company should be contracted to install a thermally (heat) activated alarm system throughout the facility. These warning devices are highly reliable and are activated by heat at a predetermined level. However, they must be in close proximity to the heat source to dependably activate. This may mean that the fire reaches later stages of progression before it sets off this type of alarm, reducing the effective response time. Fixed-temperature-line thermal detectors are recommended for barns to increase the floor area coverage at a minimal cost (Zajackowski and Wheeler, 2002).

Flame detectors are an expensive option but are the most reliable of all warning devices. Simulating the human eye, they detect the characteristic electromagnetic radiation signature emitted by flames, thus minimizing false alarms.

The standard, commercially available smoke alarm uses a photoelectric eye or ionization detector to sample the air. This style of detector gives earlier warnings but, in a barn, keeping them free of dust is necessary to avoid false alarms. Animal dander, dust, and humidity increase false alarms. Photoelectric and ionization types of smoke detectors are excellent for use in living quarters and provide very early fire detection. In a tack room and other enclosed facilities (e.g., office, lounge, living spaces, etc.) within the barn, smoke detectors of either type should be installed and maintained. These areas are commonly the origin of fires due to electrical appliances.

The fire department can often provide referrals for installation professionals familiar with livestock facilities. All of the early warning devices are ineffective if they are not connected to the 911 system, a professional monitoring service, family, neighbors, or directly to the local fire department. When properly used to alert humans, the systems provide essential time to allow fire suppression efforts and the removal of animals from the barn safely.

Water Supply

A prevalent problem for fire departments is access to an adequate water supply on the site. Many barn facilities are in rural areas of the United States and do not have fire hydrant systems, but rely on drafting from a pond instead.

The area surrounding the barn should be evaluated for emergency water sources. Ideally, a fire hydrant should be located within 300 m (1,000 ft) of the barn. Most fire departments respond to a fire with a large tanker carrying a minimum of 5,678 l (1,500 gal) of water; however, alternate water sources should be identified.

Identify ponds or canals within 300 m (1,000 ft) of the barn facility that have good, hard road surfaces leading to them (including up to the water's edge) that will support the weight of large fire trucks. If necessary, establish an agreement with the neighbor(s) to use their water supply (e.g., ponds, canals, or lakes) in case of emergency. If this is not feasible, install a *dry hydrant*:

this is a piping system leading into a large pond or lake available for fire department use. Another option is to purchase fire department float pumps that, when placed in a pond or lake, can supply up to 1,892 l (500 gal) of water per minute to a fire truck. Many facilities are installing aboveground water storage tanks with 3,785 l (1,000 gal) or higher capacities. When necessary, fire departments have used water from swimming pools. Swimming pools hold thousands of gallons of water, and fire trucks can draft or use a portable pump to remove water quickly.

If there is no water supply on site, flammable and combustible materials (e.g., hay, straw, bedding materials, cleaning supplies, etc.) should not be stored inside the barn.

RESCUE FROM A BURNING BARN

Humans First

The primary goal of responders is to ensure that human victims are identified, located, and removed from a burning structure. There may be human victims in living quarters in or above the barn; in the loft area; or inside the barn, attempting to rescue animals.

In some states, insurance is not available for barns with human living quarters above the horse stabling areas because of the significantly higher risk of fire. Dormitories, tack rooms, and other facilities used for sleeping purposes should be constructed of three-quarter-hour fire-resistant materials at a minimum and should comply with applicable provisions of NFPA Standard No. 101-1973, Life Safety Code.

Getting Animals Out Safely

Try to remain calm and alert. Think clearly, and act decisively. Notify the fire department through the 911 system dispatcher. The use of phones for the emergency call can create several problems. A call generated from a house phone (land line) to an E911 system (see Chapter 12) will not display the address of that caller's location, only the address to which the telephone bill is sent. If that house is a mile away from the barn, the firefighters will show up at the house. Using a cell phone only provides the dispatcher with the location of the cell tower to which the phone is communicating, which may be miles away from the actual emergency. The person giving directions to the dispatcher will be understandably upset and agitated. Hanging up or setting the phone down will further delay dispatch to the scene. To avoid these problems, correct address and directions to the barn can be typed on cards, inserted in a plastic holder, and tacked to the wall by the phone, making it easier and faster to give correct directions to the fire department dispatcher.

If the animals can be accessed from the outside wall of the barn, a rescue attempt is more likely to be successful. Personnel should not enter a burning building. The guilt associated with this decision can be devastating to any animal lover, but preserving human life must be the priority.

Firefighters are trained to evaluate the color and density of smoke to determine the burning conditions, but they never enter a burning structure without appropriate clothing, boots, and airway protection. Thick, black smoke tends to be produced by a lower-temperature fire, but also indicates a large area of burning inside the structure. In this instance, human safety concerns preclude any rescue attempts. Light gray or white smoke indicates an incomplete burn, which will benefit the attempted rescue of animals from the outside wall access points.

Another concern is the proximity of a water supply on scene. If there is not enough water to fight the fire, firefighters will not enter a burning structure. They will not attempt a rescue until enough water is available.

Personnel should begin to remove as many animals as possible from the immediate danger area from the outside wall access points, but should not attempt to rescue horses trapped in burning stalls. Rescue only those animals that can be safely reached. Prioritization of animals prior to a fire will allow the most valuable animals to be removed first. Remain aware of fire conditions, fire behavior, and the color of the smoke. Watch for sudden changes in wind direction or speed. A dramatic change in air temperature or humidity can cause smoke and ash or burning embers to drop around people; if this occurs, evacuate all personnel from near the structure.

The application of a blindfold is a last resort for horses that refuse to be led out of a stall in a burning building. A blindfold should be fastened in such a manner that it will fall off if the person leading the horse loses control of the animal (Figure 10.7). Inexperienced personnel should not attempt to lead animals that need to be blindfolded if there is an alternate option. If the panicked animal gets loose with the blindfold still in place, it will run in a straight line until it collides with a solid object or falls. The danger to people is obvious.

Firefighters recommend the removal of any clothing items (e.g., blankets, etc.) from animals rescued from barn fires. The animal should be hosed down from the tip of its nose to the tip of its tail. If synthetic halters or other items have melted onto the horse's skin, hose them, but allow the veterinarian to remove them. Ensure there is nothing on the animal that can burn, and consult a veterinarian for aftercare. For example, in a Midwest fire, 1 horse (of 13) survived with severe injuries that required over $30,000 in treatment (Figure 10.8). The other 2 horses rescued from the fire were covered with cinders that had fallen onto their hair

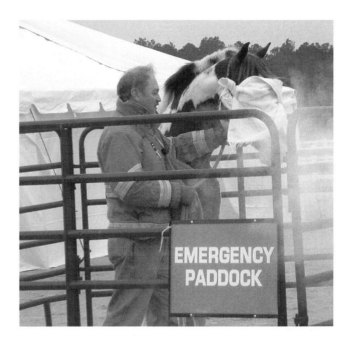

Figure 10.7 *An instructor demonstrates safe blindfold application on a horse frightened by fake smoke during a training event, tucking the ends of a towel under the edges of a halter. A blindfold is not necessary in most situations, and if applied, should be able to be quickly removed from the animal. Courtesy of Jeff Galloway.*

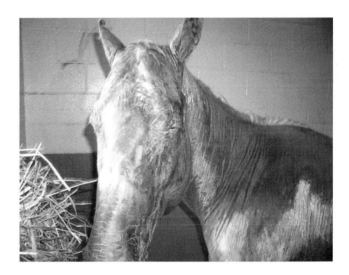

Figure 10.8 *This gelding was the only survivor of a barn fire in which most of the horses were removed from the barn, but were killed when they escaped restraint and ran back into the burning barn. At presentation to the veterinary clinic, the horse's skin and lungs were severely damaged. The horse was euthanized one year later due to squamous cell carcinoma of the burned skin. Courtesy of Nathan Slovis.*

coats, and no one realized how severely burned those horses were until later. The cinders smoldered under the hair surface and slowly spread. The horses were euthanized soon after the rescue due to the severity of their burns.

INCIDENT ANALYSIS

Some of the issues that make a large animal rescue a success or failure can be learned from a comparison of two actual incidents.

Scenario 1: At 3:15 am in Grapevine, Texas, someone driving past a barn stabling 80 horses observed smoke and called the fire department. No one was in the barn. Because this facility's owner had previously worked with their local fire department, responders knew how to locate and reach the facility. They were familiar with the basic layout, including the location of emergency paddocks. This barn used wood shavings in stalls, had an evacuation plan, and working fire extinguishers were available. Lead shanks and halters were kept by each horse's stall.

In this fire, 89% (71 of 80) horses survived—8 horses and one pony perished in the fire. The facility personnel and responders were able to rescue the remaining animals, and veterinary assistance arrived promptly.

Scenario 2: In Athens, Georgia, a fire started at 1:00 pm in a barn with 37 horses and six people present inside the barn. One person was smoking while another was handling flammable materials in the wash rack. Non-fire-retardant insulation was ignited, the fire spread into the roof insulation, and flashed over within four to six minutes. All six people ran out of the barn and opened every stall door as they left.

None of the horses left their stalls, and none were haltered and led out of the barn. The fire extinguishers in the barn were outdated, and two were nonfunctional. Obviously, there was not an enforced smoking policy. The facility had not practiced any evacuation or emergency reaction plans. These animals were standing in combustible bedding, eating combustible forage, next to combustible walls. Every dead animal found after the fire was against the outside wire wall. The bodies of the horses were burned by a fire so hot it essentially cremated the bodies; only the large abdominal organs were not consumed in the conflagration. Firefighters reported that if one touched the burned bones, they crumbled to powder. The fire was so hot that a trailer and truck parked over 25 m (82.5 ft) from the barn (with hay in the trailer) caught fire. The tires on the truck melted. In this barn fire, 35 of 37 horses died (94% mortality rate).

The primary reasons for the significant difference in survival rate between these two scenarios were proper planning and response. The first barn owner had established communication with the local fire department prior to any emergencies and had established an appropriate response plan (including a readily available halter and lead rope for each horse). In addition, personnel in the second scenario relied on the misconception that horses will run from burning barns; this was a costly mistake in this situation.

WILDFIRES

Animal owners living in areas subject to wildfires must have appropriate evacuation plans. Poor examples include owners leading horses down the street or interstate evacuation routes. The authors have seen a photograph of a person driving their car down the interstate, leading a horse from the window! This demonstrates the lengths to which people will go to attempt saving their animals and confirms that most people fail to plan ahead.

Some states have begun to address large animal rescue and evacuation more seriously. Some owners believe that horses turned loose will instinctively find shelter; this does not usually occur. The state of California now establishes veterinary triage points during wildfire disasters. Horse owners evacuate their own horses to a safe location and return to help other horse owners.

In 2006, over 10,000 large animals on pastures and ranges in the western United States were killed in wildfires. Evacuation of suburban and rural areas threatened by wildfires includes pets and large animals (Figure 10.9).

Large numbers of animals should be evacuated very early in wildfires (see Chapter 3). A significant amount of manpower and space is required to move these animals. Owners should consult emergency management and monitor the weather channels and the emergency broadcast system to determine the extent and direction of spread of the wildfire. Despite the over-

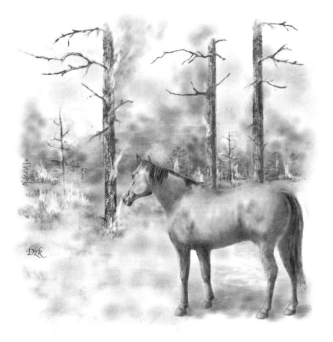

Figure 10.9 *Large animals facing wildfire scenarios have limited options available when trapped in pastures. Having an all-hazards evacuation plan is crucial to preventing losses. Courtesy of Michael Dzurak.*

whelming amount of information available on radio, television, and the Internet, each year people are unaware of the evacuation procedures and locations. Emergency managers should make these animal disaster resources known prior to the disaster whenever possible via mass communication and media releases.

Facility owners should not be stranded with their animals in danger zones under an enforced evacuation. Early evacuation avoids traffic delays, decreases travel time and allows for return trips to evacuate remaining animals. If the animals cannot be evacuated, the facility should have a shelter-in-place plan for the animals. Animals should not remain in barns during wildfires, but should instead be housed in a pasture with all combustible vegetation removed. Water and forage (e.g., grass or hay) should be provided, and each animal should be properly identified.

If trapped in a wildfire, the correct clothing can help shield humans and horses from radiant heat, burning embers, or flames. Cotton fabrics are preferable to synthetics, which will melt and cause serious burns. For humans, long pants, a long-sleeved shirt (with the sleeves rolled down), leather shoes, and goggles are advised. Sturdy leather gloves are necessary to protect hands from painful and disabling burns. Avoid synthetic (e.g., nylon or plastic) halters or lead ropes that may melt and cause serious burns to the horse or the handler. Never use nylon sheets, fly masks, or other synthetic tack or equipment during a fire. Very few items of horse clothing are fire retardant.

HORSE TRAILER AND TOWING VEHICLE FIRES

Fires in towing vehicles or trailers are difficult scenarios to address. Towing vehicle fires can be caused by overloading or poor maintenance of the vehicle. Trailer fires can be caused by poor maintenance, such as ill-maintained lubricant in wheel bearings. If the driver does not notice the sparks and fire, the tire can ignite. Sparks may be thrown into the trailer compartment, igniting hay and shavings inside the trailer. In one reported incident, a potbelly semi-trailer cattle truck was driven for more than 3 miles (4.9 km) with smoking tires and flying sparks before the driver noticed. The friction generated by the unlubricated bearings had caused so much heat that the aluminum of the trailer actually ignited, destroying the back portion of the trailer.

Other stock and horse trailer fires have been caused by the occupants of that vehicle, or a passerby in another vehicle, tossing a cigarette that lands inside the trailer. For example, a person was driving a truck towing three horses in a trailer on a New Jersey parkway. A discarded, smoldering cigarette butt landed in the front of the trailer and ignited the bedding on the floor of the trailer. The fire smoldered as the rig traveled at 100 kph (62 mph), and the smoke flowed forward into the tack compartment where dogs were housed. When the driver realized the trailer was on fire, he stopped the truck and opened the trailer doors to unload the horses. Two horses escaped and were running down the highway. Unfortunately, the four dogs were found dead. The horses ran down the parkway to the next toll booth, where personnel were able to catch them. None of the horses were injured (McKee, 2005).

Firefighters responding to trailer fire incidents protect themselves by wearing a protective, self-contained breathing apparatus (e.g., Air Pack). Any surviving animal in the trailer will be breathing toxic fumes. While one firefighting team is dedicated to fire suppression of the towing vehicle, another team unloads the horses from the trailer. This is the one scenario that breaks the cardinal rule of never unloading a horse from a trailer on the side of the road. Normally, horses are not to be unloaded beside roadways because of the chance that they might get away and run into traffic. When the horses are unloaded, it is best to lead them as far from the active traffic lanes as possible. Responders may need to cut the fence beside the interstate in order to lead the animals to a quiet place away from the highway.

ACRONYMS USED IN CHAPTER 10

AHJ	Authority having jurisdiction
NFC	National Fire Code
NFIRS	National Fire Incident Reporting System
NFPA	National Fire Protection Association
USFA	United States Fire Association

11 Ambulance and Recumbent Animal Transport

Dr. Rebecca Gimenez

INTRODUCTION

Pleasure riding, equestrian competitions, and other large animal-related activities (e.g., rodeos, shows, etc.) are associated with risk and can place considerable demands on both horse and rider in terms of fitness, skill, and concentration. When an equine injury occurs, recumbent or lame animals need to be removed safely from the incident site and receive prompt first aid. Dedicated and trained personnel work in support of the attending veterinary practitioner to deal with immediate equine or large animal emergencies and take injured animals to a safe place for treatment.

Large animals are difficult to move or transport when in sternal (on their chest) or lateral (on their side) recumbency. Their tendency to struggle in attempt to rise can lead to further injury to themselves and rescuers. Stressed cattle, llamas, and severely injured horses may refuse to stand and walk. Moving a recumbent animal may require numerous personnel to accomplish and can cause injury to the animal if not performed properly.

In certain situations, an animal may be unable to support itself on an extremity to walk or to stand in a trailer for transport to veterinary facilities. Alternatively, it may be exhibiting signs of neurological disease, shock, neglect, or other injuries that prevent normal transport. A method of preventing struggling and iatrogenic injury is to anesthetize the animal and transport it recumbent in a trailer. When correctly performed, this procedure can be safe and efficient.

CHALLENGES OF RECUMBENT LARGE ANIMALS

Early attempts to use low-wheeled tables, gates, stone boats, tarps, drag mats, or plywood for transport purposes proved impractical in the field environment, unprofessional in front of bystanders, or difficult for moving the animal long distances (Cooke, 2004). The use of a come-along to winch the strapped animal into a trailer for transport is slow and difficult and can be disturbing to the general public (Rasin, 2005).

Moving a recumbent large animal several kilometers or even 100 m (330 ft) to the closest access point of an ambulance trailer is difficult due to the weight of the animal and the friction generated; up to 14 people may be required to move the weight of one recumbent large animal (Gimenez and Gimenez, 2000). Dragging a large animal can incur injury to the animal's legs, neck, head and eyes, and creates safety concerns for the rescuers due to struggling and kicking by the animal. It can take 8–10 people to move a recumbent horse just 5 m (16 1/2 ft) even with proper equipment, especially if the animal must be pulled uphill and over soil, asphalt, gravel, or sand.

DETERMINE AN INCIDENT ACTION PLAN FOR RECUMBENT HORSES

The animal should be removed from the field environment on a field-expedient stretcher (e.g., tarp, stone plow or boat, sheet metal or plywood, gate, or transport sked) or a Rescue Glide sked and transported to a triage area or to a veterinary facility. The attending veterinarian will evaluate the animal and provide information regarding diagnostic procedures, treatment, and prognosis. If transportation to a veterinary facility is necessary, an ambulance or modified horse trailer can be used. If euthanasia is necessary, this method can also be used to move a large animal carcass for burial or disposal.

On a case-by-case basis, if they have the appropriate temperament, large animals may be encouraged to

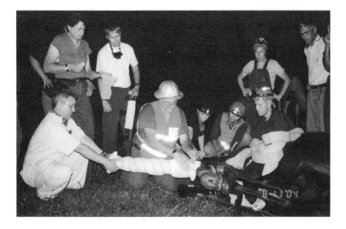

Figure 11.1 *Veterinarians and responders work to stabilize the leg of a simulated fracture patient as they apply a Robert Jones bandage in preparation for a full-limb Kimzey splint. The animal is sedated and secured to a Rescue Glide in preparation for transport. Courtesy Rebecca Gimenez.*

remain recumbent while recovering from certain diseases or injuries. The attending veterinarian will provide advice in each case. Recumbent animals are at high risk of decubital ulceration, muscle damage, gastrointestinal dysfunction, respiratory complications, nerve damage, and physiological stress. Many large animals are intolerant of prolonged recumbency and will struggle to rise, possibly injuring themselves and personnel.

Recumbent or injured animals should be evaluated and provided first aid immediately on the scene (see Chapter 17). The veterinarian may anesthetize the animal to induce recumbency and immobilization for packaging onto a sked. Extremity injuries can be stabilized with a Kimzey or field-expedient splint (Figure 11.1).

FIELD-EXPEDIENT SKEDS

The most commonly available equipment for use as a field-expedient sked is a tarp or sheet of plywood. Recumbent animals can be rolled or pulled onto the sked using webbing as an anchor for the haul, as described below.

Tarps can be folded to increase their tensile strength and thickness to protect the skin of the recumbent animal. Looping a Prusik hitch or other knot around the corners of the cloth creates handles and draws on the entire tarp during the haul. Polymer-coated tarps slide over the ground surface more easily; however, all tarps are subject to tearing and ripping when pulled over rough surfaces or obstacles.

Plywood sheeting or drag mats made of rubber materials reduce the chance of injury to the victim, but careful attention must be paid to the lip at the forward edge to prevent it from gouging into obstacles or dirt and stopping the forward motion of the sked. Handles

for the attachment of ropes may be pre-cut in the forward edge and sides of the sheet or mat to facilitate handling the equipment.

LIFTING OPTIONS

For animals accessible by vehicle, the use of a Monk's sling and Monk's Ambulance (a wheeled cart large enough to lift the animal) is possible. The animal is placed into the sling and the cart is rolled so that it is over the recumbent animal. The cart use mechanical advantage to lift the animal, and can be rolled to a safe location. This method is more commonly used for clinical cases that need minimally weight-bearing, ambulatory physical exercise during rehabilitation (Taglione, 2004).

A simple vertical lift system (e.g., figure eight sling, Becker sling, UC Davis–Large Animal Lift, etc.) using webbing around the horse and ropes to a dual overhead lift system is very effective for short-term (5–20 minutes) lifting of horses. However, the animal must be able to stand and walk away after the lift; if not, more elaborate long-term sling systems should be used (e.g., Anderson Sling, Switzerland sling, Liftex sling). These professional sling systems have been successfully used to support animals for months at a time; however, they represent a greater investment, and suspended patients require 24-hour monitoring and nursing care (see Chapter 16). In addition, moving the slung animal requires heavy-duty vertical lift equipment.

THE RESCUE GLIDE

The Rescue Glide was originally developed in 1995 by Chip Fischer and Roger Lauze of the Massachusetts Society for the Prevention of Cruelty to Animals (MSPCA) (Rasin, 2005). Virgin polypropylene sheets were used because they do not contain contaminating polymers that may compromise molding consistency and strength. Several manufacturers currently produce similar versions of this equipment using recycled plastic, which does not break under use (Blue Chip CDA Products, McCracken glide). The Rescue Glide provides a practical and efficient means of transporting recumbent, geriatric, and severely injured large animals on a plastic sked and requires minimally trained personnel to accomplish the task. The glide can be employed in response to backcountry trail accidents, trailer accidents, and structural collapse scenarios as well as clinical injuries.

Modified versions of the Rescue Glide are made of recycled high-density polyethylene or polypropylene polymer plastic (black or green, depending on the manufacturer), which does not crack or break under heavy use. The Care for Disabled Animals, Inc. product has more slip and may slide more readily over terrain.

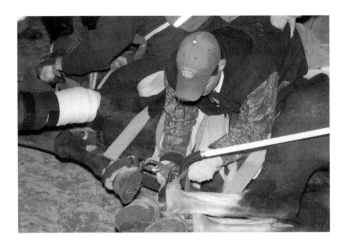

Figure 11.2 *Hobbles are attached to the animal victim's limbs. The handler should be positioned behind the animal's back, and the limbs of the animal patient should be drawn to the belly using a rope with a 2:1 pulley system. A rescuer uses a cane to assist the operational person with manipulation of the limbs. Courtesy Axel Gimenez.*

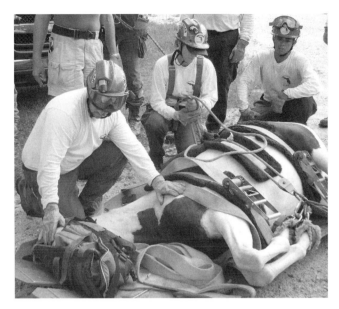

Figure 11.3 *A demonstration animal is packaged by students onto the Rescue Glide using ratchet straps to secure the animal on the sked. Note head protection and straps to hold the head down; hobbles are used to pull the animal's legs into a flexed fetal position. The protocol requires these efforts be made from behind the animal's back for rescuer safety. Courtesy of Tomas Gimenez.*

The 2.44 m × 1.44 m (8 × 5 ft) sheets of plastic feature specialty anchor points, ratchet tie-down anchor straps, and steel attachment points for winch loading into an ambulance trailer. The animal must be secured to the Rescue Glide with webbing or straps; once secured, the animal is considered "packaged" on the glide (Figure 11.2). Some instructors and professional responders prefer using 5 cm (2 in.) webbing to secure the animal onto the Rescue Glide (similar to a human patient on a backboard) because the ratchets are less reliable in rough terrain and more difficult to employ (Figure 11.3). In addition, the webbing is more easily cut and removed in an emergency (Fox, 2006). A crisscross pattern of the webbing over the animal's ribcage should be avoided because it restricts chest expansion and contributes to hypoventilation in the recumbent animal (Gimenez, 2006c).

In general, animals must be fully sedated or under short-duration intravenous anesthesia during transport on the Rescue Glide to prevent further injury to themselves or personnel. A veterinarian should be present on the scene to provide medical advice and monitor the animal's health. A conscious horse will not usually tolerate being tied down, and the use of additional personnel on the animal's neck to keep the animal from sliding off the Rescue Glide is associated with a high risk of injury. However, reports from the field indicate that this is an individual issue—some animals (e.g., geriatric, severely injured, or severely malnourished animals) have been shifted onto the glide and transported without physical or chemical restraint (Fox, 2006).

Any transport sked device should incorporate a capacity to attach the animal to the leading edge of the transport sheet or a backstop (2 m long × 5 cm diameter, or 6 1/2 ft long × 2 in. diameter, polyvinylchloride [PVC] pipe) to prevent the animal from sliding backward off the sked. Wet or sweaty animals will readily slide off the transport when being towed up a grade or trailer ramp. Providing friction surfaces on the top surface of the Rescue Glide reduces sliding; the placement of traction tape (stair tread tape) is a cost-effective method of increasing friction. Alternatively, bumpers can be placed on the upper glide surface behind the animal's hindquarters (Slusher, 2006).

Recumbent Animal Case Example

A veterinarian was called to examine a two-year-old filly found in lateral recumbency underneath a high-tensile wire fence. The filly had been trapped for up to four hours based on the observation history provided by the owner. An open, contaminated laceration with exposed bone was present on the lateral (outside surface) tarsus (hock) of the left hind limb and the left medial tibia. Joint, ligament, or tendon involvement could not be determined at that time due to severe contamination.

The horse was removed from underneath the fence with forward assist webbing, and the wound was rinsed while the exhausted horse remained recumbent without sedation. A modified Robert Jones bandage was applied; the horse rose to a standing position, but it could not support weight on the leg due to hyperflexion of the metatarsophalangeal (fetlock) joint as the result of extensor tendon damage. Based on the filly's level of exhaustion, it was determined that the horse could not support herself in a standing position for the two-hour trailer ride to the veterinary hospital. An equine ambulance was contacted.

General anesthesia was induced, and the horse was loaded onto a Rescue Glide in right lateral recumbency to avoid placing pressure on the injured left hind limb. The injured limb was not restrained. The glide and its load were pulled 60.6 m (200 ft) through a paddock by four people and pulled into the equine ambulance with a winch. A sedative was administered to the filly before departing, and real-time observation of the animal was provided via a closed-circuit camera system.

Upon arrival at the veterinary hospital, four people pulled the glide and horse out of the trailer and into an examination room. A splint was placed onto the leg while the horse was still secured to the glide. When straps were removed, the horse stood without assistance. The filly was treated and survived to become a successful broodmare.

Pros and Cons of Rescue Glide Skeds

Benefits of the Rescue Glide include reduction of the friction caused by the weight of the animal on the ground surface and a reduction in the number of personnel required to move the animal. Some manufactured products reduce friction more efficiently than others, easing the forces required to move the packaged patient (Fox, 2006). The resilient plastic is sufficiently flexible to allow it to move easily over obstacles such as logs, roots, or through ditches. The prow, or nose, of the glide is upturned to allow it to glide over obstacles, dirt, and sand. The Rescue Glide is sufficiently flexible that it curls up around the packaged animal's body, enabling it to move through a standard stall door or tight spaces as might be encountered on a trail. The Rescue Glide with its packaged patient may be attached to a winch, ropes pulled by human rescuers, or to a vehicle (e.g., all-terrain vehicle, car, etc.). The use of the glide prevents iatrogenic injury to the animal's face, skin, and eyes because the animal's entire body is on top of the plastic.

Personnel involved in placing and packaging an animal on a Rescue Glide must be properly trained to maximize safety while working around a recumbent, frightened, and injured animal. The animal must be properly secured to prevent it from struggling and rising while attached to the equipment, possibly injuring itself and/or rescuers in the process. The equipment is lightweight but large, and it must be stored flat. It has been stored in various locations in equine ambulances, including suspended from the roof or attached to the sidewalls of the ambulance. It is not recommended that the plastic skeds remain stored in full direct sun, as ultraviolet light will age the plastic and contribute to brittleness and loss of flexibility.

Practical Employment of Skeds

The Rescue Glide has been used on several occasions by paramedics for moving extremely obese human patients who do not fit on a traditional paramedic stretcher (Mayberry, 2005). It allows gentle packaging of the patient and transport using the openings as handles. As our society has grown to include morbidly obese patients, this is expected to become a common use of this piece of equipment and may represent an alternative justification for purchase by local jurisdictions.

The practical use of plastic skeds and field-expedient skeds has been demonstrated in numerous situations including severe limb injuries, neurological compromise, recumbency/inability to rise, severe neglect and malnutrition, and the recovery or removal of dead large animals. These skeds allow responders to improve their on-scene and pre-hospital care of animals in the field. The equipment is used at most race tracks and numerous equestrian events for transport of animals into ambulances. It has also been successfully employed in response to trail-riding accidents, pasture accidents, and trailer injuries.

Packaging Issues for Transport

Initial sedation or anesthesia of the animal when placed on the glide is usually necessary to facilitate the process of securing the animal to the sked. The animal's legs should be drawn close to its body in a fetal position; securing an animal in this position minimizes its ability to struggle. Once properly secured, many horses will remain immobile after the effects of sedation or anesthesia have worn off. Horses have been noted to be fully awake upon arrival at veterinary facilities, but did not attempt to move until unstrapped and allowed to stand up. Field rescue professionals report that individual animals seem to perceive that they are being helped, and after a short time, they may submit without struggle (Slusher, 2006). However, this should not be expected; due to their prey species' instincts, it is more likely that the animals will resist the restraint.

Veterinarians should be aware of the risk of cardiovascular shock, hyperthermia, and hypothermia when sedating or anesthetizing animals that will be secured in lateral recumbency for several hours. The animal's thermoregulative ability is compromised by sedation and anesthesia as well as by body position. Abdominal, thoracic, and pulmonary perfusion may also be impaired by alterations in blood pressure and distribution.

Radial, facial, or other nerve paralysis should be prevented with proper padding and positioning for transport. Radial nerve paralysis can severely compromise the animal's ability to rise and ambulate; an animal with radial nerve damage is unable to extend or bear weight on the limb without support. Severe radial nerve paralysis can be a life-threatening complication of recumbency. The risk of radial nerve paralysis is reduced by pulling the bottom limb forward so that the animal's elbow and shoulder are pulled further forward than the upper limb.

Facial nerve paralysis frequently results from halter pressure rostral (toward the nose) to or over the facial crest; affected horses exhibit a drooping lip and nose on the affected side. If minor damage is present, the condition will often resolve within 72 hours; if severe nerve damage occurs, the condition may resolve over several months or may be permanent. Proper halter placement and padding are recommended to prevent nerve damage.

Following prolonged recumbency and restraint on a Rescue Glide or field-expedient sked, geriatric or severely arthritic animals may experience difficulty rising to a standing position due to joint stiffness and discomfort. Assistance may be provided in the form of manual support or a sling to help the horse stand.

Moving the Packaged Patient

For manual transport of the patient, long ropes can be attached to the forward end of the Rescue Glide or field-expedient sked to allow personnel to pull the animal. Wrapping short Prusik loops along the length of the rope to be used as handles by rescuers is more efficient than them pulling directly on the rope.

To facilitate movement and reduce friction of the sked on surfaces, the sked can be slid over a "leap-frogged" sheet of plastic (the sheet is placed in front of the sked, the sked is pulled over the sheet, and the sheet is again placed in front of the sked; this process is repeated as necessary). Certain surfaces (e.g., wet grass, pine straw) are more slick and easily navigated than others (e.g., dry asphalt, sand, rock, dry grass). Alternatively, straw or hay can be distributed in front of the sked to make a path and lessen the resistance.

Coordination of the haul team of responders should be emphasized especially along trails or around corners to minimize further trauma to the packaged patient. This is an excellent opportunity to use bystanders and excess personnel if available. A rope assembly attached to the rear of the sked can be used as a rudder to control the sked's lateral movement while most of the haul team members are placed in front of the sked to provide pulling power. A scout may be used to determine a safe path in front of the haul team. One team member should support any injured extremity.

Many professionals recommend the purchase of a strong portable winch, which may be used in various configurations, (e.g., hand carried, hooked at either end of a vehicle or other anchor point). These winches can be powered by 12 V car power outlets or cigarette lighters, or 12 V auto batteries or (with a converter) household electrical outlet. These winches have a variety of applications in technical large animal emergency rescue (TLAER) efforts, including pulling recumbent animals from barns, ditches, trails, ravines, down slopes, etc. In addition, these winches have many

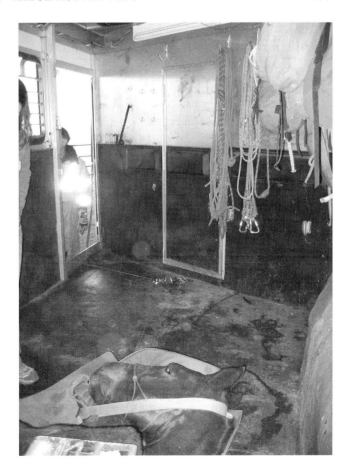

Figure 11.4 *A portable winch is attached outside the door of the equine ambulance, and pulley blocks with rescue pulleys allow the packaged patient and sked to be pulled into the ambulance. This configuration minimizes the danger of winch cable failure and injury of the patient or personnel. Courtesy of Nicole Walukewicz.*

useful non-animal-rescue applications, such as pulling an ambulance vehicle from mud or snow.

Rescue pulleys and pulley blocks (see also Chapter 14) are useful when winching or pulling packaged or dead animals around corners or out of constricted spaces (such as stalls) (Slusher, 2006). The author recommends the use of a pulley block to redirect the winch cable (Figure 11.4) inside the equine ambulance for safety reasons; this allows personnel to remain outside the large animal ambulance while efficiently winching the victim up the ramp and inside the compartment.

STANDARD OPERATING PROCEDURES FOR LOADING THE RESCUE GLIDE SKED

Equipment

There are certain pieces of equipment needed when loading the Rescue Glide.

- Two sections of webbing, 7 cm × 8 m (3 in. × 26 1/4 ft), for sliding the horse onto glide

- Two 7 cm (3 in.) ratchet straps
- Plastic Rescue Glide-type sked
- One 2 m (6 1/2 ft) long section of 5 cm (2 in.) webbing with heavy duty hook-and-loop (Velcro) fasteners
- Hobble rope, 5 m (16 ft), with a simple pulley and carabiner
- Four fleece-lined leg hobbles with two Prusik loops (see Chapter 14) and two carabiners
- Six fleece harness pads for placement between the skin and the hobbles, ropes, and webbing
- Head protection (this could also be a personal floatation device [PFD], towel, shirt, or saddle pad)
- Leg cane for handling and manipulation of the animal's legs from a safe distance

Personnel

The following personnel are needed when loading a Rescue Glide.

- Incident commander
- Animal handler (may be one of the operational personnel)
- Operational personnel (minimum of two)
- Safety officer (may also serve as animal handler or operational personnel)

Protocol for Securing a Large Animal to the Rescue Glide

The procedure requires approximately seven minutes with three trained personnel. Personnel should remain a safe distance from the animal's legs at all times, even if the animal is sedated. The person(s) securing the animal to the Rescue Glide must always have a safety buddy, a team member responsible for monitoring the person and animal and capable of pulling the person away from danger. Animals should normally be fully sedated or anesthetized for this procedure to reduce the chance of injury to personnel, but sedation or anesthesia should only be performed under the supervision of a veterinarian. A similar protocol can be applied when employing a field-expedient sked.

1. Place head protection (e.g., towel, shirt, PFD, or commercially available equine head protector) on animal's head, and pad underneath the head. Special attention should be paid to covering the eyes and preventing facial nerve paralysis by avoiding direct pressure on the animal's facial crest.

2. Using a "flossing" motion, slide the 8 m sections of nylon webbing underneath the animal to anchor points behind the front legs and in front of the hind legs (Figure 11.5). Using the cane, grasp and pass the webbing back over the ribcage so that both ends of the strap are dorsal (above or behind the animal's spine) to the animal. This provides a superior anchor point to help shift the animal onto the glide (see Chapter 15).

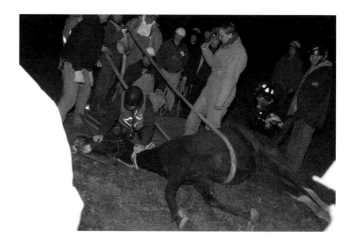

Figure 11.5 *Webbing is flossed under a recumbent horse to use as an anchor point for shifting the animal onto the Rescue Glide without rolling the animal. Note all personnel are approaching the animal from its dorsal side, staying away from the limbs. Courtesy Axel Gimenez.*

3. Place the glide directly behind the dorsal (back) surface of the animal, taking care not to let people slip on its slick surface.

4. Pull the animal onto the glide using the nylon web anchors (placed in step 2), the tail, and the mane (when available). A team member must be designated to support and move the animal's head and neck. If necessary and authorized by the on-scene veterinarian, the animal can be rolled over onto the glide while controlling the head and any injured extremities. The front legs must not obstruct the anchor openings on the glide; the anchor webbing placed around the animal's body can be used to adjust the animal's position on the glide. *Note:* Coordinate moving or rolling the animal so that any injured extremity is on the top (upper or nondependent) side of the animal for optimal perfusion and access for treatment.

5. The animal handler must keep control of the animal's head at all times, even when the animal is sedated. Placing a knee over the center of the animal's neck (avoiding the jugular furrow) and tipping the animal's nose upward (away from the ground) decreases the chance that it will stand up during the procedure. This person can monitor the animal's eyes and reflexes, respiratory rate, pulse strength and rate, and capillary refill time. An EMT, paramedic, or veterinary technician is optimally suited for this task.

6. Place one of the ratchet straps over the ribcage at the point of the withers and behind the shoulder of the front legs, and secure both ends of the strap to the glide (see Figure 11.3; Figure 11.6). The anchor must curl around the outer edge of the plastic glide and fit into the opening from the underside to prevent loss of the anchor. Apply tension on the strap until the edges of the glide start to lift. Fleece pads should be placed between the animal's body and the strap to protect its skin from the strap and ratchet.

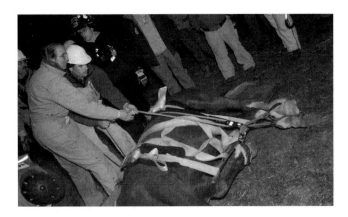

Figure 11.6 *Recumbent animals, even when anesthetized, should be handled from behind the animal's back to minimize the risk of being kicked. This rescuer is attaching the tie-down straps to the Rescue Glide. Notice the safety buddy holding onto the rescuer's belt for safety. Another rescuer is monitoring and stabilizing the animal's protected head and is in position to relay information regarding the animal's vital signs to the veterinarian. Courtesy of Axel Gimenez.*

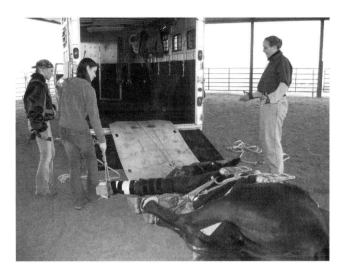

Figure 11.7 *A demonstration horse is packaged on the Rescue Glide attached to a portable winch for loading up the ramp of a type I equine ambulance. Note the injured, splinted leg is individually supported by a person. A slick sheet of plastic is placed on the ramp to facilitate this process. Courtesy of Nicole Walukewicz.*

If using 2 in. webbing to strap the animal to the glide, use a crisscross pattern from the openings to front then the back, followed by crossing over the front and the rear of the animal. The webbing must be tightened to the point that the plastic of the glide slightly curls up around the animal. This crisscross pattern, however, has been found to limit chest expansion, reducing the amount of air that enters the lungs and decreasing ventilation (Gimenez, 2006c).

7. Place a second ratchet strap over the posterior abdomen (flank) in front of the hind legs in the same manner (step 6). Apply tension on the strap until the plastic of the glide lifts slightly at the edges. *Note:* Tension on all straps should be reassessed several times during packaging and transport to ensure that they are sufficiently tight to secure the animal's position, but do not prevent chest expansion.

8. Attach one of the four hobbles to the pastern region of each limb. It is safest to attach hobbles by keeping the rescuer's body behind the animal's back and reaching over the body to work on the legs. This is the most dangerous and difficult part of the packaging process. A rope should be tied to this team member's belt during this process so that the safety buddy can pull him or her quickly away from the animal if necessary. This is less imperative if general anesthesia is used and maintained, but caution is always advised when working around large animals.

9. Using the carabiner attached to the Prusik loop, connect the bottom front leg and bottom back leg hobbles to each other. Connect the top (uppermost) front leg and top (uppermost) back leg hobbles together. *Note:* Do not connect hobbles to an injured extremity; a rope may be tied to the Prusik loop on the hobble for control of the injured extremity by a person during movement of the animal.

10. Tie one end of the hobble rope (with the pulley and carabiner) to the same opening where the front ratchet is attached to the glide.

11. Connect the carabiner to the Prusik loops on the hobbles.

12. Slide the free end of the hobble rope through the same anchor opening where the other end is tied to the glide. Place a fleece pad under the rope over the horse's chest.

13. Pull the free end of the rope through the pulley and flex all four legs to bring them as close as possible to the body into a fetal position. *Note:* Horses have an anatomical feature, called a stay apparatus, that allows them to keep their hind limbs extended (straight) without active muscle contraction—this mechanism allows the horse to sleep while standing. This apparatus effectively locks the animal's stifle in an extended position and prevents the hind limb from being flexed (bent), and it may hinder packaging on a sked. The animal handler or veterinarian may need to manipulate the horse's limb to disengage the stay apparatus. This can often be performed by swinging the limb back (behind the animal), flexing (bending) the fetlock, and applying gentle pressure toward the horse's body.

14. Tie the free end of the hobble rope to the glide to maintain the legs (bent) in the fetal position.

15. Pull the head strap from the underside of the glide through the front slit openings. Secure the head to the glide with the hook-and-loop (Velcro) strap closures.

16. The horse is packaged and ready to be moved. The straps should be regularly reevaluated for proper tension during and after movement across terrain or into an equine ambulance. Any splinted extremity

should be individually monitored to prevent it from becoming caught on obstacles (Figure 11.7).

17. At this time, electrocardiograph electrodes, a blood pressure cuff, pulse oximetry sensors, thermometer, and/or other patient monitoring equipment may be attached to the animal. Intravenous (IV) catheterization and fluid administration can be performed and maintained during packaging and transport. *Note:* Do not allow personnel to remain in the ambulance trailer with horses, regardless of the animal's position (e.g., standing, recumbent, or secured to the Rescue Glide). The animal should be monitored using a wireless camera system or by personnel in a separate compartment of the ambulance.

AMBULANCES FOR LARGE ANIMAL RESCUE

Recent developments and improvement in transportation of recumbent horses have had a profound impact on the equine insurance industry. Before these options became available and widely used, euthanasia was commonly performed on severely injured and recumbent animals.

An incident at the 2006 Preakness Stakes (Pimlico, Maryland) brought public attention to the issue of emergency transport of severely injured racehorses. The odds-favored entry, Barbaro, sustained severe fractures to his left hind limb in the early phase of the race. The stallion was transported three hours in an equine ambulance, under police and helicopter media escort, to undergo cutting-edge surgical repair to save his life. Although the horse was euthanized eight months after surgery due to severe complications, the case elevated public knowledge of equine rescue techniques and veterinary medicine.

A History of Equine Ambulance Transport

In the beginning (1868–1940), most horse ambulances were powered by a two horse "engine:" two horses were hitched to the ambulance (Figure 11.8). At that time, most equine ambulances were owned by humane organizations (e.g., Royal Society for Prevention of Cruelty to Animals, American Society for the Prevention of Cruelty to Animals [ASPCA], MSPCA, etc.) that concentrated on loading and transporting injured or overworked carriage horses on the streets of large cities.

Later, some of the first horse trailers were pulled by early vehicles for this purpose. In 1914 the MSPCA used what was probably one of the first gooseneck ambulance trailers towed by a truck. To this day, MSPCA maintains a fleet of ambulances for use at show grounds and large competition events around the United States.

Most modern equine ambulances are horse trailers (minimum two-horse capacity) or stock trailers (8 ft, or 2.4 m, wide and a minimum of 7 ft, or 2.1 m, tall) with

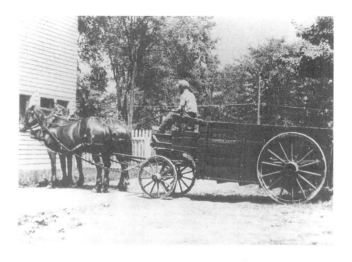

Figure 11.8 *This MSPCA equine ambulance (circa 1900) features a two-horsepower "engine" to transport equine and large animal patients for veterinary care in Boston, Massachusetts. Courtesy of MSPCA.*

removable dividers. They are outfitted with ramps or hydraulic floors to facilitate loading an injured animal or sliding animals strapped to a sked-type stretcher inside the compartment. The sked method is simple and efficient, and experienced teams can package and load an injured horse for transport in minutes.

In 1977, the Southern California Equine Foundation (SCEF) initiated a three-year development plan for an equine ambulance. Under the direction of Dr. Roy Dillon, the ambulance was specially designed for the equine athlete and cost approximately, $35,000. In association with Mr. John Kimzey, the SCEF introduced the present-day sophisticated model in 1981; the improved ambulance cost approximately $72,000, and included a tractor to haul it from track to track. A third unit was purchased in 1999, allowing the SCEF to maintain two ambulances on, and one off, racetracks. The SCEF also provides an ambulance for contingency use at the Rose Bowl parade (SCEF, 2006). The Kimzey-designed ambulance floor can be completely lowered to ground level, allowing maximum ease in loading, and incorporates a hydraulic "squeeze" apparatus to support an injured, standing horse. A winch-driven stretcher facilitates loading a recumbent animal. The unit can accommodate two standing animals.

As of publication, there are 25 of these ambulances in use across the United States. A Kimzey-designed equine ambulance was used at the Pimlico racetrack during the 2006 Preakness Stakes to rush injured favorite Barbaro to a veterinary facility three hours away. National media coverage of the event raised public awareness of the existence of this type of life-saving transportation and demonstrated the strength of the human-animal bond (Brown, 2008).

When a horse is seriously injured during competition, initial treatment and stabilization often must be performed on site, under unusual conditions, and in full view of spectators. Recognizing the sensitivity of the situation, founders of Humane Equine Aid and Rapid Transport (H.E.A.R.T.) constructed an ambulance for efficient removal of incapacitated horses from competition courses in the early 1990s. Their equine ambulances, equipped with a Rescue Glide sked, served at the 1996 Olympics in Atlanta, Georgia, and at numerous large competitions since. The show veterinarian provides treatment on site as the ambulance arrives, and ongoing first aid may be administered as the horse is transported to a facility for additional medical treatment.

By 1997, the Marion duPont Scott Equine Medical Center in Leesburg, Virginia, acquired an ambulance to provide emergency transport from incident scenes to treatment facilities. By 1998, the ambulance was present at steeplechase and point-to-point races. The custom-designed trailer is equipped with a winch that powers a sked, sling, and hoist assembly to load incapacitated animals.

In the past, ambulance owners experimented with placing an injured animal in an Anderson Sling and bringing it inside the ambulance using a rolling frame, winch system, or hydraulic overhead boom. Although these systems provided adequate support for the animal victims, difficulties were encountered in implementation. The load is subject to sway or swinging during transport, and a significant amount of overhead room was required to lift the entire animal in the sling. The system also requires a specifically built trailer that may be cost-prohibitive for many organizations or communities.

Type 1 Ambulances

Type 1 ambulances allow standing animals or recumbent, sked-packaged animals to be loaded and transported. This method has significant advantages in that it does not require as much expensive equipment (i.e., frame, lifting mechanism) as a type 2 ambulance; it is associated with less load shift and swing during loading and transport; and it does not require a custom-built trailer or vehicle. Another benefit is that this type of ambulance can be used as a horse trailer in a disaster or evacuation. With minimal changes to the layout of the ambulance compartment, it can be used to evacuate uninjured animals or to transport hay and supplies to a disaster area.

Any stock-type trailer with a ramp can be used to transport a packaged patient in a type 1 ambulance. The ramp greatly facilitates loading of the animal into the trailer. If the trailer does not have a ramp, a ramp can easily be constructed with on-site materials (i.e., plywood boards and a shovel) to allow winching or pulling of the animal into the compartment. Innovative ambulances designed by John Kimzey of Woodland, California, and Dr. Nathan Slovis and Latonna

Wilson of the Hagyard Medical Institute in Lexington, Kentucky, use a hydraulic floor that can be lowered to ground level for loading and raised for transport.

The type 1 ambulance is by far the most common type of large animal ambulance, used by large, full-service veterinary clinics, race tracks, large equine show facilities, three-day eventing competitions, steeplechases, rodeos, and other competitive events across the United States and other countries. Type 1 ambulances, based on observation of numerous examples, should share the following characteristics.

- Minimum of 2.29 m (7 1/2 ft) and preferably 2.44 m (8 ft) wide at floor level.
- Minimum of 3.66 m (12 ft) and preferably 4.57 m (15 ft) long at the floor of the ambulance for the body of the animal. The ambulance must be able to accommodate large animals averaging 15–16 hands (1 hand equals 4 in., or 10 cm) in height and 544–1,000 kg (1,200–2,200 lb) in weight. Additional room to accommodate splinted extremities is recommended.
- Minimum of 2.13 m (7 ft) and preferably 2.29 m (7 1/2 ft) height inside the trailer.
- Reflective tape or paint on the front, sides, and rear of the ambulance to prevent secondary accidents while responding to roadside emergencies. The truck and trailer should have an identification logo and amber emergency strobe lights for roadside safety. (Strobe lights may not be legal in all jurisdictions.)

Anatomy of a Typical Type 1 Large Animal Ambulance

- Overhead space (or space on interior side walls of trailer) to transport a plastic sked when not in use
- Overhead hooks for hanging IV fluid bags during transport
- Tarps or screens to allow privacy as the animal is triaged, treated, and packaged for transport
- Hooks for hanging rope bags, equipment, and personal protective equipment
- Hooks for hanging rescue webbing, rope, and equipment in bags (all bags should be clearly labeled with their contents)
- Removable dividers for separation of animals during transport or evacuation of normal standing animals (these dividers can hang on the interior or exterior side walls when not in use)
- Lightweight, portable corral panels or portable fencing
- Storage for generators, spare tires, electrical service and water source (Figure 11.9)

Type 2 Ambulances

Type 2 ambulances load and transport animals in standing position in slings. Due to the additional amount of vertical clearance required over an animal in a sling, the ambulance must be specially built with

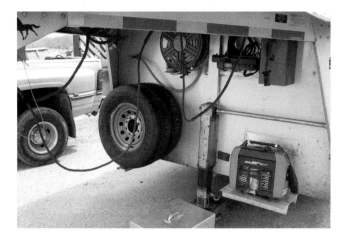

Figure 11.9 *The front of a type 1 ambulance trailer showing storage for two spare tires, electrical service (top right box), small portable generator (bottom right box), hose for water with pump and 150 l (40 gal) water tank located inside living quarters). Courtesy of Axel Gimenez.*

excess overhead height. In addition, there must be a movable frame in which to hoist the slung animal or a boom with hoisting capability extending beyond the trailer to lift the animal.

The type 2 method is excellent for transporting an animal that is unable to stand on its own but that should not be transported in recumbency due to medical concerns. An example of a type 2 ambulance includes the Moore County Ambulance, North Carolina, designed and built by Dr. Jim Hamilton and Neva Scheve of Equi-Spirit Trailers.

Equine Ambulance Business Considerations

Administrative codes in most states with horse racing boards include rules that racetrack operators must have a horse ambulance available. For example, Section 1305.110 of the Administrative Code of the Illinois Racing Board states.

> There shall be a horse ambulance at all race tracks under the jurisdiction of the Board for the safe and expedient removal of crippled animals from the track. Horse ambulances must be equipped with a screen for use when an animal must be destroyed in view of the general public, a winch to lift dead or injured animals on to the ambulance, and a removable floor or other satisfactory device for the safe loading of a recumbent horse. Said ambulance shall also be equipped with a permanently attached and locked box containing drugs solely for the use of the state veterinarians when emergency medication is required.
>
> (Amended February 15, 1974; filed February 28, 1974)

For these reasons, most racetracks have dedicated ambulances or contract for dedicated use of a private ambulance.

Horse ambulances may be minimally to fully outfitted with first aid kits, veterinary drugs and IV fluids, slings, winches, drag mats, and TLAER field equipment. The equipment required depends on the intended uses of the ambulance: private and/or public events and emergencies, emergency medical response, disaster response, neglect/starvation/abuse rescue response, or a combination of the above. Consideration should be given as to the availability of the ambulance (e.g., 24 hours and seven days a week, nights only), including coverage during vacation and holidays. Determining and clearly stating the mission of the ambulance service will prevent miscommunication within the community as to the availability of services and response.

Professionals relate that many equine patients retrieved from farms were frequently troublesome, time-consuming loaders. This can result in long delays, and some animals cannot be loaded within a reasonable amount of time. From a financial perspective, the costs of fuel, loss of income from other clients, vehicle use, and personnel time can be high; if the animal cannot be loaded, these expenses are rarely reimbursed. When transporting uninjured or minimally injured animal patients for routine or emergency care, it is recommended to inquire how well the patient loads on a trailer. It is advised to formulate a standard policy that includes a statement similar to the following: "Our policy is that, on arrival, we will spend 20 minutes of reasonable and prudent effort to load your horse, and if it refuses, or if we deem it unsafe to continue attempting to load the animal, we will retire, but we will still bill you for the one-way ambulance fee." (Slusher, 2006)

Financial and Legal Considerations

Before any ambulance can begin service, the legal and financial considerations must be addressed.

Profit or NonProfit? There are nonprofit (e.g., Blue Cross, H.E.A.R.T., MSPCA) and for-profit companies that travel to large equine-related events as a paid service to the event management. Several of these ambulance services are owned by equine veterinarians or veterinary hospitals, especially in areas with large concentrations of equestrians and equine activities. For example, the Hagyard Medical Institute uses their equine ambulance for private emergency response, private emergency medical response, and neglect/abuse rescue response, as well as for public horse sport event services. They report an excellent public response to their rescue work (Wilson, 2006).

To provide a professional and reliable service at competitive rates, many ambulance owners or services maintain the ambulance and paid staff ringside for the duration of the event, sometimes for days, weeks, or months (e.g., Rolex Kentucky 3-Day Event, in Lexington, Kentucky; horse shows in Wellington, Florida; Horseshows In The Sun, in Arizona, California, Florida, Nevada, New York, and Virginia). The MSPCA currently maintains a fleet of three equine ambulances (Cooke, 2004).

Some ambulance services respond only to emergencies within a specific area (e.g., Moore County Equine Emergency Response Unit, Moore County, North Carolina; Winston Salem Rescue Squad, Winston-Salem, North Carolina; UC-Davis Veterinary Emergency Response Team, Davis, California; Aiken County Public Safety, Aiken, South Carolina). Other ambulances are provided by veterinary schools or full-service clinical facilities, and the ambulance is specialized to provide service to their clients (e.g., Virginia-Maryland Regional College of Veterinary Medicine's Marion duPont Scott Equine Medical Center, Middleburg, Virginia; Hagyard Equine Medical Institute, Lexington, Kentucky). Privately or government-owned ambulances may contract with owners or veterinarians on an individual basis to move recumbent animals or transport animals impounded due to neglect, starvation, and abuse (e.g., Department of Agriculture, Equine Division, Georgia; Equine Outreach, Inc., Bend, Oregon).

Funding for an animal ambulance service is commonly addressed by several means. Solicitations for donations to the ambulance service are commonly used (e.g., Days End Horse Farm Rescue, H.E.A.R.T.) by 501(c)3 nonprofit organizations. An invoice is commonly provided to the animal owner following a response effort; the invoice provides an itemized list of costs incurred during the response and transportation efforts and suggests an amount for donation. Many animal owners are unaware of the costs to purchase and maintain equipment, train personnel, and conduct an ambulance service. The itemized costs shown on the suggested donation invoice educate the owner about the investment of time, equipment, and training required to provide the ambulance service. However, if the invoice is provided as a suggested donation, the owner may be under no obligation to donate money.

Numerous organizations have resorted to the use of actual invoices for their services, charging standard amounts for the response effort, staff time, equipment, and roundtrip mileage. Some units include specific items in their initial response fee, including the staff present, equipment usage, and a specified amount of time after which the fee is charged on a per hour basis. Several ambulance services accept payment in the form of cash, check, or credit card.

If an ambulance service cannot become financially viable, it will not remain available. As a professional service, it deserves a professional fee. Standard call-out fees in many areas of the country are $300–$500, and $0.65–$1.50 (minimum) per 2.2 km (1 mile) is also charged. Fees for providing standby ambulance services at equine events range from $200 to $1,000 per day, and animal owners are charged separately for services provided.

Legal Issues. Legal concerns for large animal ambulance services vary by state and are beyond the scope of this book. Persons considering establishing an ambulance service or purchasing equipment for an ambulance are encouraged to consult with an attorney and with current organizations providing ambulance services for advice concerning liability releases, training requirements, signage and emergency running lights, equipment requirements, and improvements in pre-hospital care for animals. Many of the injured animals transported from sporting events will be insured, and a method for contacting the owner and insurance company will be necessary.

ACRONYMS USED IN CHAPTER 11

H.E.A.R.T.	Humane Equine Aid and Rapid Transport
IV	Intravenous
MSPCA	Massachusetts Society for the Prevention of Cruelty to Animals
PFD	Personal Flotation Device
SCEF	Southern California Equine Foundation
SOP	Standard Operating Procedure
TLAER	Technical Large Animal Emergency Rescue

12 Communications in Veterinary Field Operations

Dr. Kathleen Becker and Tori Miller

INTRODUCTION

Successful mitigation of large animal emergencies and disasters requires a coordinated response from multiple agencies and individuals. This process begins with a complete understanding of the problem, followed by coordination with the dispatcher at the call center, and continues throughout the deployment of appropriate rescue equipment and trained personnel.

Coordination can be enhanced or hindered by the quality of the communications network as well as the communicators (people making the calls). There are four basic types of communication: between the public and emergency services, between the individual emergency service units, between emergency units and other agencies, and within emergency services under emergency and nonemergency conditions. Most large animal and other specialty rescue efforts would not be possible without initial communication with an emergency 911 dispatch system.

There are numerous communication options available for rescue teams and other organizations involved in large animal emergency or disaster response. Selection of equipment should be made only after a detailed plan is drafted regarding the specific objectives and mission established by the team. Redundancy is critical in order to provide backup systems if one system fails due to an unforeseen event. The systems should be regularly tested and evaluated. Logistics planning should include sufficient backup supplies of batteries for all equipment.

The development of an effective, coordinated, and cost-efficient communication system is not a trivial matter. For this reason, communications should always be one of the highest priorities within any organization, and this chapter will explore communication options as well as the communicator(s) involved with the 911 call.

PLANNING COMMUNICATION SYSTEMS

The communications plan should be prepared as a basic outline that can be expanded after considering many factors, such as the type of information to be transmitted, the distance between individuals, the local terrain; and the availability of existing service(s). The plan must have flexibility to accommodate the communications needs of small emergencies as well as large-scale disasters.

Establishing successful communication systems is relatively simple if planners use the P.A.C.E. (primary, alternate, contingency, and emergency plan) to develop methods of communication with all involved parties. Dwight D. Eisenhower once said, "Plans are nothing, planning is everything." If possible, maps detailing the local jurisdiction's obstacles, elevations, and key terrain features should be stored in a readily accessible manner.

Model Systems

When a rescue/disaster response team is deployed to a disaster, the team establishes a base of operations. The location of this base and its proximity to the command post will vary with the situation (Figure 12.1). The modes of communication at the base should include the following:

- Access to the standard telephone system (e.g., landline, cell phone, or satellite phone)
- Internet access
- Fax capability (including the ability to copy or scan documents)
- Very high frequency (VHF)/ultra high frequency (UHF) simplex and/or repeater radios for the intrateam network

Other forms of communication that are recommended but not always available include television and

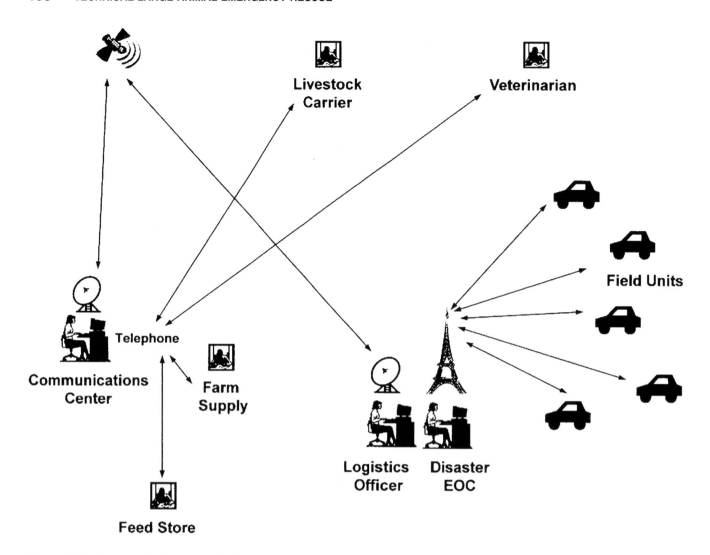

Figure 12.1 *An example of a communications plan for a local TLAER emergency. Communications links between the emergency operations center, 911 communications center, and specialty assets (e.g., veterinarian, animal handlers, alternate livestock transportation, feed store, etc.) can be accomplished by a variety of equipment, including satellite phones, radios, and telephones (mobile and landline). Courtesy of Kathleen Becker.*

radio media access and amateur radio capability, in order to communicate with local and distant resources.

Field assessment teams require fewer forms of communication because their primary line of communication is between the team and the base of operations. Recommended communications capabilities for the field teams include the following:

- VHF/UHF simplex and/or repeater radios
- Internet capability for rapid data transmission
- Standard telephone (e.g., cell phone or satellite phone) for use when the VHF/UHF repeater radios are not functioning or available.

Selection of Equipment

The selection and purchase of specific equipment represents the final step in the planning stage and should

not be performed without first developing a comprehensive communications plan.

A lack of understanding of the strengths and limitations of different systems can result in the acquisition of equipment that is inappropriate for the needs and mission of the team. High-technology equipment is not always the optimal choice. Personnel assigned to make purchasing decisions are encouraged to test the equipment; ideally, the vendor should be willing to demonstrate the equipment during a training exercise.

Determine Requirements Based on the Incident Command System

The first consideration when determining a plan is to decide who needs to communicate and why. This is affected by the situation; therefore, flexibility is necessary. It would be inappropriate, for example, for every soldier to maintain a direct line of communication with the Army Chief of Staff. In contrast, it is imperative for a small rescue squad performing a difficult high angle rescue of a horse over a 300 ft cliff to have immediate and simultaneous communication capabilities between all team members for the sake of coordination as well as safety.

To continue with this second example, safety could be compromised if the same radio channel being used by the rescue squad was also shared with the police department performing routine traffic control nearby. Lines of communication should follow and support the existing lines of incident command. Any emergency response unit, rescue squad, or disaster team formulating a large animal incident communications plan should already have a well-documented command and organizational flow chart in place.

Determine Capabilities Needed for Links

Each link on the command flowchart represents a communications link. Those links can be simple (e.g., direct verbal communication between two team members) or complicated (e.g., a disaster field hospital transmitting encrypted patient medical records to an emergency operations center located hundreds of miles outside of the disaster zone). Each communications link should be analyzed separately to determine what type of information needs to be transferred.

There are many factors that affect these links, these include but are not limited to the following:

- Area of coverage
- Local terrain
- Preexisting service
- Electrical requirements
- Battery requirements for initial setup
- Licensing
- Individual or group coverage
- Economic factors

For example, cell phone communication is a commonly available means of communication. However, the reliability of reception varies with the terrain and the proximity of transmitting towers. In a disaster situation, the towers may be damaged or not functioning. In addition, wireless networks are frequently overwhelmed in the time period surrounding a disaster. Prioritizing calls, preventing nonemergency use, and installing mobile antennas increase the function of cellular phone service and should be considered when designing the communications plan.

The ICS arose from the critical need for increased safety for fire and rescue teams. Much of this safety factor is leveraged by excellent, reliable communications capabilities. Highly reliable and rapid means of communication are imperative in potentially dangerous field environments. The emergency response plan is based on many factors, including the presence of hazardous materials (e.g., fuel containers, ammunition, fireworks, etc.), challenges associated with the local terrain, weather conditions, the presence of the animal's owner or bystanders, and traffic flow.

RESOURCES FOR DISPATCHERS

Dispatchers at the 911 call center have numerous valuable resources available, including telephone books; Internet access; computer files; and lists of personnel with specialized tools, training, or equipment. Emergency responders rely on the dispatchers to provide information and resources not readily accessible on the scene. Local technical large animal emergency rescue (TLAER) teams, state animal response teams (SARTs), and county animal response teams (CARTs) should provide their point of contact and special information to the local dispatch office for the most effective response.

Large Animal Incident Resources

The communications center should have contact information for veterinarians (large and small animal practitioners), experienced animal handlers, haulers/transporters, overnight housing facilities, and personnel trained in special rescue (such as TLAER). Contact information for sources of four-wheel drive vehicles, all-terrain vehicles, livestock panels, and watercraft should also be readily available. For example, responders may need to locate a set of corral panels at 2 am when a cattle trailer has overturned on an interstate. Similarly, responders may need to contact an experienced ostrich handler to capture a loose ostrich. A thorough and up-to-date list of resources can save vital time and effort during a response.

The allocation of resources will often depend on the number and species of animals involved. SART and CART teams can be valuable resources to the communications center. By coordinating with the incident commander and local law enforcement agencies on site, the dispatchers can arrange an emergency escort for the resources responding to the scene. In several communities, volunteers have collated the contact information and provided it to the emergency dispatchers.

There is a trend in radio service to promote equipment that is *interoperable*. For example, this term is used to describe VHF or UHF radios that allow fire department personnel to communicate directly with police. While this capability offers rapid communication on the scene of a traffic accident where teams from both agencies are present, this communication method has the potential to bypass, and thus break down, the established chain of command within each department. Bypassing the chain of command during a complex and wide-scale disaster can have severe consequences.

MODES OF COMMUNICATION

Dispatchers can advise responders by radio, mobile data terminals, pagers, or mobile phones. After determination of the specifications for each communication link, a selection of equipment can be made that best satisfies those specifications.

Data

Access to the Internet is vital; reports can be filed via e-mail, and updated maps are also readily available for download. Society has come to rely on the Internet, and a number of companies offer satellite access at reasonable cost. Data access is also offered in conjunction with satellite voice service to allow filing reports to the base of operations or to other agencies as needed. E-mail also allows personnel to communicate with their families during long-term deployments; although perhaps not vital to the direct mission, those needs should be met for the mental health of responders.

Fax

The ability to transmit an image of a document is important. Standard landline connections may not be available, but many companies provide the capability to send image files via the Internet. Therefore, a scanner connected to a notebook computer is an important accessory. If a scanner is not available, a digital camera can be used to capture an image for transmission.

Wireless Telephones

Cellular phones are ubiquitous today. They provide a readily accessible and rapid means of communication between personnel, agencies, and the emergency dispatcher. However, they also have a number of inherent limitations that may compromise their reliability when critical information must be relayed. These devices (including those that offer "push to talk" features) are completely dependent upon functioning land-based towers. Service may be available only in urban areas or along heavily traveled roadways. In addition, the towers require electrical power and a data link with that service provider's network before a call can be successfully placed. Because of these limitations, cellular phones can be useful for routine calls but may not be sufficiently dependable, especially in remote rural areas. If cellular phones are included in the communications plan, an accurate, one-page sheet listing all relevant telephone numbers should be provided to all parties involved. Alternate and backup power sources for the phones should be addressed in the communications plan.

911 Calls from Cellular Phones. Similar to landline phones, 911 calls originating from wireless (cellular or mobile phones) can provide Automated Number Identification (ANI); however, there are some differences from landline features. The provision of ANI defines Phase I wireless 911 calls. The cell phone number provided may or not be valid, depending on the status of the phone service. Wireless 911 calls make up the majority of the 911 calls received, with approximately 120 million wireless subscribers and 46,000 new subscribers added daily. According to the National Emergency Number Association (NENA), there were 140,000 wireless 911 calls placed daily in 2001. The number of wireless 911 calls per year increased from 5.9 million in 1990 to approximately 57 million in 2001.

Locational Capability. Automated Location Identification (ALI) was developed for locational purposes, a feature that greatly benefits mobile phone callers. When an emergency call is placed to 911 from a mobile phone, the dispatcher receives specific information regarding the caller's location due to triangulation of the source using cellular towers in the caller's immediate area. The information can be as exact as an address or as vague as a general area within a certain radius (called the "uncertainty factor"). The accuracy of the information ranges from 50 to 300 m and depends on the location technology used by the wireless carrier routing the call. ALI displays the address from which the call originated, the longitude and latitude coordinates from which the call was placed, or both. The provision of ANI and ALI defines Phase II wireless 911 calls.

Longitude and latitude coordinates are provided by a global positioning system (GPS). GPS was developed by the U.S. Department of Defense as a worldwide navigation and positioning tool. There are 24 satellites orbiting Earth at an altitude of over 20,000 km (12,400 miles) that serve as reference points for ground receivers. Displayed as X (longitude) and Y (latitude) coordinates, they uniquely identify any point on the surface of the earth. Computerized mapping software provides the dispatcher with an accurate location to which emergency units can respond. Ideally, units and responders in the field should have a handheld GPS device with which to determine their remote location; alternatively, the dispatcher can provide this information to emergency response personnel.

Geographical coordinates can also be provided as Universal Transverse Mercator (UTM) grid coordinates. The UTM grid was adopted by the National Imagery and Mapping Agency for military use throughout the world. This system is similar to longitude and latitude coordinates; in the UTM grid, the world is divided into 60 north–south zones (each zone spans 6 degrees longitude) and coordinates are measured north and east in meters.

Mapping Capability. Once a wireless 911 call is received by the Public Safety Answering Point (PSAP, or 911 call center), the communications center has the option to "re-bid" the call for a more current or exact location. If a wireless 911 call is automatically or manually re-bid every few seconds, and the responder is mobile, a Phase II (ANI and ALI provided) call can be mapped. The path of the caller can be tracked with an appropriate computer mapping program. NENA reported that 70% of counties in the United States have a minimum of Phase I (ANI only) service in 2005. In 2003, only 643 communication centers in the United States had Phase II Enhanced 911 (E911) service; this comprised approximately 10% of the PSAPs nationwide.

Wireless Coverage. Although some counties in the United States do not have basic 911 services, wireless carriers in all areas can deliver 911 calls from a wireless phone to the appropriate local emergency number. ANI/ALI information appears on the dispatcher's screen within approximately 30 seconds after the call is answered. Federal Communications Commission (FCC) regulations state that any wireless phone, with or without a service provider, must have the capability to make a 911 call at any time when a signal is available.

Pagers

Pagers provide a cost-effective method for simultaneous notification of all members of a rescue or response team. The most commonly used pagers are activated by a two-tone sequence transmitted from the 911 dispatch center. Once the pagers have been alerted, the dispatcher transmits the information by voice. Many pagers can automatically record the message, and others can receive and display a text message. This service is offered by several companies in the United States, often with multistate coverage, and is available to individual subscribers. The alert message is typed into a computer or encoder that automatically dials the pager's telephone number. Some companies have Web pages and allow their customers to activate the pagers and send text messages over the Internet, allowing responders on the scene to be informed of situation updates through text messaging. Pagers are easily carried and can be an excellent method to activate rescue teams on an emergency basis.

VHF/UHF Radio

Hand-held, mobile, or base station radios in either VHF (30–300 MHz) or UHF (300–3,000 MHz) are some of the most effective methods of team communication because every team member can simultaneously monitor the channel. Often used in simplex mode (direct radio-to-radio contact), the effective range for a handheld model can vary from one to several miles. Higher-powered mobile and base stations provide extended range, depending upon antenna placement and terrain.

Radio communication is the most common method of communication between dispatchers and responders and allows for essential information to be transmitted and instantly received. Prior to 1998, radio frequencies were obtained by filing an FCC license application; the license would be granted if the channel was not already in use. Currently, base stations are required to have an FCC license whereas mobile and portable radio systems are licensed under a base station license.

Cell phones and personal communications systems also operate on radio frequencies. In a trunked system, all users share the same frequency. Most emergency services operate mobile radios mounted in a vehicle or carried by hand. These units act as remote computers and are in constant contact with the base station. If more than one antenna site exists for a jurisdiction, the site with the strongest signal will dominate the radio frequency and allow transmission.

Radios are assigned a frequency of operation based on the type of service (VHF-low, VHF-high, UHF). VHF-low band frequencies tend to travel greater distances than those of higher frequencies, but they may be compromised by atmospheric conditions. UHF bands do not transmit as far as low-frequency bands, but they provide better penetration of structures.

Radios for Public Safety Response Use. The FCC has designated VHF-low band radios 39–72 MHz for public safety use. VHF-high band radios are typically used by emergency services for day-to-day communications, and 145–159 MHz bands are employed for public safety use. UHF bands are also used by emergency services for day-to-day communications, and UHF bands 400, 500, 700, 800, and 900 MHz frequencies are used for public safety communications.

Radios for Individual Use. The operation of radios in any band is strictly regulated by the FCC. Three bands are available for individual use; although these bands require no license or a simple licensing procedure, radios used on these channels must be limited in power. The three bands are Multiple Use Radio Service (MURS, VHF 151–154 MHz range), General Mobile Radio Service (UHF 462 MHz band), and the Family Radio Service (UHF 462 MHz band). FCC-compliant radios that use these bands are quite affordable and can be purchased as commercial off the shelf items.

Trunking Repeaters. Repeaters are UHF radios that rebroadcast the transmissions of handheld or mobile radios. A repeater is a remote receiver and transmitter; it receives on one frequency (the input frequency) and transmits on a different frequency (the output frequency). Mobile and base stations listen on the output frequency and transmit on the input frequency. This rebroadcast procedure extends the broadcast range up to a 50 mile (80.5 km) radius from the repeater location. The repeater antennas are often located on mountain tops, tall towers, or on top of the highest buildings in urban areas; the greater the antenna height, the farther the signal can be repeated. Conventional repeaters are being phased out and replaced by the new trunking repeaters.

Many communities have private companies that offer trunking repeater service. Trunking radios use several repeaters; different frequencies in the same band are used and coordinated by computer to allow different agencies to share the same pool of frequencies. Each agency is assigned one or more talk groups for communication. Other subscriber groups do not hear the defined group's transmissions. In this way, a number of channels are time shared by a large number of subscribers for the most efficient use of the available channels. The companies that offer this service hold the FCC license; their customers are not required to obtain a FCC license, but do pay a fee for the service. The fees charged by the companies are most often on a per radio, per month basis and are usually nominal. This type of service can be an excellent means of maintaining contact between all team members, provided they stay within the range of the repeater antenna. Systems that allow reprogramming of radio frequencies permit teams to transmit via different trunking systems based upon location.

Amateur Radio Emergency Service. Amateur radio operators, or "hams," can provide a valuable service to the community for assistance requests during routine or disaster situations. These individuals often have extensive communication capabilities and have experience using backup emergency power. The radio bands that have been set aside for amateur use range from as low as 1.8 MHz (which is just above the AM broadcast band) to several gigahertz (in the microwave transmission band). Several amateur radio organizations exist that can be of assistance to responders. The Amateur Radio Emergency Service consists of hams who can offer emergency communication service for such events as competitive trail rides for horses or endurance events. During disasters, the Radio Amateur Civil Emergency Service assists local or state governments and augments communication. During times of severe weather, "weather nets" allow amateurs to assist the National Weather Service in detecting tornados. Any of these groups can be contacted through the jurisdiction's emergency management office.

Satellite Telephones. When land-based cellular telephones are rendered unusable because of a wide-scale disaster, or if the area is too remote for reliable access, the best alternative is the use of satellite telephones. Satellite phones can provide critically needed communications without the limitations of ground-based transmitting towers.

There are two types of satellite phones. One system uses a single satellite that is in a fixed position in the sky in a geosynchronous (GEO) orbit. Because these satellites orbit at 22,000 miles (35,420 km) above the earth, any communications device must have an antenna that can remain pointed directly at the satellite. Antennas mounted on vehicles and boats have auto-locating capability, but this increases the level of technology required.

The second system uses multiple satellites called low earth orbiting (LEO) satellites, which are in constant motion much closer to the earth. The antennas required for this system are smaller than those required for the GEO system, thus increasing the portability of the units. In order for these units to function, the antenna must have unobstructed access to the sky; if these phones are used inside a vehicle, an external magnetic roof mount antenna is highly recommended. Significant expenses can be incurred by equipment purchase, activation, calling fees, and other associated charges.

Satellite Internet. Access to the Internet can be a very valuable resource during a disaster, but its use in a localized TLAER emergency may not be as vital. However, if a department uses a paging system that requires an Internet connection, Internet access is quite important. There are two systems of satellite Internet service available; these systems are comparable to those used for satellite phones.

In areas where digital subscriber line (DSL) service is not available, satellite dishes may be installed for high-speed Internet access and satellite television reception. These systems often use GEO satellite technology similar to that used for satellite telephones. Internet satellite dishes emit potentially dangerous radiation and must be installed by a licensed technician. There are units available that can be mounted on recreational vehicles or boats, but the software necessary to automatically track the satellite considerably increases the cost.

Other satellite Internet services use LEO satellites. Satellite phones with LEO technology may have satellite Internet capability. The connection speed of this system is considerably slower than GEO systems (and similar to a dial-up connection speed), but transmission of small files or e-mail is still practical.

Mobile Data Terminals

Mobile data terminals (MDTs) are computerized devices that relay information to responding emergency units and allow them to communicate with a centralized computer-aided dispatch (CAD). Today, many MDTs are ruggedized laptop computers with full data storage capabilities. Transmission of information over an MDT is accomplished via radio-related transmission frequencies rather than local area networks; therefore, the transmission speed may be slower. MDTs are available for all divisions of emergency services and are used by the majority of sheriff's offices and local law enforcement agencies that serve populations over 250,000.

RESPONSE TEAM EXAMPLES

The following three real-world examples illustrate model communication solutions for theoretical response teams, each with unique, mission-specific requirements.

Example 1: Technical Rope Rescue Squad

This 16-member specialized rescue responds to swiftwater, cave, and high-angle rescue and provides additional support for local emergency management when requested. Because the team is spread out over a wide area of Kentucky, it receives its initial dispatch through a commercial paging company with statewide coverage; all team members are simultaneously paged. Pages may originate from the county-affiliated 911 system, any team member, or an organization that requests assistance. The pagers are alphanumeric and display a message that includes information on the type of response and the staging location. Once the team is on site, the required coverage area is relatively small. The team uses a VHF simplex-frequency MURS, which provides radio-to-radio contact. If the response involves a cave rescue, a special wire line telephone system is used that can provide patient-side communication as deep as 5 miles (8 km) into the cave; this is necessary because radio waves are not effective underground. When equipping such a team, 5 miles or more (8 km) of wire line should be included in the logistics planning stages.

Example 2: County Emergency Management Team

This 25-member, volunteer emergency management team responds to a wide variety of scenarios, including lost persons, hazardous material spills, and natural disasters such as tornadoes and floods. Embedded within the team are search dogs and their handlers. This team typically responds only within their own county unless they are requested by another county with which they have a mutual aid agreement. The team is alerted using the county 911 system; their pagers are the same as those used by the fire departments, and the team has its own specific tones so that they are alerted only when requested. Once the team is alerted, the county has a VHF repeater system that allows handheld radios to be used everywhere in the response region. The frequency is a shared channel that serves both emergency management as well as the sheriff's department alternate channel. If private conversations are required, personnel use their personal cellular phones. If the team is working in a small area, they have the option of using a simplex VHF channel like the rescue squad described in the first example. Emergency management often requests the services of the technical rope team; therefore, both the rescue team and rescue squad (as in example 1) have the frequencies of the other programmed into their VHF radios for interoperability when needed.

Example 3: National Veterinary Response Team

This 40- to 60-member team responds primarily to wide-scale disasters (such as hurricanes) where the local infrastructure has been compromised. The members, distributed throughout the United States, receive a deployment alert initiated by the commander via telephone. The members report to a staging point located outside the disaster area (often in a different state). All of their treatment supplies, tentage, food, water, and communication gear must be transported into the affected area by trucks. This team depends heavily on satellite communications. Once their base of operations is established, a satellite dish is aligned to allow team command Internet access to download necessary information and send and receive e-mail. In addition, the commander carries a satellite telephone for voice communication with other agencies. Within the base of operation and fully functional field hospital, which can span several acres, personnel are linked using low-power UHF radios. An additional mission of this response team requires the deployment of small assessment teams into the community. Communication between these teams and the base of operation is accomplished with a UHF repeater or satellite telephone. The satellite telephones provide laptop computer Internet access, allowing written reports attached to e-mail to be transmitted directly from the field to the base of operations (Figure 12.2).

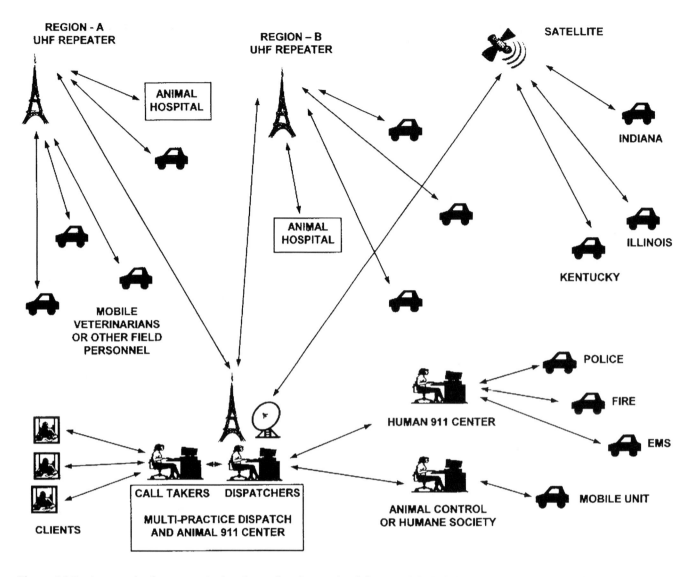

Figure 12.2 *An example of a communications layout for a large regional disaster might include a greater variety of planned communications links that take into account terrain, distance, and data transmission rate. Radios, satellite telephones, telephonic, and a variety of human links in the chain of communications at the 911 center and a special call center for animal disaster issues allows multiple TLAER incidents to be efficiently handled. Courtesy of Kathleen Becker.*

911 EMERGENCY SERVICE

"Nine-One-One, what's the location of the emergency?" The caller is frequently an emotionally distressed individual or animal owner reporting an incident with a large animal. Answering the call is the 911 dispatcher, an individual who provides a valuable link between the incident and the rescue effort. Understanding the role of the dispatcher in these calls allows large animal responders to better prepare their jurisdictions for these emergencies. Dispatchers in most jurisdictions do not have readily available information on specialty resources for large animal response and rescue efforts; a local effort to coordinate, collate, and provide this information represents the best way for interested personnel to ensure they are plugged into the local dispatch call center and emergency management.

HISTORY OF 911 EMERGENCY SERVICE

In 1967 the landline telephone was the most available means of communication for the general public. The concept of an emergency number began when the FCC met with AT&T to find a means of establishing a universal and quickly implemented emergency number. The Emergency Communications System was created in response to a mandate by the U.S. government and has significantly evolved since the number (911) was restricted by Congress to nationwide emergency use in 1968. Congress still authorizes funding pertaining to 911, wireless, and radio communications and the FCC creates the rules and regulations that govern the use of these systems.

The first 911 call in the United States was made on February 16, 1968, in Haleyville, Alabama. Since that date, 911 has become the symbol of the entire public safety communications system. Switching systems and computers route the call to the nearest public safety communications center. At the end of the 20th century, 93% of the U.S. population had access to 911 emergency services. Other countries currently use different numbers and sequences for their emergency contact system, but it has been forecast that 911 will become the worldwide emergency number.

BASIC OR ENHANCED SYSTEMS

The 911 system in an area is considered either Basic or Enhanced (E911) and is a free call from any phone. The incoming call is routed to the PSAP responsible for the area from which the call originates. The FCC maintains a Master PSAP Registry with information on PSAP names and locations. A PSAP can be a single jurisdiction (individual agency) or multiple jurisdictions (several agencies). In 2001, NENA documented 6,121 911 PSAPs in the registry, employing 97,000 public safety communications personnel. That year, NENA also reported that over 500,000 calls were made to 911 per day in the United States, totaling 190 million calls annually. Approximately 57 million (26.5%) of the calls originated from wireless phones in 2001.

When a 911 call is placed, the call is recognized by the telephone company's central office switch and routed to the 911 network. If the 911 call is placed from a Basic 911 service, it is routed to a single PSAP; this PSAP might not be the appropriate agency for the situation. A Basic 911 call is forwarded with voice communication only; the system does not provide the phone number and location of the caller. All information must be obtained verbally from the caller.

Enhanced 911 (E911) systems provide Phase I or Phase II reporting as described earlier in this chapter. The number and location information is automatically provided by the system.

Response Areas

Response areas are designated by geographic zones called emergency service zones (ESN). Each ESN is served by a specific combination of law enforcement, fire, and emergency medical services, and the databases are maintained by the servicing phone companies. Each ESN is assigned a three- or four-digit number used by the E911 system for selective routing.

Routing and Location Information

One feature that separates Basic 911 from E911 is selective routing, a process by which 911 calls are delivered to a specific PSAP based on the specific location of the caller. In the United States, 95% of 911 calls from landline phones are received by an E911 system, which provides the ability to display the caller's telephone number (indicating residence, business or mobile); name of the resident or business; house and apartment number (if applicable) and street or road name; and community or municipality name. The system also displays the date and time the call was received and the ESN to which it was routed.

The caller's address is obtained from the Master Street Address Guide (MSAG). The MSAG is a cross-reference of every assigned telephone number and subscriber address, including the block number ranges for every street in every jurisdiction served by the telephone company.

ANI and ALI functions have become standard in modern telecommunications. The telephone company maintains a database containing the subscriber's name, address, and billing information for every assigned telephone number. ANI information is relayed immediately to the 911 communications center and is displayed when the call is answered.

When the dispatcher transfers an E911 call to another agency, ANI/ALI is transferred along with the caller. Some 911 centers have the ability to automatically redial the caller upon hang-up, lock a line open for tracing purposes, or transfer calls to another agency's telephone number with a single button, which is made possible by special switches and networks used to route E911 communications.

ADVANCED FEATURES OF E911

Other resources are available to assist the public and 911 communication centers with emergency calls. These functions may provide alternate means of communication for the on-scene responder if traditional means of communications fail.

Automatic Crash Notification System and Voice over Internet Protocol

An example of an automatic crash notification system (ACN) is the OnStar system provided by some automobile manufacturers. In the event of a motor vehicle collision, a signal is initiated by an internal signal within the vehicle or manual activation by the driver or a passenger. The ACN system automatically alerts a remote monitoring station, which in turn contacts 911. A signal is initiated from inside the vehicle involved in the collision, either by an internal signal or manual push button. Once the 911 call center has been contacted, the system operator provides an approximate or accurate location of the vehicle using GPS and any additional information that has been obtained from the occupants of the vehicle.

Voice over Internet protocol (VoIP) is used on landline telephones in some businesses and residences. It is estimated that 12–15 million households will be using a VoIP service as either a primary or secondary line by the end of 2008. VoIP allows a customer to make and receive calls using traditional landline phone numbers using specialized equipment via any high-speed (broadband) Internet connection.

Language Line Services

Language line services provide foreign language translators to eliminate any communication barriers affecting the emergency call. The caller, dispatcher, and translator can be directly linked via a conference call. Not all PSAPs have this service.

Teletypewriter/Telecommunications Device for the Deaf

The Teletypewriter/Telecommunications Device for the Deaf (TTY/TDD) service was implemented for hearing impaired individuals and offers a special text telephone or computer teletype system for communication over traditional telephone lines. The caller and the 911 dispatcher use typewriter keyboards to type messages via two-way text in a format similar to that used in Internet chat rooms or by messaging services. Using TTY/TDD, the caller can contact a 911 center directly or go through a telecommunications relay service.

911 COMMUNICATION CENTERS

PSAPs can be single or multiagency centers. Some centers are responsible for emergency communications for a single agency, such as an individual police department or forestry service. Other centers provide emergency communications for multiple agencies such as fire departments, emergency medical services, forestry, police departments, sheriff offices, state highway patrol, public works, animal control, wildlife, fire marshal's office, specialty rescue teams, etc.

Communication centers can be staffed by one or more dispatchers per shift or per operator position. The dispatchers answer the incoming phone calls, dispatch the emergency responders, and enter the information into the computer or a written log. They also can assist the public at a walk-in station. Each dispatcher may be simultaneously responsible for several emergency and nonemergency phone lines, several radio frequencies and channels, and multiple response units.

THE DISPATCHER

In 2006 there were 17,876 local police departments and 3,067 sheriff offices, 49 state police agencies, and 1,481 special districts (Bureau of Justice Statistics, 2007). Of 7,195 agencies with operational communication centers, 6,706 (93%) employed fewer than 100 sworn officers, and an average communications staff of six dispatchers provided 24-hour coverage.

According to the National Fire Protection Association, there are 13,000 fire protection agencies in the United States as of 2006. Based on call volume, radio traffic, and overall workload, many 911 communication centers are understaffed. In 2003, the NENA reported that 1,296 PSAPs are staffed by a single dispatcher on duty per shift.

Scope of Dispatcher's Duties

Dispatchers for 911 are expected to process a wide range of potential emergency calls, ask appropriate questions for each situation, provide necessary instructions to the caller and relay essential information to the responding units or personnel, and demonstrate effective customer service skills with speed and efficiency. Other tasks performed by dispatchers in communications centers may include receiving and processing nonemergency calls, coordinating the activity of field units by radio, and tracking activities of emergency responders.

When the Dispatcher Answers

In larger districts a 911 call is answered by a dispatcher, or, if one is unavailable (due to other calls), the incoming call is answered by a call distributor that holds the call and automatically routes it to the first available dispatcher. In smaller jurisdictions, incoming calls are handled in the order of priority and urgency.

The dispatcher's responsibility is to obtain as much information as possible to provide the appropriate level of response. Questions might be repeated by the dispatcher or information may have to be repeated by the caller for verification purposes, such as address, phone number, and nature of the emergency.

Computer-Aided Dispatch. Some communication centers maintain written logs, and other communication centers operate using a CAD system that automates many of the daily tasks associated with the call receipt and dispatching processes. CAD reduces the time required to process calls and saves valuable time by informing the dispatcher if a second emergency responder crew is needed or if the incident is an initial call for the responding departments. Law enforcement agencies serving populations over 250,000 use a CAD system, and the complexity of the CAD program depends on the size of the public safety agency and the number of dispatchers. CAD allows entry and storage of incident information, provides chronological tracking information, and provides a comment field for any pertinent information. CAD also provides incident report numbers for more efficient filing and retrieval.

The CAD program can work in conjunction with the E911 interface. It automatically displays the phone number and address from which the call originates; the caller's name; and linked information, such as previous incidents, medical conditions, HazMat concerns, number of occupants, etc. The CAD system provides information regarding past, current, and pending incident information. Dispatchers have the capability to assign multiple units from a single agency or multiple agencies to the same incident call in the CAD.

Other advantages of the CAD system are particularly applicable to TLAER incidents. For example, once an incident is entered into CAD, the system can provide a list of suggested responding units or TLAER teams assigned to that area. The CAD is also capable of time-stamping individual entries in the narrative. Other CAD features such as mapping, address verification, and providing informational or resource files greatly benefit dispatchers.

CALL PROTOCOLS

Communication centers must act rapidly, with a high level of accuracy. Specialized computer software has been created to make the task of handling 911 emergency calls easier and more uniform. Although dispatchers do not directly participate in the response effort, they share responsibility for the safety of citizens, firefighters, police officers, and paramedics. Prioritization of responses and proper training maximizes available resources and enables agencies to match response configurations to the unique demands of the incident.

Response Codes

Specific response codes are assigned to call types and allow agencies to preassign equipment and personnel based upon local policies, procedures, and resources for a zero-minute response time; this facilitates lifesaving measures and scene safety.

The emergency medical dispatch (EMD) program and criteria-based dispatch (CBD) were developed to facilitate the decision-making process for prioritizing emergency response efforts. EMD provides medically approved triage guidelines, and CBD bases the level of response on the level of care needed by the patient and the urgency of the situation.

THE 911 CALL

The 911 call can be a critical factor in the outcome of the response or rescue effort. The caller must immediately inform the dispatcher of the location of the incident, providing detailed information when possible. An alternate phone number should be provided in the event that the initial line becomes disconnected or there is a loss of power (e.g., the cellular phone's battery depletes its charge). The caller should answer all questions, being concise and detailed while remaining calm and cooperative.

Most 911 communication centers record all phone conversations and radio traffic for future reference. Recordings can be immediately replayed and are routinely kept for a specified period of time. In general,

the 911 dispatcher will ask the caller for the following information. Depending on the nature of the call, emergency units may be dispatched before, during, or after all of the necessary information is obtained:

- Location of the incident: Information can be provided in the form of a road name, cross streets, landmark name, business name, interstate exit number, highway mile marker number, state or national park name, GPS coordinates, trail name or color, or other descriptor. The correct location of the incident avoids delays and unnecessary dispatches.
- Contact number: Provision of the phone number from which the call originates allows the dispatcher to reach the emergency caller if the call is prematurely disconnected. In Phase I and Phase II E911 systems, the phone number is automatically provided to the dispatcher.
- Victims: Information on the types of victims (e.g., animals, adult humans or children) allows dispatchers to determine the type and number of emergency personnel units that should be dispatched to the incident scene. In addition, any immediately life-threatening situations involving the victims should be provided (e.g., animal or human victims ejected from vehicles or trapped in burning vehicles).
- Number of victims: The number of human and/or animal victims allows the dispatcher to determine the number of response units necessary to address specialized rescue efforts (TLAER is considered specialized rescue).
- Scene situation: Information regarding the type of incident (e.g., motor vehicle accident, river rescue, downed livestock, loose livestock, trapped animal, etc.); the type(s) of vehicles involved in the incident (e.g., trucks, cars, tractor trailers, livestock trailers, etc.); and other details (e.g., two-, three-, or four-horse trailer, bumper pull or gooseneck, commercial liner) facilitates the formulation of an action plan for an efficient and successful rescue or response effort.
- Response: The dispatcher should be informed of special needs for trained personnel, specialized equipment or teams, fire department response, HazMat teams, emergency medical services, law enforcement, a large or small animal veterinarian, or heavy equipment (e.g., crane, backhoe, etc.). Various responders play different roles in the rescue operation.
- Accessibility: When possible, directions to the incident should be provided. This is especially important when rescues are necessary on trails. If a guide must meet the responders and direct them to the site, a meeting place should be arranged. If the scene is accessible only by small or large vehicle, all-terrain vehicle, horseback, boat, foot, or by another specialized means of transportation, the dispatcher should be notified.

HELPFUL ADVICE WHEN CALLING 911

When calling 911, keep in mind the following:

- Dial 911 only for an emergency. Use nonemergency numbers for all other routine calls.
- Make a single test call from your new phone in the local area to check that the ANI/ALI information is correct and to determine if the phone is Phase I or Phase II capable. Inform the dispatcher that it is a test call.
- When calling to report an emergency, briefly and succinctly describe the nature of the emergency. "I'm reporting ____." Stay on the line with the dispatcher. Do not hang up until the dispatcher advises you to do so. The dispatcher may keep the caller on the line while dispatching emergency units or while the units are responding in order to obtain more information or to provide lifesaving instructions.
- Stay on the phone line if the call is being transferred. A law enforcement dispatcher may answer the phone for a fire call and need to transfer the caller to the fire dispatcher.
- Let the dispatcher ask the questions. They have been specially trained to prioritize the emergency and obtain vital information. If not in a position to provide complete answers, stay on the line. The dispatcher will ask questions that can be answered "yes" or "no."
- Be prepared to describe the location of the emergency. Although E911 can display the telephone number and location of the caller, the dispatcher must confirm the displayed ANI/ALI information and may ask for more specific information.
- Be patient when dispatchers are obtaining information. The dispatchers must gather information, verify it, and enter it into a computer or written log. Emergency units are often dispatched while the caller is still on the phone with the dispatcher.
- If 911 was dialed in error, do not hang up the phone; instead, stay on the line and explain to the dispatcher that it was a mistake. In some situations, responders may still be dispatched according to protocol.
- Hanging up and trying to call back if a recording is received or the call is put on hold will only delay the call further. The call will be answered in the order of priority.

ACRONYMS USED IN CHAPTER 12

ACN	Automated Crash Notification
ALI	Automated Location Identification
ANI	Automated Number Identification
CAD	Computer-Aided Dispatch
CBD	Criteria Based Dispatch
CART	County Animal Response Team
DSL	Digital subscriber line
EMD	Emergency medical dispatch
ESN	Emergency service zones
FCC	Federal Communications Commission
FRS	Family Radio Service
GEO	Geosynchronous
GMRS	General Mobile Radio Service
GPS	Global positioning system
HazMat	Hazardous materials
LEO	Low Earth orbiting
MDT	Mobile data terminal
MSAG	Master Street Address Guide
MURS	Multiple use radio system
NENA	National Emergency Number Association
PSAP	Public safety answering point
SART	State animal response team
TLAER	Technical large animal emergency rescue
TDD	Telecommunications device for the deaf
TTY	Tele-typewriter
UHF	Ultra high frequency
UTM	Universal Transverse Mercator
VoIP	Voice over Internet protocol
VHF	Very high frequency

13 Field Euthanasia

Dr. Rebecca Gimenez

INTRODUCTION

Field euthanasia (e.g., due to trailer wreck, severe fracture during an equestrian event, on-trail accident, etc.) is a crucial part of training for responsible horse owners, emergency responders, and veterinary personnel assisting with technical large animal emergency rescue (TLAER) emergencies and disasters. Humane euthanasia renders the animal insentient and unaware of pain or any other sensations at death. It is important for responders to understand and communicate that a humane death is preferable to death by drowning or severe hypothermia or shock. When an animal cannot be rescued, or its injuries are too severe, euthanasia is often the best option.

ANIMAL WELFARE REGULATIONS

Humane slaughter laws and concerns for the welfare of commercial food animals have developed over the last several hundred years in response to growing public anxiety about the rights of animals (Leavitt and Halverson 1990). The knowledge drawn from these sources and from routine slaughter practices should be applied to field euthanasia, but extenuating or exigent circumstances in field TLAER responses may impact the course of action.

In the United States, the U.S. Department of Agriculture (USDA) is the primary federal agency responsible for animal welfare issues. The Animal and Plant Health Inspection Service (APHIS) of the USDA enforces the Animal Welfare Act in order to protect certain animals from inhumane treatment and neglect. The Food Safety and Inspection Service (FSIS) of the USDA is responsible for verifying the humane treatment of livestock, including equids, bison, and cervids, in slaughter plants. The requirements mandated by the Humane Methods of Slaughter Act (HMSA) of 1958 were extended in 1978 to all livestock slaughter facilities, including ritual slaughter facilities. HMSA, the Federal Meat Inspection Act, and the Poultry Products Inspection Act provide the FSIS with statutory authority in this area (USDA, 2004).

ON-SCENE CONSIDERATIONS

Humane physical methods must be taught to owners and fire and rescue personnel, and proper equipment must be available. The most commonly available method of euthanasia is often a firearm or projectile weapon, but use of a captive bolt device followed with a sharpened knife to induce exsanguination (bleeding out) is an effective and rapid method of euthanasia (American Veterinary Medical Association, 2002). Veterinary regulations pertaining to licensure, discharge of weapons, and the use of controlled drugs must be followed, even in emergency and disaster situations.

Euthanasia should be considered as a last-resort option. A thorough assessment of the situation, the animal's injuries, rescue options, and the safety of all personnel involved should be performed when considering the decision. Emergency responders should be aware of the importance of obtaining owner consent for euthanasia, thorough documentation of the incident, proper handling and disposal of carcasses, and proper euthanasia techniques (Baker, 2004). Knowledge of large animal behavior (e.g., flight distance, critical distance, flight mechanisms, herd instinct) is crucial to safe and effective capture, handling, triage/processing, and euthanasia on TLAER scenes (see Chapter 4). In addition, knowledge of human behavior enhances interaction and communication with the owner, bystanders, and other responders (R. Gimenez, 2005). Responders should understand and acknowledge the human response to the stressful and emotionally charged situations associated with animal incidents and disasters and plan accordingly.

The knowledge of appropriate field euthanasia is a necessary aspect of response. There have been and will be scenarios associated with emergency and disaster response where risk assessment indicates that it is not safe for humans to try to rescue the animal(s) or where medical evaluation of the animal by the veterinarian determines the animal is not salvageable. In other situations, the owner may decide they cannot afford the medical treatment necessary to preserve the animal's performance or quality of life. Other examples include obvious fatal injuries (e.g., exenteration [disemboweling] injuries and open, comminuted [fragmented] fractures) and actively drowning animals that are inaccessible to responders.

As a case in point, passersby called 911 when they observed a longhorn steer goring a llama in a field. An animal control officer and two veterinarians were dispatched to respond and evaluate the situation. When the responders arrived on the scene, the llama was disemboweled, in shock, and obviously suffering. The veterinarian recommended humane euthanasia, and the animal control agent contacted the sheriff's office to obtain the name of the property owner; however, the owner's primary residence was in another county, and repeated attempts to contact the owner were unsuccessful. Unable to make contact, the animal control agent, acting as the incident commander (IC), asked the veterinarian to perform humane euthanasia. When the llama owner arrived shortly thereafter, unaware of what had transpired, he reacted to the loss of their llama with extreme anger. At that moment, the owner was unable to perceive the futility of treatment, the suffering the llama had endured, or the risk associated with pasturing llamas and longhorn cattle on the same unsupervised premises.

Legal action was threatened by the owner but never filed, as veterinary medical records, animal control records, and the sheriff's office log confirmed that proper protocol had been followed. In that state (California), the veterinarians had acted appropriately in viewing the animal control officer as the client in the absence of the animal's legal owner and performing euthanasia at her request when deemed medically appropriate by both veterinarians. The animal control agent assumed the responsibility of communicating with the animal's owner once the veterinarians had made their verbal report (Nixon, 2006).

CONTINGENCY PLANNING

Good contingency planning is vital for public and large private events. Organizers of big public large animal activities (e.g., parades, rodeos, equestrian events, or public cattle or horse drives, etc.) need to devise a plan for emergency response, veterinary care, field euthanasia, and carcass disposal. Proper planning and execution reduces the risk of miscommunication and public outcry in the event that an incident occurs. For example, the U.S. Army Caisson platoon responsible for publicly transporting the body of a deceased president to the Capitol building has a contingency plan that addresses the possibility that the draft horses pulling the hearse wagon slip on the pavement, fall, rear, flip over backward in the traces, stampede into the crowd, collapse, or sustain severe injuries. The U.S. Army veterinarian responsible for planning each event plans an appropriate response for each event. Planning protocols should consider every worst-case scenario with a contingency plan for each event; this is especially critical when the events are publicly witnessed.

When planning and performing response and euthanasia procedures with significant public exposure (e.g., during natural disasters, parades, shows or events, racetracks), organizers should consider the attitudes and responses of the bystanders. Racetrack response teams use tarps or screens to block public view of their efforts (HEART, 2006). The author's experience has shown that using a dark-colored sheet or tarp over the animal's body after euthanasia is associated with less negative public response than leaving the body exposed; blood stains are less visible on dark sheets, and covering the body demonstrates respect and concern for the animal and its owner.

Certain euthanasia scenarios will require better scene security and control than others, particularly when well-meaning but radical or fanatic animal rescue organization members arrive at scenes such as commercial livestock hauler wrecks (particularly those haulers bound for slaughter). Some of these groups have been known to release hundreds of animals from overturned trailers and flood animal facilities or commercial farms; despite the intended mission of freeing the animals from life-threatening danger, this often further compromises the health and safety of the animal victims. The IC must take control of the scene to prevent these actions.

THE FIELD EUTHANASIA DECISION PROCESS

The following procedures should be followed when performing a field euthanasia.

- Perform a good patient medical assessment
- Document the incident with photographs or video
- Ensure good scene control and security
- Consider insurance and legal concerns
- Make a decision—should the animal(s) be euthanized?
- Choose an appropriate method
- Identify a qualified person to perform euthanasia
- Dispose of the carcass in an appropriate manner

Patient Assessment

Thorough assessment and documentation of the animal victim's medical condition are vital. If a veterinarian is unavailable, a certified/registered/licensed veterinary technician, paramedic, or an emergency medical technician may be able to perform these tasks. Veterinary technicians are highly trained medical staff, similar to nurses in the human medical profession, who work with injured and ill animals every day. In many states, a certified/registered/licensed veterinary technician is legally able to perform the examination and consult directly with a veterinarian (e.g., via telephone) for advice and protocol.

If a veterinarian or other qualified individual is not available, an emergency medical services (EMS) provider is often capable of performing a basic examination of the animal victim. In each jurisdiction, the planning for care of animals in emergencies and disasters needs to address the legal aspects of this possibility to prevent EMS personnel from being charged and penalized for practicing veterinary medicine without a license. Good Samaritan laws may be in place that can protect response personnel from legal action in an emergency or disaster; these laws vary by state or jurisdiction, and the laws affecting the area responders should be reviewed.

In cases where the animal may not be easily and safely accessed (e.g., at the bottom of a well or trapped inside an overturned trailer), the medical responder may be unable to perform a thorough assessment of the animal victim. The assessment may rely on limited visualization from a distance, audible cues (e.g., rate and effort of respiration), and intuition based on experience and the situation.

A paramedic should be able to determine the animal's respiratory rate, pulse quality, and heart rate. A basic assessment can be performed based on these findings and phone consultation with a veterinarian. All members of an animal rescue team should be skilled in basic triage, obtaining vital signs, and first aid (see Chapter 17). Care should be taken to avoid overestimation of the severity of an animal's wounds; with appropriate and timely treatment, large animals frequently recover from injuries that initially appear fatal.

The requests of the owner or their authorized agent should be considered unless that individual is incapacitated or otherwise unable to make the decision. Some incidents will not require medical expertise to realize the animal must be euthanized humanely. Examples include scenarios in which the animal sustains an open fracture or the complete loss of an extremity; eviscerations, in which abdominal contents are present outside the body cavity through a defect in the abdominal wall; and severe fractures of the animal's back or neck. The degree of pain and suffering should be considered in the decision, and the decision should be made quickly and with regard for the animal's well-being.

Documentation

The public information officer (PIO) or another responder on scene should document the incident response with good quality photographs and/or video. These rescues enhance public relations when they are efficient and successful, and the PIO office may wish to release pictures to the media. This is particularly important if the media is present overhead in a helicopter; the view from the air does not always correlate with actual events. Photographs and video should be bylined (labeled) with personnel present, techniques used, and location while these facts are fresh in the rescuers' minds. The medical status of each animal should be thoroughly documented by the medical personnel on scene (see Chapter 5).

The police and fire department reports should include information on the number of animals, injuries or deaths to animals, types of vehicles involved and other pertinent details. Documentation is important for legal and insurance reasons. When available, good photographs should be included in the documentation for educational and training purposes. Some jurisdictions limit the use of photography or consider the photographs the property of the jurisdiction.

Public attention to large animal rescues can be of great benefit to public education and funding efforts. Appropriately performed, successfully executed animal rescues represent opportunities to obtain outside funding for an animal rescue unit or team; these videos are in high demand from local TV stations, national TV shows, or animal channels. Numerous animal rescues have been locally and nationally telecast live from ground and helicopter coverage during the 2004–2006 television seasons. The live, national coverage of the transport of horse racing champion Barbaro following the 2006 Preakness Stakes exemplified the intense public interest in animals and their care—flowers and candy were sent to Barbaro from all over the world.

Scene Control and Security

If a projectile firearm is used to euthanize an animal on the scene, responders should ensure good scene control and security to prevent bystanders from being harmed from stray or ricochet ammunition, and the media should not be permitted to videotape the procedure. This is a component of good on-scene incident command system (ICS) management. A security zone should be established to prevent bystander access or interference. Vehicle security should not be overlooked, because portable equipment and veterinary drugs stored in vehicles have been stolen from response scenes (see Chapter 5).

The PIO should clearly communicate the euthanasia process to responders and bystanders (especially media), including expectations of reflexive reactions by the animal and the inability to stop or reverse the procedure once it has begun. It is the PIO's duty to explain the procedure, why the animal is being euthanized, and why the specific method of euthanasia was selected. Regardless of the method selected, any method of killing an animal can be associated with a negative public opinion. The PIO should ensure that bystanders or the media do not record the procedure, including the use of cellular phones equipped with cameras; this, too, is an important aspect of on-scene ICS management.

During the response efforts associated with Hurricane Andrew in 1992, it was necessary to euthanatize a large number of fatally wounded animals. A photojournalist with a powerful zoom lens photographed a police officer shooting a horse. The photograph appeared in the newspaper the following day with no explanation, just a photograph of a police officer aiming a weapon at a horse. This media coverage led many members of the public to believe that police officers were indiscriminately shooting horses in the affected area; as a result, concerned horse owners who had evacuated the area without their animals attempted to bypass security measures to reach their animals. Analysis of this situation emphasizes the importance of proactive communication through the PIO. Such communication would have informed the public that teams of veterinarians and officers were performing triage of affected large and small animals, and nonsalvageable animals were being humanely euthanatized; that shooting is a humane method of euthanasia.

Emphasize Safety

Projectile weapons are inherently dangerous to bystanders and to the shooter because the projectile leaving the weapon can be deadly to anything it penetrates. The shooter should be familiar with the safe operation of the weapon and ensure that the animal to be euthanized is the only target in the range of fire. The caliber of the weapon is less important than correct placement of the bullet in the brain of the animal—a bullet as small as a .22 caliber (5.6 mm) hollow point is effective when properly positioned (the exception is large ruminants; see description below). Many professionals use two to three shots to ensure death, or prefer hollow point/magnum bullets in hand weapons or shotguns for this task (Woods, 2006b). Adequate lighting is necessary to ensure proper performance. Rifles are effective for euthanasia, but they are less desirable because they can be difficult to aim properly and often use high-velocity rounds that may increase the risk of ricochet or bystander injury.

Captive bolt equipment should also be treated as a weapon. The device uses a small explosive charge to force a 10-cm (4-in.) steel rod into the animal's brain. The rod is then retracted back into the device. A captive bolt may be a safer choice for non-law enforcement personnel than a projectile weapon but training is required for proper use, and it is not appropriate in

some scenarios (such as an overturned livestock trailer) (see Chapter 21).

The proper handling of firearms is necessary for safe discharge of a weapon, but does not eliminate the dangers associated with their use on TLAER scenes. On July 4, 1972, two California Highway Patrol officers provided on-scene assistance at the site of an accident involving a horse trailer. The horse trapped in the trailer was severely injured, and the owner requested the officers euthanatize the horse. The officers entered the trailer and fired three shots. One of the bullets ricocheted off the trailer and struck and killed one of the officers (ODMP, 2006).

In the above incident, it is likely that three shots were fired because the officers did not properly position the firearm to penetrate the animal's brain. It is possible that the officers were unaware of the appropriate site for bullet placement or the caliber of the weapon was insufficient to penetrate the animal's skull. From a TLAER standpoint, other concerns involve personnel entering the trailer with the increased risk of injury or death associated with the presence of two responders in the trailer with the animal. In addition, many modern trailers are made of lightweight aluminum; if a bullet penetrated the trailer wall, bystanders or responders could be injured or killed.

Consider Legalities and Insurance

Insurance Concerns. With good documentation, a police report, and a veterinarian's statement, most companies will honor the insurance policy on insured animals. In some cases, an owner may request the animal be euthanized when it may have a good prognosis; the veterinarian on the scene can provide advice on these issues. Some insurance companies require notification or a second opinion before honoring a policy. This may be difficult to obtain in an emergency situation. In Canada, it is illegal for an insurance company to demand a second opinion if obtaining that opinion prolongs the suffering of an animal (Woods, 2006b).

Look for Emergency Information. On vehicular incident scenes, responders should look for emergency stickers and information about the animals in the vehicle. Many animal owners have been educated to place emergency contact information regarding the owner and their animals in their truck and trailer. This information often includes contact information for the veterinarian, the name of an individual authorized to make decisions related to the animals, the name of the next of kin, and possibly a euthanasia consent form. Some proactive owners complete a legal document and place it in the trailer, giving any local responding veterinarian authorization to do whatever needs to be done; some statements provide a monetary spending limit for treatment and authorize euthanasia if the costs of treatment are expected to exceed that amount (Cole, 2006). When owners provide this information, they facilitate the efficiency of the response effort and appropriate treatment of the animals in their absence.

The response community has encouraged the use of in case of emergency (ICE) contact numbers saved in the cellular phone contact list for emergency use. Veterinarians have encouraged designating ICE numbers specifically for owners' animals, with names such as "ICE (horse)" or "ICE (llama)," with a contact number for the animal's assistance. This allows responders to rapidly contact an individual who is authorized to provide for that animal's needs if the owner is incapacitated.

In most jurisdictions, the owner is the only individual with the legal authority to direct the euthanasia of his or her own animal; in special situations, the law enforcement or animal control officer on the scene is authorized to make this decision on behalf of the owner (as the "owner apparent") to prevent suffering. If the owner is not present or is injured or incapacitated, his or her agent (a person with legal permission to make decisions for the owner) may give authorization to euthanatize an animal. When euthanasia is necessary, the process should be explained to the animal owner (or the owner's agent) and permission to euthanatize the animal should be obtained before the procedure is initiated.

Are Animal(s) Going To Be Euthanized?

Once the decision is made to euthanatize an animal, the procedure should be performed as soon as practical. A telephone consultation with a veterinarian may be all that is necessary to make the decision; at other times, the owner may request euthanasia of the animal. If the owner is deceased or en route to the hospital and cannot make decisions for the animal, another individual will have to make that decision. Depending on the jurisdiction and the availability of a veterinarian, animal control officers or law enforcement may need to make that decision.

The American Association of Equine Practitioners offers the following euthanasia guidelines for horse owners to consider when making decisions about their animals. These criteria may also assist the emergency responder on scene when making decisions regarding euthanasia. These guidelines are applicable to any large animal in emergency and clinical scenarios (AAEP, 2004).

- Is the animal's condition chronic, incurable, and resulting in unnecessary pain and suffering? (*Note:* There is often little doubt as to pain and suffering and the need for humane euthanasia to relieve current and future suffering on emergency scenes.)
- Does the animal's condition present a hopeless prognosis for life?

- Is the animal a hazard to itself, other animals, or humans?
- Is the animal constantly and in the foreseeable future unable to move unassisted, interact with other animals of the same species, or is the animal exhibiting behaviors that may be considered essential for a decent quality of life?
- Will the animal require continuous medication for the relief of pain and suffering for the rest of its life?

Horses and downer cattle that are unable to rise and stand unassisted may not be loaded, transported, and/or unloaded at an abattoir or slaughter facility; they may only be euthanized immediately or loaded with veterinary authority for treatment purposes (Federal Register law; USDA). In addition, horses may not be loaded in a cattle livestock (double-decker) transport for any reason (Federal Register law; USDA).

Choose a Method of Euthanasia

The method of euthanasia should be chosen based on availability of equipment, trained personnel and the situation. The American Veterinary Medical Association (AVMA) Guidelines on Euthanasia (available at: http://www.avma.org/issues/animal_welfare/euthanasia.pdf) used the following criteria to evaluate euthanasia methods: "Ability to induce loss of consciousness and death without causing pain, distress, anxiety or apprehension; time required to induce loss of consciousness; reliability; safety of personnel; irreversibility; compatibility with requirement and purpose; emotional effect on operators and observers; compatibility with subsequent evaluation, examination or use of tissue; drug availability and human abuse potential; compatibility with species, age and health status; ability to maintain equipment in proper working order; and safety for predators/scavengers should the carcass be consumed." (AVMA, 2007) These same principles should be considered by emergency personnel on scene when selecting a method of euthanasia with or without a veterinarian present.

If euthanasia cannot be performed safely (i.e., without significant risk of injury to personnel), it may be necessary to let a dying animal expire on its own. The primary task of a good risk assessment is to prevent the injury of personnel during the animal euthanasia procedure.

What Really Happens to the Animal? The object of euthanasia is to induce unconsciousness and immediate death in the brain and nervous system of the animal. Brain death is not the same as heart and lung (organ system) death. The heart and lungs can continue to function for minutes to hours in an animal whose brain is destroyed (King, 1989). Some animals will paddle with rudimentary leg movements, and the heart may continue to beat; these are reflexive responses of the nervous system to the shock of brain destruction. These will eventually slow and stop. All animals will draw deep breaths (one or more) as the carbon dioxide level in their blood increases: These are called agonal breaths. These agonal breaths may occur many minutes after the animal's brain is destroyed; they can be disturbing to uninformed owners, who may incorrectly assume that the animal is still alive and is suffering. Those performing the euthanasia procedure should assure personnel on the scene that the animal is rendered instantly insentient and is no longer suffering.

EUTHANASIA

The definition of *humane euthanasia* is to render the animal insentient (AVMA, 2007), unconscious, and unaware of pain or of its surroundings. It cannot feel or sense pain and cannot react to pain. Euthanasia is the scientific name for humanely killing an animal; the word *euthanasia* is derived from "eu," good, and "thanatos," death. A "good death" is one that occurs with a minimum of pain and suffering.

Various organs die at different rates if lethal injectables are not administered; the lungs may continue to expand and the heart may continue to beat; the skeletal muscles may twitch or contract in response to a stimulus for several minutes to hours; and the smooth muscle of the gastrointestinal tract can still exhibit peristaltic contractions for hours after death. Personnel on the scene should realize that muscle twitching (fasciculation) and hyperextension of the back and limbs (ophisthotonus) will occur as reflexive responses to death, and do not indicate consciousness or pain. Agonal breathing (terminal breaths) may occur reflexively. These reflexive pathways occur in the spinal cord (and not in the brain). An animal with a destroyed brain can still exhibit movement due to spinal cord reflexes; the possibility of this movement persists until the spinal cord has died and the reflex arcs are lost.

With some methods of euthanasia, the animal's heart may continue to beat, and its lungs continue to expand despite brain destruction (as determined by fixed and dilated pupils and the lack of a corneal reflex). These methods should be accompanied by another method of ceasing these reflexes (e.g., bilateral pneumothorax/thoracotomy or exsanguination). Any corneal response (eyelid blink or eye retraction) when the eye is touched with a finger indicates a need for firing another bullet or implementing an alternate method of euthanasia (Wright, 2005).

Large Animal Euthanasia

According to the AVMA Guidelines on Euthanasia, there are four acceptable methods of euthanasia for large animals (AVMA, 2007). The Humane Slaughter Association, USDA, and the U.S. Public Health Service ascribe to these recommendations.

The four accepted methods of euthanasia include chemical and physical methods. Chemical methods of euthanasia, also known as lethal injection, are preferred by most U.S. owners. Approved physical methods of euthanasia include projectile weapons, penetrating captive bolt, and exsanguination (fatal bleeding) of an unconscious animal. Physical methods are considered conditionally acceptable, especially in natural disasters or in TLAER emergencies when another method is not immediately available, and are used with appropriate restraint to ensure correct placement of the weapon (AVMA, 2007).

Chemical Methods—Lethal Injection. Lethal intravenous injection with an overdose of a barbiturate anesthetic (for example, sodium pentobarbital alone or in combination with phenytoin, which may be followed by a potassium salt) is the most commonly accepted and performed method of euthanasia in the United States. The barbiturate anesthetizes the brain and the salt is cardio-toxic (i.e., it stops the contraction of the heart muscles) (Jones et al., 1992). Chemical euthanasia is rapid and may be less emotionally traumatic to personnel on the scene. Chemical euthanasia must be performed by a veterinarian or euthanasia technician (animal control and humane officers); possession and administration of the barbiturate requires a Drug Enforcement Agency license (AAEP, 2004).

The jugular vein is the preferred site for administration of the lethal injection. However, the jugular vein may not be accessible (e.g., if the animal is trapped inside a trailer or down in a well). It may be necessary to sedate the animal heavily via the tail vein or an intramuscular injection with a dart or jab stick (Gimenez and Gimenez, 2002).

Chemical euthanasia may be associated with delayed or incomplete euthanasia in animals with compromised circulation (e.g., cardiovascular or septic shock), severe trauma, or internal hemorrhage (bleeding). It may be difficult or dangerous to administer the chemicals to ambulatory animals unaccustomed to human handling (e.g., commercial cattle, bulls, or injured or wild horses). These are situations where a firearm may be the only choice (Woods, 2006a). When large numbers of animals must be euthanatized, the supply of euthanasia solution may be inadequate (Nenni, 2006).

When possible, an indwelling jugular catheter should be placed. The catheter allows consistent access to the circulatory system for the administration of medications and intravenous fluids during transport. In addition, it facilitates euthanasia if it becomes necessary. Large volumes (100 cc or more) of euthanasia solution are required for euthanasia of large animals; an indwelling catheter ensures access to the vein and reduces the risk of incomplete administration of the solution.

Aggressive, fearful, or wild animals should be sedated prior to catheter placement and intravenous administration of the lethal injection solution. This decreases the risk of injury to personnel; relaxes the animal for the procedure; and minimizes the risk that the lethal injection is administered perivascularly (outside of the vein), which may be associated with incomplete euthanasia and delayed death (AVMA, 2007). Severe hypotension (low blood pressure) and vasodilatation, which may occur in animals with cardiovascular shock or animals that have been administered acepromazine, impairs the delivery of the drug to the brain and may increase the difficulty and time of the euthanasia procedure. As a general rule, healthier animals with good cardiac output succumb to chemical euthanasia more rapidly than compromised animals. The PIO should educate personnel regarding the possibility that a severely compromised animal may not die as quickly as is desired.

Chemical euthanasia is often not practical in field situations. Most U.S. animal owners accept chemical euthanasia for animals, and many have a cultural bias that shooting an animal is inhumane. Others object to euthanasia by firearm based on the noise (gunshot) the procedure generates. However, euthanasia by firearm may be the most practical method when large numbers of animals must be euthanatized or there are concerns about secondary poisoning. Ethical deliberation and exigent circumstances must be addressed, and a decision must be made in a timely manner.

Secondary Poisoning Concerns. Chemical euthanasia is not a viable euthanasia option if the animal carcass is intended for consumption by humans or other animals or if the carcass cannot be immediately removed from the scene. Lethal injection with a barbiturate generates barbiturate residues in the animal's tissues and can potentially poison animals and raptors that scavenge the body (Booth, 1988). Once an animal has been euthanatized, the carcass cannot be left aboveground; it must be buried or incinerated (Figure 13.1).

Most incidents of secondary poisoning have been caused by both intentional and unintentional failure to properly dispose of a barbiturate-tainted carcass, leaving it exposed to animal scavengers. In recent years at least 139 eagles have been poisoned in this manner (USFWS, 2002). One scavenged cow carcass in British, Columbia, Canada, was responsible for 26 eagle deaths. Veterinarians and owners have been fined for violations (Otten, 2001).

Veterinarians and livestock owners have been charged with violations of the Migratory Bird Treaty Act (MBTA), the Bald and Golden Eagle Protection Act (BGEPA), and the Endangered Species Act (ESA). Penal-

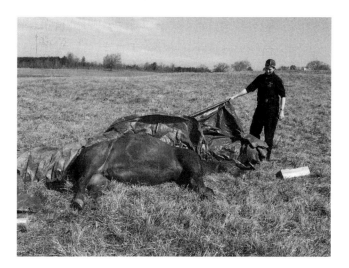

Figure 13.1 *This horse was chemically euthanatized by a veterinarian using injectable euthanasia solution. The animal was covered with a tarp to prevent the possibility of secondary poisoning to wildlife that might scavenge the carcass before burial. Courtesy Tomas Gimenez.*

ties imposed by the U.S. Fish and Wildlife Service (USFWS) are based on the circumstances surrounding a poisoning incident and vary on a case-by-case basis. The laws provide for imprisonment and substantial fines for criminal violations. Criminal penalties can approach $250,000 per individual or $500,000 per organization under MBTA and BGEPA and may include imprisonment for up to two years and forfeiture of vehicles and equipment under some circumstances. In civil cases, maximum fines range from $500 to $25,000 under ESA and up to $5,000 for any violation of BGEPA.

To determine whether a case falls under USFWS jurisdiction, for information on law enforcement and liability issues, or if a dead animal is found, contact the regional USFWS Law Enforcement Office (regional offices are located in Portland, Oregon; Albuquerque, New Mexico; Fort Snelling, Minnesota; Atlanta, Georgia; Hadley, Maine; Denver, Colorado; and Anchorage, Alaska). To determine whether a case falls under the jurisdiction of the state wildlife agency, for state and local assistance with dead wildlife, carcass issues, or other wildlife-related questions, contact the nearest office of the state's department of fish and wildlife, fish and game or other wildlife agency in the state. The U.S. Geological Survey National Wildlife Health Center maintains a partial database of secondary pentobarbital poisoning cases.

For information on medical treatment of poisoning victims, the National Animal Poison Control Center of the American Society for the Prevention of Cruelty to Animals provides a fee-based service for emergencies and other cases of poisoning. For information call 1-888-426-4435 (1-888-4ANIHELP).

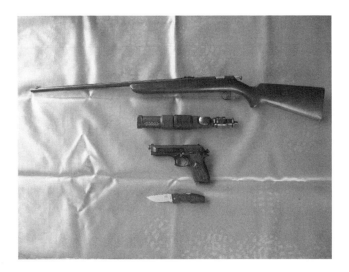

Figure 13.2 *From top to bottom: .22 caliber rifle; captive bolt stunner; 9 mm handgun; sharp knife. These all represent appropriate physical methods of euthanasia of large animals. There are specific requirements for each animal species to achieve maximum brain destruction. Courtesy of Tomas Gimenez.*

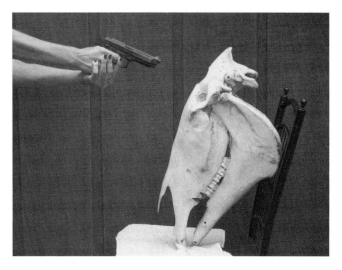

Figure 13.3 *The photograph shows the approximate 90-degree angle of projectile weapon placement in reference to the skull of a horse. Using this angle will minimize the chance of ricochet of the bullet fragments off the skull surface or exiting the skull after penetration. Courtesy of Tomas Gimenez.*

Physical Methods. Physical methods (Figure 13.2) involve firing a projectile weapon (e.g., firearm, pistol, rifle, shotgun) or captive bolt to the animal's head. These techniques are preferred for euthanasia of a calm, sedated, or humanely restrained animal by a professional trained in the method (AAEP, 2004).

Firearms and captive bolts are very efficient when used by an individual trained in the use of such equipment. The muzzle of the weapon should be fired at an angle and location (Figure 13.3) to penetrate the brain, causing destruction of the brain and rendering the animal immediately insentient. Animal handlers should ensure that the animal does not fall on the operators or themselves, and if inside a commercial liner, that the animal does not crush them between the wall and the animal. Horses will often fall forward suddenly when stunned with the captive bolt. The operator should remain a safe distance and to the side of the animal when euthanatizing a standing animal with a physical method. The use of a captive bolt in livestock trailer incidents should be secondary to a firearm for this reason (Woods, 2006a).

After a fully loaded cattle trailer in Texas overturned onto its right side, responding sheriff's deputies were required to shoot 20 fatally injured cows trapped in the trailer or strewn along the side of the road. The remaining cattle were loaded into another trailer for transport, this was an appropriate response.

A number of bullet calibers can be used, including a rifled slug fired by a shotgun (410 gauge or larger) and rifles (including .308 [7.8 mm] and .223 [5.7 mm]) aimed 2–5 cm (1–2 in.) or greater distance from the skull. The smaller caliber .38 (9.7 mm) police service revolver or .22 caliber (5.6 mm) long rifle bullet may render the

animal unconscious, but may not be lethal to other organs and may require multiple shots or exsanguination (bleeding out) subsequent to shooting. Although a rapidly and readily available means of euthanasia, the use of a firearm may be aesthetically unpleasant for the owner. In addition, the release of a projectile(s) by a rifle or shotgun poses a potential danger to animals and humans in the vicinity (Wright, 2005).

A common misperception about euthanasia with a firearm is the public belief that an animal can be killed if it is shot between its eyes. Shooting large animals is an efficient and humane method of euthanasia; in many European countries, horses and cattle are routinely euthanatized by shooting or captive bolt. Close examination of Figure 13.3 reveals that shooting an animal between its eyes does not result in brain penetration by the bullet; instead, the bullet penetrates the paranasal sinus cavities, resulting in hemorrhage and severe pain. There are numerous anecdotal reports of law enforcement officers and cowboys firing multiple shots into animals' skulls without successfully killing the animal. Knowledge of the appropriate landmarks of the skull will prevent these unprofessional incidents.

Although Figure 13.3 exhibits a horse skull, other large animal skulls are anatomically similar. The preferred site for the projectile or captive bolt is located by drawing lines between the base of each ear and the contralateral eye (i.e., lines drawn from the right ear to the left eye and from the left ear to the right eye); the animal's brain is located underneath the intersection of the two lines (Figure 13.4). On horses, the projectile or captive bolt should be aimed approximately 1–2 cm (0.5–1 in.) above the intersection of the lines. Lipstick,

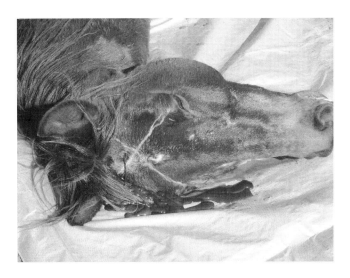

Figure 13.4 *A horse was euthanatized with a physical method of euthanasia and shows the appropriate position of the landmarks for aiming the weapon. An "x" was made with white chalk to ensure proper positioning of the firearm for instantaneous brain death. Courtesy Tomas Gimenez.*

a marker, or chalk can be used to physically mark the location to avoid misinterpretation.

If a veterinarian is not present and the decision is made to euthanize the animal, euthanasia should be performed by an individual with training in the discharge of firearms (e.g., law enforcement or military personnel). There are two scenarios where a police officer can legally fire their weapon without inciting an investigation, target practice and euthanatizing an animal.

When educating an officer on the landmarks of where to shoot the animal, they should be instructed to aim at an 80- to 90-degree angle (see Figure 13.3) to the skull so that any bullet fragments will lodge into the neck, minimizing ricochet. The officer should not stand directly in front of the animal and should wait until the animal is still. Handheld weapons should not be placed against the animal's skull; they should be fired from a 2–8 cm (1–3 in.) or greater distance. Shotguns should be fired from approximately 25 cm (10 in.). If possible, the animal should be haltered and restrained by an animal handler standing directly behind the shooter (Woods, 2006a).

The captive bolt is used in the slaughter process because it induces instantaneous loss of consciousness. When performed properly, it is rapid, leaves no chemical residues, and is a similarly efficient alternative to lethal injection. The muzzle of a captive bolt must be placed in direct contact with the animal's skull. Captive bolts can be difficult to use on livestock downed in a trailer due to movement of the animals' heads, and the close proximity required to fire the captive bolt may place personnel at risk of injury if the animal lunges forward (Woods, 2006a). Smaller animals, such as

llamas and some pigs, may be easier to handle and euthanatize with a captive bolt. Extensive training and practice are needed to effectively use a captive bolt, and preventative maintenance must be performed to ensure the weapon will fire when used (AVA, 1987).

Numerous veterinarians in the United States perform euthanasia using a .22 caliber (5.6 mm) handgun, with two bullets placed approximately 2 cm (1 in.) apart; this method is less costly than chemical euthanasia, and some veterinarians are proficient with the method and comfortable with its use. Others use it as a backup method to lethal injection. On a draft horse or bovids with over 1 cm (1/2 in.) of skull thickness, a larger caliber weapon is necessary. Most law enforcement officers carry 9 mm or .45 caliber (11.4 mm) ammunition; these are often sufficient for euthanatizing a horse, but are probably insufficient for euthanatizing a large bull or a boar. A shotgun (410 gauge or larger) is the preferred weapon for many professionals who respond to livestock incident scenes (Woods, 2006).

In some countries, the use of manually applied blunt trauma to the head is considered unacceptable, and in some U.S. states (such as Florida) it is a third-degree felony punishable by a $10,000 fine (Shearer and Nicoletti, 2002). In other states, the exceptions to the above physical methods are piglets under three weeks of age or under 6.5 kg (14 lb) and newborn calves. This method involves striking the animal on the top of its head with a heavy, blunt object such as a 1.2-kg (2 1/2 lb) hammer with a striking face of 2 × 2 cm (1 in. × 1 in.) for piglets or 4 cm × 4 cm (2 in. × 2 in.) for calves (Hides, 2002). The blow should be administered at the same site described for shooting or captive bolt penetration (Woods, 2006b).

Livestock Liner Euthanasia Standard Operating Protocol. This standard operating protocol is that published for brand inspectors (official agriculture representatives) in Canada and is recommended by the author for consideration by other professionals and team members performing field euthanasia in emergency or disaster situations (Woods, 2006a).

- Responder must be authorized or receive authorization to euthanize an animal as per the applicable laws.
- Responder selects the safest and most effective choice for euthanasia on a trailer or liner accident scene.
- Responder must be trained and experienced in firearm use.
- Responder must be trained to safely and effectively euthanatize an animal, knowing the correct point of entry for each species of animal, and be aware of species-specific hazards: for example, horses may lunge forward when shot and bison are best shot in the side of the head to lessen the chance of ricochet.

- Remove all mobile livestock possible from the compartment before shooting the downed livestock.
- Earplugs must be worn when firing a weapon within the confines of the trailer.
- A .22-caliber (5.6 mm) rifle with hollow point bullets is the most effective firearm to use for most animals; when shooting larger animals such as large bulls, bison, or boars, a larger caliber weapon should be used.
- Do not place the muzzle of the weapon flush to the head; rifles should be held approximately 5–15 cm (2–6 in.) away from the point of entry, shotgun 25–30 cm (10–12 in.) away, pistols 2–8 cm (1–3 in.) away.
- Work in conjunction with law enforcement and traffic control to stop the flow of traffic when discharging the firearm.
- Ensure everyone on the scene is behind the line of fire before shooting; bystanders should be kept well away from the scene.
- If someone is in the trailer to assist the shooter (i.e. holding a flashlight or halter), she or he must stand directly behind the shooter.
- Immediately prior to discharging a firearm, a warning must be yelled out to everyone on the scene (i.e., "fire in the hole").
- Ensure the animal is dead before proceeding to next downed animal by performing eye test and/or bleeding the animal out.

Emotional Aspects of Euthanasia to Consider. Exposure to dead or severely injured people is an unfortunate but expected aspect of emergency response, and personnel develop individual coping strategies to address the evoked emotional response. However, most responders will admit that injured children and animals evoke stronger emotion and mental stress because they perceive that animals and children are innocent and placed in harm's way by others. Killing animals is an unpleasant task and can be distressing to responders.

Responders and owners may benefit from mental health debriefing to allow verbal expression of their emotions and concerns after the incident. Veterinarians and their staff encounter death more frequently than do their human medical counterparts and often must induce an animal's death at the owner's request. Based on these experiences, veterinarians are often good resources for compassionate handling of concerned personnel.

The observers and the owner should be prepared for the procedure and informed of the possible events (e.g., movement, agonal breaths, etc.). Many owners do not wish to observe the euthanasia process, while others refuse to leave the animal's side and may place themselves in danger. The owner should be made aware that euthanasia is permanent and the animal will be dead; euphemisms such as, "putting it to sleep," "the shot," or "putting it down" should not be used.

Human psychological responses include grief at the loss of life, guilt for causing the accident, an ethical struggle with the implications of ending an animal's life, and anger at responders for being unable to save the animal's life. These feelings are normal and should be expected (AVMA, 2007). The PIO and veterinarian should be active in the process and discuss quality of life and end of life issues with the owner, bystanders, and responders that express concerns.

If a projectile or captive bolt weapon is to be used for euthanasia, the personnel performing the procedure should be assured that they are serving the best interest of the animal by ending its suffering. Although some view projectile euthanasia in an emotionally detached manner as being similar to hunting, most responders find it emotionally stressful to shoot a companion animal at close range.

Firing the Weapon. Personnel selected or who volunteer to perform the field euthanasia should be educated about the considerations and proper method of euthanasia. They should approach the animal slowly and let the animal relax as it becomes accustomed to the presence of a human. They should not stand directly in front of a standing animal, as it might fall on them when shot. The weapon should be carefully and slowly placed at the appropriate distance away from the hair and bone at the landmark, aimed, and fired. Animals may move or toss their heads, especially if the muzzle of the weapon touches the animal's skin or hair; consistent aim and visualization of the target area is important. The angle of entry is important to ensure fragments lodge in the neck and to prevent ricochet inside enclosed spaces. Each species has appropriate species-specific landmarks and angles to use as guidelines, and responders should review them. Shotguns should be used from approximately 25 cm (10 in.) away from the skull, and captive bolts should be placed in direct contact with the skull. Rifles should be used from a comfortable distance away for the safety of the sharpshooter.

In some states, it is technically illegal to shoot a horse for any reason. These laws were enacted to prevent support of the horse slaughter industry, but may complicate the euthanasia process in emergency scenarios.

Captive Bolt. The captive bolt, also called a *humane killer* or *stunner*, should be used by an experienced and trained operator. Even though the projectile does not extend more than 10 cm (4 in.) from the muzzle of the device, it is still a dangerous weapon powered by blank cartridges (.23 cal, 5.8 mm). However, it does not require a license or permit and can be legally transported in a vehicle. When used properly, a captive bolt will stun the animal by destroying its cerebral hemisphere and/ or brainstem; the animal must be exsanguinated (bled out) or a pneumothorax induced by bilateral thoracotomy to induce death and complete the euthanasia procedure (AVMA, 2007). The captive bolt is the most common method of large animal euthanasia in European countries and Australia (AVA, 1987).

The captive bolt has a 10 cm (4 in.) steel rod (the bolt) that projects from the barrel of the weapon when fired, but it is considered safer than other weapons because it does not fire a projectile. When fired, the bolt penetrates the skull of the animal, driving fragments of the skull into the brain and destroying it; the animal will drop immediately. Individual weapons are fired by a powder charge. Modern slaughter houses use air-powered captive bolts to stun animals prior to exsanguination (Thurmon, 1986). Similar to projectile weapons, the captive bolt has a safety and a trigger to release in preparation for firing.

An animal may move its head to avoid contact with the muzzle of the weapon when it touches the animal's hair and skin. Because the bolt is 10 cm (4 in.) long, the muzzle must be in almost direct contact with the skull to ensure adequate penetration.

Exsanguination. The term exsanguination refers to the act of draining or losing blood. Exsanguination can be performed by cutting open a large blood vessel (e.g., jugular vein, cranial vena cava, aorta, etc.) and is **not** an acceptable method of euthanasia unless the animal has already been rendered unconscious (Figure 13.5). This procedure is commonly performed in slaughterhouses after the animals have been stunned with a captive bolt. However, the procedure results in the release of approximately 20 l (5 gal, or 4% of the animal's body weight) of blood from an adult horse or cow, depending on the size of the animal. This will make the rescue scene grisly and provide a slipping hazard.

Exsanguination of an animal can evoke a negative emotional response from personnel and bystanders; if performed, the animal and the anticipated area of blood accumulation should be covered with dark sheets. Unconscious, exsanguinating animals are capable of violent, involuntary muscle movements that can inflict serious injury (Shearer and Nicoletti, 2002).

One method of exsanguination in the stunned animal is the chest stick procedure, which is intended to prevent arterial blood from reaching the animal's brain as the blood drains. A sharp knife is used to create a 15 cm (6 in.) skin incision overlying the jugular furrow and trachea at the base of the neck. The knife is then inserted into the chest cavity at the thoracic inlet, and the major vessels are severed above the heart (Hides, 2002).

For the neck stick procedure, a deep incision is made underneath the jaw (in the throat area) from the point

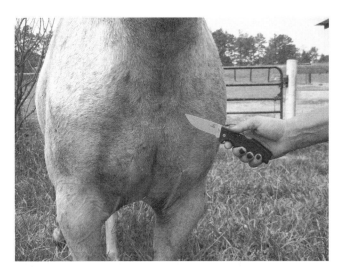

Figure 13.5 *Exsanguination should only be performed on animals that have been rendered brain dead by a primary method of field euthanasia (e.g., projectile weapon). A sharp knife should be inserted at the bottom of the neck (at the site pointed to on this live animal) and used to cut the large veins and arteries near their junctions with the heart. Courtesy of Tomas Gimenez.*

of the jaw below one ear to the other ear, cutting deeply to sever the jugular veins, windpipe, and carotid arteries (Shearer and Nicoletti, 2002).

The aorta can be severed with a scalpel or small blade via a rectal approach; this method should be performed by a veterinarian. The veterinarian holds the scalpel or blade in his or her hand while inserting the arm in the animal's rectum; a dorsally directed (upward) cut is made in the posterior vena cava and/or iliac veins and the animal's posterior aorta/iliac arteries, allowing the blood to pool inside the abdominal cavity. The blood will remain and clot within the abdomen, preventing a visible blood pool.

Bilateral pneumothorax induces death by allowing air to enter the chest cavity and collapsing the lungs. A knife is used to incise a large hole in the chest wall between the ribs on each side of the animal's thorax. This procedure is also called a bilateral thoracotomy (Figure 13.6).

Exceptions to Humane Euthanasia. The euthanasia method chosen should cause as little pain and distress as possible. Shooting an animal in the heart or abdomen will not instantaneously induce brain death and will cause pain and distress; for those reasons, the methods are not considered humane. However, on emergency scenes there may be extenuating circumstances where an acceptable means of euthanasia cannot be performed due to the risks of human injury or death. For example, a llama escaped a sport utility vehicle at an interstate rest stop in Alabama and was running loose in the parking lot. Law enforcement officers informed the owner that the llama would be shot if it could not be

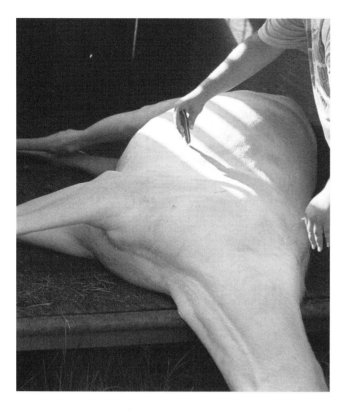

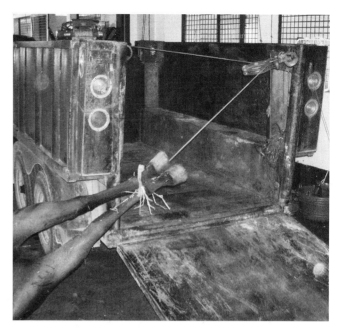

Figure 13.7 The use of pulley blocks and a winch is effective for moving a dead large animal for transport from the scene. A dark-colored sheet should be used to cover the animal if the process will be performed within sight of the public. Courtesy of Tomas Gimenez.

Figure 13.6 A veterinarian induces pneumothorax with a bilateral thoracotomy by cutting a large hole between the ribs to eliminate negative pressure in the thorax and collapse the lungs. This must be performed on both sides. Courtesy of Tori Miller.

caught and approached highway traffic: this decision was based on the high risk of human injury that would result from vehicular collisions caused by the loose animal. Even a highly skilled marksman would have been unable to shoot the moving animal in the brain; therefore, the officer would have had to shoot the animal to stop its progression, then fire a fatal shot from closer range.

Make Sure the Animal Is Dead. The animal's death must be verified, preferably by a veterinarian, before disposing of the carcass. Animals should be evaluated for swallowing, chewing, or tongue movement; jaw muscle tension when the mouth is opened; audible or palpable heart contraction; normal, rhythmic breathing; tension in neck muscles; or blinking or eyeball retraction in response to corneal pressure (Hides, 2002). If any of the responses listed are observed, the animal might regain consciousness. Thus, a secondary method of euthanasia should be applied (Shearer and Nicoletti, 2002).

Most veterinary and agricultural professionals use a simple rule of thumb in the field: if the animal does not have a heartbeat or is not breathing after five minutes, the animal is dead (Hides, 2002). A secondary method of euthanasia (e.g., exsanguination, bilateral

thoracotomy) is recommended to ensure death of the animal, and the corneal reflex should be absent.

Carcass Disposal. For many people, watching an animal's carcass being winched into a truck evokes a stronger negative emotional response than watching the euthanasia procedure. The practical concerns of euthanasia do not stop at the death of the animal. Appropriate and legal disposal of the animal's carcass should be included in the response and euthanasia plan. If the animal is ambulatory, it may be possible to load it onto a trailer before euthanasia so the body can be readily transported after death has been confirmed. If this is not possible, a method of lifting or dragging the body will need to be devised (see Chapter 15). In general, it is illegal to leave a carcass exposed for scavenging, especially if lethal injection residues are in the carcass (Figure 13.7).

Burying an animal carcass is often possible, unless there is permafrost, a blizzard, high water table, or it is forbidden by local laws. However, the proper disposal of multiple carcasses presents a larger challenge. Personal protective equipment may be necessary for personnel and is especially important when there is a risk of disease. Incineration, group burial, and composting methods may be used.

Appropriate disposal of the carcass by incineration, composting, rendering, or burial must be accomplished in accordance with local laws and availability of equipment, and the method used may depend on the mass

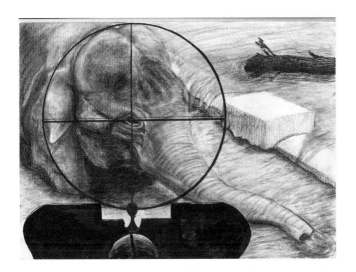

Figure 13.8 *During the 2002 flooding of the Prague Zoo, Kadir the bull elephant had to be humanely euthanatized by a sharpshooter when the panicked elephant refused to follow instructions from zoo keepers and began to drown as the floodwaters rose within his enclosure. This illustration shows an imaginative example of how this scenario would appear. All remaining elephants and over 1,200 other animals were successfully evacuated from this 500-year flooding event in an exceptionally well-organized disaster evacuation. The 8,000 kg (17,600 lb) carcass of this animal represents a significant disposal challenge. Courtesy of Julie Casil.*

of the carcass (Figure 13.8). Carcass disposal regulations and requirements vary among cities, counties, and states, as do agencies that administer and enforce them. When developing a mass animal fatality contingency plan, responders should consult federal, state, and local agricultural, environmental, and public health authorities (including the USDA, APHIS, and the state's depart-ment of agriculture). Environmental regulators that focus on solid waste handling and disposal include the EPA, and state and local departments of ecology, environmental health, environmental management, solid waste management, or other similar agencies.

The state veterinarian and other public health regulators (such as the state department of health or public health and board of animal health) can provide advice on the public and animal health aspects of carcass disposal and burial. Land-grant university cooperative extension services may also have information on carcass disposal methods approved for the local area. It is important to remember that regulations change, especially with growing concerns over agricultural biosecurity and environmental protection.

ACRONYMS USED IN CHAPTER 13

APHIS	Animal and Plant Health Inspection Service
AVMA	American Veterinary Medical Association
BGEPA	Bald and Golden Eagle Protection Act
EMS	Emergency Medical Services
ESA	Endangered Species Act
FSIS	Food Safety and Inspection Service
HMSA	Humane Methods of Slaughter Act
MBTA	Migratory Bird Treaty Act
IC	Incident Commander
ICE	In case of emergency
ICS	Incident command system
PIO	Public Information Officer
TLAER	Technical Large Animal Emergency Rescue
USDA	United States Department of Agriculture
USFWS	United States Fish and Wildlife Service

14 Rope Rigging and Mechanical Advantage

Dr. Tomas Gimenez

INTRODUCTION

A basic knowledge of rope rigging and equipment as used in heavy rescue is important in an effective technical large animal rescue. It is not the intention of this chapter to cover all aspects of rescue rope knot tying and rope rigging, but rather to introduce some foundation concepts that will help the reader better understand the capabilities of rope rescue and to stimulate further reading and training. The large animal victim in technical large animal emergency rescue (TLAER) incidents is several times larger than the human victims to which the rope rescue riggers are accustomed; this presents challenges that must be overcome with increased mechanical advantage and heavy-duty systems.

In this chapter, the term *software* refers to the ropes, cord, and webbing used in rope rescue. The term *hardware* refers to the carabiners, pulleys, rigging plates, etc.

This chapter introduces some of the rope rescue equipment available and the techniques most commonly applied to TLAER. Several sources of rope rescue rigging equipment and training can be found on the Internet, and excellent resources on aspects of rope rescue are available for those interested in learning more about this subject.

SAFETY IN ROPE RESCUE

By far the most important aspect of rope systems in heavy rescue is safety for the rescuers and for the animal victim. Before attempting to use any type of rope system in an incident, rescuers should attend practical hands-on training in rope rescue. Rope rescue equipment should be used only in accordance with the manufacturer's recommendations. It is more important to understand the physics of the different components of

a rope system than it is to learn how to assemble a specific system. Understanding the physics of a system gives the rescuer the flexibility to modify and customize a system to suit the particular environment and conditions of an incident.

Always use rescue-quality equipment in TLAER rescues. One of the few aspects that the rescuer can fully control is the purchase of high-quality, dependable equipment. The stronger the equipment used, the greater its ability to support the victim. The safety factor quotient is a ratio of the maximum strength of the equipment to the load placed on the system. The equipment should be rated in excess of the expected load and stress that will be placed on it in order to increase the safety factor ratio. The use of rope rescue systems should include an understanding of strength, rope, cord, webbing, knots, software, and hardware.

STRENGTH AND SAFETY

When purchasing carabiners, rope, or any type of webbing from a commercial manufacturer, the equipment should be labeled with information on its strength. This information may be expressed as the following:

- LBF = Pounds of force = breaking strength
- MBS = Maximum breaking strength
- MTS = Maximum tensile strength
- SWL = Safe working load
- WLL = Working load limit; roughly a 10:1 or 15:1 safety factor ratio for humans is required
- kN = kilonewton (1,000 Newtons: a newton is a unit of force, obtained by multiplying mass and acceleration)

TLAER uses the same heavy rope rescue rigging equipment as that used for humans. However, because large animal victims are many times heavier than human victims, the safety factor ratio is decreased when using the same equipment (NFPA, 2000).

Measure of Strength under Impact

The force with which a falling object (called the load) contacts the ground or reaches the end of the rope after a free fall is a combination of the load's mass (commonly used as weight or mass) and the acceleration caused by gravity ($9.81\,m/s^2$). This combination of mass (weight) and gravitational acceleration at impact is known as the maximum impact force and is expressed in a unit of force called a newton. A static mass of 1 kg on the ground contains 9.81 (normally rounded to 10) newtons. Thus, 1 kilonewton (kN) corresponds to a static mass of 100 kg (220 lb).

As an example of maximum impact force, an 80 kg (176 lb) person coming to a sudden stop after a free fall of 5 m (16 1/2 ft) generates a maximum impact force of 4 kN (4 tons). Studies performed by the U.S. Air Force have shown that the human body can only withstand a maximum impact force of 12 kN (1,226 kg) or less without causing severe body malformation or death. Large animals can be expected to be no different in the ability of their tissues and skeletal components to withstand this impact force.

Sudden Impact Forces. In the rescue environment, the kilonewton gives the best measure of the strength of rescue equipment when subjected to sudden impact force generated by the load and the gravitational force it generates. Rescue rope such as 12.7 mm (1/2 in.) low-stretch kernmantle rope will stretch 2%–3% under a 1 kN force (Table 14.1).

Calculations of force are made using the following equation.

Impact force equation:

$$F = \mu g + \mu g \frac{\sqrt{1 + 2fK}}{\mu g}$$

where:

F = impact force in newtons
G = gravitational acceleration = $9.81\,m/s^2$
K = elongation characteristics of the rope (Young's modulus; this figure is unique to the rope used and is a ratio of the change of stress with strain)

Table 14.1 Strength of some rescue components.

Component	kN	Kg
Low-stretch kernmantle rope (12 mm)	40	4,086
Prusik cord (8 mm)	20	2,043
New England Tech Cord (5 mm)	22	2,270
Webbing (25 mm)	20	2,043
Steel carabiner	72	7,246
Brake tube	44.44	4,540

Note: Strength measured in kilonewtons (kN).

f = fall factor (obtained by dividing the length of the fall by the distance from the falling load to the anchor point)

For example, consider a 100 kg animal suspended by low-stretch kernmantle rope (modulus 1.5) 6 ft above the bottom of a hole. The anchor point is 2 ft from the animal, and the animal falls 4 ft. The fall factor is 4 divided by 2, or 2. The impact force sustained by the rope would be 1,059 N (1 kN).

It is important to note that this equation assumes that the rope absorbs all of the force associated with the fall. In addition, it does not account for the presence of knots (which absorb energy) or hardware. However, it can provide an estimation of the impact force sustained by the rope.

Minimum Breaking Strength

MBS is commonly used to express the strength of rescue software and is also used to calculate the safety ratio of the equipment to the load (Figure 14.1). The strength and elongation of various rescue software varies with the selected system (Table 14.2).

COMMON COMPONENTS IN TLAER ROPE RESCUE

In general, the same components are used for TLAER incidents as for human incidents, but the mechanical advantage must be increased to move the load. Components must be strength rated to support the large animal's mass, or that of a large object such as a horse trailer, that is being stabilized or moved.

Rope

The most common type of rope used in TLAER is nylon, 12.7 mm (1/2 in.) diameter, low-stretch kernmantle

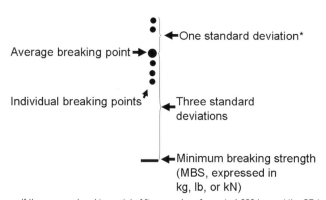

If the average breaking point of five samples of rope is 1,000 kg, and the SD is 100 kg, then the MBS for that rope is 1,000-300 = 700 kg

*Standard deviation (SD) = Range of deviation from the mean.

Figure 14.1 *The calculation of (MBS) of rescue components is based on testing of actual components by product manufacturers. Courtesy of Tomas Gimenez.*

Table 14.2   Strength and elongation of rescue software components.

Name	Material	Diam.	MBS*	Elongation (%)
Kernmantle low-stretch ("static")	Nylon	12.7 mm	4,086 kg	6–10
		1/2 in.	40 kN	
		16 mm	5,675 kg	4.5
		5/8 in.	55 kN	
Kernmantle high-stretch ("dynamic")	Nylon	11 mm	2,270 kg	20–35
		7/16 in.	22 kN	
Sterling high tenacity ultra-low stretch, static	Polyester	12.7 mm	4,622 kg	2.0
		1/2 in.	41 kN	
		16 mm	5,993 kg	1.7
		5/8 in.	51.1 kN	
Water rescue rope	Polypropylene	10 mm	1,636 kg	
			8.45 kN	
Tubular webbing	Nylon	25 mm	1,816 kg	
		1 in.	17 kN	
Flat webbing	Nylon	25 mm	2,724 kg	
		1 in.	26 kN	
Prusik cord	Nylon	8 mm	1,305 kg	
			12 kN	
Prusik cord	Nylon	9 mm	1,440 kg	
			26 kN	
New England Tech cord	Armid/polyester	3 mm	2,270 kg	
			22 kN	
Accessory cord (pilot cord)	Nylon	3 mm	184 kg	
			1.8 kN	
Accessory cord	Polyester	3 mm	270 kg	

*Minimum breaking strength.

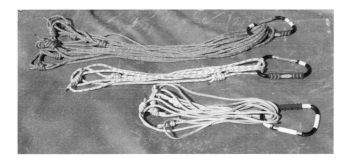

Figure 14.2   *Rescue cord in lengths of 1.5, 2.1, and 2.7 m (5, 7, and 9 ft) are used to make preknotted Prusik loops and are maintained in the cache for use on scene. A color code is used internally to differentiate short, medium, and large loop sizes. Courtesy of Axel Gimenez.*

rope. The fibers (kern) of the rope run lengthwise and are protected by an outer sheath (mantle). Lengths less than 33 m (109 ft) have minimal value in TLAER rope rescue, and 100 m (330 ft) lengths are preferred. Dynamic kernmantle ropes exhibit up to 35% elongation when loaded; these ropes are designed to absorb the forces of a fall by elongating and absorbing energy. Dynamic ropes are not appropriate for use in TLAER scenarios. Static kernmantle ropes do not elongate appreciably when loaded.

The working end of a rope is the section used to tie a knot or form a rigging, whereas the standing end is not used. The running end is the free end of the rope.

A bight is a U-turn of the rope on itself and is a component of knots.

Cord

Cord, 8 mm (3/8 in.) in diameter, is used to make Prusik loops, which have multiple uses as handles, brakes, holds, and backups. The diameter of the cord should be 70% or less of the diameter of the rope it is intended to grab for friction brakes. A variety of these loops of various lengths should be preassembled and stored for ready access during incidents (Figure 14.2).

Webbing

Tubular 25.4 mm (1 in.) webbing has numerous uses in TLAER but is most commonly used to attach the rope system to a bombproof anchor (that is strong enough to support several times the weight of the load) to prevent damage to the rope itself (Figure 14.3). Segments of fire hose may be used in a similar manner. The high abrasion resistance of webbing makes it excellent for anchoring rope systems. A typical webbing loop is made by tying both ends of a single length of webbing with a water knot.

To tie a water knot, begin with a simple overhand knot in one working end (the knot resembles a pretzel). Take the working end of the second line through the first overhand knot, retracing the original path in the opposite direction. Make sure all lines are laid neatly next to each other and there are no folds or twists in the knot. Tighten the knot by pulling the standing

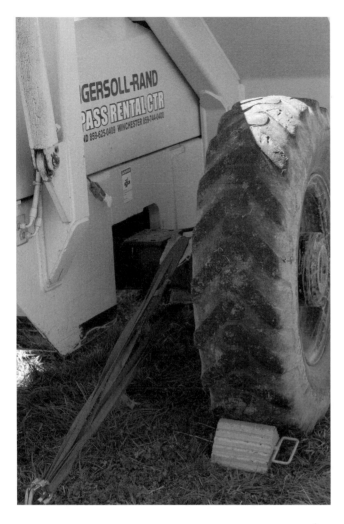

Figure 14.3 *Webbing, 12.7 mm (1/2 in.), is used to attach a rope system to an appropriate bombproof anchor. Note that a section of fire hose is wrapped around the axle before the webbing is attached to protect the webbing from friction and abrasion. The wheels are chocked, and the ignition key is removed to prevent accidental movement of the anchor. Courtesy of Axel Gimenez.*

Table 14.3   Fire hose size based on diameter or width.

Diameter (cm, in.)*	Width (cm, in.)**
2.5, 1	3.8, 1 1/2
3.8, 11/2	6.3, 2 1/2
4.4, 1 3/4	7.6, 3
6.3, 2 1/2	11.4, 4 1/2
7.6, 3	13.9, 5 1/2
12.7, 5	20.3, 8

*With water.
**Empty.

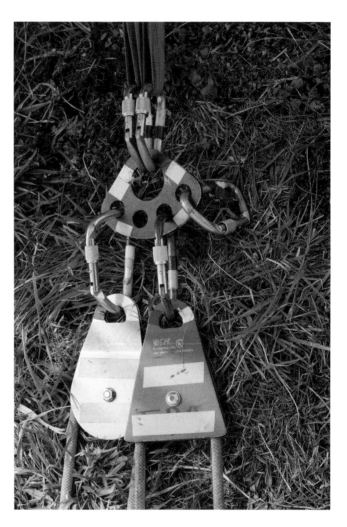

Figure 14.4 *On the left is a simple pulley, and on the right is a Prusik-minding pulley as part of a 9:1 mechanical advantage system. The carabiners connect the pulleys to the gathering plate, and additional carabiners connect the system to the anchor. Brake tandem Prusik hitches have not yet been built into the system in this photo. Courtesy of Axel Gimenez.*

ends of the lines. This knot is simple to tie and is very solid, it is difficult to untie once it has been loaded.

Fire Hose as Webbing in TLAER. Fire hose is an extremely useful source of rescue software in TLAER. When a fire department finds any defects in the hose, regardless of size, the entire section of fire hose is discarded. However, the strength of the webbing component of the fire hose is not adversely affected by small holes, and the discarded fire hose sections function well as sections or loops for TLAER (Table 14.3). The ends of fire hose section can be sewn into loops using a heavy duty sewing machine such as those found in saddle or leather shops. Stitching performed in a close zigzag fashion over a 15 cm (6 in.) or longer section of hose is stronger than an "X"-shaped stitch. Stitching should use heavy-duty stitching materials.

Hardware

All hardware should be of rescue quality, and it is generally obtained from manufacturers of equipment for rope rescue. Equipment purchased from hardware stores or sporting goods stores are not rescue quality and are unsuitable for TLAER use (Figure 14.4).

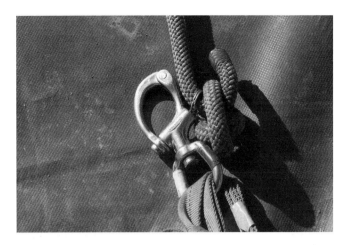

Figure 14.5 *The snap shackle is a crucial safety device used as a quick release mechanism for simple vertical lifts, allowing the quick release of the animal from the overhead spread bar and lifting mechanism as the animal's limbs contact the ground. Courtesy of Axel Gimenez.*

- Locking steel carabiners 9 cm (3 1/2 in.) in length (29 kN; 2,724 kg strength rating) are some of the most useful and used items in rescue. A normal TLAER rescue cache will include 25–30 steel carabiners of various sizes. Larger gate carabiners are useful when linking heavy webbing loops to each other, round slings to webbing, or heavy webbing to rope.
- Extra-large steel locking carabiners 26 cm (10 in.) in length (41 kN strength rating) allow the appropriate distribution of mass (load) to the equipment. These carabiners are heavier duty than those used for rock climbing.
- Rescue swivels, 9 cm (3 1/2 inch) in length (36 kN, 3,632 kg strength rating) allow easy rotation of the victim that is suspended from a rope system without twisting or binding the rope system.
- Stainless steel snap shackles 89 mm (35 cm) in length (29.42 kN; or 3,003 kg strength rating) allow for quick disconnection of the spread bar and overhead equipment from the vertical lift large animal sling. As soon as the animal's legs touch safe ground following a simple vertical lift, these can be opened to quickly free the animal from the equipment (Figure 14.5).
- Single rescue pulleys (6.4 cm [2 1/2 in.], 36 kN strength rating)
- Double rescue pulleys (6.4 cm [2 1/2 in.], 36 kN strength rating)
- Prusik-minding pulleys (6.4 cm [2 1/2 in.], 36 kN strength rating)
- A gathering plate (rigging plate) (36 kN strength rating) allows multiple hardware components to be connected to the same anchor.
- A steel heavy-duty brake bar with six bars can be used as a friction device to control and ease the descent of a load such as a large animal victim or a horse trailer.

- A brake tube. Like the brake bar, the brake tube is a very efficient friction device used to control and ease the descent of a load such as a large animal victim or a horse trailer.

CARE OF RESCUE EQUIPMENT

Rope rescue equipment must be properly maintained to preserve maximum strength and performance during an incident. All software and hardware should be permanently marked to ensure return to the owner or team. It is common on live rescue scenes for multiple jurisdictions or teams to respond, and poorly marked equipment may not be returned. A unique color scheme is commonly added to all equipment to allow rapid identification. Hardware should have small pieces of reflective tape added to minimize the chance of loss, especially in the dark; during breakdown of the scene and collection of the equipment, shining a flashlight across the incident area will detect lost or dropped equipment marked with reflective tape.

Software Care

Rope, cord, and webbing should be stored dry in bags or other suitable containers that protect them from prolonged exposure to ambient light and humidity. Responders should avoid stepping on ropes or cords, as their weight will force dirt particles through the sheath (mantle) of the rope into the rope fibers (kern) and weaken them due to the dirt's abrasive effect. Rope should not be stored with tight knots in place because it will permanently reduce the strength of the rope.

Rope should not be coiled into the storage bags to decrease tangling and twisting. It should instead be "flaked"; this is performed with gloves by holding the edge of the bag with the thumb and index finger of one hand and using the rest of the hand as a channel for the rope. The other hand pulls sections of rope and "flakes" or drops short sections of rope into the bag. The rope should occasionally be settled at the bottom of the bag by shaking the bag against the ground. Once the rope is flaked into the bag, a simple figure eight at the end of the rope allows responders to easily locate the leading end. A rope that has been flaked in a rope bag will be very easy to pull out, and it will not become tangled.

Dirty rope, cord, and webbing can be washed with a mild detergent, rinsed thoroughly, and hung to dry in the shade or placed in a dryer at very low heat. All ropes, cord, and webbing should be thoroughly inspected after cleaning for any signs of wear; if wear is detected, the equipment should not be used in a TLAER rescue. In particular, rope should not be used again for a rescue after it has been subjected to the stress of a shock load (catching the maximum impact force of a weight) in an incident.

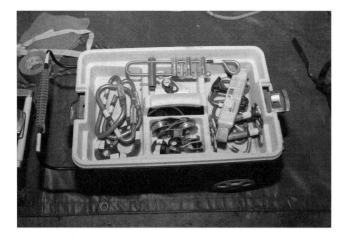

Figure 14.6 *This photograph shows an example of a suitable storage box for rescue hardware. The box organizes the equipment, protects it from damage, and provides quick access on the scene. The far-left compartment contains large gate carabiners and rigging plates. The compartment at the top of the photo contains a six-bar break bar, and the one at the bottom contains two single pulleys and rescue swivels. The right compartment contains additional carabiners, edge protectors, and a lanyard. This box has wheels and is constructed of lightweight plastic; underneath this top tray are additional strings of carabiners and pulleys. Courtesy of Axel Gimenez.*

Hardware Care

Rescue hardware (e.g., carabiners, pulleys, etc.) should never be dropped on the ground and should be inspected after every use for any signs of malfunction or deformation. Rescue hardware should never be repaired after it has been damaged; it should be destroyed to prevent reuse or permanently marked for use in non-live victim training. Rescue hardware can be stored in bags or boxes to prevent rusting or damage (Figure 14.6).

On-Scene Care: Staging Tarps

At the scene of an incident, all rescue equipment should be placed on a tarp known as a staging tarp when not in use. The use of a staging tarp protects the equipment from damage and decreases the risk of equipment loss. Additionally, the equipment can be laid out in a readily visible manner to allow rescuers to select from the cache easily as they assemble a system. Tarps may also be used for covering equipment during precipitation (e.g., rain or snow), covering carcasses, and as field expedients to move victims (see Chapter 11).

COMMON RESCUE KNOTS

The number of different types of knots developed during the last few thousand years is overwhelming, and there are entire collections of books dedicated to knots for a multitude of different purposes. Fortunately, knowledge of a few knots will enable most rope rescue procedures used in TLAER situations.

Table 14.4 Loss in strength of 12.7 mm (.5 in.) kernmantle rope or webbing when tying various knots.

Knot	Strength at Knot (kg)	Loss in Strength (%)
Double fisherman's	3,631	21
Figure 8 bend	3,922	19
Figure 8 loop	3,886	20
Double figure 8 loop	4,004	18
In-line figure 8 loop	3,632	25
Butterfly	3,632	25
Bowline	3,259	33
Water (12.7 mm webbing)	1,389	36

From: Dave Richards. 2007. Knot Break Strength vs. Rope Break Strength. Rescue Response Gear Newsletter. The Cordage Institute, Sugar Land, TX.

Basic Concepts of Knot Anatomy

It is important to understand a few basic concepts that apply to all knots, particularly those used in rescue situations and systems.

- A knot will always reduce the strength of the rope by a certain factor (Table 14.4).
- There are basically two types of knots. Knots that tend to remain tight are called *inherently tight*, for example the figure nine and figure eight knots on a loop. Knots that tend to become loose without applied tension are called *inherently loose*, for example the bowline knot. For obvious reasons, it is preferable to use inherently tight knots in TLAER rope rescue systems. Within the special operations technical rescue community, some operational personnel and instructors will use both types of knots, but it is recommended that TLAER responders use the inherently tight knots.
- After making a rescue knot, one should "dress the knot." Dressing the knot involves ensuring that the portions of the rope in the knot don't ride over top of each other, but are parallel to each other. A knot that is twisted and not properly dressed weakens the rope more than a properly dressed knot and will be extremely difficult to untie once a load has been applied.

Practice at Home

The figure eight, fisherman's knot (used to make Prusik loops), and water knot are fundamental knots that are necessary for several rope rescue procedures. Regular practice of these knots is essential; knot-tying skills should become second nature to TLAER responders. During an incident is not an appropriate time to learn how to make these knots.

THE FIGURE EIGHT KNOT

The figure eight is the most common and useful rescue knot in TLAER. The figure eight knot on a loop is one of the strongest knots used in rescue (Figure 14.7). Additionally, it can be used to make an emergency rope halter (see Chapter 4). This knot retains approximately 65%–75% of the strength of the rope and is very easily untied.

THE FIGURE NINE KNOT

The figure nine knot begins similar to a figure eight knot, but adds an additional half turn to the knot (Figure 14.8). The figure nine knot can be used in any rescue operation where the figure eight knot would be used. The figure nine is stronger than the figure eight knot and retains 70%–85% of the strength of the rope. The figure nine knot is also very easily untied.

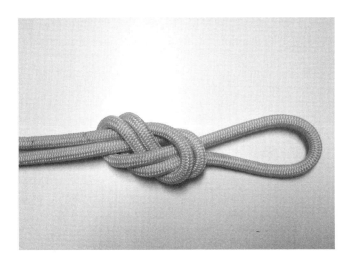

Figure 14.7 *The figure eight knot on a loop is inherently tight and is the most commonly used rescue knot in TLAER. This photograph demonstrates a properly dressed knot, which makes the knot stronger and easier to untie after a load has been placed upon it. Courtesy of Tomas Gimenez.*

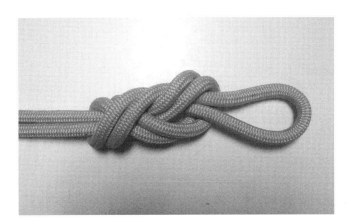

Figure 14.8 *The figure nine knot on a loop as shown is also an inherently tight knot, features greater strength than the figure eight, and is easier to untie. It is tied in a fashion similar to the figure eight knot, but includes an additional half turn of the rope. This knot is correctly dressed. Courtesy of Tomas Gimenez.*

THE PRUSIK LOOP

The Prusik loop is made with cord and has many different applications in large animal rescue. It is formed by tying a double fisherman's (or double mariner's) knot on a 7–8 mm (3/8 in.) diameter cord. For specialty applications such as placement around an extremity, larger Prusik loops of wider diameter (12.7 mm, or 1/2 in.) rope may be used (see Chapter 15).

To tie the double fisherman's knot, the two working ends of the rope are placed overlaying each other and facing opposite directions. The end pointing away from you is wrapped twice around the other line, making an "x" on the rope. The working end is then fed through the wraps beneath the "x" and pulled tight. The set of ropes is then rotated, and the same procedure repeated with the opposite line. The standing ends of the ropes are then pulled away from each other to draw the knots together.

THE PRUSIK HITCH

The Prusik hitch is used to connect the rescue line to a hardware component (e.g., pulley, rigging plate, etc.). It will slide on the rope when not subjected to a load, but will grab the line as soon as a load is placed on the hitch. The holding strength of this Prusik hitch is 1,135 kg.

The Prusik hitch is formed by wrapping the Prusik loop cord three times around the larger rope and passing the knotted end back through the loop (Figure 14.9). The Prusik loop must be soft and have a diameter of 70% or less than the diameter of the rope around which it wraps to obtain the hitch effect. Responders should maintain an assortment of ready-made Prusik loops of three different sizes, small (1.5 m, or 5 ft),

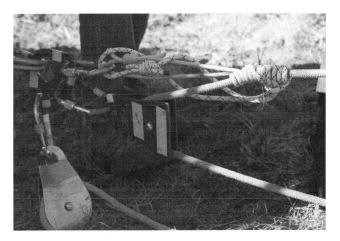

Figure 14.9 *This photograph demonstrates tandem Prusik hitches acting as a friction brake (on the upper right) holding the load on the lifeline of a 9:1 system. These Prusiks must be minded by a person wearing gloves or a Prusik-minding pulley as depicted here. Courtesy of Tomas Gimenez.*

medium (2.2 m, or 7 1/4 ft) and long (3 m, or 10 ft). These lengths refer to cord length from end to end before making the loop. Using different color cord for each loop size facilitates their use and allows quick recognition by the technician.

WHAT IS MECHANICAL ADVANTAGE?

If a rope system is to be used to move a load, the responder can achieve various degrees of mechanical advantage by passing the rope around pulleys placed between the load and the anchor. A mechanical advantage allows movement of a load using only a fraction of the effort needed to move the entire weight of the load. It does not necessarily imply the use of mechanized power equipment to achieve that work; simple rope pulley systems may be used to provide a mechanical advantage.

Mechanical advantage is expressed as the ratio of the force that performs the useful work to the force applied. For example, a 5:1 mechanical advantage system used to lift a 500 kg animal allows the 500 kg weight to be lifted with only 100 kg (one-fifth of 500 kg) of force applied to the system.

Although less force is necessary to move the load, more line must be pulled through the system to achieve movement of the load. For example, in a 3:1 system, the load on the system will be one-third the original weight but will require three times the length of rope to move the same distance. *Note:* When the beginning of the rope is attached to the anchor, the mechanical advantage ratio will be even (2:1, 4:1, etc.); when the beginning of the rope is attached to the load, the mechanical advantage ratio will be odd (3:1, 5:1, 7:1, etc.)

Types of Mechanical Advantage Systems

The type of mechanical advantage system to be assembled will depend on the following:

- Load weight
- Available personnel (it is estimated that a healthy adult can pull an average of 23 kg, or 51 lb)
- Terrain
- The availability of bombproof anchors

Type I Systems

In Type I systems, a static pulley is attached to the anchor. This pulley changes the direction of the force from (b) to (a), but the force required to lift the load does not change. Mechanical advantage is expressed as the ratio of the force (F) needed to move the load to the full weight of the load (L). In this case the force-to-load ratio (F : L) is 1 : 1 (Figure 14.10).

Type II Systems

In Type II systems, a second and moving ("free") pulley is placed between the static pulley and the load and

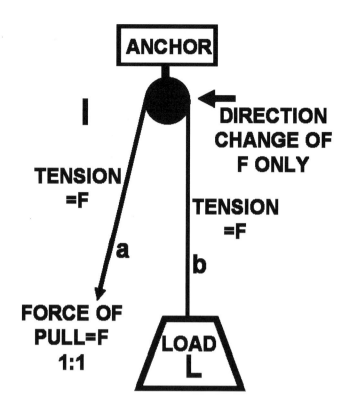

Figure 14.10 *A Type I system provides a 1:1 ratio with a change of direction but does not provide any mechanical advantage to the rescuers moving the weight of a large animal. Courtesy of Tomas Gimenez.*

will move toward the anchor when force is applied to the end of the rope (Figure 14.11). In this example, two segments of rope, that is, the anchor to moving pulley (c) and the free pulley to static pulley (b), share an equal amount of the load (L); in this case, each segment bears one-half of the load. The ratio of (F) to (L) is 2:1. If the load weighs 20 kg (44 lb), a force of 10 kg in (a) will be sufficient to move the full load. In reality, a force somewhat greater than 10 kg must be applied to overcome the friction (although small in magnitude) between the rope and the pulleys.

Type III Systems

Type III mechanical advantage systems have the following characteristics:

- The beginning of the rope (line) is attached to the load (L) instead of the anchor.
- Segment (a) of the rope also shares the load.
- All three segments of the rope (a, b, and c) each move toward the anchor, and each segment bears one-third of the load.

Therefore, a force slightly greater than one-third of the load applied to segment (a) will move the entire load, which gives this system a 3:1 mechanical advantage ratio (Figure 14.12).

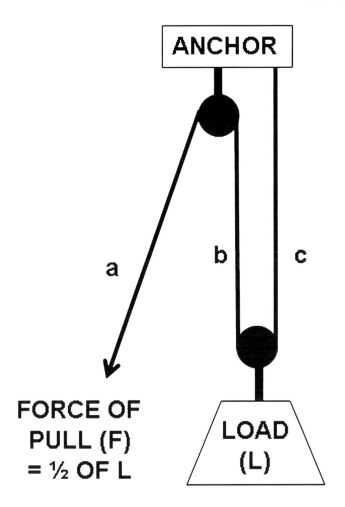

Figure 14.11 *A Type II system provides a 2:1 ratio with the least mechanical advantage that can be achieved by having one pulley that allows the movement of the (b) and (c) segments of the rope toward the anchor. Courtesy of Tomas Gimenez.*

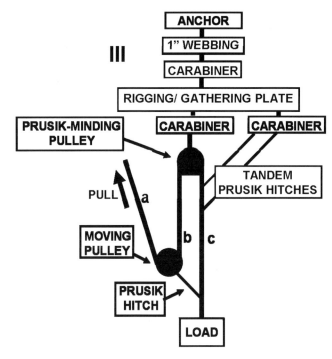

Figure 14.12 *A Type III system provides a 3:1 ratio with a moving pulley that allows the movement (due to the Prusik hitch) of all segments of the rope (a), (b), and (c) toward the anchor. This diagram lays out all components of a typical rope system for a Z-rig system commonly used in human rescue. For TLAER scenarios, this Z-rig will be compounded to generate greater mechanical advantage for the increased weight of the victim. Courtesy of Tomas Gimenez.*

This system resembles the shape of the letter "Z," hence the name *Z-rig* is commonly used to describe these 3:1 systems. The Z-rig is the mechanical advantage system of choice in human rescue based on an average human weight of 85 kg (187 lb). Using a Z-rig, two to three rescuers can easily lift a human victim. In large animal rescue, however, it is necessary to assemble systems that will provide a greater mechanical advantage, that is, ratios of 9:1 to 15:1.

Common Rope Systems Used in TLAER

The heavy loads (animal victims) lifted and moved using rope systems in TLAER scenarios necessitate the use of 9:1 and 15:1 ratio systems to allow the loads to be moved with small numbers of personnel.

The 9:1 System. The 9:1 system is assembled by attaching two Z-rigs or 3:1 systems in a piggyback manner. The first Z-rig bears one-third of the load. The second Z-rig pulls one-third of the load placed on the

first Z-rig (i.e., one-third of one-third of the load), which is one-ninth of the total load, for a 9:1 ratio.

The 15:1 System. The 15:1 system is a combination of a 5:1 and a Z-rig. This type is considered a compound system. The Z-rig pulls one-fifth of the load. The line of the Z-rig is pulled toward the anchor and therefore bears one-third of a fifth, or one-fifteenth, of the total load. The 15:1 system allows rescuers to pull very heavy loads with limited personnel. For example, two to three rescuers can pull an 800 kg (1,760 lb) animal with this system.

ADVANTAGES OF ROPE SYSTEMS

Rope rigging allows the rescuer to assemble a variety of rope systems that move or lift a heavy load in the absence of power equipment and with limited personnel. A rope system or mechanical advantage system has the following advantages over power equipment (e.g., winches or cranes):

- Portable: Rope systems can be carried by personnel to any location.
- Lightweight: Rope systems are very lightweight compared to power equipment.

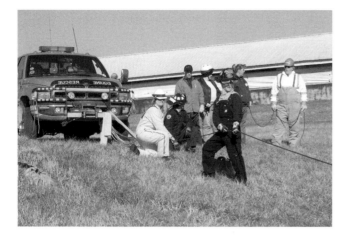

Figure 14.13 *Firefighters and volunteers use a descending brake tube friction system to control manipulation of an overturned horse trailer. In this photograph, the weight of the load has not yet been transferred onto the lifeline, thus it is slack. A chocked vehicle's welded winch frame is being used as the anchor point for this system, and all operational personnel are wearing gloves. Courtesy of Axel Gimenez.*

- Powerful: Rope systems can be assembled that will lift a heavy draft horse (1,000–1,500 kg, or 2,200–3,300 lb) with only two to three rescuers.
- Gentle: Unlike power equipment, rope systems allow slow and gentle movement without sudden stops and jerks. Manual control provides "feel."
- Versatile: Rope systems can be assembled that adapt and function efficiently in any rescue environment where moving or lifting a large animal is necessary (Figure 14.13).

ASSEMBLING A ROPE RESCUE RIG

The basic components needed to assemble a mechanical advantage system include:

- Rope: The most commonly used rope is 12.7 mm (1/2 in.) kernmantle rope. When part of a rope rescue rig, the rope is called a *line* or *lifeline*.
- Prusik loops
- Pulleys (single, double, triple, Prusik-minding): The Prusik-minding pulley has a flat side facing the load. When the rope is pulled and the load moves toward the anchor, the Prusik hitches will slide on the rope when they make contact with the flat side of the pulley, preventing them from being caught or pulled through the pulley.
- Steel carabiners
- Rigging/gathering plates (steel or aluminum plates): Rigging and gathering plates allow placement of up to five components between the rope system and the anchor.
- Webbing loops: Loops of 25 mm (1 in.) webbing are used to link the rope system to the anchor (Table 14.5).

Table 14.5 Standardized color codes for 25.4-mm (1 in.) webbing.

Color	Total Length (m)
Green	1.5
Yellow	3.5
Blue	4.5
Red	6.0
Black	7.5

From: R. Lipke. 1997. *Technical Rescue Guide*, Conterra, Inc., Bellingham, Washington.

- Strong, bombproof anchor(s): An anchor must be sufficiently strong and secure to support several times the weight of the load (e.g., fire apparatus, large truck, large live tree, heavy construction equipment, etc.).

CONTROLLING THE DESCENT OF A HEAVY LOAD

Whether the scenario involves a large animal vertical lift descent or a horse trailer being overturned or manipulated, it is often necessary to lower a load in a very gentle, careful, and slow manner. This descent is often controlled using friction of the rope against itself or a metal hardware friction device. There are a number of friction devices used in rope rescue; equipment choice is based on weight of the load, size and weight of the device, ease of use, etc.

Friction Devices

For light loads (such as average-weight humans), there are friction techniques and equipment such as the Italian or Münter hitch, the figure eight, or the rappelling brake bar that are safe and appropriate for descending and rappelling these loads. Friction devices that use rope-on-rope friction can destroy the rope for future rescue use, especially when used for heavy loads.

Descending Brake Tube

When friction is used to control the descent of heavier loads (e.g., trailers or large animals), it is better to use heavy-duty friction devices such as the 6-bar brake or the brake tube. After using different types of friction devices over the years, the authors prefer the descending brake tube for controlling the descent of heavy loads. The descending brake tube is very strong, easy to use, and can generate enough friction to control the descent of loads weighing several thousand kilograms. The descending brake tube is the most appropriate device for controlling heavy descending loads such as a horse trailer. The more turns of rope around the brake, the greater the control of heavier loads. Using this device, one person can control the descent of a trailer being overturned (Table 14.6).

Table 14.6 Brake tube holding strength when using 12.7-mm (1/2 in.) kernmantle low-stretch rope.

Turns around Brake Tube	Holding Strength kN
4	2.5
5	5.0
6	7.0
7	12.0

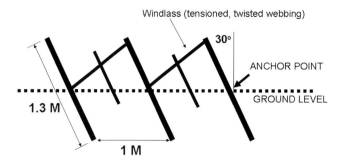

Figure 14.14 *Schematic of the picket anchor system. The picket stakes (3) are driven into the ground at a 30-degree angle away from the load and a wound webbing windlass connects each picket stake into the system, offering increased strength by the increased number of stakes. Courtesy of Tomas Gimenez.*

ANCHORS

Tensionless or High-Strength Hitch

The function of the tensionless or high-strength hitch is based on surface friction and increases with the diameter of the anchor. The more rope turns around the anchor, the stronger the hitch.

Picket Anchor System

Picket anchor systems are used when no other suitable bombproof anchors (e.g., large trees, heavy equipment, etc.) are available (Figure 14.14). Such a scenario in TLAER incidents might require an anchor for stabilization of a trailer on the grassy shoulder of a road. Two people are needed to build a picket anchor system.

The holding strength of the picket anchor system is 816 kg (1,800 lb); however, its security is also determined by the type of soil in which it is built. In good soil, such as a standard loamy soil, 100% of the anchor's holding strength is preserved. In a clay and gravel mix, 90% of holding strength is preserved. In coarse sand, the holding strength is decreased by 50%. This is a 1:1:1 anchor that does not provide a mechanical advantage; it simply allows a strong anchor to be emplaced in a particular position. Pickets are more secure during gradual pulls than during sudden shock loads. Increasing the number of pickets in the system increases the holding strength of the system.

Picket Components
- Picket: the stake driven into the ground to support a load
- Forward picket: the picket located closest to the load
- Lashing material: 25 mm tubular webbing used to link pickets to each other
- Windlass: lashing material between pickets is threaded from picket to picket, and the windlass passes from the top of one picket to the base of the picket behind it

- Deadman: in picket anchor systems, a deadman is an object (e.g., heavy pipe, tree trunk, etc.) placed horizontally between two picket anchor systems and used to support the load

Other Suitable Anchors

Rescuers may use a truck wheel or truck axle as an anchor. The vehicle should be parked with the axle pointing toward the center of the load, the ignition key removed, and wheels of the vehicle chocked. The webbing should be passed around the anchor through the tire wells or around the entire tire and axle. Heavy vehicles are preferred, such as fire apparatus, excavators, tractors, forklifts, or one-ton pickup trucks. If the frame or hitch of a vehicle is used as an anchor, as when using a wheel or axle, the vehicle must be securely chocked and ignition key removed.

In appropriate terrain, extremely large boulders may be used as anchors by wrapping protected fire hose or other webbing around the entire boulder.

Unsuitable Anchors

Telephone and power poles may be rotten and are not recommended as anchors. Fence posts and small or dead trees are similarly poor choices for anchors. The bumper of a vehicle should not be selected for an anchor; in general, the attachment of a bumper to a vehicle is not sufficiently strong to bear a heavy load.

ACRONYMS USED IN CHAPTER 14

kN	kiloNewton
MBS	Maximum Breaking Strength
TLAER	Technical Large Animal Emergency Rescue

15 Manipulating the Animal Victim—Basic Rescue Techniques

Dr. Rebecca Gimenez

INTRODUCTION

The typical large animal victim can be thought of as a 500–1,000 kg (1,100–2,200 lb) object that must be moved, lifted, shifted, or dragged without damage to the animal or injury to the rescuers. There are a limited number of directions in which an animal can be moved: up (vertical lift), down, forward, backward, horizontally, or laterally (to the side). Additional challenges include the victim's temperament and its inability to understand human speech, directions, or the intentions of responders.

Large animal victims can be safely and effectively moved from most situations by using simple methods. A review of public and private videotaped rescues has revealed a lack of knowledge of simple equipment commonly and locally available to facilitate large animal rescues (Gimenez et al., 2003). The stress responses and size of the large animal must be taken into account and might require specialized rescue methods to accommodate its greater weight and powerful reactions.

LET THE VICTIM ASSIST ITSELF

When possible, responders should use techniques that allow the animal itself to provide the propulsion force necessary to escape the entrapment with the guidance and assistance of the human rescuers. The forward assist is the best example of this concept. By placing a sling around the animal's body (Figure 15.1), the animal can still use its head and neck to balance itself, and move its limbs to free itself of the entrapment (Fox, 2005). Other manipulation methods should use the skeletal strength of the torso (e.g., ribcage, pectoral and pelvic girdles) to the advantage of the rescuers. In general the head, neck, or legs are unsuitable anchors for pulling an animal out of an entrapment. A review

of reported and video-documented rescues has revealed that although the animal may survive the initial rescue, iatrogenic soft tissue injuries of the lower limbs, head, and neck incurred reduce the animal's long-term prognosis.

Give the Animal Room

Large animals require a larger area than humans to maneuver; vehicles, equipment, and personnel should not be permitted in close proximity to the incident. The animal handler(s) should be provided with sufficient area to move the animal a safe distance from the incident scene. Most handlers of large animals request a 15 m (50 ft) diameter, obstacle-free area around large animals; this is often unrealistic on an incident scene, but should be considered to maximize safety for both the animal victim and responders. In a learning (practice) environment, personnel must be in close proximity to learn and practice the techniques, but proximity can be dangerous on an actual scene with an unpredictable and excited animal (see Chapter 4).

Training Should Be Realistic

Training for large animal incidents should simulate the realistic environment as closely as possible. The use of live, trained large animals for demonstrations and hands-on work is recommended. However, there are scenarios that are too dangerous for live animal use in training simulations: a realistically weighted mannequin or carcass can be used in these training scenarios. Some teams have purchased or made a mannequin that simulates the weight, size, and flexibility of an animal. A veterinarian or animal control officer may coordinate the donation of a dead animal for training purposes.

A dead cow carcass in the water allows an introduction to the weight and buoyancy of that animal. A dead horse carcass can be donated for practice in extricating

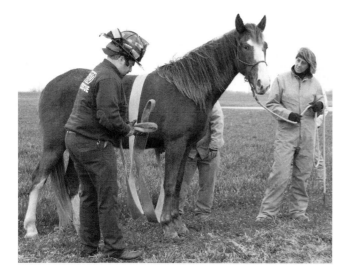

Figure 15.1 *Students practice placing a forward assist around the body of a demonstration horse, feeding the free ends between the front legs. The animal handler is standing to the side in a safe position. Animals may act surprised when the webbing is pulled out in front of them because they cannot see well underneath their chests. This method is excellent as a backup plan for animals being led out of difficult terrain; if they should fall, the rescuers will already have an anchor point in place. Courtesy of Al Filice.*

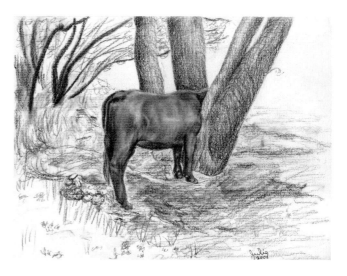

Figure 15.2 *Although the scenario appears simple, this cow with its head stuck in a tree illustrates several challenges to TLAER. If a chainsaw is used to cut one limb, the noise will likely frighten the animal, increasing the risk of responder injury. Performing a vertical lift requires specialized equipment and a lifting mechanism. It is also important to note that this animal may not be accustomed to human handling or the placement of a halter and may be difficult to contain once freed from the entrapment; alternatively, she may demonstrate aggression toward her rescuers. Courtesy of Julie Casil.*

it from an overturned trailer, well, or ravine, etc. If possible, a local veterinarian (encouraged to join as a response team member) should perform a necropsy on the animal afterward to highlight the areas of interest to rescuers (e.g., jugular vein, trachea, skull, and placement of the brain, lower limb structure, etc.).

TYPES OF ENTRAPMENT REQUIRING MANIPULATION OR VERTICAL LITF

Hung on an Obstacle

A large animal trapped halfway over a gate, fence, board, tree limb, or similar obstacle is a common rescue scenario. An animal may become entrapped when it tries to escape an enclosure or while playing. A corollary of this type of rescue is the animal that gets its head or other body part trapped in the crotch of a tree (Figure 15.2), kicks through an object and hangs by a limb, rears and puts a foot through a small trap, or is lying on top of an object with its legs above the ground.

A simple approach is the foundation of a successful and efficient rescue. The following scenario (Figure 15.3) illustrates this point. A horse was trapped hanging halfway over a fence, and the weight of the horse made it impossible to lift its limbs clear of the fence. The responders were horse owners who self-organized quickly designating an animal handler who approached and calmed the horse; an operational responder who brought a reciprocating saw to cut the board on the fence; another operational responder who turned off

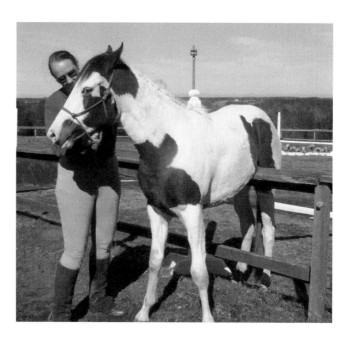

Figure 15.3 *This filly attempted to jump out of an arena when chased by another horse and misjudged the height of the fence. The owner is calming the horse while another rescuer brings a reciprocating saw to cut the board obstructing her movement. Power to the electric fence has been disconnected. Courtesy of Tomas Gimenez.*

the electricity to the fence and took photographs; and a safety officer/incident commander who directed the operation and kept bystanders out of the way during the rescue. The board was cut, and the horse freed uninjured. The keys to the successful rescue included the use of an appropriate tool, a simple approach, and an organized effort.

Other simple options to consider include unbolting, cutting the fence, or disassembling a pipe corral. In another example, a horse became hung on a pipe corral in Felton, California. Rescuers were concerned that the horse would become entangled in the lower rails, and possibly fracture a limb, if the top rail of the corral was removed. To address this concern, they removed the bottom corral rails first and backed the horse instead of leading it forward as another responder lowered the pipe section to the ground. When the animal is backed up under control it is less likely to bolt (surge forward) when its rear feet contact the ground. The jaws of life (hydraulic rescue tools) were used to cut the pipes; this tool is quiet but creates sharp points, so the animal's limbs were padded prior to cutting the pipe (Fox, 2006).

In another incident, a barn manager noticed a Warmblood mare lying down in her stall. On closer inspection, she realized that the mare's hind limb was entrapped between the bars of the stall. The mare was lying with the trapped limb at a strange angle with most of the animal's weight hanging from that leg. The animal, exhausted from struggling all night, was exhibiting signs of shock. The stall bars were cut from the other side of the wall to release the leg. The mare was loaded immediately for transport to veterinary facilities and survived (Gimenez, 1998).

Unfortunately, there is a corollary to this type of incident that is very common and rarely survived by large animal victims, that is, when the animal has impaled itself or has been gored by a sharp object (e.g., fence posts, T-posts, limbs, heavy farm equipment, or the horns of cattle). These animals struggle and may manage to dislodge themselves, but often sustain life-threatening or fatal injury (including evisceration, hemorrhage/exsanguination, punctured lung, cardiac trauma, etc.). These injuries often necessitate field euthanasia (see Chapter 13). If the animal is impaled but salvageable, first aid on the scene includes cutting off the impaling object close to the animal's skin, packing the wound, and transporting the animal for immediate veterinary care.

Cast Animals

There are several pieces of emergency rescue equipment that can be adapted to assisting an older or arthritic horse to rise. The choice of equipment used depends on the location of the recumbent animal; a down horse in an open pasture is more easily assisted than one in a stall. Animals of all species and ages can become trapped on their backs; horses may become trapped ("cast") in this manner in a stall or on ice in a pasture. As stated in previous chapters, it is important to keep personnel away from the limbs. The animal should

be assessed for injuries, particularly of the entrapped limbs, prior to assisting it to rise.

A simple option involves pulling the cast animal away from the wall by flossing a rescue strap or webbing around the animal's girth and pulling it horizontally using the strap or webbing, the mane, and possibly the tail (Fox, 2006). Rolling a cast animal increases the risk of injury to the animal and the rescuers.

Rolling Procedure. A cast animal can be righted by looping or twisting a soft cotton rope over the lower (down) limb at the junction of the rear hoof and the pastern and pulling the rope in a slightly cranial direction (toward the head) at about a 45-degree angle to the body until the horse rolls over and is able to rise. If there are two or more people present, both lower legs can be looped with rope to pull the animal (Figure 15.4). Caution is advised when performing this procedure in a trailer or stall, as the animal will often struggle and flail its limbs as it rolls and rises. It is recommended that the ropes be of sufficient length to allow the rescuer(s) to be outside the stall when pulling.

There are several equine slings available for lifting recumbent or injured animals (see Chapter 16). If the animal is recumbent due to arthritis, neurologic disease, starvation, or other medical conditions, rolling or raising the animal provides short-term resolution. A "stretcher" or "stone boat" sked, such as the Rescue Glide, can be used to transport animals from the pasture to a sheltered location, barn, or veterinary facilities via ambulance trailer (see Chapter 11). The Rescue Glide provides a safe and efficient method of securing the patient ("package" the animal) for transport. Some animals may need to be sedated by a veterinarian to reduce the risk of injury to the animal victim or

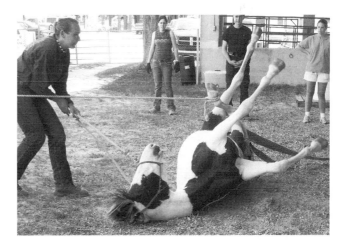

Figure 15.4 *In a demonstration, a long cotton rope is slipped around the pastern on the dependent (bottom) rear limb of a cast horse. The horse was rolled by two people pulling at a 45-degree angle over the animal's head and supporting the head with a taut lead rope as it rolls over. Personnel should remain a safe distance from the horse, especially in close quarters. Courtesy of Tori Miller.*

personnel. In other cases, responders have successfully moved a recumbent animal patient on the Rescue Glide without any sedation, hobbles, or packaging. Geriatric and medically compromised animals may experience less detrimental effects (mental and clinical) without physical and chemical restraint and usually tolerate this transport method. (Fox, 2006).

Trapped in Mud, Unstable Ground, or Ice

An animal trapped in mud, unstable ground, or ice requires specialized equipment and personal protective equipment for rescuers because of the additional hazards presented by water or threat of entrapment. The partial vacuum (suction) of mud can be overcome by use of the Nikopolous needle and air and water injection next to the extremities of the animal during a horizontal haul or vertical lift. Various appliances such as webbing for the forward assist, Hampshire slip, or backward drag configurations may be used to access an anchor point on the animal in the rescue environment. Recent technological improvements in equipment and methods for surface ice rescue of humans can be applied to large animals (see Chapter 7).

Animals Trapped in Confined Spaces

Large animals are commonly trapped in overturned horse trailers (see Chapter 9), farm equipment and culverts, under fallen trees or collapsed barns, and in ditches or trenches, wells or manure pits. These scenarios may require responders to consider specialized aspects of stabilizing the scene (e.g., air quality monitoring, shoring trenches to prevent collapse, shoring to prevent overhead collapse) before accessing the animal victim, and are beyond the scope of this book. On these scenes, bystanders or untrained responders should consult with emergency response professionals before allowing any person to enter the rescue environment. Trench collapse, inadequate ventilation, overhead collapse, and animal-induced injuries have contributed to deaths of responders annually.

Placing an appliance of webbing onto animals in these confined space incidents is often the simplest approach to removing the animal to safety. An operational person should approach and place webbing as an anchor point for the use of a forward assist, Hampshire slip, or backward drag. If only the extremities are accessible, hobbling the lower legs is an appropriate method of getting an anchor point for haul systems.

Trapped on Steep Terrain or Cliffs

Numerous reports of large animals slipping off riding trails (horses) or pasture (cattle and horses) have been documented by the author. In most cases, the animals are uninjured; in the remaining cases, the injuries sustained tend to be fatal and require immediate field euthanasia. Medical stabilization may be the first priority for these animals before attempting rescue. For

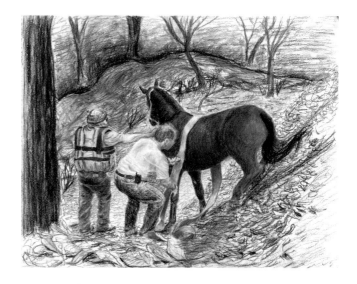

Figure 15.5 *A horse trapped in steep terrain is ready to be led out by responders, but as a backup plan the forward assist webbing is being emplaced around the animal's thorax. If the animal slips farther down the cliff, rescuers will have a prepositioned anchor point on the animal to assist it along the trail that was cut to lead it out. Courtesy of Julie Casil.*

example, a horse that slipped off a trail in the mountains of Tennessee in 2002 was found in dorsal recumbency (upside down) trapped between a tree and a large boulder. Due to darkness and inclement weather conditions, rescuers were forced to abandon the animal until the following morning. When a team of rescuers hiked 10 km (6.2 miles) up the mountain to reach the animal early the next morning, the animal had managed to extricate itself overnight and was standing on the trail, apparently uninjured. The horse was led to a trailer and transported immediately to a veterinary clinic, where it received extensive medical treatment for hypothermia and dehydration.

The use of a forward assist to support the animal as it is led out on a trail to safe ground is recommended (Figure 15.5). Cutting a trail for the animal is the most simple response scenario, despite the additional time it may require. Responders should remember that leading the animal down the terrain profile may be easier than bringing the animal back up to where it started.

Alternatively, these scenarios have required vertical lift equipment (see Chapter 16) and in appropriate circumstances, a helicopter sling load may be considered (see Chapter 18).

GENERAL RULES FOR MANIPULATION OF LARGE ANIMALS

Find a Way to Use the "Motor"

A large animal needs freedom to move its head and neck to balance itself; the weight of the head and neck acts as a fulcrum and as the "steering axle." An animal that is healthy should not be prevented from using its legs or head and neck to climb a hill, thus providing the drive axle or "motor" (propulsion and power) to rescue itself with only guidance from the humans. The torso is the best site for placement of forward assist, backward drag, and vertical lift configurations.

No Ropes on the Legs. Tying an animal's legs compromises its ability to balance and move, prevents the animal from assisting in its own rescue, and increases struggling and anxiety. However, it is a very common scenario in videos and photos of animal rescues reviewed by the authors. The lower limbs are sensitive to pressure injuries and have minimal soft tissues underneath the skin, thus increasing the risk of iatrogenic injury associated with tying the limbs.

In one California response using early technologies, ropes were placed around the pasterns of a large horse lying on the roof of an overturned two-horse straight-load horse trailer and attached to the winch of a tow truck. Despite sedation, the horse violently fought the ropes and pressure, immediately stood up inside the horse trailer, and backed itself out into the roadway. Fortunately, the animal was protected by a horse blanket and shipping wraps and suffered no injuries. This and other similar attempts have shown that the extremities make poor anchor points for equipment and line haul.

There are scenarios where rescuers may have no other option but to use the limbs as anchors. In another rescue a 750 kg (1,650 lb) prize Angus bull had fallen 22 m (72 1/2 feet) down a rock-sided sinkhole in South Carolina, and the only part of the animal accessible to rescuers was the animal's hind limbs. Using hobbles and padded Prusik loops (Figure 15.6) around the long

bones and pasterns of the rear limbs, the bull was successfully lifted straight up and out of the hole by a large crane. The veterinarian had to remove the straps with no containment or physical restraint of the dazed animal, but the animal had not sustained injuries. Support of the head and neck for these lifts is important to prevent iatrogenic injury. When the animal is lifted in the dorsally recumbent (on it's back) position, it is important to provide support to the head to avoid overextension of the neck. When the animal is in cranial recumbency (head down) and one or both hind limbs are used as anchor points for lifting, it is not possible to provide support to the head.

No Ropes on the Head or Neck. As stated previously, the heads and necks of large animals are not suitable or safe anchor points or handles for dragging or manipulation. A good rescue should prevent an uninjured animal victim from becoming a casualty of the rescue effort. Large animals use their heads and necks— approximately 10% of body weight in a horse, or 50–75 kg (110–165 lb)—to balance themselves by moving them up and down or laterally (to the sides). Rescuers should avoid immobilizing the head and neck with appliances; a halter and lead rope is excellent for guidance, support, and restraint to prevent the animal from becoming loose but should not be an attachment point for rescue equipment (see Chapter 6).

Rather, the torso should be used as the anchor for equipment (e.g., webbing or slings) for the rescue. The rib cage and pelvis are stronger and closer to the animal's center of body mass. The lower limbs are easily traumatized because of the comparative lack of muscle and soft tissue interposed between the skin and the nerves, blood vessels, tendons, and ligaments of the lower limb.

Increase the Surface Area

One rule of large animal rescue is to maximize the surface area of the equipment or appliance in contact with the body of the animal to minimize the pressure placed by the webbing, ropes, or attachment points on the animal's tissues and muscle. This can be accomplished using field-expedient padding (e.g., T-shirt, towel, flat piece of fire hose webbing, etc.) or specialty padding (e.g., tarps, fleece, or foam padding, larger diameter rope, extra wide webbing) between the animal and the equipment. In addition, minimizing the time of contact between the equipment and the skin and body tissues will also reduce injuries.

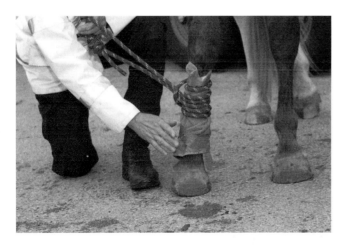

Figure 15.6 *A 3 m (10 ft) Prusik loop can be attached to an extremity in incidents where the limbs must be used as handles to manipulate or move the animal. Padding in the form of a T-shirt or towel is recommended, as are as many wraps of the loop as possible around the limb. Courtesy of Axel Gimenez.*

SIMPLE TOOLS AND EQUIPMENT FOR MANIPULATION OF THE ANIMAL

Webbing

The most commonly used rescue tool on TLAER scenes is a 6-to 9 m (20–30 ft) section of 10 cm (4 in.) webbing,

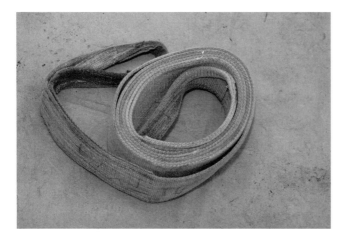

Figure 15.7   *About 7–9 m (23–30 ft) of sewn 10 cm (4 in.) webbing with loops on each end constitute the most valuable and flexible piece of TLAER equipment. It may be used for the backward drag, Hampshire slip, forward assist, as an anchor point in a modified vertical lift, etc. Courtesy of Axel Gimenez.*

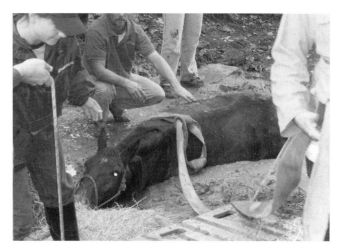

Figure 15.8   *The Nikopoulos needle allows webbing to be pulled underneath the chest of this animal stuck in mud. The webbing is applied in a lark's foot configuration (modified Santa Barbara sling). The owner authorized sedation of the animal, so it was offered alfalfa hay to keep it distracted until all equipment was emplaced, then it was sedated for removal. Courtesy of Tori Miller.*

also called a rescue strap, developed by Tim Collins (Figure 15.7). Discarded fire hose can be used to create a rescue strap by cutting off the ends and sewing loops of various sizes and lengths. This tool may be used as an appliance on the animal in forward assist, backward drag, Hampshire slip, or simple vertical lift configurations.

Webbing can also be used to protect ropes and other pieces of webbing at anchor points and across sharp edges, as padding for the animal, or as the anchor on the animal's body. Webbing of various lengths and widths for rescue use may be locally available.

When an animal is trapped in dorsal recumbency, only the lower limbs are accessible as an anchor point for lifting the animal. In this case, commercially available hobbles can be used around the pasterns for a rapid lift to safe ground. The majority of equine surgical facilities use pastern hobbles and an overhead hoist system to move anesthetized horses for short distances without injury. In the absence of hobbles, a triple wrap Prusik hitch made with 12 mm (1/2 in.) kernmantle rope can be placed around the pastern and cannon bone on each leg. This will increase the surface area of the rope by a factor of 12 and minimize injury. Protective material (e.g., shipping boot, sweatshirt sleeve, etc.) should be placed between the Prusik hitch and the skin.

The head and neck should always be supported by a halter and lead rope held by a responder or secured (but easily released) to the lifting mechanism. Allowing the head to hang during lifting can cause overextension of the neck and injuries of the cervical (neck) region, skull, or face.

Nikopoulos Needle

Developed in the United States by Dr. Tomas Gimenez in collaboration with Dr. Dino Nikopoulos of Shelby,

North Carolina, this equipment has been modified to improve its efficacy in rescue response. This tool is a 2 m (6.6 ft) section of 12 mm (1/2 in.) stainless steel tube bent into a "c" shape, with a steel loop at one end and a garden hose connector welded to the opposite end. It acts similar to a suture needle to drive webbing or a pilot line underneath an animal deeply entrenched in mud or unstable ground. The strop guide is not generally suitable for this purpose because the curvature of the guide is too shallow; the curve of the Nikopoulos needle closely follows the curve of the animal's thorax or abdomen (Figure 15.8). This allows rescuers to approach a recumbent animal from a dorsal (back) position and feed ropes or straps of webbing under and around the animal's body.

Procedure.   To use the Nikopoulos needle, a garden hose is connected to its adapter, and water is allowed to flow through the device and exit the loop end. An operational person stands behind the animal's back, out of the range of the feet and head. The loop end of the needle is pushed into the mud from the rescuer's side and passed underneath the animal, following the contour of the chest or abdomen. Water flows continuously through the needle during this procedure to create a path through the mud to facilitate the needle's passage. Due to the curve in this tool, when pushed down and under an animal (either directly behind the withers or in front of the hips, or both), the free end will be forced underneath and around the animal through the mud or ground surface, and upward on the opposite side of the animal. If the needle encounters an obstacle such as a leg or log, the end of the needle is slightly redirected and gently pushed until it passes without resistance (Figure 15.9).

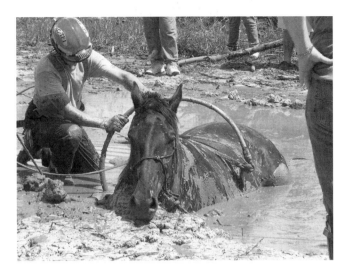

Figure 15.9 *The Nikopoulos needle is used like an oversized suture needle to pass a pilot cord underneath the animal. This allows operational personnel to pull webbing around a large horse trapped in mud and configure it for a vertical lift or horizontal haul. Courtesy of Tori Miller.*

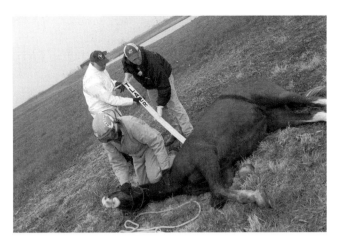

Figure 15.10 *Students practice pushing the strop guide under a recumbent animal to safely and easily pull or push rope or webbing around the torso of the animal. Courtesy of Axel Gimenez.*

Once the loop of the needle appears from underneath the animal, a pilot line of rope, 2 cm (3/4 in.) webbing, or the rescue straps can be attached. The needle is then threaded in the reverse direction, following the curve of the needle, and pulled back underneath the animal to place rescue webbing in the Hampshire slip, backward drag, or forward assist methods.

Strop Guide

Developed by the Hampshire Fire Brigade, United Kingdom, the strop guide is made of 2 m (6.6 ft) long by 7 cm (3 in.) wide by 3 mm (1/8 in.) thick, cold rolled steel. A t-bar handle is attached at one end and the opposite end is rounded, with a cut slit to accommodate 12 mm (1/2 in.) nylon web. The guide's curve closely approximates the curvature of one side of a large animal's torso (Figure 15.10). The strop guide allows rescuers to approach a recumbent animal from behind its back and easily feed straps or webbing underneath it. The tool is especially valuable for placing webbing around animals lying near the surface of mud or unstable ground.

Procedure. To use a strop guide, an operational person should stand behind the animal, out of range of its feet and head. The rounded end of the strop guide is lubricated with petroleum jelly (or obstetrical lube), then pushed underneath the animal directly behind the withers or in front of the hips (Figure 15.11). Due to the natural curve in the tool, the free end will be guided underneath and around one side of the animal's body to a point past the animal's limbs, and the length of the guide ensures that the free end of the guide clears the animal's hooves. The straps or a rope pilot line is

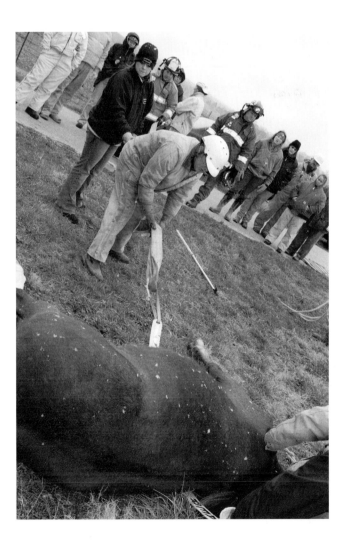

Figure 15.11 *Once under the torso, a pilot of webbing is attached to the strop guide, which can then be pulled back underneath the horse to attach webbing for a horizontal pull. Courtesy of Axel Gimenez.*

attached, and the guide is pulled back underneath the animal for emplacement in the Hampshire slip sideways drag, backward drag, or forward assist.

Mud Lance

Also developed by the Hampshire Fire Brigade, the mud lance is constructed of stainless steel tubing (1.5 m by 12 mm, or 5 ft by $\frac{1}{2}$ in.), with a garden hose connection welded at the top end. This tool is used to insufflate air or water into the mud around the extremities of animals to break the partial vacuum (suction) before extraction (see Chapter 7). The piercing applicator, used by many fire departments to pierce through sheetrock and spray water on the other side of the wall, may also be used as a mud lance.

BASIC METHODS OF MANIPULATION

"Flossing" of Webbing

In certain scenarios it might be easier to "floss" a segment of webbing underneath the animal to establish an anchor point (i.e., for pulling the animal onto a sked, using a forward assist or backward drag, etc.). This can be accomplished from the hind end or the front end.

Procedure. To use the flossing technique, a 5 m (16 1/2 ft) section of fire hose, webbing, or rope is laid on the ground next to the animal's front or hind end. There should be at least two people at each end of the webbing or hose. The animal's tail (or head) is lifted slightly while the teams slip the webbing underneath its hind end (or head and neck) (Figure 15.12). The teams move toward the center of the animal and pull

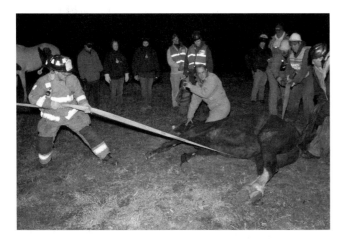

Figure 15.12 *Flossing webbing under the recumbent or trapped animal is an excellent way to feed rope or webbing around the animal's torso. Here, two teams work together to floss webbing from the rear end of the animal toward the withers to place an anchor point for a horizontal pull. Courtesy of Axel Gimenez.*

rhythmically, first one team then the other, to floss the webbing underneath the animal until it is threaded to an anchor point (e.g., immediately behind the withers and forelimbs or immediately in front of the pelvis and hind limbs).

Using webbing around the body as an appliance facilitates manipulation of the animal onto a drag mat (such as the Rescue Glide), movement to a location where it can rise unassisted, or as a backup anchor around the animal in case other equipment fails. Any size webbing can be introduced with 2 cm (3/4 in.) webbing placed as a guide. Rescuers keep their angles flat to the ground as they floss the webbing, pulling as gently as possible to avoid friction burns of the animal's skin (Fox, 2006).

Forward Assist

The forward assist method was originally developed by Tim Collins of Santa Barbara, California, and used by Cpt. John and Debra Fox of Felton, California. The forward assist method uses a rescue strap of webbing over the top of the animal's torso (behind the withers) and threaded between the animal's front legs to allow human rescuers to assist the animal with forward movement. These techniques can be used on standing and laterally or sternally recumbent animals, as well as on animals trapped in mud or tight spaces (e.g., collapsed barns, etc.).

Procedure. Using a 15 m (50 ft) section of 12–15 cm (5–6 in.) webbing with loops sewn at each end, operational personnel approach the animal on each side and floss the webbing underneath the animal. For animals in lateral recumbency, the strop guide may be used to place the webbing on the dependent (down) side of the animal.

The webbing is wrapped around the animal in one of two configurations. In the basket configuration, one end of the webbing is wrapped around the animal's chest at the level of the withers, and both ends of the webbing are threaded evenly between the front legs and in front of the animal (Figure 15.13). In the lark's foot, (also called choke or cinch) configuration, one end of the webbing is wrapped around the animal's chest at the level of the withers (caudal or directly behind the shoulder blades of the animal), fed through the loop in the other end of the webbing, and threaded between the front limbs of the animal. Unlike the basket configuration, this configuration tightens around the animal's body and will not slip over the limbs to allow the animal to slide out of the webbing. However, this configuration is recommended only for preventing catastrophic loss of the animal during a horizontal haul (Figure 15.14) out of unstable ground or for vertical lift from small holes, because it places significant pressure around the ribs and sternum of the animal.

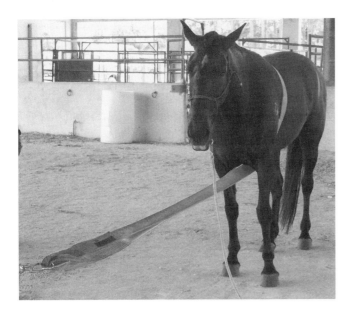

Figure 15.13 *In this demonstration, 9 m (30 ft) of webbing has been emplaced around the animal's chest and the free ends fed threaded between the front legs to a pulling system for a forward assist. Note the lead rope is for guidance and restraint only. Courtesy of Tori Miller.*

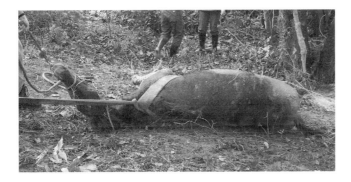

Figure 15.14 *The use of 9 meters (30 ft) of lark's-footed webbing around this animal's chest demonstrates that even this unsedated animal will not struggle while there is pressure from a steady pull on the chest. The animal was pulled 5 m (16 1/2 ft) out of mud by manual methods. Upon release of the pressure, the animal immediately rose. Courtesy of Tori Miller.*

The free end(s) of the webbing is (are) attached to a manual or mechanical rope system for the line haul. To prevent the animal from stepping on the webbing or the attached rope system, a loop can be placed around the lowest part of the neck (similar to a martingale) to hold the webbing out of the way of the moving limbs.

Note: These configurations should never be used with a mechanical (winch) or motorized (vehicle) pull device. Similarly, they should not be used if the animal is trapped underneath an obstacle (e.g., tree limb, barn wall, etc.) or entrapped in mud without the benefit of air or water injection to break the suction effect of the mud on the animal's extremities. Both configurations

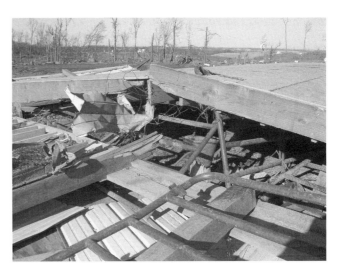

Figure 15.15 *A tornado destroyed this barn, and there may be horses trapped alive under the debris. Rescuing animals from confined spaces such as this requires a plan and simple methods of horizontal pull such as backward drag or forward assist. Courtesy of Joseph Stokely.*

place pressure on the animal's chest during the forward assist, and animals have been asphyxiated or have sustained rib or chest injuries when excessive pressure is placed (as in that generated by motorized devices or strong pulling against mud suction). If an animal's chest cavity has been compromised by the entrapment or incident, an alternate means of moving the animal is recommended to avoid further injury. The veterinarian on the scene should monitor all equipment applications and provide recommendations according to the situation and existing injuries; the rescue straps can be reconfigured if necessary (Fox, 2006).

Backward Drag

Developed by Tim Collins and used by Cpt. John and Debra Fox, this method allows the rescuer to emplace a web appliance around the hindquarters of an animal to drag it backward out of the entrapment. This technique can be used on laterally and sternally recumbent animals as well as animals trapped in tight spaces (e.g., horse trailer, collapsed barns, etc.; Figure 15.15) without compromising the safety of rescuers. The pelvic area of a large animal is very strong and provides an excellent anchor point for the webbing. One problem with the backward drag is abduction (spreading) of the hind limbs as the pelvis is pulled; this may allow the webbing to slide over the tuber coxae (the prominence on the outside of the pelvis that anchors the webbing in front of the pelvis) and slip off the animal. However, rescuers should avoid tying the distal hind limbs together because this places significant strain on the limbs and hip joints. Operational personnel may need to adjust the angle of pull to prevent slipping of the webbing (Fox, 2006). There are few scenarios the author can

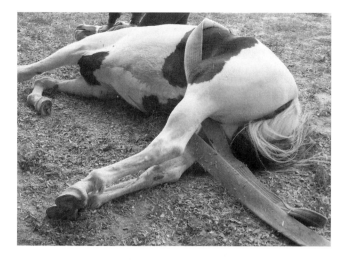

Figure 15.16 *To accomplish a backward drag, the webbing is flossed under the animal to the level of the pelvis and the free ends pulled back between the rear legs to a pulling system (manual or rope system preferred). Courtesy of Tori Miller.*

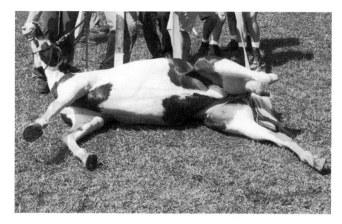

Figure 15.17 *Close-up view of the webbing placed around the dependent (downside) pelvis of a demonstration horse in preparation for the Hampshire slip method for a sideways drag. Courtesy of Claudia Sarti.*

imagine where this method would be used on a standing animal, except perhaps one that refuses to leave a horse trailer or culvert.

Procedure. To perform a backward drag, a 15 m (50 ft) section of 12–15 cm (5–6 in.) webbing with loops sewn at each end is flossed around the animal in either the basket or lark's foot configurations.

In the basket configuration, one end of the webbing is wrapped around the animal's abdomen at the level of the flank or hips, and both ends are passed evenly between the rear legs behind the animal. On a recumbent animal, this can be accomplished by the flossing method described above (Figure 15.16) or by using the strop guide to place the webbing on the dependent (down) side.

In the lark's foot configuration, one end of the webbing is wrapped around the animal's abdomen at the level of the flank (cranial or directly in front of the animal's pelvis), fed through the loop in the other end of the webbing, and threaded between the rear legs and behind the animal. The free end(s) of the webbing is then attached to a manual or mechanical rope system for the line haul or vertical lift. An alternative to this is the Hampshire slip method for a sideways drag (Figure 15.17).

This method should not be selected as a primary extrication method except in situations where an animal falling out of the appliance would result in catastrophic injuries. It is sufficient as a backup system for a vertical lift where the only anchor point consists of hobbles on the animal's rear legs. This method places significant pressure on the animal's abdomen and should be employed for the shortest time possible.

Removal of Animals from Trailers. This application of the backward drag was developed by Cpt. John and Debra Fox to allow placement of webbing on a recumbent large animal entrapped in an overturned trailer or similar enclosed space (e.g., culvert, collapsed barn) without requiring the rescuers to enter the space with the animal. Webbing is introduced into the trailer and placed around the animal using long poles passed through natural openings in the trailer walls, doors, or windows. The webbing is flossed under the animal from the outside of the trailer into the forward assist or backward drag configurations, and the haul system attached.

Sideways Drag (Hampshire Slip)

Developed in Hampshire, United Kingdom, to allow rescuers to safely pull a large animal over the ground surface of mud on tidal flats, this method has numerous uses in other scenarios to safely manipulate an animal's body. If webbing straps are emplaced around an animal and traction is applied, the animal's body acts as a natural pulley and rolls over, driving the limbs into the ground and increasing resistance to the pulling effort.

The sideways drag method uses the animal's limbs to provide pressure on the webbing, preventing the pulley action and maintaining the animal in a position with its limbs facing away from the system; this allows rescuers to efficiently and safely pull the animal. This technique relies on the tendency of an animal's body to become distorted when laying on a flat surface. The straps are placed around the dependent (down) limbs and drawn underneath the body; as the webbing is pulled, the animal is partially lifted (P. Baker, 2006).

Procedure. To use the sideways drag, two pieces of 7 m (23 ft) long webbing are pushed under the animal from behind its back at the spinal column, toward its belly

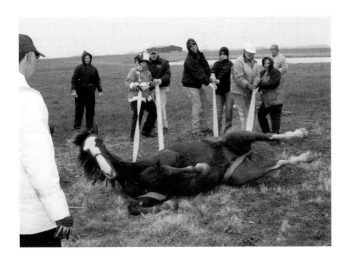

Figure 15.18 *In the Hampshire slip or sideways drag, two pieces of webbing are worked under the animal's body. One free end is pulled between the front legs and underneath the neck, and the other between the hind legs. Courtesy of Tori Miller.*

(ventral abdomen), at the midpoint of its body (from head to tail) using the flossing method, the strop guide, or Nikopoulos needle. Using a cane or other method to lift the animal's legs, one strap is pulled back through and between the front legs and underneath the animal's head and neck; the other strap is pulled backward between the rear legs and passed to the rear of the animal (Figure 15.18). A pulling method (manual or rope system) is attached to the four free ends of the webbing, and the animal is pulled so that its back (spinal column) is the leading edge of the animal's body.

Note: If the animal is pulled on an abrasive surface (e.g., asphalt, gravel, sand, etc.), the abrasive effects can be ameliorated by placement of a tarp underneath the animal, spreading hay or straw over the drag route, or use of a drag mat, sked, or inflatable rescue path.

Tail Tie

The authors strongly discourage pulling a large animal by its tail, regardless of the circumstances associated with the rescue. Pulling an animal by its tail can cause severe injuries. The authors are aware of a scenario where a horse was pulled by its tail; the tail as avulsed (separated) at the level of the coccygeal vertebrae, exposing the spinal canal and pelvic cavity. The horse was euthanatized due to the severity of the injury.

Barrel Tie

This method may have limited use in rescue to immobilize cattle. Although not commonly used, the technique is described here for information. This tie begins with a simple loop around the neck of the animal that is then placed in a barrel pattern around the animal's

chest, then posterior abdomen. When the free end of the rope is pulled backward, the animal will lie down and remain immobilized as long as pressure on the rope is maintained.

In the United Kingdom, this tie method is used on dairy cattle to allow students to practice TLAER methodologies on unsedated animals during training sessions (P. Baker, 2006).

Hobbles

Hobbles provide anchor points on the animal's limbs when there is no other option available. Because the rescuer must be in close proximity to the animal's limbs to place the hobbles, this procedure is associated with increased risk of injury; animals should be approached from a safe position by a rescuer wearing head protection (i.e., hard hat). The veterinarian may opt to anesthetize or sedate the animal before attachment of the hobbles to limit movement of the animal victim.

This equipment is used commonly in veterinary hospitals to vertically lift large animals in dorsal recumbency for surgical procedures and is locally available through horse tack vendors or veterinary supply companies. Hobbles should be made of heavy-duty leather or webbing with fleece or padding to protect the skin of the pastern or cannon bones of the extremity to which it is attached.

Extensions of the Arm

Tools that provide extensions of the human arm to introduce webbing or manipulate ropes and webbing around the animal's extremities should be considered to prevent injuries to rescuers. Other uses for these poles may be to shove webbing under overturned trailers, across water obstacles, or to apply an emergency rope halter to an animal's head. Canes can be used to physically manipulate the extremities of an animal.

Poles may include lightweight aluminum poles such as golf ball retrievers, human extensible walking canes, painting poles, or pike poles used by the fire service.

LUBRICATION

One major factor encountered in all of the procedures described in this chapter is that of friction. In addition to moving the victim's weight, the rescue procedure must overcome the resistance offered by friction during the rescue. Therefore the use of lubrication between the victim and the underlying surface will facilitate the rescue. Examples of effective lubricants are obstetrical lube (carboxy-methylcellulose) or liquid detergent. In any case the lubricant should be water soluble because oil-based lubricants will damage rescue equipment.

16 Manipulating the Animal Victim—Vertical Lift Techniques

Dr. Rebecca Gimenez

INTRODUCTION

Due to their prey instincts, weight, and sensitive nature, large animals present challenges to removal from entrapment in mud, swimming pools, septic tanks, or steep ravines. Vertical lift is one of the most commonly required techniques for movement of large animals when a horizontal pull is not possible; it can be performed with locally available equipment and webbing. The use of slings to lift and suspend trapped, geriatric, or injured animals has resulted in the successful rescue of many horses. Technological advancements have been made, (Figure 16.1), but there are also simple field-expedient sling systems that can be assembled on scene from appropriate materials.

Typical lifting equipment (i.e., cranes) may be difficult to bring to the scene: for that reason A-frames and tripods are discussed in this chapter. Alternatively, mechanical rope systems may be employed (see Chapter 14). These methods may also be necessary for lifting recumbent, neurologically impaired, or ataxic animals in clinical scenarios. With prolonged recumbency, animals are at significant risk of developing respiratory, muscular, neurological, gastrointestinal, and psychological disease, as well as skin and soft tissue injuries (see Chapter 20). The use of the UC Davis-Anderson Sling is well suited for long-term clinical support and helicopter rescue scenarios (see Chapter 18).

EARLY ATTEMPTS AT LIFTING ANIMALS

Canvas slings have been used since 1450 AD (or earlier) to lift large animals onto transport ships for war or exploration. Columbus' crew used slings to lift the animals onto their ships for transport to North America. The militaries of many countries used these techniques well into the 20th century, and even today U.S. military units use helicopters to move pack animals into areas that are difficult to traverse except on foot.

In 1898, as documented in Howard-Smith's (1912) *The History of Battery A*, the troops loaded hundreds of artillery horses and mules onboard the transport *Manitoba*, en route to Puerto Rico during the Spanish-American War. Two journal entries illustrate the challenges.

> Friday, August 5. To-day we loaded mules and horses. We had to sling the mules and killed one that dropped out of the sling.
>
> Sunday, August 14. Helped unload the horses, they had to be swung from the ship 35 feet from the deck and would kick like mad in mid-air.

In 1875, the American Society for the Prevention of Cruelty to Animals developed a horse rescue sling for supporting a debilitated animal in a stall. The challenge has always been that large animals are frequently uncooperative victims and may struggle violently against the sling restraint. Improvements in materials and technology have led to the development of a wide variety of sling systems (some species specific) for large animals.

TYPES OF SIMPLE WEB AND ROPE SLINGS AND SLING SYSTEMS

Simple web and rope slings use material wrapped around the body mass of the animal in various configurations to support the animal's weight and balance it during a short (5–15 minute) lift. These slings are not designed for long-term support of geriatric or injured animals, but rather are used to lift the animal out of entrapment or up onto its feet so that it may walk.

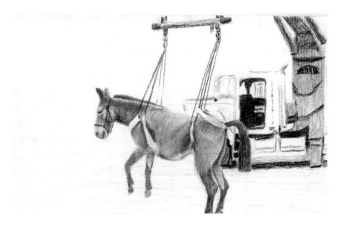

Figure 16.1 *Research and development into methods of simple vertical lift using locally available webbing (i.e., on a responding fire truck) has determined that support of the chest, sternum, and abdominal area is sufficient for equids, which do not have anatomical features to maintain secure placement of a strap across the hindquarters. It is obvious that the strap does not provide support for this mule. However, the rear strap is important in cattle for vertical lift. Courtesy of Julie Casil.*

Figure Eight Rope or Web Sling

A rope or web figure eight sling was the standard for use on large animals for many years by several rescue and humane groups, and it is still used today by many responders. Live demonstration testing of the method on horses (T. Gimenez, 2000) revealed that the technique was difficult for responders to learn and uncomfortable for the animals compared to more advanced sling systems. Other instructors and responders have noted that this sling remains a viable rescue option and offers the benefits of a low lift point and security without requiring tension. For this reason, it has been used to successfully lift many uninjured but entrapped animals from situations where dropping the animal could be catastrophic. Adjustments to the knot to increase security and decrease bulk place the "handle" over the animal's spinal column and allow easy adjustment of the fulcrum. Proficiency is developed with practice; the sling must be symmetrically applied, and the rope, webbing, or fire hose section must be positioned so it rests in the "deep pockets" of the animal's body (i.e., regions where the animal's anatomy forms a concave area that reduces the risk of slippage; an example is the animal's abdomen immediately in front of the hind limbs) (Fox, 2006). Applying the sling in mud is extremely difficult, but several responders and instructors prefer this method for recumbent animals because it is safer for the rescuers. For example, in Alabama this sling was used successfully to remove cattle from entrapment by two people using a tractor with a boom.

The figure eight sling consists of 30 m (100 ft) of 2.5 cm (1 in.) cotton rope or webbing or 2.5–4 cm (1–1 1/2 in.) wildland fire hose webbing wrapped around the animal's neck and body to support the entire body.

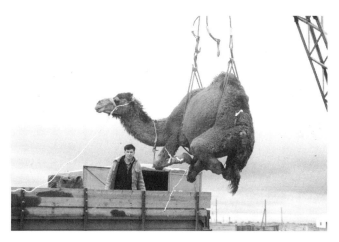

Figure 16.2 *This camel is being lifted in preparation for transportation in a vehicle in Turkmenistan. Ropes passed over the back of the animal and secured to the limbs force them to remain flexed so the animal cannot stand, and remains in a kushed position in the back of the truck. Courtesy of Dr. Bernard Faye.*

When the sling is complete, it provides support to the pelvic (hindquarter) and pectoral (chest) areas of the animal for the lift by encircling all four quarters of the animal. When tied properly and securely, the animal can not fall forward or backward out of the sling. The sling will always pick the animal up on its feet and can be adjusted to pick up the front or rear of the animal first. This is the only simple sling that, once secured on the animal, can be left in place without restricting the animal's ability to stand, walk, lie down, or rise (Fox, 2006).

Camel Rope Sling

Camels in Asia and the Middle East are commonly lifted into trucks or other transport using hobbles and a rope sling that maintains the animals in a kushed position (Figure 16.2) while lifted and keeps them kushed during transport. The rope is a hobble on the legs that passes over the animal's back and prevents it from rising while in a vehicle. This type of sling works well on camelids due to their anatomy, but is not recommended for any other species.

Field-Expedient Rope/Web Slings

The author has observed numerous attempts to perform vertical lifts of large animals using other methods, including simple ropes or webbing placed behind the hindquarters (instead of around the abdomen or between the legs), cargo netting, and canvas slings. Several were ineffective, others were dangerous to the rescuers or victim, and others were extremely complicated to emplace on the animal. In several cases, the animal was dropped or slipped out of the sling, usually in a backward direction. A good sling system must be able to maintain animals inside the appliance despite their weight and tendency to struggle. Training to ensure correct application of the sling systems is recommended for all types of slings.

Homemade and Inexpensive Slings. There are several vertical lift or support slings (EquiSling, cowsling, Monk's Sling and Ambulance, E-Z Up Sling, Liftex Sling, etc.) available through the Internet, ranging in price from $700 to $1,600. Most of these slings are not intended for long-term support of the animal; they are designed for short-term use to lift the animal. None of these slings are recommended for use in helicopter operations, although several have been used successfully for lifting anesthetized animals. It is important to note that several of these slings are not intended for use on all species.

Many homemade, field-expedient, or inexpensive slings support most of the animal's weight on a belly band, which can compromise respiration and place significant pressure on the animal's abdominal organs. This is often acceptable for short-term lifting and support, but is unsuitable for a long-term lift. Other slings prevent the movement of the head and neck; if the animal panics and throws its head, it can literally jump or flip forward out of the sling. Some slings do not support the rear quarters of the animals and have allowed animals to slip backward out of the sling. It is particularly important to support cattle with a strap or webbing behind the hindquarters because their weight distribution differs from that of horses or llamas (Slessman, 2006). Several manufactured slings evaluated for use by the author did not properly distribute the animal's weight; others did not balance the load, allowing the animal's body to tilt within the sling. The worst placed all of the lift pressure in the center of the animal's abdomen, allowing the animal to easily slip out of the appliance forward or backward.

Veterinarians have expressed concern with decreased venous return from the animal's head, neck, and legs if webbing or ropes are improperly or too tightly applied. If a rescue is prolonged, focal pressure points may develop that contribute to myopathy, neuropathy, cardiovascular, respiratory, or gastrointestinal effects (Taylor et al., 2005). Heavy-duty webbing, rope, or hose capable of lifting over 500 kg (1,100 lb) must be used. Field-expedient web slings can be locally produced with access to heavy-duty stitching equipment or made from lengths of retired fire hose (see Chapter 20).

SIMPLE VERTICAL LIFT WEB SLING SYSTEMS

A simple vertical lift web sling system is highly successful in lifting animals from various rescue environments (e.g., mud, water, ice, pools, septic tanks, ravines, etc.) where the rescuers have access to the animal's front and hind ends. There are several versions of simple web slings available that lift the hind and front ends of the animal simultaneously. However, none of these systems are recommended for lifts longer than 15–30 minutes in duration or for vertical lifts if responders do not have access to the front and hind ends of the animal victim. Personnel must be trained in proper use of the vertical lift web sling system to maximize safety when working with a trapped or recumbent frightened animal. Sedation or anesthetization of the animal is often essential for proper application of the sling and prevention of struggling and further injury to the animal or the rescuers.

Becker Sling

In 2000, Dr. Kathleen Becker adapted homemade equipment to produce a manufactured sling for use by rescue groups and individuals. This sling has numerous safety features as well as components that have been tested for shear and tension strength. It has been used on recumbent, geriatric, and mud-entrapped animals. The Becker sling consists of 15 cm (6 in.) minimum width heavy-duty webbing straps with sewn loops on each end, Prusik loop connectors, and steel attachment points for use with a vertical lift system (Figure 16.3). This sling features quick-release snap shackles to allow

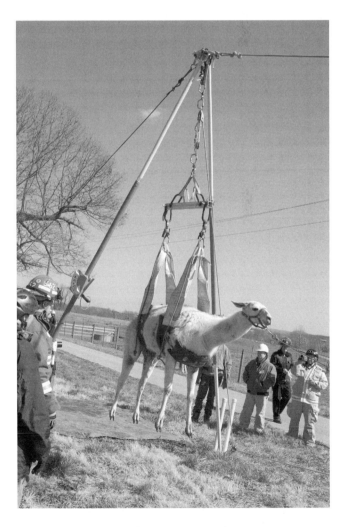

Figure 16.3 *A llama is lifted using the A-frame overhead lift system. The animal's weight is well distributed in a Becker-type simple web vertical lift sling. Courtesy of Axel Gimenez.*

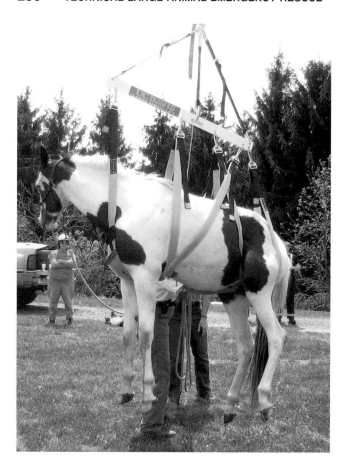

Figure 16.4   *This demonstration horse is shown in the Large Animal Lift designed at UC-Davis. This device is based on the concept of the figure eight web sling. Courtesy Tomas Gimenez.*

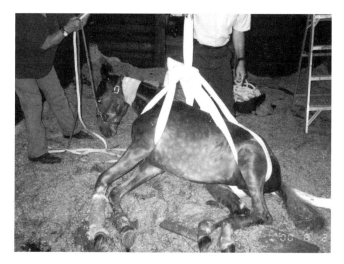

Figure 16.5   *An extremely ill young horse was lifted to its feet in a stall environment using a wildland fire hose version of the figure eight sling. Notice the sling supports the body at the junction of the limbs and the body. Courtesy of Rebecca Gimenez.*

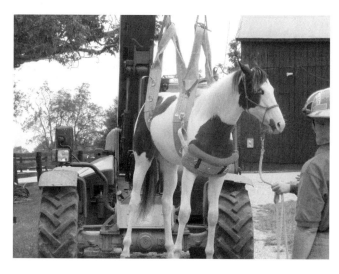

Figure 16.6   *A close-up of the Becker sling shows the use of padding between the webbing and the animal to provide comfort and increase the surface area. In some field scenarios (e.g., mud, recumbency, etc.), the padding may not be practical. Courtesy of Axel Gimenez.*

rapid release of the animal once it reaches solid ground. The protocol for employment of this sling is described below.

Large Animal Lift

In 2004, a University of California at Davis College of Veterinary Medicine team, under the leadership of Dr. John Madigan, designed a sling system called the Large Animal Lift. This sling is a modification of the rope figure eight sling and is available for equine practitioners and emergency response professionals for clinical and rescue use. The sling can be placed on a recumbent animal and supports the animal using its musculoskeletal system (Figure 16.4).

Fire Hose Slings

These slings are field expedients and provided the original inspiration for the Becker and figure eight slings (above). Several versions have been successfully used: retired fire hose sections with sewn loops on the ends; fire hose tied into loops; and sections of strapping used for loading trucks. It is similar to the Becker sling, with wide straps for increased surface area and two lift points above the animal (the chest and the pelvis). (See the Becker sling protocol below.) The fire hose web version of the figure eight sling uses 4–6 cm (1 1/2–2 1/2 in.) wildland hose to provide support to the animal (Figure 16.5 and Figure 16.6).

Liftex Sling

The Liftex sling is widely used in veterinary hospitals to support horses with severe musculoskeletal trauma or neurological injury (Figure 16.7). It has been used prior to surgery for support during induction of anesthesia and during transport from the induction/recovery stall to the surgery room or recovery pool. It has been successfully used to assist recumbent animals to

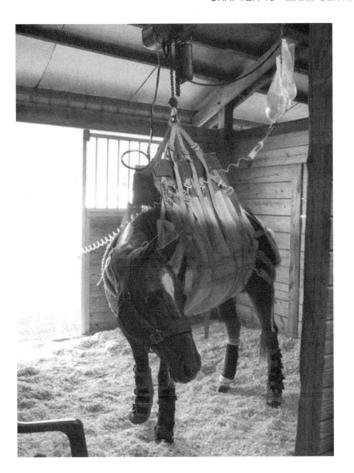

Figure 16.7 *A quarter horse mare exhibiting weakness due to West Nile virus infection is supported by a Liftex sling. The mare's weight is supported, but not suspended, by the sling. Courtesy of Dr. Kimberly May.*

stand and to lift animals out of ravines or other entrapments. The sling design prevents the large animal from falling or backing out of the sling and is adjustable to fit animals of different sizes. The fulcrum of suspension from the lifting rings can be adjusted to promote sternal or abdominal support, with the lift point located at the withers. This sling is challenging to place on a recumbent animal or one trapped in mud or water.

Sling-Shell System

The sling-shell recovery system was developed at the University of Berne, Switzerland, specifically for assisting horses during recovery from anesthesia. This system is placed on the patient while it is recumbent. When the horse is sufficiently awake from anesthesia, it is lifted in the sling into a standing position. The apparatus consists of two customized glass-fiber-enhanced plastic shells that fit adult horses (280–685 kg, or 616–1,500 lb) and are connected to each other by a short girth. One shell matches the contour of the animal's chest, and the other shell fits around the ventral thorax caudal to (behind) the elbows. The sling-shell supports the animal's weight without causing pressure damage

to soft tissues or impairing respiratory expansion of the rib cage. Transverse girths passing in front of and behind the hind limbs support the hindquarter. The use of this sling for technical large animal emergency rescue (TLAER) incidents is unreported. However, in a study of anesthetized horses, recovery in this sling system was well tolerated in 72% of 104 horses, minor complications were observed in 22% (23) of the horses, and 6% (6) of the patients did not tolerate the sling despite sedation with xylazine.

Recovery Sling

This sling system maintains an animal in caudal recumbency ("dog-sitting" position) for anesthetic recovery and was developed at the Large Animal Clinic, Veterinary Faculty, at the University of Zürich, Switzerland.

UC Davis-Anderson Sling

The UC Davis-Anderson Sling was originally intended for clinical use in long-term surgical recovery cases and clinical management of recumbent horses, but it has become the industry standard for helicopter operations with equines because of its demonstrated safety margin, design, and strength. However, with all its accessories and pieces, this sling is a significant investment for a TLAER team. The sling was developed by the late Charles Anderson, Richard Morgan, and Dr. John Madison.

The UC Davis-Anderson Sling has been successfully used for helicopter operations in a large number of emergencies and training demonstration flights, and it is the only equine sling recommended by rescue professionals for this purpose. The U.S. Army, Coast Guard, and Marines have used this sling to assist with emergency rescues and to transport mules for desert military operations and training.

In a recent study, horses identified at high risk for recovery-related injuries or complications following general anesthesia and surgery were recovered in a UC Davis-Anderson Sling, and the results of their clinical experience were reported. Twenty-four high-risk horses (32 recovery events) were evaluated for safety and efficacy for anesthetic recovery in the sling (Taylor et al., 2005). Twenty-three of 24 horses (96%) recovered safely and successfully from general anesthesia (31/32 recovery events) without clinical evidence of neuropathy, myopathy, or other injury to the horse or surgical site. The use of the UC Davis-Anderson Sling in clinical setting requires at least three people trained to correctly apply the sling and use a fixed hoist system. The researchers noted that no recovery method is failsafe. Risks to the horse while in the sling appeared minimal but could include equipment failure, injury to the surgical site, catastrophic failure of the surgical site, abrasions caused by the sling's straps, or injury from struggling and resisting the sling (Taylor et al., 2005).

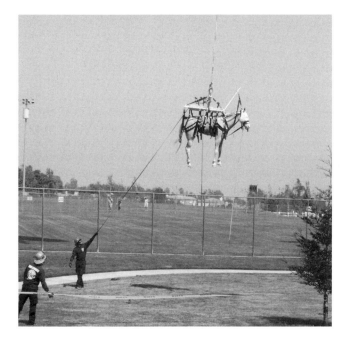

Figure 16.8 *A demonstration animal is subjected to a practice lift in the UC Davis-Anderson Sling, using a crane to simulate a helicopter lift. The limb supports for the sling are usually unnecessary in TLAER rescue scenarios. Courtesy of Axel Gimenez.*

The UC Davis-Anderson Sling is designed to transfer much of the weight of the animal to cross straps underneath the pelvis and sternum. In clinical use, the leg straps are also attached to further distribute the animal's weight, but the straps are not necessary for rescue lifts. The animal is attached to the soft part of the sling by straps encircling its barrel (so that it cannot jump or throw itself out of the sling) and supports the skeletal system with broad mesh panels and cross straps to prevent respiratory compromise, focal pressure points, or excessive abdominal pressure (Taylor et al., 2005). A steel overhead counterbalance frame with 18 attachment points (Figure 16.8) allows proper weight distribution, head and neck support, and uniform stability and support of the animal's body (Taylor et al., 2005).

Although the UC Davis-Anderson Sling is the safest sling for long- or short-term vertical lift purposes, it is not as practical to emplace on an animal below ground level, where a rescuer would have to get in the hole with the animal to place it. It isn't practical to use when animals are trapped deep in mud or water, where the sling parts will become wet and heavy, or when animals are contaminated by hazardous material (HazMat), or where an easily cleaned or disposable webbing system is desirable. The sling's cost limits its availability in many locales. Alternative slinging systems (e.g., Becker sling, Large Animal Lift, etc.) have been used for these types of scenarios when a vertical lift is required.

VERTICAL LIFT CONSIDERATIONS

A large animal should be sedated during vertical lift to prevent further injury to itself or attending personnel during this procedure. Sedation should be performed by a veterinarian. The protocol presented in this book is specifically for the Becker sling, but it is similar for other versions of vertical lift web slings and is applicable to other equipment. Please refer to the instruction booklet that accompanies the sling for the specific details of its application and use by the manufacturer.

The simple vertical lift sling systems, in conjunction with appropriate lifting equipment, provide safe and suitable means of short-term vertical lift of large animals. Use of this equipment allows practicing veterinarians to improve their emergency on-scene and prehospital care of horses in the field. Benefits of the simple vertical lift web sling systems include simple application, low cost, and good efficacy. The technique makes the animal feel completely entrapped so that it will hang quietly during the lifting procedure.

Personnel must be trained in the use of vertical lift web slings to maximize safety working around a trapped or recumbent frightened animal. Initial sedation or light anesthetization of the animal is often essential to allow it to be strapped in the sling and to prevent struggling and further injury to itself or to rescuers.

Many vertical lift web systems (especially the Becker and similar field expedient slings) appear to place significant pressure on the abdominal area of the animal; however, abdominal, thoracic, and pulmonary perfusion have not been significantly impaired in actual rescues or in the demonstration animals lifted in this manner (for 2–12 minutes) in training scenarios (Gimenez, 2006a). Pregnant mares have been successfully lifted using this equipment and technique. Contact pressure is minimized by using wider straps for the lift and increasing the surface area of the contact points on the animal. The Becker sling and the large animal lift, in conjunction with appropriate lifting equipment, provide safe and suitable means of short-term vertical lift of large animals.

VERTICAL LIFTS OUT OF HOLES

Before attempting to rescue a large animal from a hole, the reader should be aware of the fact that any hole deeper than 91 cm (3 ft) and deeper than it is wide constitutes a trench. Trench rescue is a specialty area in rescue because of the inherent risk of trench collapse and the potential for severe injury or loss of life. Rescue of large animals from trenches should be performed in collaboration with emergency personnel trained in trench rescue.

Front End Presentation (Caudal Recumbency)

An animal with its hindquarters entrapped in a hole presents significant challenges to rescuers. Examples include a horse in a small ice hole, a pony 4 m (13 ft) down a well and submerged in 1 m (3 ft) of water, a horse that fell through the decking of a bridge, a draft horse that fell into a hole in a culvert, and a cow that slipped to the bottom of a narrow ravine. These animals cannot be vertically lifted by the front and hind ends simultaneously with the simple vertical lift web sling systems because the rump is below the ground level and cannot be accessed to emplace equipment or webbing.

For this situation, webbing is emplaced around the animal's chest and anterior abdomen at the level of the withers in a lark's foot/cinch forward assist configuration (see Chapter 15). Rescuers have reported that performing the vertical lift while manually rolling the animal onto its side is effective. The webbing puts pressure on the chest; usually, the animal will initially struggle once or twice but remain quiet as long as pressure is maintained on the chest. As soon as the pressure is released, if not sedated, the animal will rise, often rapidly. It may be necessary to sedate the animal immediately before the lift, and long ropes from the halter held by rescuers on two sides of the animal facilitate control.

If vertically lifted from out of a small hole, the animal must be lifted far enough for the pelvis (hips) to clear the edges before moving the animal away from the hole; moving the animal prematurely increases the risk of pelvic or hind limb fractures. When the animal is set down on the ground, the hole must be covered so the animal (or a rescuer) will not fall into it, and the animal must be set down a safe distance from the hole. If the animal must be dragged over the ground once out of the hole, responders should use tarps or other protection to cover the ground surface and prevent injury.

Hindquarters Presented (Cranial Recumbency)

There are scenarios where the animal's front end has fallen into a hole, ravine, or entrapment, and the only accessible parts of the animal's body are the hindquarters and pelvis. Examples include a horse that fell head-first into a culvert; a bull at the bottom of a 25 m (82 ft) deep sinkhole, and a horse hanging by one hind limb from a railroad trestle 6 m (20 ft) over a creek. Prusik loops and hobbles may be placed on the hind limbs, or webbing may be placed around the pelvis in a lark's-footed (or cinched) configuration of the backward drag (Figure 16.9). Animals should be sedated for this procedure to avoid injury to the limbs and/or back. The head and neck should be allowed to hang in a natural position when setting the animal down after the lift. The animal handler should maintain control of the

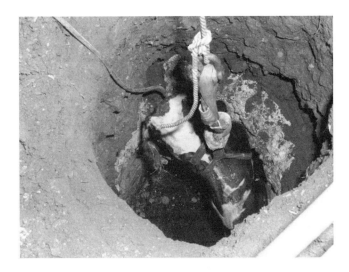

Figure 16.9 *A calf is lifted from a hole by the only part of its body that was accessible—the pelvis. The backward drag sling is placed in a cinched or lark's-footed configuration to prevent the animal from slipping out of the sling. This is considered a last resort method, as it places extreme pressure on the animal's abdomen and hind limb musculature and skeleton. Courtesy of Paul Baker.*

animal's halter and lead rope; alternatively, if no head restraint is used, the animal should be set down inside confinement (e.g., portable corral panels).

Animal Upside Down (Dorsal Recumbency)

Under normal circumstances, the lower limbs should not be used as anchor points for lifting an entrapped animal. However dorsally recumbent animals present the exception to this rule. When using this method, the rope pressure should be distributed as widely as possible, and a minimum of two lifting (anchor) points (the use of four lifting points is preferred) should be used. A UC Davis-Anderson Sling frame or spread bar are useful devices for this lifting procedure. The UC Davis-Anderson sling frame allows distribution of the load to all four limbs and supports the head and neck. The animal must be sedated for this procedure to prevent struggling and injury when the animal has been freed from the entrapment but is still secured to the rescue equipment.

For example, in Maryland responders found a horse trapped in dorsal recumbency in a ditch in the middle of a pasture. Rescuers chose to use hobbles on the horse's pasterns and perform a vertical lift (Figure 16.10). Hobbles were placed on the sedated animal's legs and connected to the UC Davis-Anderson Sling frame. To protect the horse's neck and head, it was tied in a normal head-down position. This method allowed the legs to be lifted in a normal position to balance the load and provided support for the head and neck. The obvious danger associated with lifting an animal by its limbs is the close proximity to the hooves required to emplace the hobbles and lift system.

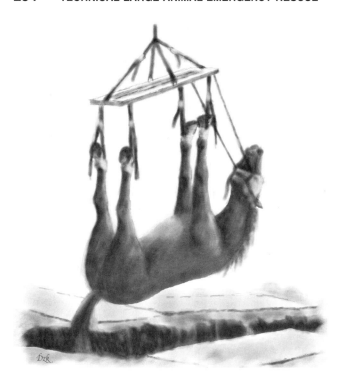

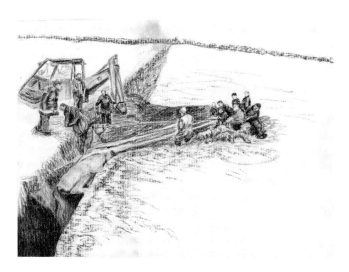

Figure 16.11   *A horse trapped on its side in a ditch is pulled out using webbing around its chest after heavy equipment increased the accessibility to the animal. Trench rescue considerations must be addressed in these scenarios. Courtesy of Julie Casil.*

Fig 16.10   *A horse found upside down in a trench presented all four feet to rescuers from Days End Farm Horse Rescue, who used hobbles and the frame of the Anderson Sling to lift the animal. The head and neck of the animal are appropriately supported in this rescue. The animal must be sedated when this method is used. Courtesy of Michael Dzurak.*

Increasing contact area between the rope and the animal victim is vital to preventing injury to the animal's limbs. Webbing is preferred over rope because of its larger surface area, and padding (e.g., shirt, cotton, or other padding materials) should be placed between the rope or webbing and the animal's skin (see Figure 16.6).

Pronation of the animal to a normal standing position can be accomplished by attaching hobbles to the front legs and pulling the chest, head, and neck over the animal's hindquarters. The head must be supported and maneuvered in the same direction, but the main force of the rotational pull should be placed on the hobbles and not the head and neck. In an illustration of this concept, in California a horse landed upside down on top of its rider in a narrow trench. The person appeared uninjured and insisted that responders rescue the horse. This scenario emphasizes that the rescue focus should be on the human victim because the rescuers spent several hours trying to figure out how to remove the animal without injuring the trapped rider, bringing in equipment and a helicopter to remove the patient once extricated. The animal's front feet were eventually hobbled and it was pronated (rotated over the hindquarters) by pulling on the hobbles and head/neck; as this was completed, the

rider was removed from the trench. (*Note*: Paramedics have pointed out that the rider should have been immobilized before she was removed from the trench.) The horse was helicopter-lifted in a UC Davis-Anderson Sling to the trailhead for transport. In retrospect, the edges of the trench could have been partially knocked down to build a ramp over which the animal could walk. Other potential solutions include digging out the ditch on one side of the animal, rolling it over, and allowing it to rise (Figure 16.11).

In a similar scenario, a horse fell into a concrete ditch and landed on the bottom in dorsal recumbency. The veterinarian on the scene placed a web nylon halter on the head, attached a chain to the ring, and pronated the animal onto its feet. Although this method was successful, the use of motorized forces applied directly to the head and neck is associated with a high risk of injury. As stated previously, the hobbled limbs should serve as the anchor points for the pronation effort.

Trenches pose significant danger due to the tendency of the sides to collapse or cave in (Figure 16.11). Trench rescue is a specialty rescue area within the emergency response professions and requires specific knowledge and training. Techniques for shoring and minimizing vibration near the trench and specialty equipment required for trench rescue are beyond the scope of this volume. For example, plywood should be placed along the edge of the trench to distribute the weight over the ground surface. Human safety is a primary factor in any trench-related rescue, and professional responders must use caution when personnel enter the area surrounding the trench. There are numerous resources that discuss trench rescue.

When lifting a dorsally or caudally recumbent animal, the animal's head and neck must be supported. If an animal's neck is unsupported and in an abnormal position, overstretching can cause severe head and neck injuries. The head should be supported in a normal or lowered (grazing) position.

SPECIAL CONCERNS FOR VERTICAL LIFTS

Septic tank drainage and other Hazmat concerns on scene should be handled by trained, certified HazMat personnel (see Chapter 19). All personnel should use extreme caution when assisting an animal in a water environment because swift or flood waters rescue require training and certification. Emergency personnel should not attempt to assist animals in concrete ditches, canals, and flumes until the public works department has been notified to redirect possible floodwaters. Mud and unstable ground rescues require specialty equipment but rarely require vertical lift, although it is an option if the operator can access the animal safely. Air and water injection around the animal's legs will greatly facilitate extrication from mud (see Chapter 7).

System Components

When constructing a system that will be loaded (e.g., with an animal victim), it is vital to consider the strength ratings of all components of the system. In addition, an extra safety factor is added to prevent system failure. In human rescues, the safety factor is 15:1, indicating that a 272 kg (600 lb) load should have a system rated to 4,082 kg (9,000 lb). While this level of safety is ideal, its application in TLAER is often impractical due to the great weight of the victim and expense of equipment. Therefore, a reasonable compromise must be made.

For example, the components of the Becker sling system have been tested for maximum working loads or breaking strengths to the ratings listed below:

- Master oval link: maximum load 6,895 kg (15,200 lb)
- Prusik loops made with 12 mm kernmantle rope (using a doubled configuration): 8,164 kg (18,000 lb) maximum breaking strength (MBS) each loop
- Shackles: maximum working load 4,536 kg (10,000 lb) each
- Aluminum spread bar: 9,798 kg (21,600 lb) breaking strength (total load equally divided on both ends). *Note*: A steel spread bar was originally considered for this sling, but testing on the aluminum bar demonstrated a sufficient safety factor such that the manufacturer offers only aluminum due to its light weight and ease of machining and finishing
- Body slings (basket configuration): Nominal 9,072 kg (20,000 lb) maximum load

The term *working load* or *maximum load* is that load which a part can typically sustain safely on a daily basis (with periodic inspections for damage). *Breaking strength* is that load which will cause immediate failure. A part should never sustain a load that approaches or approximates the equipment's breaking strength.

LIFTING EQUIPMENT

It is not always necessary to lift a large animal victim. A horse stuck in dry mud in Ohio was extricated using a excavator bucket available on the scene to pull away and loosen the mud. The animal was able to get up after the mud was removed. This method is associated with a higher risk of injury to the animal and rescuers; therefore, the animal was sedated as the excavator was used. The use of heavy equipment is not recommended if there is a better option, because the noise may frighten the animal and the operator must be extremely careful not to injure the animal. Typical motorized heavy lifting equipment that can be used in incidents includes cranes of various sizes, tractors, all-terrain forklifts, and wreckers.

The nonmotorized A-frame uses mechanical rope or winch systems to swing out over a load, lift it, and slowly move it back to safe ground. Important considerations in its use include the objective of the rescue, load size, terrain, and accessibility. Although motorized equipment generates noise that may stress the animal, this must be weighed against its ability to quickly extricate the victim.

The lift equipment must have enough throw and distance to raise the animal out of the hole high enough to ensure that the animal's limbs clear the edges of the hole (or trench, etc.) (Figure 16.12). Because most lifts will involve lifting the animal out of a belowground level hole or ravine, the equipment must be able to reach very high in the air or have a pulley system to maximize the lift distance over the animal. Any lift equipment with a boom and pulley system for the cable can be used. Responders should be aware that the animal load may swing like a pendulum into equipment or personnel.

Wreckers are generally poor choices for large animal lifting equipment for several reasons. A hydraulic "foot" must be anchored directly behind the tow truck to balance the boom for a lift. The foot often becomes a physical obstruction to rescuers; it is often in close proximity to the animal and equipment and may increase the risk of injury. Also, the wrecker may not be able to drive with the load attached.

For long-term clinical cases, physically lifting the animal on a daily or hourly basis is accomplished using a tractor with a boom or a high-clearance ceiling and beam rated to support the weight of the horse, sling and pulley system, or chain hoist lifting mechanism. Tractors allow easy access and movement of the slung

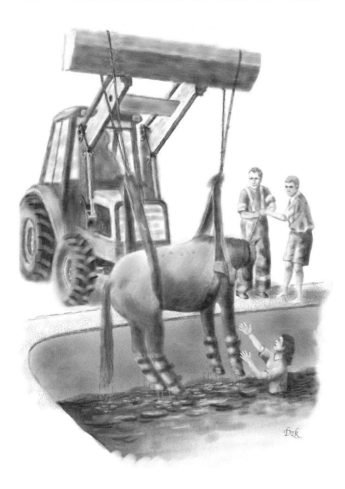

Figure 16.12 *This horse is being lifted out of a pool by heavy equipment in a vertical lift with fire hose webbing. This pool did not have a shallow end with steps to allow easy rescue. Note the unsafe position of the person in the water with the animal and that the equipment has almost reached its maximum height. Shortening the dead space between the bucket and the animal would prevent that problem. Courtesy of Michael Dzurak.*

animal unless it is in a confined space or stall. Chain hoists and pulley systems are usually fixed and difficult to deploy in the field due to lack of an appropriate overhead anchor. These systems are suitable for fixed use in a stall or barn area designated for management of disabled horses.

A-FRAME LIFT

The A-frame concept is commonly used in human rescue scenarios. It was first applied to large animal rescue scenarios by the Norco Fire Department in California. An aluminum Airshore A-frame/tripod was modified for large animals by purchasing sections to increase the height and width of the frame. This equipment readily supports a load of 1,400 kg (3,080 lb). The A-frame was designed specifically for removing animals from situations (e.g., wells, cliff sides, concrete flumes, pools, etc.) where cranes or heavy equipment could not

safely access the scene and where helicopter sling-load operations were not indicated, practical, or available. The author contracted for a custom-made steel A-frame to provide the same capability with greater load capacity.

Standard Operating Procedure for Lifting Large Animal Victims

An added advantage of the A-frame or tripod is the absence of vibration (as produced by motorized equipment) during trench rescue efforts.

Conditions for Using an A-Frame and Tripod. The following conditions for using an A-frame or tripod for lifting large animals apply.

- The equipment must be easily disassembled, carried manually to the incident location, and assembled on site.
- The equipment must provide sufficient width and height to allow the animal victim to clear the edges of the entrapping area (e.g., hole, trench, flume, etc.). Up to 2.5 m (8 1/4 ft) of additional vertical height may be required.
- The equipment should easily support weight up to 1,361 kg (3,000 lb).
- The equipment should be able to pivot in either direction (A-frame) or remain stationary (tripod) over the entrapped animal and the site.

Personnel. Personnel needed for a rescue using an A-frame or tripod are the following:

- Animal handler
- Operational personnel (four to six)
- Safety officer (SO)
- Veterinarian familiar with the species involved and with the incident command system

Equipment. The author's custom-made steel A-frame consists of the following parts.

- Base plates (two): 25.4 cm × 25.4 cm × .95 cm (10 in. × 10 in. × 3/8 in.) with attachment points for the bottom sections, chain, and a carabiner, with a 1 in. hole at each corner. The outside end of each plate must rest 5 cm (2 in.) off the ground.
- Top plate (one): 25.4 cm × 25.4 cm × .95 cm (10 in. × 10 in. × 3/8 in.) with attachment points for the top sections, one anchor point on either side, and an anchor point in the center.
- Bottom sections (two): 1.8 m (6 ft) of 4.7 mm (1 7/8 in.) outer diameter (OD) seamless, unthreaded steel pipe (ASTM schedule 80), with a three-point hitch ball welded on one end of each section (to attach an end plate).

- Center sections (two): 2.13 m (7 ft) × 5.95 mm (2 3/8 in.) OD seamless, unthreaded steel pipe (ASTM schedule 80).
- Top sections (two): 1.8 m (6 ft) × 4.7 mm (1 7/8 in.) OD seamless unthreaded steel pipe (ASTM schedule 80).
- Steel stakes (4): 1.9 cm (3/4 in.) × 91.4 cm (3 ft) steel.
- Chain: 3.6 m (12 ft) × .95 cm (3/8 in.) chain.
- Shackles (two).
- Pins (two): 12.7 cm (5 in.) × 1.9 cm (3/4 in.) pins with handle and cotter pin (for connecting bottom section to base plate).
- Pins (six): 12.7 cm (5 in.) × 1.25 cm (1/2 in.) pin with handle and cotter pin (for connecting sections to each other and to top plate).
- Large sledge hammer.
- Wood boards (two): 1.22 m (4 ft) long, 4.44 cm × 9.53 cm (1 3/4 in. × 3 3/4 in.), with a notch cut on one end of each board (to support the assembled top sections).
- Polyvinyl chloride (PVC) pipe sections (four): 5 cm (2 in.) × 60.9 cm (2 ft), with caps (four each) to cover the stakes for safety.
- Inclinometer.
- Kernmantle rope (two): 46 m (150 ft) × 12 mm (1/2 in.), low stretch.
- Kernmantle rope (two): 61 m (200 ft) × 12 mm (1/2 in.), low stretch.
- Components for assembling a 9:1 mechanical advantage system, for example, carabiners, pulleys, Prusik loops, webbing, etc.
- Components for assembling a 15:1 mechanical advantage system, for example, carabiners, swivels, pulleys (including one triple pulley and one double pulley), Prusik loops, webbing, etc.
- Components for assembling a friction system using a brake tube (for example, carabiners, Prusik loops, webbing, etc.)
- Secure anchors (three), or the components for assembling a picket anchor system.
- Simple vertical lift web sling or field-expedient sling (one).
- Rescue swivels (two): 4,082 kg (9,000 pound) MBS.
- Spread bar (one) with snap shackles (two).

A-Frame Procedure

Because of the complexity of the A-frame system, the rescuers should obtain practical training on the assembly and use of an A-frame. The information contained here is intended as an introduction to the system and does not replace proper training.

A-Frame Assembly. The A-frame and all rope systems should be completely assembled and ready for operation before placing the simple vertical lift web sling or field-expedient sling on the animal. All components of the A-frame should be laid out on the ground and systematically assembled using the appropriate pins.

1. The base plates should be located no less than 60 cm (2 ft) from the hole (or trench, etc.).
2. Ensure the elevated side of the base plates faces the outside of the A-frame legs.
3. The bottom and top sections should slide no less than 18 cm (7 in.) into the middle section.
4. The chain is connected to the base plates by shackles, with a distance between the base plates of 3 m (10 ft).
5. In the custom A-frame, the distance from the ground level to the top plate is 4.9 m (16 ft).
6. Secure the base plates to the ground by driving two steel stakes through the outside holes of each plate. The depth to which the stakes are driven into the ground depends on the solidity and soil composition of the ground. In dry clay or rock-based soils, it will be sufficient to drive half the length of the stakes; in sandy soils, at least three-quarters of the length of the stakes should be driven into the ground. The stakes should be covered with safety covers (PVC pipe) to prevent injury.
7. Once the A-frame is fully assembled, the top is raised off the ground and supported with the two wood boards. Personnel should not be allowed to walk underneath the A-frame.
8. Attach the inclinometer to the A-frame so that it will indicate the degrees of inclination from the vertical when tipped over the hole.
9. Place or select two secure anchors on both sides of the A-frame at a 90-degree angle from it. The anchors should be placed directly across from each other (at a 180-degree angle). A third secure anchor is placed to the side of the anchor for the 9:1 mechanical advantage rope system.
10. Assign a team to each of the rope systems: the 9:1 mechanical advantage system, the friction system, and the 15:1 mechanical advantage system.
11. With a 46 m (150 ft) rope, assemble a 9:1 mechanical advantage system, and place it from the closest secure anchor to the A-frame's top plate.
12. With the other 46 m (150 ft) rope, assemble a friction system, and place it over the hole passing from the other secure anchor to the A-frame's top plate.
13. Using the 61 m (200 ft) rope, one triple pulley, and one double pulley, assemble a 15:1 mechanical advantage system, and attach the triple pulley to the A-frame's top plate.
14. Attach the bottom double pulley to the spread bar, placing a swivel between them.

15. Attach a single pulley to one of the base plates with a swivel or two carabiners between the plate and the pulley.

16. Pass the 61 m (200 ft) rope through the single pulley (from step 15 above), and assemble a 3:1 (Z-rig) system between that pulley and a third secure anchor located to the side of the 9:1 anchor to complete the 15:1 compound system. *Note*: A rope system with a smaller mechanical advantage may be sufficient in some cases, based on the weight of the animal to be lifted.

Making the Lift. Once the A-frame is in place and all rope systems are assembled, the animal is secured in the vertical lift sling and hauled out of the entrapment.

1. If indicated, administer sedative to the animal.
2. Have the SO inspect the A-frame and all rope systems.
3. Using manual power on the mechanical advantage rope system, remove the slack from the friction system and raise the A-frame until it reaches the vertical plane (0 degrees of inclination).
4. Hold the A-frame at the vertical position with the 9:1 mechanical advantage and friction systems.
5. By slowly feeding rope on the 9:1 system, increase the degree of inclination of the A-frame over the hole (or trench, etc.) until the top plate is directly above the animal to be lifted, but not beyond 35 degrees of inclination. Inclination beyond 35 degrees will transfer the load weight from the A-frame to the anchors and increase stress on the rope systems.
6. Secure the 9:1 system in place with the tandem Prusik brake.
7. Place the sling system on the animal, leaving a halter with an attached lead rope on the animal.
8. After consulting with the veterinarian, lower the spread bar, connect it to the sling, and proceed to lift the animal *without hesitation*.
9. Lift the animal until its feet have cleared the ground surface by a minimum of 20 cm (8 in.).
10. Secure the lifting rope system with the tandem Prusik brake.

Bringing the Victim to Safety

1. The animal handler should grasp the lead rope and rotate the animal until its long axis (the spinal column) is in line with the 9:1 and friction systems and at a 90-degree angle to legs of the A-frame. (This will ensure that the animal will clear the legs of the A-frame while it is being pivoted toward the 9:1 system; Figure 16.13.) *Note*: It is very important to avoid any sudden movement of the A-frame that

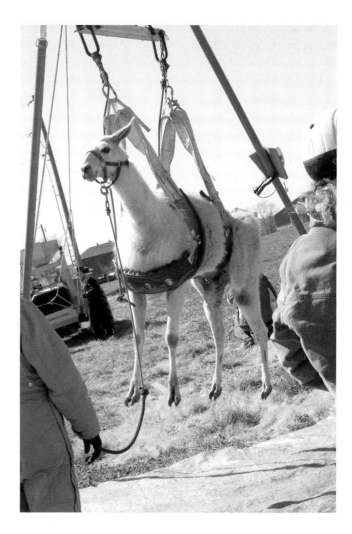

Figure 16.13 *Using the modified A-frame to lift a llama in a Becker sling during a demonstration shows the animal handler in a safe position to the side of the animal in preparation for set down and the operational person approaching from the opposite side. Courtesy of Axel Gimenez.*

could swing the animal's weight against the frame's legs. This impact would subject the A-frame to a shock load that could cause system failure.

2. Pivot the A-frame toward the 9:1 mechanical advantage rope system.
3. Once the A-frame passes the vertical point, the friction system is used to control and slow the descent of the A-frame until the animal's feet are in contact with the ground, and a designated member of the rescue team simultaneously releases both snap shackles or the SeaCatch on the spread bar by forcefully pulling both lines (Figure 16.14).
4. The animal handler leads the animal away from the A-frame to allow removal of the sling and medical examination by the on-site veterinarian.
5. The A-frame is lowered and all equipment disassembled and stored.

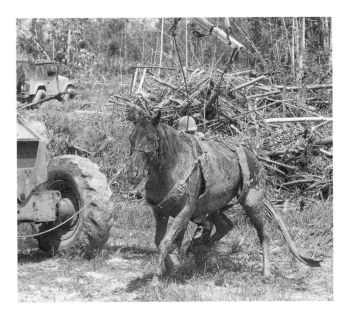

Figure 16.14 *As soon as the animal's feet contact the ground, one operational responder should pull the snap shackles to release the animal from the overhead gear and heavy equipment. The animal handler should remain to the animal's side and at a safe distance as the animal may lie down or jump forward. Courtesy of Axel Gimenez.*

BECKER SLING PROTOCOL FOR VERTICAL LIFT

Prior to using any vertical lift system, rescuers should consult the manufacturer's instructions for use. The Becker sling is a simple device and is included in this chapter as an example of a sling system that can be constructed on-scene using fire hose or webbing materials for a field-expedient version (Higdon, 1998).

Materials and Equipment

Materials and equipment necessary for a Becker sling vertical lift include the following:

- Fire hose webbing (two): sections 1 m (3 1/2 ft) in length and 8.5 cm (3 1/2 in.) or wider, with sewn loops. *Note*: Alternatively, heavy-duty webbing may be purchased for this purpose. Foam or fleece padding should be added to provide comfort for repeated or prolonged lifting of clinical patients but may not be practical in many field rescue scenarios or mud.
- Chest restraint (one): 1 m (3 1/2 ft) section of 10 cm (4 in.) fire hose webbing or western cinch with ropes attached. A similar hindquarter restraint is necessary for cattle and zoologic species.
- Spread bar (one): 6 cm (2 in.) square aluminum tubing 1 m (40 in.) in length with four steel anchor shackles placed 10 cm (4 in.) apart at each end.
- Prusik loops (two): loops formed from 12 mm (1/2 in.) kernmantle rescue rope.
- Large steel gate carabiners (two).

- Snap shackles (two): 2,722 kg (6,000 lb) MBS or SeaCatch.
- Head protection and blindfold for the animal (e.g., a towel or shirt).
- Overhead rope system, crane, wrecker, rough terrain forklift, winch system, tripod or A-frame rescue system, with minimum 3 m (10 ft) boom clearance.

Protocol for Securing the Animal in the Becker Sling

This procedure requires five minutes with three trained personnel.

Note: Stay clear of the animal's legs at all times (even when the animal is sedated). The operational personnel securing the animal in the appliance should always have an escape plan. Animals should be fully sedated or even anesthetized for this procedure to reduce the chance of injury to personnel, based on consultation with the veterinarian.

1. Place a halter on the animal for guidance and restraint and head protection on the head, and/or a blindfold. Operational personnel should attach the spread bar and shackles to the overhead lifting equipment away from the entrapment site. The animal handler should remain in a safe position depending on the situation (e.g., not directly in front of the animal or in the hole with the animal).
2. Slide a 1.8 m (6 ft) section of webbing underneath the animal immediately behind its front limbs.
3. Gather the sewn loops of webbing with a doubled Prusik loop connected to a carabiner.
4. Repeat step 2 and 3 with another 1.8 m (6 ft) section of webbing in front of the hind limbs. Many animals will resist pressure in the flank and groin area and may kick or buck in response to contact (Figure 16.15). The rear webbing piece can be placed farther forward (cranial) on the abdomen until the lift is initiated. *Note*: Use care to keep the webbing cranial to the sheath and penis of male horses. Due to their anatomy, the sheath and penis of male camelids and cattle will be underneath the webbing; the use of wide webbing and adequate padding is recommended to prevent injury.
5. Attach the chest restraint to the appropriate buckle on the front piece of the webbing, at approximately the point of the shoulder. Ensure that the webbing will not ride up too high and put pressure on the trachea, or drop so low that it is underneath the pectoral muscles (Figure 16.16).
6. If lifting cattle or zoologic species, be sure to use a hindquarter restraint similar to the chest restraint. Their balance point is different from that of horses, and they may slip out of the back of the sling without hindquarter support. The webbing should pass below the point of the hip, below the

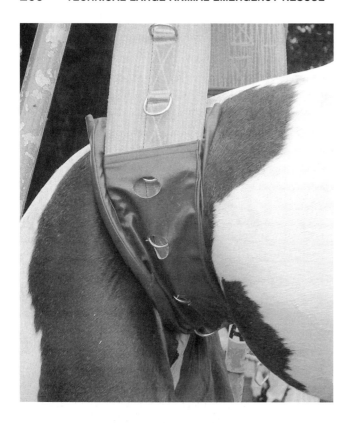

Figure 16.15 *The support of the animal's abdomen by the wide webbing of the Becker sling demonstrates how the abdominal contents move out of the way due to the pressure of the webbing. This does not injure animals during short-term lifts. Courtesy of Tori Miller.*

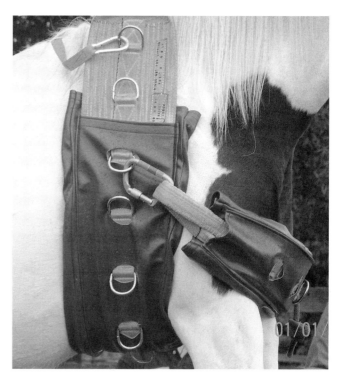

Figure 16.16 *The attachment of the breast collar support to the main chest/sternal webbing of the Becker sling is shown here. Thick foam padding is used to increase the surface area in contact with the animal's skin. D-rings provide numerous attachment points for the breast collar. Courtesy of Tori Miller.*

hindquarters, and attach to the rear abdominal webbing.

7. Bring the lift equipment to a location above the animal. Quickly connect the carabiners to the snap shackles on the spread bar shackles. Slide the rear webbing in front of the rear limbs (and attach hindquarter restraint in cattle), and prepare to make the lift when directed by the incident commander.

8. Make the lift in one smooth motion. Jerking or snatching the load may contribute to component failure or injury to the animal. Most unsedated animals will struggle for a short period when the feet leave the ground and pressure is applied, but then hang quietly until their feet contact the ground again. Operational personnel and the animal handler should remain a safe distance from the animal.

9. Disconnect the snap shackles with one motion, separating the animal from the heavy equipment, and allow the lift equipment to move out of the area away from the animal. Some animals will lie down when set down, but they may jump up rapidly when they realize they are back on solid ground. *Note*: Use of a blindfold should be considered on an individual basis, and it should be applied so it will fall off if the animal gets loose.

SLING EFFECTIVENESS

The practical use of simple vertical web lift systems has been successfully demonstrated in numerous situations and with other large animals in live rescue situations (Figure 16.17). The equipment continues to evolve in response to results and challenges encountered during field use. The authors have collected 39 examples (e.g., videos, photographs, witness accounts, etc.) of use of these slings in live rescues that were effective, meaning that the animal was safely set down at the end of the rescue. Data regarding the long-term health consequences has not been collected.

No lifting system is perfect: they each have advantages and limitations. No sling system is ideal for all situations. The importance of proper training for the different sling systems cannot be overstated. One animal in California was dropped from an inappropriately configured sling on the first lifting attempt with a helicopter: however, modifications of the sling allowed successful rescue of the horse. In another scenario, an animal fell backward out of the Becker sling when inappropriately attached (Fox, 2006). Two video accounts revealed improper application of a UC Davis-Anderson sling on horses, and in one case an animal fell from the sling due to the incorrect application (Fox, 2006).

For example, a pregnant mare fell into a water flume approximately 4 m (13 ft) deep, with approximately

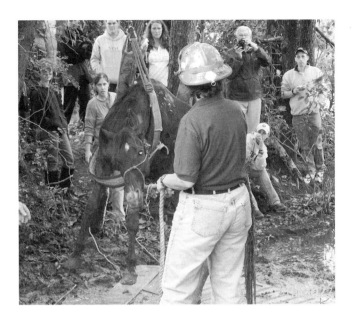

Figure 16.17 *An unsedated horse is vertically lifted from a deep mud entrapment using short sections of fire hose with sewn loops. Although the animal is calm and not struggling, the animal handler is standing in a safe position to the side of the animal while supporting the head with tension on the lead rope. A large number of bystanders and media have assembled in the background very close to the scene. Courtesy of Tori Miller.*

1 m (3 1/2 ft) of standing water at the bottom. The rescuers opted to perform a vertical lift of the standing mare. Webbing and ropes were used to sling the front of the mare with support to the chest and sternum. Another sling was emplaced behind and around the hindquarters of the mare. Despite sedation, the mare struggled at approximately the pinnacle of the lift; the hindquarter support slipped. The mare slipped backward out of the sling and back down into the hole, landing on her back in the water. The mare was able to stand up again in the tank. The sling was reapplied, but the hindquarter support was secured to the front support and the animal was further sedated. The animal survived its rescue. The authors are aware of several other unsuccessful rescue attempts (via witness accounts) using various forms of slings or nets with various species.

Training scenarios using live demonstration animals (horses or llamas) in the Becker sling have been performed by the authors for emergency responders and veterinary personnel on over 200 occasions since 1995, through 12 improvement evolutions of this equipment. In each scenario, a trained demonstration animal is secured in the Becker sling by students. The animal is then pulled by rope or winch systems with an A-frame out of the scenario's rescue environment (e.g., swamp, ravine, hillside, or other significant terrain feature). Each of these training scenarios has been successful and has resulted in no injuries to demonstration animals or personnel. The UC Davis-Anderson Sling has been similarly employed on over 100 occasions.

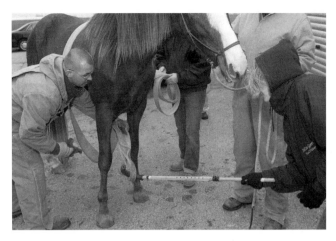

Figure 16.18 *Canes and extensions of the arm are used to manipulate the webbing around animal's hooves and legs. Courtesy of Axel Gimenez.*

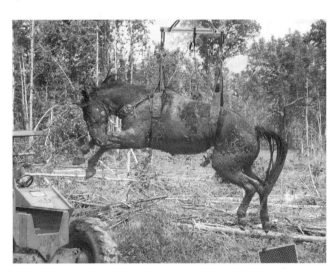

Figure 16.19 *Animal handlers should remain in a safe position at all times when working with large animals. This animal struggled only once, but note how far its feet come forward. When an animal fights in a sling or other equipment that has been applied, their struggling is a panic reaction and they exert significant physical effort as shown here. Equipment and slings used for TLAER must be excellent quality and overrated for the load to absorb the dynamic forces placed on them without failure of the system. Courtesy of Tori Miller.*

SAFETY AND HEALTH CONCERNS

Vertical lifts of large animals can present significant safety hazards. As has been stated previously numerous times, the manipulation of limbs should be performed by equipment employed as extensions of the arm (Figure 16.18). While suspended, the animal's limbs present risk of injury to responders within range; proper attention to safe distances and personal protective equipment are critical (Figure 16.19). In addition, all equipment and materials should be functional, well-maintained, and sufficiently strong to support the animal's weight.

The responding veterinarian should be cognizant of the potentially increased risk of cardiovascular or hypovolemic shock when combining sedation with rescues. Because the animal has often been entrapped for several hours (or more), it may be necessary for the veterinarian to provide first aid prior to sedation and extrication. This is especially important when a thorough physical examination is not possible prior to sedation.

ACRONYMS USED IN CHAPTER 16

ASTM	American Society for Testing and Materials
HazMat	Hazardous materials
MBS	Maximum breaking strength
OD	Outer diameter
PVC	Polyvinyl chloride
SO	Safety officer
TLAER	Technical large animal emergency rescue

17 Large Animal Field Emergency Medicine

Dr. Janice Baker

Between animal and human medicine there is no dividing line—nor should there be. The object is different but the experience obtained constitutes the basis of all medicine.

Robert Virchow, father of
20th century pathology

INTRODUCTION

Providing first aid to a large animal in a field emergency incident or backcountry wilderness presents numerous challenges rarely encountered when responding to a human incident. Large animals are medically fragile and subject to severe stress in response to the situation (Figure 17.1). When injured or entrapped, these animals are unlikely to perceive the human responder as their rescuer. Unlike human victims, they are likely to react instinctively by struggling to escape the approaching "predators." Thus, the responder must maintain an egress opening and escape route away from the animal at all times.

The basic first-aid principles of attending to airway, breathing, and circulation (ABC) can be adapted for use on horses and other large animals, with some additional important considerations. This chapter strives to provide a basic overview of the most common injuries that can be expected on technical large animal emergency rescue (TLAER) incident scenes and how first responders might assess and provide first aid to animals. Detailed information on veterinary care of large animals is available in other texts.

Responders should strive to provide improved standards of prehospital care to large animals in emergency incidents by becoming trained in basic large animal first aid and accumulating a cache of appropriate, basic veterinary medical supplies to use on the scene (Figure 17.2). In the field environment, especially following a disaster or mass casualty event, responders should triage animal victims and perform euthanasia on the *expectant* (fatally injured or death imminent) patients. One of the benefits of triage is the conservation of resources (materials and personnel) for treating victims that are more likely to survive.

Preparedness for Medical Emergencies and Disasters

Particularly after a large-scale disaster, conditions may be chaotic and dangerous. Services society takes for granted, such as electricity, phone service, clean running water, and access to human or animal health care, may be disrupted. The emergency response system may quickly be overwhelmed and unable to send assistance, as was observed during the September 11, 2001, terrorist attacks, Hurricane Katrina, and the London and Madrid train bombings. Local veterinary service may be overwhelmed if the incident occurs in an area with a small number of veterinarians providing care for a large number of animals. Additionally, if the veterinarian is personally impacted by the emergency or disaster, assistance may not be available for several hours to days following a disaster. Significant loss of veterinary equipment or facilities can lead to prolonged discontinuation of service. Animal owners should be prepared to care for their own animals in a disaster situation—a responsibility of ownership.

As an example of the challenges that might be encountered associated with a minor disaster, a large complex of thunderstorms developed during a large, organized trail ride with over 100 horses and riders in Missouri in 2005. Over 10 cm (4 in.) of rain fell on the area in a short period of time, and the storms were associated with dangerous lightning and wind gusts in excess of 80 kph (50 mph). No human injuries were reported, but the emergency equine response unit's

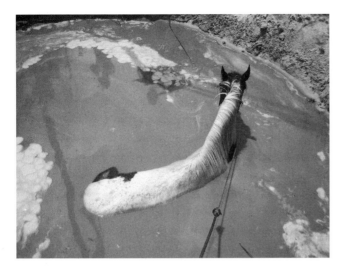

Figure 17.1 *A horse trapped in a muddy hole in a remote location on a camping trip represents the challenge of providing good field medical care to large animals and the value of preparedness for such emergencies. Although removing this animal from its entrapment using a forward assist is relatively simple, the medical status of the animal may quickly decline after the rescue is complete. Courtesy of Tomas Gimenez.*

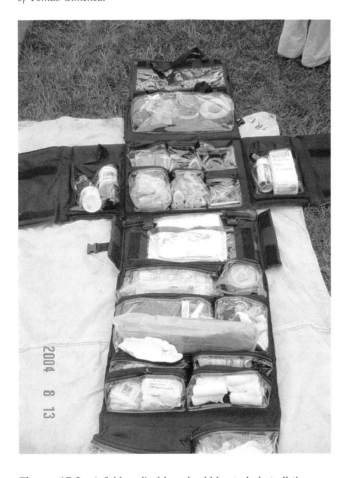

Figure 17.2 *A field medical bag should be stocked at all times; after every use, the bag should be inventoried and restocked. Ensure that expired pharmaceuticals are retired and fresh ones added, and consider security for drugs in the bag. Contents of the bag should emphasize the use of commonly needed and sensible products. Courtesy of Tori Miller.*

(EERU's) staff veterinarian examined, triaged, and treated over 40 horses with injuries ranging from a splinter in the eye to a large chest laceration. The following day, several horses were evaluated and treated by EERU staff for dehydration and exertional rhabdomyolysis ("tying up") because the animals lacked the physical conditioning to traverse the thick mud for long distances. The staff noted that most horse owners were not prepared to handle many of the first aid situations, and they implemented educational efforts with the ride organizers to advise horse owners of helpful emergency preparedness tips such as proper conditioning of their horses, the importance of electrolytes and hydration, and maintaining equine first aid kits.

Similarly, veterinary and animal-sheltering groups responding to a large-scale disaster may have limited medical supplies, and the volume of animal patients in need of care may limit what can be done for an individual animal. Basic first aid may be all that can be provided before responders must proceed to the next site.

Chaotic disaster and emergency situations are usually associated with three common problems: persons operating above their scope of care in veterinary medicine, persons providing substandard care when standard alternatives are available, and persons offering free services in the name of "humanitarian aid" despite the presence of functioning veterinary practices in the area. Professional emergency responders should be aware of these concerns and strive to prevent them on emergency scenes.

Field-Expedient Materials

The term *field expedient* refers to materials easily used, improvised, or created for use in a field environment. For example, a llama in South Carolina with a severe hind limb injury sustained on a trail walk was bandaged and splinted with materials fashioned from two T-shirts, local vegetation, duct tape, and thick wooden branches. Regardless of the situation, a solid grasp of basic first aid techniques combined with creativity and ingenuity will go a long way in field environments and possibly save the life of an animal or human.

The best approach to veterinary emergencies in the field environment is proper emergency planning. First-aid kits for the barn and vehicle, emergency/disaster kits for the home and vehicle, and personal survival gear carried by an individual are important components of hazard and contingency planning. Despite proper planning, situations will arise where the responders have to improvise field-expedient materials and methods.

STANDARD OF CARE IN FIELD ENVIRONMENTS

Regardless of the situation, veterinarians, veterinary technicians, emergency medical personnel, and nonmedical horse handlers must work within their scope of care and provide the best standard of care possible in a field or prehospital setting. When available, materials should be used in a manner consistent with their manufacture and intended use. Field expedients should be used only when the appropriate materials are not available and the injury must be treated immediately. For example, a non-life-threatening wound should not be sutured with makeshift materials (e.g., thread, fishing line, etc.) if the animal can receive quality standard of care wound repair within a reasonable time after the injury is sustained. Proper field first aid in such a case would consist of cleaning and dressing the wound and administering antibiotics and anti-inflammatory medication (if necessary).

Expired medications should not be used if nonexpired, suitable medications are available within a reasonable time period. Owners, bystanders, and other responders should not use expired medications or field-expedient materials to avoid seeking care from a licensed veterinarian.

Free Veterinary Services

Veterinary services are a very common source of humanitarian aid following disasters, civil conflicts and wars, and for underdeveloped countries. Nongovernmental organizations specializing in animal sheltering and veterinary care, faith-based veterinary organizations, and the military commonly offer free veterinary services to areas in need. These services are provided by these groups to assist animals and animal owners during stressful periods. An unintended consequence of these humanitarian efforts is that they may divert much-needed income from the local veterinarians.

There is often a compulsion to vaccinate horses and other livestock following a disaster (especially those disasters involving water, e.g., floods and hurricanes) in anticipation of animal disease outbreaks. Aside from dermatitis and diarrhea, infectious disease outbreaks in animals have not been documented following disasters in the United States. With the exception of the 1975 Red River flooding incident, disasters have not increased the spread of arboviruses (such as the eastern equine encephalitis virus, western equine encephalitis virus, Venezuelan equine encephalitis virus, and West Nile virus) (Nasci and Moore, 1998; Watson et al., 2007) The administration of tetanus toxoid vaccines is often warranted due to the prevalence of skin wounds following disasters, but no-cost vaccination for other diseases is unnecessary and may negatively affect the local veterinary practices' income.

There are situations where gratis (free) animal vaccinations are appropriate. Shelters accepting stray animals with unknown vaccination histories may require vaccination of incoming animals in order to protect other animals. It is recommended that groups interested in providing assistance during these situations contact the local veterinary community to determine what services are needed. Assistance can be provided in the form of unpaid volunteers to provide labor and case management or donations of medications, vaccines, or supplies.

LARGE ANIMAL PATIENT ASSESSMENT

Assessment of the animal patient begins with a visual survey of the animal and does not require a medical degree. First aid for humans in the field or an emergency environment is considered *wilderness medicine*, and in a disaster environment it is called *disaster medicine*. The expertise and concepts of these specialties can be applied to large animal incidents, but it is unlikely that someone with medical expertise is first on the scene for large animal emergencies.

First responders should appraise the general appearance and demeanor of the animal and report their observations to the veterinarian by telephone or when they arrive on the scene. The animal's demeanor can indicate the severity of injury or shock; an animal that is quiet, hanging its head, minimally responsive to stimuli, and reluctant to move may be exhausted, severely injured, or in an advanced state of shock. Rapid or labored breathing can indicate fear, shock, thoracic (chest) trauma, stress, or other conditions. A respiratory rate per minute can often be obtained by watching the steam from the nostrils in cold environments or by observing chest expansion or nostril flare. An animal that is shivering or sweating may be showing signs of environmental stress. An animal that is obviously non-weight bearing or favoring one or more limbs may have sustained soft tissue (e.g., tendons, ligaments, nerves, muscle, joint tissue, etc.) or bone injury.

The presence of blood, open wounds, visible bone, or impaled objects should be noted. If blood is observed, it should be determined if the animal is actively bleeding; if active bleeding is present, the rate (e.g., trickle, moderate flow, arterial spray, etc.) should be noted. These observations can be critical when determining how quickly the animal needs medical treatment compared to other injured animals or humans on the scene (triage) and to assess the prognosis of the animal (Figure 17.3).

Especially in mass casualty situations (e.g., overturned cattle liner, stampeding loose animals hit by cars, etc.), the responders should focus their resources and attention on the human or animal victims that can benefit from their assistance. If consent for euthanasia has not yet been obtained, administering pain-relieving medications or sedatives within the scope of care or on the instruction of a veterinarian may make the animal more comfortable until euthanasia can be performed. A common misconception is that administering pain medications to severely injured animals may

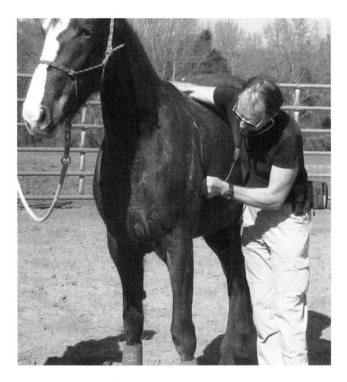

Figure 17.3 *Animals should be triaged in a primary survey for evidence of immediate life-threatening injuries using the principles of ABC. Here a veterinarian is determining a horse's heart rate. Courtesy of Rebecca Gimenez.*

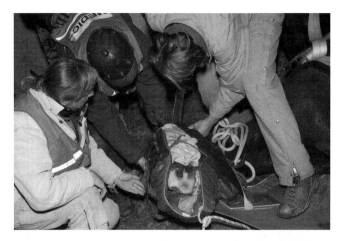

Figure 17.4 *The head and neck of a recumbent animal allow responders access to many of the parameters necessary for evaluation of the patient. Heart rate, pulse quality, respiratory rate, and mucous membrane color are excellent indicators of the animal's medical status and can be assessed from a safe position behind the animal's head. Courtesy of Tori Miller.*

mask their pain and cause them to further injure themselves; the degree of pain relief provided by most medications will not render the animal free of pain. Aside from the ethical implications associated with the failure to provide appropriate pain relief; persistent, severe pain may cause the animal to struggle enough to worsen its injuries and sustain additional injuries.

PRIMARY SURVEY

When the incident commander or other authority (perhaps the only person present in on-farm emergencies) determines that it is safe to approach the animal, responders should focus on life-threatening injuries as part of the primary survey of the scene. Many injuries appear worse than they actually are; it is important to develop an understanding of what constitutes an immediately life-threatening injury.

Basic first aid for humans and animals is built around the concept of ABC. Addressing these three areas facilitates the treatment of most immediately life-threatening injuries or conditions. Problems affecting the airway (the structures through which air passes from the environment to the lungs), breathing (the effort to take breaths), and circulation (e.g., heart beat, bleeding, blood volume, blood pressure, blood flow, and the ability of blood to carry oxygen to the tissues)

must be addressed first in what is called a primary survey. Much of the initial assessment can be performed from a safe position behind the animal's head (Figure 17.4). When responders have performed the necessary interventions to assure the function of these aspects, they are able to address other injuries and conditions in a secondary survey.

Situations arise when the ABC order must be rearranged to address a potentially life-threatening problem. For example, an animal may appear relatively normal but is profusely hemorrhaging (bleeding) from a limb wound. Although the hemorrhage is addressed in the "C" portion of the ABC approach, it should be addressed here first. If the animal is also having difficulty breathing, direct pressure should be applied to the bleeding wound as the horse's respiratory problems are assessed (Figure 17.5).

A secondary survey may address conditions such as lacerations and wounds with minimal or no active bleeding. Although limb injuries (including fractures) and gastrointestinal conditions (such as severe colic) may also be life-threatening, they are not considered immediately life-threatening unless they result in obstructing breathing efforts or severely hemorrhaging. Addressing the ABCs in the primary survey, conducting a secondary survey, and suggestions for field-expedient materials applicable to these situations are described here. If a veterinarian is present, he or she may or may not have appropriate medical materials and methods to deal with the injuries.

Airway

Airway in ABC refers to the unobstructed pathway through which oxygenated air passes from the environment to the lungs. The airway is usually divided into

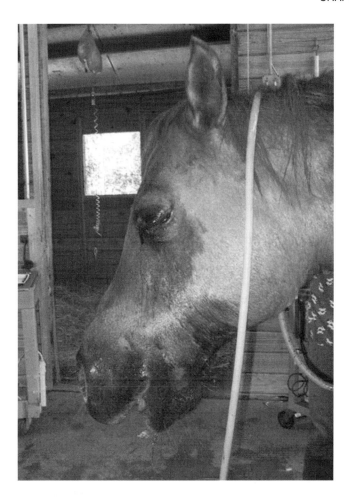

Figure 17.5 *This quarter horse gelding exhibits severe swelling caused by a rattlesnake bite to the horse's head. Due to the severe swelling, the animal was unable to breathe through its nostrils and nasal passages. An emergency tracheotomy was necessary before further assessment could be performed. Although the swelling subsided with aggressive treatment, the gelding died several days later due to venom-associated cardiac (heart) failure. Courtesy of Dr. Kimberly May.*

the upper airway—nose and nasal passages/mouth, pharynx, larynx (voice box), and trachea—and lower airway—bronchi, bronchioles, and other smaller airways within the lungs. The airways are frequently assessed by evaluating the animal for obvious disruption of the airway (e.g., swelling, lacerations with openings into the airways, bleeding, etc.), head and neck position, detectable airflow from one or both nostrils, altered respiratory effort (e.g., increased or abnormal effort), mucous membrane color, respiratory noise, or coughing.

In large animals, upper airway problems are more likely to be helped with basic first aid than lower airway problems. The primary method of first aid addressing the lower airways is the provision of supplemental oxygen and ventilation.

In general, it is abnormal for a large animal to attempt to breathe through its mouth. A partial or complete obstruction (blockage) of the airway prevents oxygenated air from reaching the lungs. Obstruction can result from swelling or physical blockage (e.g., feed, mud, aspirated gastric content, or a foreign object). Conditions that can result in partial or complete upper airway obstruction include, but are not limited to, the following: snakebite-induced or allergic (bee sting, etc.) hives or swelling of the nose and face; swollen lymph nodes due to *Streptococcus equi* infection ("strangles"); esophageal obstruction ("choke") compressing the trachea or causing aspiration of materials from the esophagus; iatrogenic (responder-induced) injury (e.g., an animal pulled with a rope around its neck); or trauma associated with the entrapment or emergency situation.

Aspiration of fluids such as stomach contents, water, or mud can occur, causing pneumonia and lung damage. Other common causes of aspiration include forcing water into a horse's mouth with a hose and force-feeding orphans milk products with a syringe. Regardless of the cause, the inability of air to pass through the upper airways is immediately life-threatening. Immediate care is required to provide an open airway to allow oxygenated air to reach the lungs. The situation, location, and severity of the obstruction, and the medical provider's scope of care guides what materials can be used to provide an airway.

A large animal with a partially blocked airway will usually lower and extend its head and neck. Nostril flare may be evident and abnormal respiratory noise may be heard. The animal may appear distressed, and there is often an obvious increase in respiratory effort. In some cases, it may be difficult to determine if the animal has an airway obstruction or lung disease. Animals in severe septic shock due to enteritis, severe intestinal obstruction, intestinal devitalization, choke, or systemic disease may also exhibit this posture and behavior due to lack of tissue oxygenation.

Horses are obligate nasal breathers; the anatomy of their pharynx does not allow mouth breathing unless the soft palate is dorsally (upwardly) displaced. Thus, any swelling in the nose or face may block their airway. At the first indication of swelling, passing a relatively firm tube in their nasal passage may preserve an open airway. The tubing must be firm enough to avoid collapse under mild pressure, but soft and smooth enough to prevent physical trauma or undue discomfort to the animal. Soft plastic tubing such as nasogastric tubes or orotracheal tubes (used for anesthesia) can be cut to approximately 6–8 in. (15–20 cm) lengths and carried in a first-aid kit for this purpose. Garden hose can also be used as a field expedient for this purpose. Nasopharyngeal airway tubing for humans is generally too small, short, and soft for use in large animals for this purpose.

Asphyxiation Death. A complete blockage of the airway at any location will lead to asphyxiation in a matter of five minutes or less. Asphyxiation is not considered a humane death. As the animal is asphyxiating, it will struggle violently and become extremely dangerous to anyone close to it. Eventually the efforts to breathe will cease after the agonal breaths (spontaneous, erratic gasping breaths) occur as the animal dies. These breaths usually signal the end of respiratory effort and impending death, but they may continue for a few minutes after the detectable heartbeat has ceased (see Chapter 13).

Emergency Tracheotomy. Tracheotomy is a procedure performed to create an external opening into the trachea to bypass the upper airway above the site. Animals with obstructions below the tracheotomy site will not respond to tracheotomy. Ideally, the procedure should be performed by a veterinarian or trained veterinary technician.

Although it can be a life-saving procedure, there are inherent risks associated with performing a tracheotomy. If performed incorrectly, it can cause serious injury. Vital structures in close proximity to the trachea include the esophagus, common carotid arteries, external jugular veins, and vago-sympathetic nervous trunk. The individual providing veterinary care to the horse must be absolutely sure a tracheotomy is necessary and must be trained to perform the procedure. The procedure is included here for informational purposes only; it is not the intent of the author to teach nonveterinary or nonmedical personnel to perform the procedure.

In an ideal situation, the skin overlying the cranial (upper) half of the ventral neck ("strap") muscles and trachea is prepared by clipping or shaving the hair and performing a surgical preparation with povidine–iodine, chlorhexidine, or other surgical preparation scrub solution. Local anesthetic (e.g., lidocaine, mepivacaine, etc.) is injected in a vertical, linear pattern underneath the skin overlying the trachea at the junction of the upper one-third and lower two-thirds of the neck. *Note*: the trachea is readily palpable in the cranial (uppermost) portions of the neck and becomes less palpable as it courses underneath the muscles to the thorax.

In an emergency situation, it may not be possible to perform these preparatory steps. Clipping the hair requires clippers or shaving materials. Cordless clippers are available and recommended components of an emergency kit; the clippers must be charged with an electrical adapter, and a spare battery is recommended. Disposable razors may be suitable if the area is thoroughly soaked with water and heavily lathered with soap or water-soluble surgical lubricant, lotion, or sunscreen. Any substance used as a shaving lubricant should be thoroughly cleansed from the skin prior to skin incision. Coarse hair quickly dulls disposable razors, increasing the difficulty and time required to prepare the site; manually shaving the area is often too time-consuming in an emergency situation, delaying a life-saving procedure.

The skin is incised in the center of the locally anesthetized area, and the underlying muscles are bluntly separated on the midline of the neck to expose the trachea. The incision should ideally be made with a sterile, surgical scalpel blade; other instruments such as a very sharp multipurpose knife or scissors can be used if there is no other option. Large animals' skin is tough, and it may be difficult to create an appropriate incision with knives or scissors.

Following exposure of the trachea, a controlled incision is made parallel to the tracheal rings (i.e., horizontal) and in the membrane between two rings. The cartilaginous rings of the trachea must not be incised. An initial stab incision into the trachea creates an opening into the airway; once the opening is established, forceful expirations in a dyspneic animal may spray blood and mucus outward and decrease the view of the area. Sterile or clean absorbent materials (e.g., surgical gauze, clean cloth, sanitary pads, etc.) should be available to allow removal of the expectorated material.

To maintain patency of the airway, a tube is placed in the tracheal opening. Self-retaining tracheostomy tubes made specifically for large animals are available through veterinary supply vendors. The device must be inserted so the tube is angled downward (toward the lungs). Nasal tubes, stomach tube sections, garden hose segments, a handle from a one-gallon jug or 10–12 cc syringes (with plungers and the luer [needle] end removed) can be used as emergency tracheotomy tubes when proper materials are not available. If prepared ahead of time, the cut edges of syringes or hose tubing should be smoothed with sandpaper or filed to smooth the edges and decrease tissue trauma. These materials can be irritating and traumatic to the tracheal tissues and should be replaced by a standard, commercially made equine tracheotomy tube as soon as possible.

The tube should be secured to the neck to prevent advancement too far into the trachea. The flanges on the plunger end of a syringe prevent losing the syringe in the tracheal lumen and can be used to secure the syringe to the neck. If the tubing or syringe is advanced too far into the trachea, it can cause tracheal trauma or obstruction. The tracheotomy should be cleaned as necessary to remove debris and fluid to preserve the patency of the tracheal opening.

Nasal Tubes. If tubing is prepared as part of a first-aid kit, clothesline or 5–50 parachute cord can be secured in a loop through one end to act as anchors to tie or secure it to the halter. Following a snake bite or other conditions where significant swelling is present or likely to occur, one tube is placed in each nostril. Shorter tubing (15 cm [6 in.]) protects the soft tissue structures rostral (in front of) the bony support of the nasal cavity, while 20 cm (8 in.) or longer tubing provides support and airflow farther into the nasal passages.

Nasal tubes are passed in a manner similar to nasogastric or nasotracheal tubes, but they do not reach the pharynx or larynx. In horses, caution is advised when passing a tube; passage of the tube in the dorsal (upper) section of the nasal passage can impact the ethmoid turbinates and cause significant hemorrhage. Tubes should always be passed into the ventralmost (lowest) portion of the nasal passages (i.e., along the floor of the nasal passage). Tubes can be kept in place as needed; the tubes will usually fall out or can be removed manually when the swelling subsides. Tubes should be placed far enough into the nasal passages to provide support to the soft tissue structures, but the outer ends should be clearly visible and secured to prevent loss into the nasal passages, pharynx, or trachea.

Breathing

The "B" in ABC represents *breathing*. While *airway* refers to the physical passages through which air passes to and from the lungs, breathing is the effort of taking in air (e.g., inhalation [inspiration] and exhalation [expiration]) and the exchange of gases within the lungs (i.e., exchange of oxygen for carbon dioxide in the blood). Parameters assessed to evaluate breathing function include mucous membrane color, respiratory effort and noise, nasal discharge, and respiratory rate. An animal can have a patent (open) airway but poor or no breathing. Lack of breathing or difficulty breathing can be caused by many different illnesses and injuries. With few exceptions, most of these problems are difficult to improve or resolve with basic first aid. The responder should take steps to minimize the animal's stress and keep it quiet and unmoving while assessing possible explanations for the problem.

Compromised breathing can result from conditions such as primary lung disease, trauma, and chronic illness. Cranial or central nervous system trauma can inhibit (prevent) transmission of the "message" to breathe from the brain to the diaphragm and other muscles of the thorax (chest). Thoracic trauma resulting in fractured ribs can compromise the physical effort of breathing. Pneumothorax, the presence of air within the chest cavity and around the lungs (e.g., from lung puncture, penetrating wounds, etc.), prevents the generation of the negative intrathoracic pressure necessary to inhale (inspire). Prolonged difficulty breathing from pulmonary disease or injury can exhaust the diaphragm and intercostal (between the ribs) musculature.

Due to the large size of horses and other livestock, manual or "rescue breathing" is not effective in adult animals over approximately 75 kg (165 lb) without the assistance of an appropriately sized mechanical ventilator; foals, calves, and small ruminants may be exceptions (see below). If the reduced or absent respiratory effort is caused by severe trauma or systemic illness, the prognosis for that animal is poor. In a field environment, especially following a disaster, those animals should be triaged as expectant (death imminent), and humane euthanasia or allowing a natural death should be considered.

Rescue Breathing. Rescue breathing, as performed during cardiopulmonary resuscitation of humans, is generally not effective in large animals due to their large size and lung volumes. Without the help of mechanical ventilators, responders cannot force enough air in at a sufficient pressure to adequately inflate the lungs of a horse, cow, or llama. Foals, calves, and small ruminant animals may benefit from rescue breathing. If other illness or injuries are causing breathing compromise, it is unlikely they will survive without intensive medical care.

In witnessed asphyxiation cases (e.g., submersion in ice water, rope entanglement, anesthesia or sedation overdose, nonbreathing neonates, etc.), rescue breathing or mechanical ventilation may be successful. To revive an animal that has been submerged it should be laid on its side with its head and neck below the rest of its body to allow drainage from the lungs. It is important to note that an abnormally low body temperature may result in an extremely faint heartbeat that often requires veterinary experience and a high-quality stethoscope to auscult (detect by listening).

Pulmonary Edema. Pulmonary edema refers to swelling and fluid accumulation in the lungs. Smoke and chemical inhalation, aspiration of water, lightning strike, and heart failure can cause breathing compromise due to pulmonary edema. The presence of pulmonary edema restricts or prevents the exchange of oxygen from the air for waste gases from the blood. As a result, the animal's blood cannot deliver sufficient oxygen to its body tissues. If supplemental oxygen is available, an oxygen mask for humans can be held to the animal's nose if tolerated. Alternatively, an oxygen line can be placed in the nasal passages and secured in place with suture or tape. Humidified oxygen (i.e., the oxygen gas is passed through sterile water to add moisture) should be used when available; unhumidified oxygen can have a desicating (drying) effect on the tissues of the nasal passages and airway. Oxygen from emergency medical services sources should not be depleted for use on an animal unless an immediate replacement of the oxygen supply is available, in case it is needed for a human patient.

Penetrating Thoracic (Chest) Wounds. Penetrating thoracic (chest) wounds can be the result of impalement by objects (e.g., branches, fencing materials, windborne debris, etc.) or projectiles (e.g., gunshot wounds). Normal inhalation (inspiration) begins with the generation of negative pressure in the chest cavity; the ribs are pulled outward, and the diaphragm is pulled toward the abdomen, creating a suction effect that brings air into the airways and lungs. If the negative pressure cannot be generated, air is not pulled into the airways. The entry of air into the chest cavity from a wound negates the negative pressure and prevents lung expansion (inflation) and breathing. This condition is referred to as *pneumothorax* and is immediately life-threatening if it affects both lungs.

Assessment of the depth of wound penetration may be difficult. If air can be heard entering or exiting the wound or foamy blood is observed entering and exiting the wound as the animal breathes, the thoracic cavity has been penetrated. Any wound over the chest cavity that is more than a superficial laceration or abrasion should be treated as if it is an open, penetrating chest wound until proven otherwise by a veterinarian.

The wound should be carefully packed and/or covered with gauze or other absorbent material and covered with an impervious or waterproof material to prevent air from entering the wound and chest cavity. The air-proof and waterproof material is most important, but any type of material or cloth can be field expedient. A plastic garbage bag, gallon-sized kitchen storage bag, or other similar material may be used. Tape does not often remain adhered to the animal's hair coat, but elastic, leg bandages, duct tape, or other tape can be used around the chest to hold the wound dressing and tape in place. Penetrating chest wounds require immediate veterinary care. The animal's vital signs and respiratory effort should be carefully monitored. Potential complications of penetrating thoracic wounds include asphyxiation death, hemorrhage, cardiac (heart) injury, pneumonia, esophageal rupture, pneumothorax, pneumomediastinum (air within the partition separating the two halves of the chest), and pleuropneumonia/pleuritis (infection and inflammation of the lungs and the membrane lining the thoracic cavity).

CIRCULATION

Circulation refers to the ability of the blood and blood vessels to carry oxygen to the body tissues. It may be compromised by hemorrhage (bleeding) as well as cardiac (heart), blood volume, and blood pressure abnormalities. Parameters used to assess circulation include heart rate, pulse quality, blood pressure, extremity temperature, mucous membrane color, and capillary refill time (CRT).

Cardiac injury can result in ineffective contraction and failure (insufficiency) to pump blood into the blood vessels. Preexisting cardiac abnormalities (e.g., valvular conditions, arrhythmias, etc.) may increase the risk of cardiac insufficiency in a stressful emergency situation.

Blood pressure is the pressure exerted by the blood on the blood vessel walls as it flows through the vessels and is a factor in determining how much blood reaches the body's tissues. An animal must maintain a minimum blood pressure to deliver oxygen-carrying blood to the tissues. Hypotension (low blood pressure) can result from true hypovolemia (low blood volume) or relative hypovolemia (the overexpansion of blood vessels relative to blood volume). True hypovolemia can result from hemorrhage, dehydration, or blood/fluid loss into body cavities. Relative hypovolemia often results from venous dilation secondary to the administration of sedatives and anesthetics (particularly phenothiazine tranquilizers, such as acepromazine). Pulse quality indicates a subjective measure of the strength and consistency of an arterial pulse palpated on the face or extremity. A weak, thready pulse quality indicates poor perfusion and low blood pressure.

Bleeding

Noncritical wounds in large animals may falsely appear critical due to the presence of blood (Figure 17.6). A 500 kg (1,100 lb) horse has approximately 40 l (10 1/2 gal) of blood (8% of body weight in kilograms). Signs of hypovolemic/hemorrhagic shock occur when approximately 30% (12 l, or 3 gal) of blood volume is

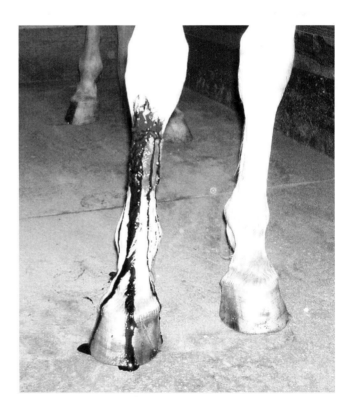

Figure 17.6 *Large animals can sustain wounds that appear severe due to considerable hemorrhage (bleeding) but are actually minor, non-life-threatening lacerations. This injury bled significantly but did not require sutures. Courtesy of Tomas Gimenez.*

lost. Signs of weakness or dehydration may be observed in animals with lesser amounts of blood loss.

The most life-threatening circulatory emergency is acute (sudden and severe) hemorrhage. The most effective measure to control hemorrhage is the application of direct pressure to the area. If available, gauze or other bandage material should be packed into the wound and solid pressure held on the material for several minutes or until bleeding appears to be controlled. The vessels of the lower limb are easily compressed with direct manual (finger or hand) pressure.

Tourniquets are rarely necessary; if necessary, a tourniquet can be improvised from materials such as belts, bandage materials, reins, lead ropes, or T-shirts. Continuous pressure should be maintained for several minutes before the wound is reassessed; removal of the pressure dressings or bandage material may disrupt blood clots and stimulate additional hemorrhage. If blood continues to seep up through the initial bandage or dressing, additional bandage material should be applied over the first bandage. Wound exploration and ligation or clamping of blood vessels should only be performed by a veterinarian.

Household or field-expedient materials can be used for pressure dressing or bandages if veterinary medical products are not available. In fact, most commercially available equine first aid kits do not contain enough bandage material to control severe bleeding. Diapers, sanitary pads, kitchen or bath towels, and clothing (especially nonsynthetic materials) are suitable for this purpose. In the field, a saddle pad, shipping boot, or T-shirt may be useful. If no other material is available, handfuls of leaves or thick grass have been used; these materials will contaminate the wound with dirt or other organic material, but concerns regarding sterility are often outweighed by concerns regarding blood loss. The animal can then be transported to a veterinary facility for care.

Pressure bandages can be held in place with standard leg bandaging material. Wounds on the face tend to bleed profusely due to the thin and highly vascular soft tissues covering the skull; bleeding is usually easily stopped with direct pressure. An elastic bandage placed lightly on the head, avoiding pressure on the nostrils, can hold a facial pressure bandage in place.

Dehydration

Dehydration can occur quickly due to diarrhea, sweating, heat stress, exhaustion, and water deprivation. Young animals of all species are especially susceptible to dehydration and can die quickly if not appropriately treated.

The level of dehydration can be roughly estimated by looking at the skin, eyes, and mucous membranes. If the skin over the neck or shoulder is "tented" (i.e., pinched or pulled away from the body to resemble a tent shape), it should return to its flat orientation within 1–2 seconds. Dehydration causes loss of fluid from the skin and makes the skin less elastic, so it does not quickly return to its pretented position. However, other factors, such as age and nutritional status, may affect this response. Experience assessing many different animals, normal and diseased, will improve one's skills with this assessment method. The eyes of severely dehydrated animals may appear sunken; the eye itself will appear sunken within the bony orbit.

Fluid Therapy. Fluid therapy refers to the administration of specific fluids via an intravenous catheter or other routes. Intravenous fluid administration is the most rapid and effective method for treating dehydration-induced hypovolemia. Intravenous catheters should only be placed by veterinarians, veterinary technicians, or veterinary-trained human emergency medical personnel. Similarly, only these qualified persons should attempt to administer fluids by nasogastric tube. Nasogastric administration of fluids and electrolytes may be a good option for a veterinarian in a disaster situation or underdeveloped area where intravenous fluids are not readily available. Large amounts (frequently in excess of 40 l, or 10 1/2 gal) are often required to rehydrate a large animal; it is usually not practical to carry this amount of fluid in a first aid or hand-carried field kit.

When possible, it is recommended that animals not be allowed to eat or drink until veterinary approval has been obtained. However, in a disaster or emergency situation where veterinary care is not immediately available, the animal should be offered clean water to drink (if available). Allowing a hot animal to drink water will not cause laminitis ("founder") or colic.

SECONDARY SURVEY

Once life-threatening injuries or conditions have been addressed through the ABC process, the secondary survey allows responders to assess and treat other wounds such as nonbleeding limb injuries and lacerations.

Vital Signs

Basic vital signs include body temperature, pulse rate, and respiratory rate (TPR) and CRT. A stethoscope assists in the assessment, but it is not absolutely necessary. Responders should record the measurements they obtain and inform the veterinarian of their findings when they arrive or via telephone consultation.

Heart Rate. To obtain the animal's heart rate, the stethoscope is placed over the chest between the animal's "elbow" and body wall to auscultate the heartbeat. Alternatively, the responder can palpate the pulse of the facial artery as it courses over the jaw. Several methods can be used to obtain the heart rate: the number of beats in 60 seconds can be counted to give the heart rate in beats per minute (bpm); the number of beats counted in 30 seconds can be multiplied by 2 to give the rate in bpm; or the number of beats counted in 15 seconds can be multiplied by 4 to give the rate in bpm. If any heart rhythm abnormalities (arrhythmias) are auscultated, the heart rate should be obtained over one full minute.

It is important to note that large animals, particularly horses and some cattle, may have more than two audible heart sounds. In humans, two sounds are heard; these sounds are often called "lub-dub" sounds and represent the sounds associated with the closure of the heart valves. Large animals' hearts are significantly larger in size compared to human hearts, and one or two sounds may be auscultated in addition to the two lub dub sounds. One of these sounds is a whooshing sound as blood fills the ventricles of the heart, and the second is the sound as atrial contraction pushes blood into the ventricles. It is important to count the heart rate by counting the same sound as is it repeated.

Respiratory Rate. The number of breaths per minute is easiest to obtain at a distance by watching the expansion and relaxation of the chest or the breaths condensing in cold air. If present, nostril flare may also be a good indicator of respiratory rate. Alternatively, a hand can gently be placed on the animal to feel the chest excursions. If a stethoscope is used, the preferred sites of auscultation are over the ribs or the trachea. This rate should be determined over the course of one full minute.

Body Temperature. Body temperature is most commonly obtained with a rectal thermometer. Digital thermometers register temperature more quickly than traditional glass–mercury thermometers and are associated with less risk of breakage (Figure 17.7). Digital thermometers purchased for use on large animals should be labeled as "fever" thermometers on their packaging; thermometers of other types do not reach the temperature levels necessary for animals. Aural (ear) thermometers are not suitable for use on large animals. Lubrication (e.g., petroleum jelly, water-based lubricants, or saliva) facilitates insertion of the thermometer.

Obtaining the rectal temperature of an unfamiliar animal is associated with a risk of injury. The animal should be approached as described in Chapter 4, and the responder should maintain contact with the animal as he or she gradually approaches the animal's hindquarters. The responder should stand close to the animal and beside the hind limb (if the animal kicks, it will generally kick straight behind itself). The tail should be gently lifted or pushed to the opposite side, and the thermometer should be gently inserted. If a thermometer is not available or the risk of injury does

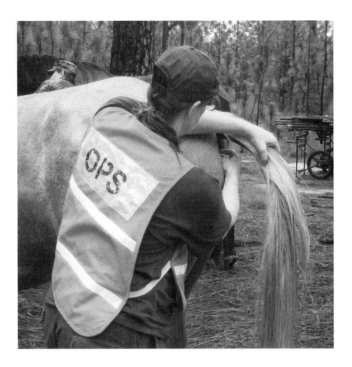

Figure 17.7 *A veterinarian takes the rectal temperature of a horse in a field scenario. The TPR data are crucial for medical personnel to evaluate the medical status of the large animal. Courtesy of Tomas Gimenez.*

not justify the procedure, the animal should be assessed by feeling the skin for obvious heat, cold, sweat, or lack of sweat.

Capillary Refill. Mucous membrane color and CRT can be beneficial in determining the perfusion and hydration status of an animal. The animal's mucous membranes, or gums, underneath the upper lip should be pink, moist, and covered in clear saliva. Pressing a finger firmly on the membranes for one second will press the blood out of the capillaries (called *blanching*). When pressure is released, the area should return to a normal pink color within one to two seconds. Prolonged CRT (three seconds or longer) may indicate poor perfusion of blood to the body tissues due to hypotension (low blood pressure). As mentioned above, poor blood pressure could result from excessive hemorrhage, dehydration, or systemic illness.

Dry mucous membranes can indicate mild dehydration. Pale mucous membranes can indicate anemia (decreased red blood cells) or poor perfusion due to excessive bleeding, shock, or hypotension. Bright pink-orange mucous membranes often indicate septicemia (toxins circulating in the blood). Dark, brick-red mucous membranes are often seen in severe shock or sepsis, colic with intestinal obstruction, or animals with intestinal perforation. A blue hue to the mucous membranes often indicates a lack of oxygenation. Purple or purple-black membranes indicate fatal shock or sepsis and often immediately precede death.

General Wound Care

When possible, wounds should be cleaned to allow assessment and reduce contamination and infection. Actively hemorrhaging wounds should not be cleansed or should be cleansed very gently prior to the application of a pressure bandage.

Wounds should be cleaned with mild soap and clean water, or dilute wound disinfectant solutions specifically made for use on animals or humans. Water or saline solutions are safe for most wounds, and large-volume lavage (flushing) may be necessary to remove debris. Mild soap and water, dilute povidine–iodine solution or scrub, or dilute chlorhexidine solution or surgical scrub should be used to cleanse the wounds. Hydrogen peroxide, iodine, or household cleaning solutions should never be used to clean wounds because the substances induce severe damage to the tissues and impair wound healing.

Studies have shown that the most beneficial initial treatment of open wounds is thorough irrigation with water, which physically removes debris and contamination from the wound. This thorough washing and physical removal of contaminants protects wounds from infection better than topical antimicrobials or antibiotic therapy alone. A minimum of 7 psi pressure is recommended for effective wound lavage, and pressures of 10–15 psi are very effective (Stashak, 1991). In a field situation, lavage solution can be delivered using an 18-gauge needle attached to a 35 cc or 60 cc syringe (being careful to avoid needle contact with the animal's skin). For large wounds, the wound can be sprayed with a hose while gently rubbing the wound with gauze or other material to loosen debris. Care should be taken to avoid driving contaminants deeper into the wound or separating tissue layers. The wound should be covered with a clean bandage to provide protection from flies and other contamination, and veterinary care should be sought as soon as reasonably possible.

Despite their claims, lanolin-based wound salves and ointment-type wound remedies found in tack shops, feedstores, and agricultural supply catalogs are minimally effective in fighting infection, and they may actually trap bacteria in the wound. Prescription and over-the-counter triple antibiotic ointments and creams (bacitracin-neomycin-polymyxin) can help protect the wound from infection and have minimal negative effects on wound healing. Commercial fly-repellant ointments may be of benefit in protecting the wound from flies but should not be applied directly to the wound; the wound should be covered with a dressing or bandage as described previously, and fly repellant ointment sprayed around the edges and over the top of the bandage or dressing.

Lameness and Limb Injuries

Lameness can be caused by a variety of problems, and the overall treatment differs greatly depending on the cause. However, in a field environment, basic first aid procedures are the same for most causes of lameness.

The animal should be safely approached (see Chapter 4) and restrained for examination and to prevent it from further injuring itself. The limb should be examined for swelling or obvious deformity. The animal's posture or the presence or absence of swelling does not often clearly indicate the diagnosis. Animals will often toe-touch on the affected limb regardless of the site of injury, and an animal with a hoof abscess (generally a non-life-threatening condition) may exhibit the same posture and lameness as an animal with a fracture.

First-aid for obvious or suspected fractures or severe ligament or tendon injuries should focus on immobilizing the limb and keeping the animal quiet and calm. Open wounds on the limb should be cleaned and covered and hemorrhage controlled if necessary. Splints and bandages can be made of many materials found in the field, as long as the responder adheres to the principles of splinting and bandaging.

Bandaging and Splinting. Bandages are intended to protect wounds, provide pressure (to stop hemorrhage and/or limit swelling), and protect exposed tissues. Splints are intended to allow limited weight bearing on injured limbs and to prevent further injury to the affected limb. Three basic principles of bandaging and splinting extremities apply to most limb injuries: (1) protect or pad pressure points of the limb, (2) ensure effective length of the splint or support bandage, and (3) avoid placing elastic materials directly on the skin. If these three basic principles are followed, many different materials can be used to make an effective bandage or splint.

The level of pain associated with severe musculoskeletal injuries may make the animal fractious and difficult to restrain. Adequate stabilization with a splint will often decrease the animal's stress and pain and facilitate restraint.

Pressure Points. Bony contours or protruding areas become pressure points because they sustain increased pressure by the bandage or splint. In addition, there is usually minimal protective soft tissue covering these areas. Pressure sores resulting from excess pressure and abrasion by bandages or splints can be extremely painful and cause secondary lameness or infection. Specific areas at risk of pressure sores on the forelimbs include the coronary band and heel bulbs, fetlock, carpus (knee)—especially over the accessory carpal bone on the back of the limb, and the olecranon (elbow). In the rear limbs, the coronary band and heel bulbs, fetlock, and tarsus (hock) are susceptible to pressure injury. Tendons of the lower extremities can also be damaged by excessive pressure from bandage material. Placing "donut" dressings over pressure points

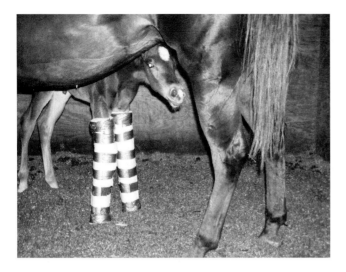

Figure 17.8 *A foal with PVC field-expedient splints on both front legs features modified Robert Jones bandages. The splints extend above and below the joints that demarcate the injury (in this case the cannon bones). Courtesy Rebecca Gimenez.*

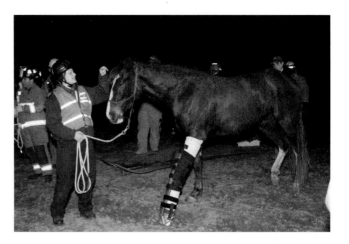

Figure 17.9 *A horse in a training demonstration stands up with the Kimzey Leg Saver Splint applied to a front leg and supported by a modified Robert Jones bandage underneath the splint. The animal can walk on this splint, although the Rescue Glide was used to transport the animal for a long distance to the ambulance in this scenario. Courtesy of Axel Gimenez.*

under bandage material and splints can reduce direct pressure on these areas. To make a donut dressing, a hole is cut in the center of a thick dressing; the hole should be the same size as the area to be protected, and the dressing should be sufficiently thick that the area does not protrude through the cut hole. Adequate padding must be placed between pressure points and splints; this is especially important in areas underlying the ends of the splint. If regular bandage material is not available, cloth, a T-shirt, or other such material can be used for padding.

Before applying a splint, thick padding should be placed over the pressure points of the extremity. A bandage is applied underneath the splint to provide additional protection for the pressure points. Many natural (e.g., limbs, etc.) and manmade materials (e.g., polyvinyl chloride (PVC) pipe, wooden boards, rebar, etc.) can serve as field-expedient bandages and splints for horses and livestock. Around the extremity, a modified Robert Jones bandage consists of several inches of padding and might be made of saddle pads, leg wraps, foam insulation, clothing, or vegetation (Figure 17.8).

Splint Length. The length and location of the splint are important factors in its efficacy. Splints that are too short, too long, too loose, or placed incorrectly on the limb can induce additional injury or worsen existing injuries. The length of the splint is determined by the site of the injury, but the splint should typically extend from the ground surface to one joint above the joint closest to the injury: for example, an appropriate splint for a metacarpal (cannon bone) injury extends from the ground to the elbow. Splinting techniques to address specific injuries are beyond the scope of this chapter and are addressed in veterinary texts.

If standard veterinary materials (e.g., Kimzey Leg Saver Splint) are not available (Figure 17.9), splints and bandages can be made from a variety of materials in the vicinity, provided responders adhere to the principles described above (Figure 17.10). A T-shirt filled with grass or leaves can make a sufficiently padded field-expedient leg wrap underneath a splint. Sturdy branches, wood fencing, or pipe can be employed as splinting materials. Sections of 10 cm (4 in.) diameter PVC pipe (white plumbers' pipe) cut lengthwise into three pieces are commonly used by veterinarians for splinting limbs because the pipe can be cut to any specified length. In addition, these sections are lightweight, sturdy, and portable.

Elastic Materials. The placement of elastic materials directly on the skin should be avoided or, when necessary, performed with caution. Elastic bandages applied tightly around an extremity can cause excessive pressure, decreasing blood circulation to the skin and underlying tissues. Tendons and ligaments can also be damaged from this pressure.

Elastic materials are often used for pressure bandages or temporary bandages when other materials are not available. However, these bandages should ideally be applied and monitored by a veterinarian or veterinary technician.

Hoof Injuries and Protective Bandages

Hoof injuries are common events following large-scale disasters such as hurricanes or floods. Excessive wetness of the hooves and ground debris increase the risk of hoof abscesses, hoof bruises, penetrating foreign bodies, and heel bulb or coronary band lacerations.

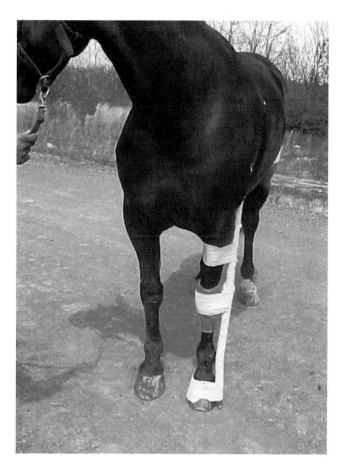

Figure 17.10 *A horse that was trapped in harness and dragged in a wagon accident demonstrates field-expedient splinting of the front leg. Responders improvised a splint using a sturdy limb cut from a tree. Courtesy of Rebecca Gimenez.*

Open wounds on the hoof or coronary band should be flushed with clean water and dilute antimicrobial or disinfectant solution appropriate for use on animals, as described above. The decision to remove penetrating objects from the hoof depends on the situation and should be made by a veterinarian. If the object is removed, the site of penetration should be marked on the hoof and the angle and depth of penetration should be carefully noted and recorded. The wound should be cleaned with water or saline; antiseptic solutions should be avoided in the event that synovial structures (joints or tendon sheaths) are involved.

It is often advised to leave penetrating objects in place until radiographs (x-rays) of the hoof can be obtained to determine what internal structures may be affected. If the object is left in place, the limb should be padded so that the object will not be driven deeper into the hoof. Alternatively, the protruding surface/end can be cut off to a point above the hoof surface, and the hoof marked to allow easy detection of the object. The prognosis for these conditions depends on the depth and angle of penetration and the involvement of anatomic structures within the hoof. Possible com-

plications include hoof abscess, septic osteitis (bone infection) of the third phalanx (coffin bone) or distal sesamoid (navicular) bone, septic navicular bursitis, infection of the collateral cartilages, sepsis (infection) of the tendons or ligaments within the hoof, and sepsis of the distal interphalangeal (coffin) joint. The hoof should be padded with clean material—clean or sterile 4 × 4 gauze is ideal, but cotton, folded diapers, or sanitary pads also provide sufficient padding. A folded T-shirt or leaves or grass packed into a sealable plastic sandwich bag have also been used as field-expedient padding.

The hoof should be protected with a water-resistant bandage over the padding. Commercially made hoof boots (e.g., EasyBoot, etc.) are available and suitable for this purpose, but several different sizes must be available to ensure a proper fit. Duct tape is readily available, inexpensive, and well suited for an easily constructed and durable hoof wrap. Twelve strips of duct tape approximately 30 cm (12 in.) long are cut. Six of the strips are overlapped by approximately 1 cm to create a square sheet of tape approximately 28 cm × 28 cm (11 in. × 11 in.). The remaining six strips are placed in the same manner perpendicular to the first set to create a double-layered square of duct tape. An 8 cm (3 in.) slit is cut at each corner diagonally toward the center. The center of the sheet is placed over the padding on the sole of the hoof, and the free corners are wrapped around the hoof to secure the bandage in place. Several additional strips of duct tape can be used to encircle the bandage for added security and protection from water.

LACERATIONS AND OPEN WOUNDS

Lacerations and open wounds can pose problems with assessment and triage because of their deceptive appearance. Wounds over joints, tendon sheaths, chest, or abdomen should be considered potentially serious unless it is obvious the wound does not completely penetrate the skin. Responders should consider the animal's overall appearance and vital signs, the degree of lameness, and other factors before deciding a wound in these areas is non-life-threatening.

Wounds over Joints or Tendon Sheaths

Wounds over joints or tendon sheaths can penetrate into the joint or sheath, causing septic arthritis (infection of the joint tissues and bone) or septic tenosynovitis (infection of the tendon sheath and tendon). Animals with penetrating injuries may exhibit minimal lameness for several days after the injury; if the joint or sheath is open, the fluid produced by the inflamed structure will leak from the wound and prevent the pressure that causes pain and lameness. As the wound heals and seals the entry to the joint or tendon sheath, the fluid accumulates within the structure and causes severe pain and lameness. Immediate veterinary attention is needed for any injury involving a joint or tendon sheath. It is always best to consult with a veterinarian about these wounds. Severe septic arthritis or tenosynovitis is generally associated with a poor prognosis. Possible complications of penetrating joint injuries include septic arthritis (joint infection), septic osteomyelitis (bone infection), septic physitis (infected growth plates), and chronic osteoarthritis. Possible complications of tendon sheath penetration include septic tenosynovitis (tendon sheath infection), tendon damage or rupture, and tendon adhesions. Chronic lameness is a common sequela of these conditions.

Wounds Over the Thorax

Lacerations on the chest or trunk (thorax) may penetrate into the chest cavity and cause pneumothorax or severe infections. The wounds should be covered with an occlusive bandage as described above, and the animal should be assessed and treated by a veterinarian as soon as possible. If it is obvious the wound does not penetrate the chest, it should be cleaned with mild soap and water or a dilute disinfectant solution made for wound cleaning as described above.

The wound should not be closed with staples or sutures except by a veterinarian or other health care provider in special circumstances. Skin closure without proper debridement, cleaning, and closure of underlying tissues can trap bacteria and fluid in the wound and increase the risk of infection. The cleansed wound should be covered with a clean dressing or bandage to protect the wound from dust, flies, and other contamination. The dressing can be stapled in place with skin staples, a bandage encircling the chest, or stent bandage. A stent bandage is created by placing several large loop sutures on all sides of the wound, approximately 5 cm (2 in.) from the wound edges; a dressing is placed over the wound, and string or other cord is laced through the loop sutures over top of the dressing like a boot lace to hold the stent in place.

Wounds over the Abdomen

Horses are very susceptible to peritonitis (inflammation of the lining of the abdominal cavity). Bacteria introduced through the wound or leaked from punctured bowel can cause infection and severe inflammation within the abdomen. Perforated, torn, or punctured bowel will usually cause sepsis, shock, and death within hours of the injury. Contamination without intestinal damage is associated with a longer clinical course, but often results in peritonitis, septic shock, and death. Immediate medical and/or surgical intervention is often required to decontaminate the abdominal cavity. The resulting inflammation often results in adhesions or scarring in the abdomen that increase the risk of subsequent intestinal obstruction, entrapment, or devitalization. Penetrating abdominal wounds in horses in

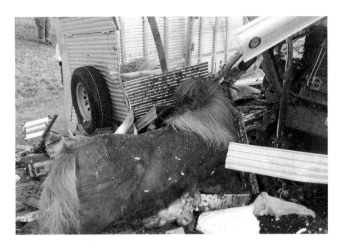

Figure 17.11 *This horse was eviscerated in a trailer incident in which a semi-tractor and trailer impacted a horse trailer being pulled by a 40-foot motorhome. The horse was immediately euthanatized on the scene. Another horse and the truck driver were also killed in this incident. Courtesy Douglas Kane.*

TLAER scenarios are often considered expectant, and euthanasia is performed (Figure 17.11). However, similar injuries in ruminants are usually associated with a better prognosis.

Large abdominal wounds with bowel protruding from the wound (evisceration) is usually a fatal condition for horses for the reasons already mentioned, but cows and other ruminants may survive following appropriate veterinary treatment. The protruding intestines should be contained in wet bandage material or cloth, or in a plastic bag or bowl with a small amount of water or saline solution to keep them moist. If the healthy intestines can be easily placed back into the abdominal cavity without excessive pain or distress to the animal, it is often the best course of action; bowel outside the abdominal cavity is at higher risk of injury and desiccation (drying). Noticeably torn and leaking bowel should not be replaced into the abdomen. If the wound clearly does not enter the abdomen, cleaning and dressing the wound as described with chest injuries may be sufficient until veterinary help is available.

EYE INJURIES

Eye injuries are common in large animals following natural disasters; blowing debris easily penetrates animals' corneas. Entrapped or recumbent animals are likely to sustain eye injuries from thrashing and hitting their heads on the ground or other objects. If the animal is still trapped or unable to rise, placing protective covering over their head will help prevent further injury. Neoprene head protectors are ideal, but other suitable materials include vest-style human water personal flotation devices (life jackets). These devices provide skull protection and, depending on the size, the arm holes may be positioned over the eyes to allow

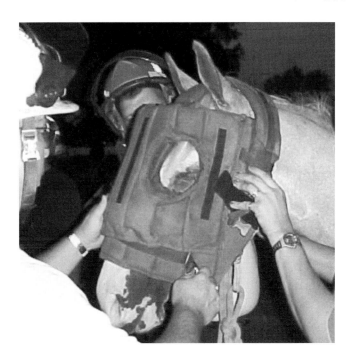

Figure 17.12 *In many large animal scenarios, providing head protection for the animal can prevent iatrogenic injuries, especially in confined areas or when animals are recumbent. Protection can range from a specialty device such as this commercially available head protector to field expedients such as a towel, human personal flotation device, or T-shirt. The eyes of sedated and anesthetized animals should be protected. Courtesy of Houston Park.*

the animal to see (Figure 17.12). A folded blanket or pillows taped to the head can also be used.

If tolerated by the animal, the eyes should be lavaged (rinsed) with saline or bottled or clean water to remove debris. A gentle spray from a syringe or bulb syringe (or field expedients such as a turkey baster or squeeze bottle) can be used to lavage the eyes. Ointments or creams should not be applied to the eyes unless they are specifically labeled for ophthalmologic use or unless the use of nonophthalmic preparations is directed by a veterinarian. Ophthalmic preparations containing steroids should be avoided unless directed by a veterinarian; steroids can impair corneal healing and increase the risk of corneal damage if scratches or lacerations are present.

If there is obvious damage to the eyeball itself or the tissues surrounding the eye, the eye should be covered, taking care not to actually touch the eye with the protective covering. A Styrofoam cup, cut down to a depth of several inches, can be placed over the eye and held in place with a bandage around the head. An excellent improvised eye covering that conforms well to the large animal head is a brassiere. Underwire, B- or C-cup padded bras hold their shape and offer superior padding and protection, and they can easily be included in animal first aid kits. Maternity brassieres with detachable cups allow for examination/doctoring of the eye

without removing the brassiere. When applying a brassiere for eye protection, the back strap of the brassiere is passed around the jaw and buckled at the throatlatch. The shoulder straps are placed over the ears to hold the brassiere in place with the cups over each eye. The cup can be cut away from the uninjured eye to allow the animal to see.

If an eyeball has been popped out of the eye socket, it should be gently rinsed with saline or clean water. It is unlikely that the horse will tolerate replacement of the eye into the socket; the procedure is very painful. Forcing the eyeball back into the socket will increase damage to the eyeball and eye socket. If the eyeball cannot be replaced into the socket easily, it should be covered as described above to protect it and should frequently be rinsed to keep it moist. If the optic nerve is not damaged, the animal may retain sight in the eye.

Eye injuries are extremely painful; animals with these injuries may not eat or drink due to pain. If it is within the provider's scope of care, or if directed by a veterinarian, nonsteroidal anti-inflammatory medications (e.g., phenylbutazone, flunixin meglumine, etc.) should be administered to relieve some of the pain and swelling.

COLIC

Colic is a lay term used to describe abdominal pain. It may occur as the result of a large number of conditions. An in-depth discussion of colic is beyond the scope of this text; for those interested in learning more about the subject, multiple veterinary and lay texts are available. However, the condition is included in this chapter due to its prevalence.

The clinical signs exhibited by an animal with abdominal distress vary with species, the structures involved, and the severity and duration of the problem. Ruminants tend to display more subtle signs of distress, including depression, anorexia, arched back, reluctance to move and abnormal defecation (stool passage). Horses can display these same signs, but more violent signs may also be observed. Additional clinical signs that may be exhibited by horses include exaggerated flehmen reactions (curling the upper lip), abdominal distention (bloating), looking or biting at the flanks, pawing, kicking at the abdomen, backing into corners, stall walking, recumbency, and rolling. Horses with severe abdominal pain are often uncontrollable and may pose a significant safety risk to humans.

Basic first aid for colic generally involves the administration of analgesics (pain relievers) and laxatives. Medications such as flunixin meglumine (Banamine), dipyrone, ketoprofen, or *N*-butylscopolammonium bromide (Buscopan) should not be administered except on the order of a veterinarian. Although these products do not mask pain, as some myths promote, they should be administered after a baseline examination has been performed.

Veterinarians and veterinary technicians are trained to be extremely careful when passing nasogastric tubes to administer oil or other fluids into the stomach; if the tube is inadvertently passed into the trachea or is not passed into the stomach, fluids can be aspirated into the lungs. For that reason, no one other than trained veterinary personnel should attempt to pass a nasogastric tube or administer anything through a nasogastric tube.

Any animal exhibiting signs of colic should receive immediate veterinary attention. Treatment for colic varies with the cause of the problem and is beyond the scope of this text.

FIRST AID OF DOWNED, RECUMBENT, OR ENTRAPPED ANIMALS

Basic first aid as covered previously in this chapter also applies to entrapped animals or those unable to rise for various reasons. The responder should understand the physiologic problems of entrapped animals; specific treatments should focus on maintaining the animal's body temperature, hydration, and preventing it from further harming itself (see Chapter 20).

Regardless of the reason an animal has become recumbent, anyone not specifically providing emergency veterinary care (e.g., injection, emergency tracheotomy, or other specific procedure) should remain a safe distance from the animal. Only personnel essential to the focused, purposeful treatment of the animal should be near the animal. This should include a safety buddy if there is only one person providing veterinary care.

A typically unsafe scenario is the responder or veterinarian entering a stall with a recumbent horse (Figure 17.13) and numerous bystanders crowding the doorway of the stall. This situation is dangerous because the

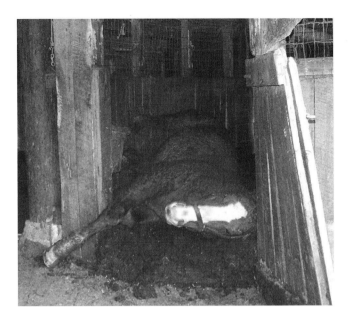

Figure 17.13 *A recumbent horse in a stall is a common on-farm scenario and presents significant safety concerns. Personnel entering the stall should have a clear path out of the stall in an emergency. Courtesy of Rebecca Gimenez.*

bystanders have effectively shut off the veterinarian's (or responder's) escape route. The safety officer or public information officer should take control and instruct bystanders to remain clear.

ACRONYMS USED IN CHAPTER 17

ABC	Airway, breathing and circulation
bpm	Beats per minute
CRT	Capillary refill time
EERU	Emergency equine response unit
PVC	Polyvinyl chloride
TLAER	Technical large animal emergency rescue
TPR	Temperature, pulse, and respiration

18 Helicopter Operations

Dr. Rebecca Gimenez

INTRODUCTION

Large animal short-haul helicopter rescue involves suspending a rescue cable under a helicopter, connecting and lifting an animal victim from the rescue site, and flying it (unattended) the shortest possible distance to safe ground for transfer to a ground vehicle equine ambulance (Figure 18.1). The technique is considered relatively simple for human rescue because it is associated with a short period of risk for the crew and aircraft, but annual training and expertise are required (Segerstrom, 2002). When large animals are added to the equation, the risk increases due to unpredictable behavior and increased weight as compared to human rescues.

Helicopter sling loading has been performed to relocate large animals trapped in remote, inaccessible areas (e.g., floodwater, steep ravines, etc.) during a disaster or emergency or targeted for removal from extreme terrain. The procedure requires significant planning, resources, and personnel training for safe employment, and it is **not** recommended except in extreme circumstances. Any consideration of helicopter operations is high risk and a last resort technique. There are many simpler, cheaper, and less dangerous options available for rescuing a stranded large animal in most situations (see Chapters 15 and 16). Recent scenarios using this technique were reported by the incident commander (IC) to be the only option other than euthanasia of the animal victim (Lauze, 2006; Olari, 2006).

Over the last 15 years, much time and effort has been devoted to the dilemma of large animal sling load lifts for emergency rescue by helicopter (UC-Davis Veterinary Emergency Response Team, U.S. Marine Corps, technical large animal emergency rescue [TLAER], etc.). Improved equine slinging equipment, heightened awareness of safety considerations, and use of the inci-

dent command system for on-scene leadership have significantly decreased the risk of accidents.

The inclusion of a helicopter in any operation increases the risk, but there are legitimate uses of helicopters in TLAER; examples include extreme terrain and floodwater. The proper considerations for safety and operations as well as specialty techniques and a standard operating protocol (SOP) for employment are included here. These include a focus on sling loading operations, with mention of herding, net-gunning, and euthanasia using a helicopter as a platform for firing. Although most localities will not have the equipment discussed here, familiarity with this chapter will increase responders' capabilities to assist with a large animal rescue attempt using locally available assets. In addition, the information supplied is expected to assist providers when making decisions for risk assessment purposes.

HISTORY OF LARGE ANIMAL SLING LOADING USING HELICOPTERS

In 1991, Charles Anderson and Dr. John Madigan (of the University of California-Davis College of Veterinary Medicine [CVM]) reported their development of a prototype sling to support the skeletal system and distribute a large animal's weight. That same year, the team received an urgent call for the rescue of five mules and a horse stranded in the Sierra Madre range (Madigan, 2005). A volunteer rescue team was quickly assembled to test the sling in this unconventional situation. The test environment was ideal because the animals were uninjured, the skies were clear, and the weather conditions were mild. All five animals were successfully airlifted 4 miles to solid ground, introducing a new option for rescuing large animals. Since that time, the UC Davis-Anderson Sling has been used in numerous rescue operations throughout the country (Anderson, 2004).

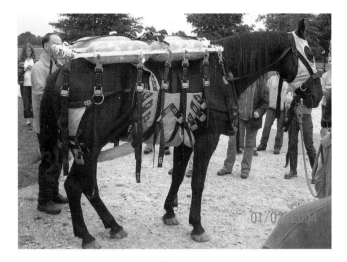

Figure 18.1 *In a training scenario, the UC-Davis Anderson Sling has been applied to a horse and is prepared by students for a demonstration lift by crane. The lower leg supports of the sling system are not necessary for helicopter lift. Courtesy Rebecca Gimenez.*

In 1992, capture operations of large zoologic animals were advanced when a helicopter was used to sling load a rhinoceros from the Umfolozi Wilderness Area of Africa. These animals are considered endangered species and are also extremely dangerous. Management policy prohibited the use of vehicles in the wilderness zone, so conventional capture methods were not possible. After the rhinoceros was successfully darted by a shooter in a smaller helicopter, a powerful helicopter capable of lifting in excess of 3 tons (2,700 kg) was directed to where the animal had fallen. A net was dropped, and a ground crew positioned the rhinoceros in the net. The helicopter returned to hoist the animal, airlifting it directly to recovery vehicles miles away. With modern technology, rhinoceros mortalities during moving operations and while in the holding pens have declined to less than 1%.

Since 1991, helicopters have been used to lift live horses using the UC Davis-Anderson Sling in numerous successful rescues conducted by the following organizations:

Massachusetts Society for the Prevention of Cruelty to Animals (1 rescue)
University of California-Davis -Davis College of Veterinary Medicine (more than 25 rescues)
Alta Loma and Rancho Cucomonga, California (1 rescue)
Louisiana State University (LSU), College of Veterinary Medicine (2 rescues)
Massachusetts Disaster Animal Response Team (2 rescues)
Idaho Mountain Search and Rescue Unit (1 rescue)
Live animal demonstration of TLAER (6 rescues)
Horse mannequin demonstration of LAR (8 rescue)

Other helicopter lifts of anesthetized animals using rope slings or cargo nets have been successfully performed in Britain (2, cattle), in Scotland (5, cattle), and the United States (1, horse).

EXAMPLE OF HELICOPTER SLING LOAD DURING FLOODS

In 2001, 12 horses were stranded on a 2-acre section of land by rising floodwaters in Pineville, Louisiana. The Rapides Parish Office of Emergency Preparedness contacted veterinarians, students, and technicians from the LSU CVM to execute airlifts and barge transportation in coordination with the U.S. Coast Guard. Following an on-site planning meeting and briefing, the volunteers formed three teams: one team prepared 2 animals for transportation by helicopter sling load; one team anesthetized and transported 10 recumbent animals on a barge; and the final team recovered the animals and conducted the medical examinations (Haven, 2006; Pettifer et al., 2002).

This rescue effort was complicated by the challenge of gathering horses that were not halter-broken or accustomed to human handling and that were frightened by the presence of helicopters and personnel. To decrease stress and anxiety for the horses, the veterinarians heavily sedated and blindfolded each horse before it was lifted by the helicopter. The combined effort enabled the school to better understand the sling's capabilities and gave the Coast Guard firsthand experience airlifting large animals from disaster situations. Prior to the rescue effort, the LSU CVM used its UC Davis-Anderson Sling extensively in the equine hospital but had not previously used the equipment in a disaster setting.

The Coast Guard coordinated the airlift with three pilots and four crew members. To lift the 500 kg (1,100 lb) horses the pilots minimized the helicopter's weight by removing fuel and limiting the time available for the operation. The animals were lifted 15 m (50 yards) above obstacles such as power lines and over a distance of 2 km (1.2 miles) to dry land.

It should be noted that the team assigned to transport 10 animals on a barge across the floodwaters was able to complete its mission in the same time required to complete two helicopter lifts. None of the horses sustained injuries during either phase of the rescue operation. After being relocated from the flooded area, the animals were triaged, and one horse that had sustained skin abrasions from a barbed wire fence was treated by veterinarians (Haven, 2006).

SUGGESTIONS FOR IMPROVEMENTS TO PREVIOUS STANDARD OPERATING PROTOCOLS

Viewing videotapes of previous large animal helicopter rescue attempts worldwide demonstrated many critical safety offenses by rescuers, pilots, and the general public. Observed incidents and safety concerns included the following: the web strap from the cable to the frame became wrapped around personnel; failure to disconnect snap(s) from the frame as the helicopter lifts off after delivery of the animal; up to 15 personnel under the hovering craft at one time; incorrect application of the sling on the animal; no tag line; loss of the drogue chute; up to four people simultaneously giving signals to the pilot; lack of correct personal protective equipment (PPE) on ground personnel; and personnel shocked by the static electricity conducted by the steel cable.

From these experiences a critical assessment of each scenario was conducted by pilots, safety officers (SOs), and ground personnel to devise an improved SOP that aggressively minimizes the number of people under the helicopter, addresses safety concerns, and shortens the time that people are under the hovering craft to less than 30 seconds. The improved SOP is presented in this book.

If the UC Davis-Anderson Sling is not available, the use of wide webbing with consideration of contact surface area on the animal's body is particularly important. The World Society for the Protection of Animals reported the unsuccessful attempts of helicopter crews to rescue cattle trapped in volcanic lava flows and mudslides in El Salvador and Guatemala; the crews were not breaking the suction of the mud when using the cable from the helicopter to lift the animals. Due to the powerful suction effect of the mud, the animals were cut in half as the cable tightened around their bodies.

In one video provided to the author, Australian cowboys used a helicopter to lift wild adult cattle by roping one leg, two legs, or the horns, lifting them by the rope and setting the cattle down into a waiting truck. It was reported that the cattle were on national park lands and otherwise marked for destruction. The amount of damage done to the animal's extremities and any accidents (e.g., dropped cattle, sling load failure, etc.) were not reported in the video clip.

The "lessons learned" evaluations after the helicopter lift of five horses stranded by floodwaters following Hurricane Floyd (1999) in North Carolina showed that the protocols in use at that time did not sufficiently address the safety of the rescuers on the ground, and changes were necessary to increase the safety of what is already a dangerous activity. At that time, the protocol provided for the helicopter to bring the frame to the animal in the water, with the soft part of the sling already attached by ground personnel. The helicopter was instructed to hover in place approximately 36 m (120 ft) above the animal while ground personnel securely attached 18 buckles to the overhead frame and made adjustments (Baker, 2000). During one of these lifts, the pilot was required to hover in that position

for over four minutes as three ground personnel and one team member in a small boat worked underneath the craft in the hurricane-force winds generated by the helicopter rotors. Although not completed due to the SO's risk assessment at the emergency operations center, one team of rescuers considered performing a night helicopter rescue of a horse from the flood zone, this is not reccomended.

There have been suggestions to sling load animals inside a large animal trailer; this is not recommended due to structural concerns with the configuration of the standard two-horse trailer and a shifting live load. If an appropriate loading box with configuration to prevent escape or load shift was available, animals could be loaded into the box and the entire assembly transported by an appropriate-sized helicopter without requiring the application of a sling on the animal (Ranson, 2002).

OVERALL RISK ASSESSMENT

A significant concern for professional emergency responders is the ever-present danger associated with helicopter operations, irrespective of technique. It is a common point of contention whether helicopter assets should be used for animal victims. In a disaster situation, helicopter assets should be prioritized to assist with saving human lives and may not be available for animal rescue despite prior planning and coordination; this may influence the responders' choice of treatment, rescue, or euthanasia.

Technological improvements in rotary-wing aircraft, equine slings, and improved SOPs related to their use have allowed consideration of these techniques today (Gimenez and Gimenez, 2002a). Since 1991, a review of news reports and personal communications with the author reveals that over 50 documented large animal helicopter lifts have been successfully completed (Gimenez, 2006c).

The importance of safety cannot be overstated for helicopter operations, especially when incorporating various civilian, law enforcement, military, and aviation personnel into the operation. Specific considerations for an on-scene risk assessment are discussed later in this chapter. In a real situation, most personnel will not have had time to read the SOP or have any experience actually lifting an animal with a helicopter. Those personnel experienced with helicopter lifts should act as the SO for the operation and advise the IC (Ranson, 2006).

The Media Effect

As large animal owners develop increasingly close and emotional relationships with their animals, their expectations of the rescue capabilities of veterinary and emergency rescue professions also increase. Owners expect rescuers to save their large animals from what would previously have been considered impossible scenarios. Helicopter rescues always generate media attention, and the public may be misled into thinking that it is the only safe way to rescue large animals. For example, on December 13, 2000, the *Swindon Advertiser* (United Kingdom) reported that Royal Society for the Prevention of Cruelty to Animals rescuers were receiving special awards for a helicopter lift of a steer owned by a television personality out of a ravine. In the article, the firefighters noted that the animal slipped out of the canvas-type sling three times before they were able to correctly apply it. It is possible that there were rescue methods that would have been as successful but associated with less risk of injury to personnel and the animal victim.

Dress Correctly

The minimum PPE for rescue ground teams includes hearing protection, long sleeves and pants, well-fitting full goggles, and a helmet with a chinstrap. This equipment prevents ocular (eye) and dermal (skin) injuries from airborne debris in the rotor wash and skull injuries from flying or dropping debris. All jewelry should be removed to prevent neck chains, earrings, or rings from becoming caught in lines and possibly causing loss of a body part.

Perform the Assessment First

Triage of animals by the assessment or field rescue teams must be completed prior to a helicopter lift. There have been situations where animals rescued by helicopter sling load operations had to be euthanatized moments after touchdown at the landing zone (Baker, 2000). If the animal has life-threatening injuries, the decision to euthanatize the animal should be made immediately and well before mobilizing resources for a helicopter lift.

Choose Safe Equipment for the Animal

One of the few factors that responders can control on the scene is proper equipment. The author recommends that only the UC Davis-Anderson Sling be used for helicopter sling load operations with large animals. The safety record of this equipment has been excellent, despite video evidence (two incidents) and pictures showing incorrect application in some successful rescues. The sling is well tolerated by the animal victims; therefore, the SOPs in this chapter are based on its use.

Canvas slings, other livestock slings, cargo nets, and rope slings are not designed to accommodate the weight and aerodynamics of sling loading and may slip or fail. For this reason, these slings can present significant risks for the animal and rescuers. Many slings not designed for helicopter lift place excessive pressure on the animal's diaphragm or might be prone to slipping, especially if the victim is recumbent when placed in the sling. If one of these slings must be used, inducing general anesthesia prior to performing the lift procedure is recommended to prevent struggling or movement of the live load in equipment that is otherwise unacceptable and might not adequately support the load.

It is critical to ensure a patent airway when an animal is lifted in a cargo net. Large carnivores (e.g., bears, lions, etc.) and large exotics (e.g., rhinoceros, elephants, etc.) are commonly transported in cargo nets as part of management and wild capture procedures, but this method can result in mortality (Caulkett and Cattet, 2002). Slinging can induce hypertension (increased blood pressure) and hypoxemia (low blood oxygen levels). Flexion of the animal's neck can produce partial or complete airway obstruction and worsen the hypertension and hypoxemia, increasing the risk of death. Ideally, an anesthetized carnivore should be transported with its head and neck extended and its body positioned in sternal (chest down) or dorsal (back down) recumbency to facilitate the animal's respiratory effort. A stretcher-type sling can facilitate this positioning for carnivores (Cattet et al., 1999).

Numerous cargo net rescues of sedated or anesthetized cattle (34 total rescues) have been reported through the media worldwide. An intensive literature and Internet search generated no data as to injuries or deaths associated with these practices or the effect of body position on the outcome of the rescue. (See also the discussion of net gun operations near the end of this chapter for information regarding cargo net transport of burros.)

PILOT CONCERNS

Rigging and weight of the live load is critical to the pilot. The type of sling and the clevis fastener must be capable of supporting a significantly greater weight than the actual load because gravity (G) forces on a load increase its relative weight. These increases in G forces are exerted during climbs and turns. A qualified individual should review the load arrangement prior to every load, especially if using a nonrecommended sling or cargo net. The weight of the load is important.

In ground effect (IGE) and out of ground effect (OGE) are conditions that affect the engine power necessary to maintain a constant altitude (hover). In IGE conditions, the downwash of air from the helicopter's main rotor pushes against a hard surface (i.e., the ground) and helps produce lift force; the helicopter is able to hover with less engine power. In OGE conditions, there are no hard surfaces to rebound the rotor downwash; therefore, more engine power is required to maintain a constant altitude. Most external sling loads are considered OGE conditions.

The lifting ability of any helicopter varies with altitude (elevation) and temperature. The higher the temperature and/or higher the elevation, the less weight a helicopter can lift. For example, a Bell UH-1 series Iroquois (Huey) helicopter might be capable of lifting a 500 kg (1,100 lb) horse near the coast on a cool day, yet be unable to lift the same load in the mountains on a hot day (Ranson, 2006).

The pilot should perform careful computation of performance data, weight, and balance prior to initiation of the operation. Wrecking an aircraft due to weight-induced loss of anti-torque capability or droop of the rotor is terminal to the rescue effort and may kill or injure people and crew. A helicopter should never be required to hover any higher than is necessary to clear the rotor system and fuselage, because the higher the hover height, the more power required (Bazzarre, 2006). In addition, higher altitudes increase the difficulty in maintaining hover position by using visual cues necessary to detect movement fore, aft, laterally, and vertically. The difficulty is markedly increased during night conditions despite the use of night vision devices.

A drag chute is attached to the sling frame to orient the animal's hindquarters into the wind during flight. Efforts to prevent oscillation facilitate maneuverability and streamline the load to prevent spinning.

The live load must be carried at a sufficient altitude to clear obstacles (e.g., trees, towers, ridgelines, etc.). Unfortunately, there have been cases where human live loads have accidentally impacted obstacles while suspended 10–30 m (33–98 ft) or more below the aircraft. There is no data available regarding this occurrence with live animal loads, but the likelihood exists.

Pilot Responsibilities

The pilot is a crucial link to scene safety. At a minimum, he or she should do the following:

- Perform a thorough face-to-face operational briefing with all ground personnel. The briefing should include the sequence of events, a communication check with ground crews at the lifting and landing sites, and a review of maneuvers, hand/arm signals, commands, and emergency procedures (Figure 18.2).
- Personally check the cargo hook-apex fitting-cable attachment for the sling load or harness for the net gun.
- Visually determine that personnel and equipment are secured in the aircraft and discuss terrain considerations with crew and ground personnel.
- Demonstrate an ability to properly communicate with ground personnel. It is recommended that one flight crew member remains on the ground with each ground team (lifting site and landing site) to facilitate communication.

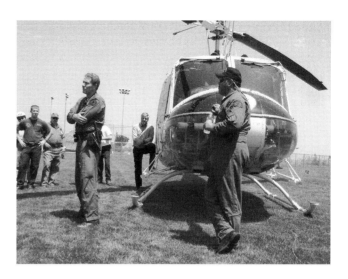

Figure 18.2 *The pilot should hold an operational briefing with all air and ground personnel, including a safety briefing on behavior around helicopters, before commencing a live sling load of large animals. Courtesy Tomas Gimenez.*

- Maintain positive control of the aircraft while demonstrating proper power management during sling loading or net gun operations.
- Demonstrate awareness of animal behavior in relation to helicopter operations, especially net gun and herding targets. Aerial Capture, Eradication and Tagging of Animals (ACETA) certification is preferred.
  Note: ACETA certification includes aerial capture (net gunning, darting, chemical immobilization); eradication (euthanasia by use of firearms), and marking (use of paint ball gun or similar device) where a helicopter or airplane is used as a shooting platform. An evaluation of pilot skills is required for certification by an inspector. Four pilot operations are identified in this task: (1) animal herding; (2) animal eradication; (3) animal marking and darting; and (4) net gun. Applicants must exhibit knowledge of technical points with the Department of the Interior (DOI) ACETA Handbook and demonstrate techniques in a practical test with live or simulated animals to include understanding of animal behavior (OAS, 2000).
- Demonstrate a thorough understanding of emergency procedures including aircraft mechanical problems, weapon safety considerations, net gun malfunctions, and shooting harness failure, as applicable to the operation.

Helicopter Requirements

The U.S. DOI updated their recommendations for helicopter performance in 2006. These recommendations require that the helicopter used meet the minimum performance in at least one of the following categories:

A. Sea Level to 1,219 m (4,000 ft) density altitude (DA). Hover OGE at 1,219 m DA.

B. Above 1,219 m to 2,133 m (7,000 ft) DA. Hover OGE at 2,133 m DA.

C. Above 2,133 m to 2,743 m (9,000 ft) DA. Hover OGE at 9,000 feet DA.

D. Above 2,743 m DA. The aircraft must meet Hover OGE performance for the highest anticipated DA (OAS, 2000).

Helicopter Sling Load Equipment

To perform sling loading, the following equipment should be available:

- Helicopter with appropriate sling load capacity and trained crew.
- UC Davis-Anderson Sling with steel overhead frame and all ancillary equipment, modified with brightly colored boat bumpers on frame (see section below), minus leg supports.
- Cable assembly (24.4 cm [10 in.]) steel ring, 30.48 m (100 ft) steel cable, 6.1 m (20 ft) web, large steel hook, 6.1 m brightly colored web tag safety line or 45.72 m (150 ft) Kevlar cable instead of steel cable.

Modifications to the UC Davis-Anderson Sling for Helicopter Sling Load Operations. Recommended modifications to the UC Davis-Anderson Sling's metal frame include bolting boat bumpers onto the metal frame and a system of color coding to facilitate rapid attachment of the hooks to the overhead frame. The boat floats serve two purposes: (1) if the frame falls into the water or mud, it will float and can be easily seen and recovered; and (2) the floats allow the frame to be easily

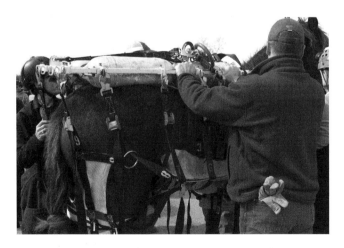

Figure 18.3 *The use of boat floats allows the UC Davis-Anderson Sling to be set onto the animal's back and all adjustments attaching the soft part of the sling system to be made before vertical lift equipment or a helicopter is brought overhead. Minimizing the number of personnel and the time spent under the helicopter are crucial aspects to safety. In this SOP, only one hook must be attached before the animal is lifted. Courtesy Axel Gimenez.*

and comfortably rested on the animal's back while attaching all the buckles from the soft part of the sling to the frame (Figure 18.3). Painting the floats reflective orange helps the aircrew to see them (Figure 18.4). Color coding the buckles and hooks allows personnel to quickly recognize incorrect attachment of buckles and hooks to the frame.

The overhead frame should be kept with the soft part of the sling at the lifting location to allow the animal to be prepared for the lift. A one-hook connection between the helicopter cable and the sling can be used to perform the lift, based on the SOP change presented in this book and tested in live demonstrations. To deliver the sling to the lifting location, all parts can be carried in the helicopter. For this reason, it is prefer-

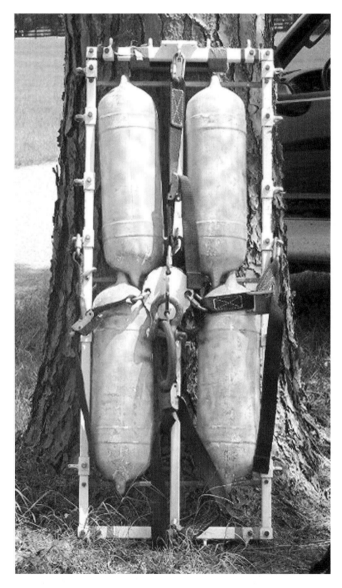

Figure 18.4 *The overhead frame of the UC Davis-Anderson Sling with modifications as suggested by a helicopter pilot instructor, including brightly painted (orange) boat floats and color coding of sling system hook attachments to the frame. Courtesy Tori Miller.*

able to maintain all sling components in a large, lidded and marked box.

All sling loading operations should be performed in accordance with the U.S. Army manual *Multiservice Helicopter Sling Load: Basic Operations and Equipment* (FM 10-450-3, www.quartermaster.army.mil).

The leg supports that attach to the soft part of the UC Davis-Anderson Sling are not necessary for helicopter sling load operations. These leg supports are designed for and crucial to medical or clinical patients requiring long-term support (days to months). In the hospital setting, the UC Davis-Anderson Sling is used primarily to provide support or assistance to hospitalized horses that cannot stand alone, specifically for rehabilitating equine patients with laminitis (founder), fractured limbs, and neurologic conditions (Taylor et al., 2005).

Sedation Protocol for Horses

Animals to be sling loaded should be sedated to increase their cooperation, yet sufficiently alert to be able to support their own weight plus the weight of the UC Davis-Anderson Sling; ideally, the animal should be minimally or nonreactive to the approaching helicopter, yet able to support its own weight when delivered to safe ground. If the animal is prematurely sedated or anesthetized in water scenarios, its head will need to be supported until the lift is attempted. When the animal is set down at the landing location, it is preferable that the animal land with its rear end into the wind to allow it to flex its hind limbs and ease its body onto the ground.

LSU veterinarians reported that effective titration of sedatives for helicopter sling load operations was best accomplished through an intravenous (IV) jugular catheter. Prior to catheter placement, LSU personnel sedated two horses with intravenous xylazine hydrochloride (0.4–0.5 m g/kg IV) or detomidine hydrochloride (8–10 µg/kg IV) (Pettifer et al., 2002). Administration of an additional dose of xylazine hydrochloride (0.4–0.5 mg/kg IV) immediately prior to placing the blindfolded horse in the UC Davis-Anderson Sling produced an appropriate level of sedation without excessive ataxia (incoordination). As the helicopter approached, another dose of 0.4–0.5 mg/kg xylazine hydrochloride (0.4–0.5 mg/kg IV) was sufficient to prevent reaction to the noise and wind associated with the hovering helicopter. A final dose of xylazine hydrochloride (0.25 mg/kg IV) proved effective in reducing the reaction to lift and transport of approximately 5–10 minutes duration. Researchers reported that xylazine hydrochloride was more effective than detomidine hydrochloride, possibly because of the shorter onset time and duration of action exhibited (Pettifer et al., 2002). It should be noted that these doses were effective for animals that were not accustomed to human handling; the doses may need to be adjusted for indi-

vidual animals and situations and should be administered by a veterinarian.

Clemson University researchers reported success using a blindfold and detomidine hydrochloride (8–10 µg/kg IV) for a calm, trained, nonstressed animal in four live helicopter lifts for demonstration purposes (Gimenez, 2006b). The administration of sedatives (e.g., xylazine hydrochloride, detomidine hydrochloride, medetomidine hydrochloride, etc.) is not innocuous; these drugs are capable of inducing changes in cardiovascular and respiratory function. If the animal victim is compromised by injuries or illness due to its situation, sedation or anesthesia can increase the risk of decompensation and death. The veterinarian must weigh the benefits of sedation or anesthesia with the risks when making the decision to administer sedatives and anesthetics. Several veterinarians or rescuers assisting with actual lifts reported using minimal sedation in the animals lifted due to concerns with hypothermia (two animals), shock (one animal), overexposure (one animal) and dehydration (two animals). The dose and type of sedation chosen in these cases was not reported. Sedation protocols for other live large animals and exotics have not been reported; responders should consult with a large animal veterinarian in all sling loading scenarios.

STANDARD OPERATING PROTOCOL FOR HELICOPTER SLING LOAD OF A LIVE LARGE ANIMAL

Performance of this procedure is not timed; the emphasis is on safety. Trained personnel can conduct the entire protocol in less than two hours. The UC Davis-Anderson Sling should be applied according to the manufacturer's recommendations. The protocol here may be applied to other field-expedient sling systems, although their use for helicopter operations is not recommended.

Personnel Requirements

Two ground teams are required in addition to the helicopter aircrew. The lifting team remains with the large animal victim to attach the sling and overhead frame to the animal in the rescue environment (e.g., floodwater, mud, precipice, deep snow, etc.). The landing team is deployed at a preselected landing zone (LZ) to connect the cable and web strap with the hook to the helicopter prior to the lift operation and later to receive the large animal and disconnect it from the helicopter cable.

The minimum number of trained personnel for each team is as follows.

Lifting Team:
Animal handler (one)
SO (may also function as communications officer) (one)

Communications officer (preferably crew chief) (one)

Sling operator (on one side of large animal) (one)

On-site IC (may also function as animal handler) (one)

Landing Team:

Animal handler (one)

SO (may also function as communications officer) (one)

Communications officer (preferably an aircrew member with a radio) (one)

Sling operator (one)

On-site IC (may also function as animal handler) (one)

TEAM RESPONSIBILITIES

Landing Team Responsibilities–Initial

The landing team selects a LZ based on safety for the helicopter and aircrew. Preferred LZs include mowed pastures at least the size of a football field with no overhead obstructions (e.g., telephone lines and poles, antennas, etc.). There must be a minimum clearance of 10 m (33 ft) from any power poles, trees, or other obstructions. There must be a minimum clearance of 40 ft from a cliff or rock face.

The LZ should be cleared of all small objects such as cans, bottles, boards, and limbs to prevent foreign object damage (FOD). FOD occurs when an object is sucked into the air intakes of the helicopter engines and can cause engine failure and a fatal crash. The helicopter's rotor wash will force small objects and sand into the faces of any ground personnel; correct PPE must be worn.

The landing team should provide the aircrew with the 911 address or GPS (global positioning satellite) coordinates of the LZ site. GPS coordinates can be obtained from a cellular phone with GPS capability or from a GPS device and should be provided as latitude and longitude or in Universal Transverse Mercator grid coordinates (see Chapter 12). The geography will appear very different on the ground than it does from the air. The crew may or may not be familiar with the area; following a disaster, known landmarks may be unrecognizable or absent. The use of conventional landmarks is not recommended. Ground personnel reporting their location and choosing an LZ should use GPS coordinates.

A 2.5 m (8 1/4 ft) length of yellow caution tape should be attached to a nearby branch, tree, or other anchor to act as a wind sock and give the pilot an indication of the wind direction at ground level.

The helicopter will land in the LZ. Ground personnel should not be allowed to approach the helicopter without the pilot's permission. This SOP should be provided to the aircrew. An operations meeting should be held, and all safety and planning considerations should be discussed before attempting the lift. Time spent in the planning phase maximizes safety and efficiency of the rescue.

The steel (or Kevlar) cable and webbing should be stretched on the ground facing the helicopter, with the steel ring nearest the helicopter. The aircrew attaches the steel cable by its ring to the apex fitting underneath the belly of the helicopter; the 10.16 m (33.3 ft) web with hook for attachment to the sling is attached at the other end of the cable. If a backup strap is used to prevent accidental load loss, it should be attached at this time. It is possible for some aircraft to ground taxi under very little power and position the belly of the aircraft over the load cable so that a crewmember can reach down and attach the aircraft hook to the cable ring. The pilot can then maneuver over the load for the lifting operation (Bazzarre, 2006).

For this SOP it is preferred that one member of the aircrew be brought by vehicle or boat to the lifting team's location to serve as the safety and communications officer. If possible, another aircrew member should remain at the LZ with the landing team as the communications officer for set-down. These personnel should have direct radio communication with the pilot. Hand and arm signals are not safe alternatives, but very high frequency (VHF) radios are acceptable. When possible, a fly-over should be performed and good communications established with the lifting team before attempting the lift.

Lifting Team at Large Animal Victim's Location

The lifting team should include an aircrew member and have the UC Davis-Anderson Sling and the overhead frame with them to place on the large animal victim. In extreme terrain where these components are heavy or cannot be transported with the lifting team, the helicopter can deliver them to the lift team site. However, the team should not attempt to emplace the sling while the helicopter hovers above them; the exposure of the lifting team underneath the helicopter should be kept to a minimum. The empty sling and frame are easily transported underneath or inside the helicopter.

The soft components of the UC Davis-Anderson Sling should be placed on the animal. All buckles and straps should be correctly attached before attempting the lift (Figure 18.5). The veterinarian should be consulted for sedation of the animal; in most cases, the animal should be heavily sedated to prevent movement of the sling load. For large animals entrapped in water, sedation may cause the large animal to collapse underneath the surface of the water. In these situations, sedation may be reduced, avoided, or administered immediately before the helicopter lift is made (Haven, 2006) when the animal's weight is supported

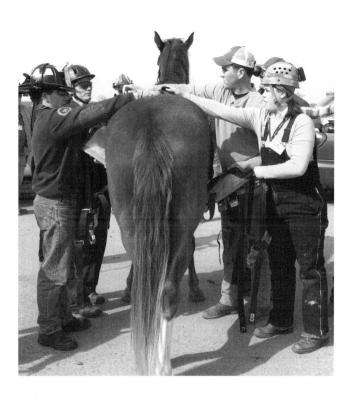

Figure 18.5 *Application of the UC Davis-Anderson Sling requires practice to develop efficiency and coordination by the operational personnel. It is possible for a trained team to emplace this sling on a recumbent animal. Courtesy Axel Gimenez.*

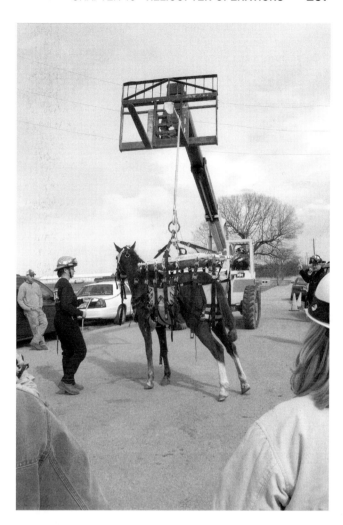

Figure 18.6 *In a training scenario, a demonstration animal in an UC Davis-Anderson Sling is lifted by a crane to simulate helicopter sling loading. The animal handler is the last person to get out from under the overhead lift, after one operational person attaches the hook from the lift equipment or helicopter to the ring above the steel frame. Courtesy Axel Gimenez.*

in the sling. Immediately prior to lift, ear plugs and a blindfold should be emplaced. The steel overhead frame (with floats) is placed on top of the animal's back. The 18 attachment points of the soft portion of the sling should be connected and last minute adjustments made to balance the load.

It is preferred that the communications officer be a flight crew member who remains on the ground with the lifting team and communicates with the pilot via radio.

The SO should monitor the position of the cable and, if necessary, use a rod to prevent the slack in the cable from becoming caught on the sling or wrapping around personnel during descent, attachment, and ascent. The SO should have a full view of all personnel and should have a pre-established hand and whistle signal for stopping the operation at any time. The noise generated by the helicopter prevents effective vocal communication. Ideally, the lifting team will be experienced in emplacing the UC Davis-Anderson Sling.

A veterinarian should administer chemical restraint to the animal, timed to take full effect as the team attaches the hook to the frame and the helicopter performs the lift. All connections should be checked a final time before the lift is initiated.

The helicopter should arrive and hover at approximately 31 m (100 ft) over the large animal victim,

allowing the load hook to be attached to the steel overhead frame of the sling. The animal handler and one sling operator (one on each side) remain with the animal until the load hook is connected (Figure 18.6).

The IC gives the command to lift the animal to the communications officer, who relays the command to the pilot. All personnel leave the area underneath the helicopter as soon as the large animal's feet leave the ground. The lead rope should remain attached to the halter and the SO should stabilize the load with the hanging 6.1 m (20 ft) web tag line until the sling load is lifted out of reach.

Landing Team at Large Animal Landing Zone

On the order of the IC, the communications officer signals the helicopter pilot to descend to the set-down point within the predesignated LZ and set the large animal on the ground while hovering at approximately

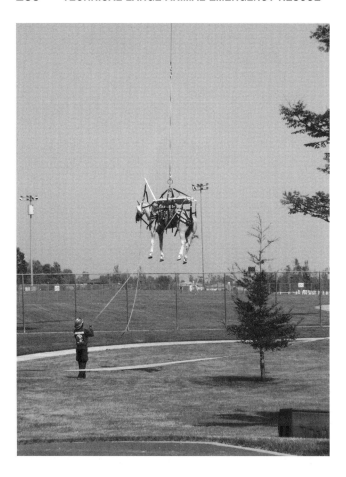

Figure 18.7 *The SO grasps the tag line as the sling loaded animal descends, minimizing the chance of spin or pendulum swing. The animal is blindfolded to minimize stress and to protect the animal's eyes from injury. Courtesy Tomas Gimenez.*

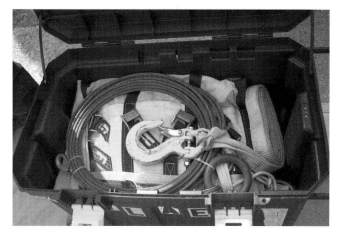

Figure 18.8 *The UC Davis-Anderson Sling, cable assemblies, and webbing should be stored in a dry location out of sunlight to maintain the integrity of the stitching and fabric used in the sling. In this example, a wheeled large box with handles is used to store all the equipment related to the sling system. Storing a humid or wet sling will mold and rot the stitches. Courtesy Axel Gimenez.*

31 m (100 ft). The animal handler should grasp the lead rope while the SO grasps the tag line web to stabilize the load as it descends. No other personnel should be close to the set-down point (Figure 18.7).

One of the design features of the UC Davis-Anderson Sling is that it allows the animal's hind legs to maintain a correct position for landing rear-end first to prevent facial injuries, broken extremities, etc. Once the large animal is set down on the ground, it should be allowed to stabilize itself; some animals will lie down, and others will attempt to stand. Although the nylon web strap should eliminate the need to ground the load, care must be taken by rescue personnel to avoid handling the steel cable as it is lowered to a reachable height. The aircraft may lower its position to allow the metal portion of the cable assembly to rest on the ground away from the large animal and rescuers to prevent the buildup of static electricity.

One team member should be designated to release the hook from the metal frame of the sling by disconnecting the hook from the sling frame and stabilizing the hook with an attached 3 m (10 ft) tagline until the hook clears everyone's head as the helicopter ascends.

The hook should not be allowed to swing freely after it is disconnected from the sling; if uncontrolled, the hook will act as a 40 m (132 ft) long pendulum and can cause severe head trauma despite the appropriate PPE.

On the order of the IC, the communications officer signals the helicopter to move away from the set-down point and land the craft at a safe distance to disconnect the cable assembly. Alternatively, after placing the load on the ground, the helicopter can move to the side (usually the left side) and release the cable assembly. A good helicopter crew will never release the sling from the aircraft when directly over the load. Cargo can be damaged by a clevis or cable assembly dropped from a helicopter; in addition, humans and animals underneath the aircraft could be seriously injured or killed (Ranson, 2006).

The sling frame and sling can then be removed from the large animal and stored for future use (Figure 18.8). The veterinarian should assess the animal prior to transport to the nearest veterinary hospital.

INITIAL RISK ASSESSMENT

The use of a helicopter in an equine rescue operation should be the absolute last choice in any scenario. Sling loading operations are extremely hazardous to personnel underneath the aircraft, and intensive training and practice are required to perform sling-load operations in a safe, efficient, and successful manner. In any rescue scenario (including human rescue) where the flight crew becomes endangered for any reason or the helicopter experiences in-flight difficulty, the pilot will drop the sling load, regardless of whether it is a bale of alfalfa or a live animal load. The lives of the human rescuers will always take precedent over that of an animal victim. Risk assessment is crucial for all aspects of any helicopter operation; it is necessary to consider all of the possible problems that might be encountered.

Select the Correct Size Helicopter

As part of risk management, the safety margin of a helicopter's sling load should be considered and pro-rated based on age of the craft and safety factors. Sling cargo weight must not exceed the lifting capacity of the helicopter. When considering the safety ratio for a live large animal sling load, the greatest sling load capacity available should be chosen. Payload is the amount of weight that the helicopter can carry inside the helicopter and is different from the sling load capacity (the weight a helicopter can carry underneath its belly).

Appropriate common types of helicopter include the Bell UH-1 series Iroquois (Huey) and the Sikorsky UH-60 "Black Hawk." As a helicopter ages it will be assigned a reduced sling load capacity, or it might be retrofitted to increase the capacity; this rating cannot be determined by visual inspection. Lifting an average-sized horse in a sling approaches the maximum weight capacity of a Huey, with a sling load of 750 kg (1,650 lb); a larger sling load capacity rating increases safety. An appropriate rotary-wing aircraft must be used with a minimum sling loading capacity of 1,000 kg (2,200 lb) for lifting an average 500 kg (1,100 lb) large animal (two times the weight to increase the safety margin). This must be coordinated prior to the lifting operation. Most news and civilian helicopters are not rated or certified to attempt this procedure.

Retrofitted aircraft may be capable of carrying larger loads. According to the helicopter's pilot, a retrofitted UH-1 (Huey) from San Bernardino County, California, has a sling load capacity of 3,628 kg (almost 8,000 lb, or 4 tons).

Realistically, the only helicopters suitable for lifting large animals are the UH-1 (Huey) and the UH-60 (Black Hawk); the majority of these craft are in military service. Any helicopter smaller than a UH-1 is impractical for lifting large animals. Any helicopter larger than a UH-60 is too large and creates additional safety concerns (Ranson, 2006). Both the Huey and the Black Hawk have one "main rotor" system. The two blades of the Huey generate less rotor wash. The four blades of the Black Hawk provide additional lift, but generate hurricane-force winds on the ground.

This SOP refers to single rotor aircraft. The Boeing CH-47 Chinook has two main rotor systems and can lift 9,071 kg (20,000 lb) but causes excessive rotor wash for the animal and ground personnel (Ranson, 2006).

Communication. Communication between the aircraft and the ground crew is crucial to the risk assessment. The optimal plan includes the presence of a crew chief on the ground with direct communication with the craft. The pilot cannot see the ground team or the sling-loaded large animal underneath the helicopter and must rely on excellent directions from a crew chief, who relays all signals and communications from the IC to the pilot. As a backup or alternate plan, a civilian VHF aviation handheld radio for communication with the helicopter is acceptable because military and civilian helicopters have VHF aviation radios. They are relatively inexpensive. The VHF radio must be an "aviation VHF" radio, not a police band radio. Spare batteries should be available (Ranson, 2006).

Communication between the lifting and landing teams and the IC should be established and tested before initiation of any sling loading operations.

Maneuver Room. During the risk assessment phase, it must be determined if a helicopter can safely maneuver in the rescue environment. Trees, antennas, and phone and electrical lines will prevent the helicopter from approaching a sufficient distance to perform the sling load operation. The best use of helicopter and boat resources in a floodwater scenario may be to deliver feedstuffs and fresh water to animals stranded on dry land until the water recedes and the animals can walk or be led or driven to dry ground.

Scene Security. Areas used for landing zones, preparation of equipment, and the rescue site should be secure. The general public and media should remain a safe distance from the operation. Helicopter operations can endanger people on the ground.

Night Operations. Night rescue operations with helicopters are not recommended due to significant safety risks for ground personnel. Although many pilots are trained in the use of night vision devices and regularly perform night operations, darkness multiplies the danger for the ground crews. Instead of attempting night rescue, the animal should be made as comfortable as possible, provided with forage and fresh water; the rescue crew should wait until daylight to attempt rescue. If the animal cannot be stabilized or maintained until daylight, it should be euthanatized in place.

Safety Concerns Around Helicopters. Major hazards with helicopter operations include overloading, incorrect use of or poorly maintained slinging equipment, blown debris or equipment, and protruding vegetation or terrain that may snag loads. Pilot fatigue, lack of personnel training, miscommunication between parties involved (especially between the pilot and ground personnel), and marginal weather conditions increase the risks associated with sling loading. To prevent accidents, all parties must follow safe slinging procedures and be fully alert and well briefed, with mutual responsibilities clearly understood.

Helicopter rescues tend to draw crowds. For example, the Sheriff's Department of San Bernadino County, (California, agreed to perform a live sling load training session in association with the Alta Loma Riding Club and Rancho Cucomonga Fire Department in 2003. The decision was made to perform the operation in the Rancho Cucomonga city park because it is an open grassy area with no power lines. The helicopter landed for the safety briefing and discussion; within minutes, almost 200 bystanders had gathered.

Ground personnel must be familiar with safety procedures around helicopters to minimize the chance of injury and must establish scene security to prevent bystanders from approaching the helicopter or personnel. Naive as well as knowledgeable and experienced persons have been decapitated by helicopter rotor blades (Bazzarre, 2006). A helicopter should never be approached without permission from the pilot or crew. When approaching a helicopter, personnel should approach at a 45-degree angle to the nose of the aircraft.

The helicopter rotor blades generate hurricane-force winds downward that can sandblast personnel and equipment, overturn small boats in the water, and forcefully blow debris, endangering ground personnel and the victim. FOD presents a significant danger to personnel and to the helicopter; the rotor wash can pick up and throw a sheet of plywood, or an object as small as a hat can enter the engine and destroy the helicopter (Ranson, 2006). A heavily weighted hook should be used on the lanyard dangling from the helicopter; fatal accidents have occurred when unweighted lanyards have struck the helicopter tail or main rotor during flight.

Flight crews might be concerned about carrying the empty UC Davis-Anderson Sling frame underneath the aircraft due to concerns that it could fly back into the tail rotor. The empty sling can be transported inside the helicopter until needed (Ranson, 2006).

A sling load builds up static electricity immediately upon takeoff. If a steel cable is used, it must not be touched without well-insulated gloves. The 3 m (10 ft) insulating webbing section should always be used between the steel cable and end hook. The accumulated static electrical charge is strong enough to knock down a person. Kevlar cables do not transmit the static charge to the load and are suitable for sling load use. Alternatively, a shepherd's hook can be used as a grounding rod before the load touches the ground and before touching anything metal on the sling load (clevis, hook, frame) (Bazzarre, 2006).

Emergencies with the Helicopter. In case of emergency, pilots are taught to open the cargo hook and drop the load if necessary to save the aircraft and its occupants. If possible, the pilot will try to set the load down and land the aircraft. To prevent accidental release of the cargo hook, a load release backup subsystem (Heli-Strap) can be used as specified by the Federal Aviation Administration in the *Code of Federal Regulations*.

If a mechanical problem or malfunction occurs, the pilot will usually attempt to go left and forward of the current position to take the helicopter away from the ground personnel underneath the aircraft. Due to the nature of their design and aerodynamics, during loss of power or engine malfunction, the craft will drift to the left as it descends (Bazzarre, 2006). However, the reality is that when a helicopter goes down, it tends to fall out of the sky with minimal control; personnel on the ground should abandon the victim and run to the right of and away from the helicopter as fast as possible. Personnel on the ground should be cognizant of the helicopter's position at all times in case of a crash. This is one of many reasons to maintain a wide safety zone of at least 200 m (660 ft) surrounding the helicopter (Bazzarre, 2006).

NET GUN CAPTURE OPERATIONS

Ground-based net gun capture operations are discussed as an effective means of capture and restraint for numerous exotic animals (see Chapters 6 and 7). The use of helicopters as net gun shooting platforms has been demonstrated to be a safe, economical, and humane method of capturing wild burros (but not horses) if the helicopter safety considerations discussed in this chapter are implemented. It has been speculated that net gun capture of cattle would be effective for small groups trapped in remote areas or rising floodwaters if a ground-based alternative was not available. The use of helicopters as shooting platforms for chemical capture (with darts), followed by sling loading of the animal in a cargo net, has been widely used by wildlife officials.

Animal Safety Concerns

Helicopter net gun capture techniques have been associated with unacceptably high mortality if not properly managed. Net gun operations have been used to capture wild burros in Arizona since its initial demonstration and evaluation in November 1992, when 44 wild burros near Temple Bar, Arizona, were successfully captured and relocated. Representatives of the Bureau of Land Management, National Park Service, International Society for the Protection of Mustangs and Burros, Wild Horse Organized Assistance, Nevada Wild Horse Commission, and a veterinarian were present. Of the 44 animals captured, 42 were safely transported to the Kingman Corrals and 2 died (4.5% death loss). No negative aftereffects were reported from the net gun capture or from transport in a (cargo net) sling under a helicopter (USDOI, 1998).

In July 1993, the Las Vegas District used the net gun technique to capture 118 wild burros from the Gold Butte Herd Management Area. The animals were slung underneath a helicopter to Temple Bar and transported to the Kingman Corrals. Of 118 burros captured, 25 died (21% death loss). Deaths in the corrals were attributed to severe stress brought on by extreme heat at the time of capture as well as to the stress of being captured and transported to the corral facility.

The Kingman, Arizona, capture crew used net gun capture techniques to capture wild burros in Arizona in a limited capture role. The Phoenix, Arizona, field office removed 115 wild burros from an island in Lake Pleasant. Under these operational conditions, two deaths (1.7% death loss) were reported. For reference, the expected death loss from traditional capture methods of feral animals is 2%–4%.

Consider All Options

Net gun capture can be used if concerns can be mitigated in order to make it safer and humane; otherwise, this method can be associated with high mortality rates. Traditional capture techniques (e.g., Judas animals, bait trapping, helicopter herding, etc.) should always be considered before net gun capture is chosen. The net gun technique may be more effective for small, widely dispersed populations; specific target animals with no access by vehicle or wrangler; or when specific concerns for animal safety exist (e.g., animals trapped on an island in rising water, etc.). Net gun capture is a tool that may be employed in combination with traditional capture techniques or as the primary capture technique if it is the only feasible option. The net gun capture technique with these mitigating measures is approved in the United States for the capture of wild burros only. Net gun capture has not been evaluated for the capture of wild horses (USDOI, 1998).

Operational Guidelines

Personnel involved in sling operations must be trained in external load/long line/remote hook procedures. A minimum 8 m (26 1/4 ft) line for cargo net sling load operations should be used, and a 37 m (122 ft) long line is preferred.

When possible, an observer with the ability to communicate with the pilot should be placed in a location that will allow an adequate view of the operation.

Minimize Stress and Injury

Steps should be taken to minimize the stress and injury to the burros when the net capture method is used.

- Burros should be herded by the pilot to an up-hill grade to slow them from a full run at capture (to minimize facial and skull injuries to the netted animal).

- Netted burros should be blindfolded until removed from the net at the unloading site. Foals should be sling loaded separately from adults. Areas where animals are lowered by the helicopter to the ground should be free from rocks, debris, etc. (*Note:* FOD is a significant safety issue for animals, ground crew, and helicopter.)
- The time the netted animals spend on the ground should be minimized. Disposable nets that can be cut free should be used to minimize the time that an entangled animal is immobilized.
- The captured animals must be moved to a temporary or permanent holding facility with shade and water available within eight hours of capture. Net gun operations should stop if the ambient temperature at the capture site equals or exceeds 37.8°C (100° F).

Darting and Euthanasia

For animals that must be chemically captured using darts or for humane euthanasia of trapped large animals with no hope of rescue, a helicopter is an appropriate shooting platform for trained sharpshooters versed in the techniques of projectile firearms for these purposes (see Chapter 13). In one study, combinations of etorphine hydrochloride and xylazine hydrochloride in varying dosages were tested for their efficacy as immobilizing agents on 16 recently captured feral horses. The results of these trials led to the use of a standard combination of 5.5 mg of etorphine hydrochloride, 150 mg of xylazine hydrochloride, and 3 mg of atropine sulfate in a 7 ml dart syringe for field capture. This combination was administered by dart gun from helicopters to capture 87 free-ranging feral horses from approximately 80 bands. Five mares died at the time of capture, and the remains of three other mares were found near the site of capture four months later. Blood samples collected from each animal and analyzed for hematologic variables, concentrations of urea, and glucose yielded values comparable to domestic "hot-blooded horses." Serum cortisol concentrations (4.7 ± 0.4 µg/dl) were comparable to values from undisturbed captive animals. Therefore, it was concluded that the dart capture technique did not induce significant stress or physiologic changes in the darted animals. Approximately 48 minutes of helicopter time were required per horse captured. The cost per animal captured was $159 for helicopter time and $66.70 for drugs and darts (Seal et al., 1985).

An in-depth treatment of the subject of chemical capture is beyond the scope of this book. (See Chapter 6.)

ACRONYMS FROM CHAPTER 18

ACETA Aerial capture, eradication and tagging of animals

CVM	College of Veterinary Medicine	LSU	Louisiana State University
DA	Density altitude	LZ	Landing zone
DOI	Department of the Interior	OGE	Out of ground effect
FOD	Foreign object damage	PPE	Personal protective equipment
G	Gravity	SO	Safety officer
GPS	Global Positioning Satellite	SOP	Standard operating protocol
IC	Incident commander	TLAER	Technical large animal emergency rescue
IV	Intravenous	VHF	Very high frequency

19 Decontamination of Large Animals

Dr. Lisa Murphy, Dawn Slessman, and Bob Mauck

INTRODUCTION

Certain large animal rescue situations may involve the release of chemical, biological, or radiological agents, resulting in the subsequent contamination of large animals. An example is the exposure of an entire herd to floodwaters containing fecal material from a facility's manure pit or septic tank and various potent agricultural chemicals routinely stored and used by livestock producers and farmers. Overturned trucks or livestock trailers may result in animals covered in excrement, gasoline, and other automotive fluids. In addition to suffering direct effects from these substances, animals can also pose a risk to human health and the environment by physically transferring contaminants as they move from place to place. For these reasons, decontamination may be needed for individual animals or larger groups and herds.

Decontamination is the process of removing harmful materials and reducing their concentrations to the lowest quantity possible in order to reduce the potential for negative health effects. There are many opinions in the field of emergency response regarding where the responsibility of hazardous materials (HazMat) decontamination exists—or whether it is even required—for animals. Emergency responders may feel that it is not their responsibility to rescue and decontaminate animals affected by chemicals involved in a release, yet other emergency response personnel insist that any life saved or assisted is a positive accomplishment. This issue presents several new problems that consistently arise: what equipment is required for performing animal decontamination and what are the differences between animal decontamination and that of human victims? Most human evacuation shelters or facilities do not allow animals, with the exception of working or service animals.

Many domesticated animals are not bathed or handled on a regular schedule or by unfamiliar personnel, presenting handling challenges. In addition, many decontamination methods involve handling and procedures that are unfamiliar to the animals and may induce panic responses. The decontamination handling methods presented in this chapter are generally consistent with the manner in which veterinary medical personnel handle and examine animals to reduce risks for first responders and personnel performing decontamination.

DEFINITIONS

Gross decontamination indicates the removal of as much of the contaminating agent as possible to save the victim. This is often restricted to external (skin) decontamination.

Technical decontamination is a thorough decontamination process performed on the victim. This is a more time-consuming process and may involve decontamination of internal organs by various means.

INITIAL GOALS AND OBJECTIVES

Human safety is the most important consideration when making decisions about contaminated animals. The welfare of the affected animals must be considered the next priority.

The first objective is to minimize further exposure to the suspected toxicant (Galey, 1996), especially if decisions regarding decontamination have not yet been determined. Immediate actions that benefit the affected animals while minimizing direct human–animal contact are the removal of point sources (e.g., stopping a leak from a vehicle or pipeline) and the provision of alternate food and water supplies if existing feeds and water have been contaminated. If an entire animal group can be safely moved with minimal risk of animal escape or injury and limited human exposure, relocation to an adjacent or nearby uncontaminated area, such as a fenced pasture, barn, warehouse, or other enclosed structure, should be considered.

Making the Decision to Decontaminate Live Animals

Decisions regarding decontamination of animals that have survived an initial event will be largely driven by the known or suspected agent(s) involved. If a zoonotic disease (a disease transmitted from animals to humans) or highly toxic chemical is involved, the risk to human health may be deemed too great to proceed with an animal decontamination operation. Veterinarians and hazardous materials specialists should be consulted, especially when particularly rare or valuable animals (including police or military horses) have been affected (Figure 19.1).

Depending on the incident and the toxicant involved, some animals may require medical stabilization or life-saving interventions before decontamination can be accomplished. A veterinarian should assist in triaging all animals to determine the best course of action. Humane euthanasia should be considered for severely affected animals that are unlikely to survive their injuries or the stress of decontamination, as well as for animals that are too fractious for personnel to safely handle. Even experienced animal handlers may be critically maimed or injured by a frightened or aggressive large animal contaminated with substances that can similarly affect a human.

Environmental concerns and their related legal and jurisdictional issues must be addressed before animal decontamination can commence (Figure 19.2). Of particular importance are the disposition of the extremely large volumes of contaminated wastewater that will be generated by bathing the large animals and the disposal of dead and euthanized animals. In addition to the potential human health risks associated with the handling of decaying carcasses, the presence of chemical, biological, and radiologic agents may require treating dead animals as hazardous waste. Local, state, or federal environmental authorities should be consulted.

Should Live Animals Be Decontaminated?

Many jurisdictions have teams that specialize in handling HazMat situations; they can identify an unknown type of material leaking from its container, stop or contain the leak, and decontaminate the exposed humans, providing medical attention if necessary. However, many first responders and HazMat teams are not familiar with procedures to decontaminate pets, livestock, or wild animals exposed to the same materials. In addition, there are currently no universal veterinary standards of care available for animal decontamination.

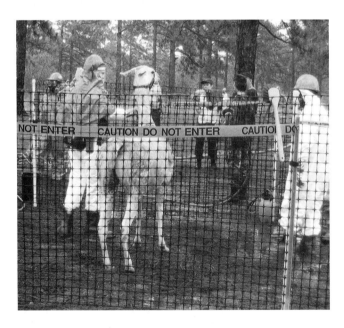

Figure 19.1 *Decontamination of large animals requires trained personnel, personnel protective equipment, decontamination equipment, and large amounts of water. Excellent animal handling skills are crucial to allow operational personnel to safely approach and work on the animal. Courtesy of Tomas Gimenez.*

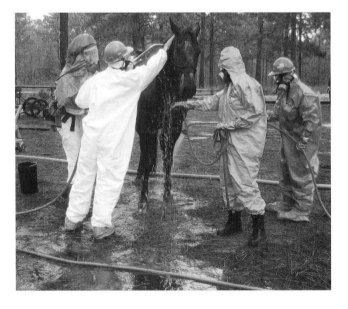

Figure 19.2 *During a training scenario in 2005, veterinary medical assistance team and special medical assessment team-veterinary members decontaminate a police horse with water and stiff brushes. For this practice scenario, soap was not used, and the water was allowed to drain into the sand of Ft. Bragg, North Carolina; in a real chemical incident, the runoff should be contained for later treatment. Courtesy of Tomas Gimenez.*

Although veterinarians and veterinary technicians are trained and equipped to address the medical treatment of the animals, a team of highly trained responders must be available to handle technical animal decontamination in HazMat incidents. The animal decontamination team can work concurrently with the human decontamination line and perform similar decontamination procedures.

In the fall of 2004, a train derailed in Graniteville, South Carolina, and released a large quantity of chlorine gas. Chlorine gas reacts with water (or the moisture present on a human's or animal's mucous membranes) to form hydrochloric acid, which can cause serious injury and death. Hundreds of people were evacuated and decontaminated by HazMat teams, and several human and animal deaths occurred due to this incident. This affected a large residential area, and small companion animals and some livestock were located in the hot zone (contaminated zone). These animals did not receive the same treatment or care that their owners were afforded. Several concerned animal response groups and veterinary personnel responded to the incident, but none had the proper training or equipment to perform technical rescue, decontamination, and treatment. HazMat personnel provided feed and water to animals trapped in the hot zone, but several animal fatalities resulted from the lack of preparedness.

The concept of animal decontamination is not new within the animal industry or emergency response services. Urban search and rescue teams regularly decontaminate their search-and-rescue dogs after training and missions. Local, state, and federal agencies have been performing this service on a variety of species affected by the spills or release of hazardous materials on water and land for the past 50 years.

The most memorable example is the 1989 *Exxon Valdez* incident. The oil tanker ran aground on Bligh Reef in Prince William Sound (Alaska). The tanker's hull split open, releasing approximately 11 million gallons (41.8 million liters) of oil. The oil created an eight-mile (12.9 km) oil slick and contaminated over 1,300 miles (2,080 km) of coastline. According to the U.S. Environmental Protection Agency (EPA), *"The spill posed threats to the delicate food chain that supports Prince William Sound's commercial fishing industry. Also in danger were ten million migratory shore birds and waterfowl, hundreds of sea otters, dozens of other species, such as harbor porpoises and sea lions, and several . . . whales."* Over 250,000 seabirds, 3,000 otters, 300 harbor seals, 250 bald eagles, and 22 orcas were killed; in addition, significant damage was done to the salmon and herring egg deposits.

Mounted police horses are regularly decontaminated as part of good grooming protocols, sometimes daily. Service animals are also commonly decontaminated after visiting hospitals, hospices, and other locations with high concentrations of people and/or animals; in addition, they may be decontaminated prior to the visits to reduce the chance of transmission of zoonotic diseases. Animals removed from mud, septic tanks, or pools may need immediate decontamination and drying of their hair.

Special Considerations

Following food animal exposure to certain chemicals (such as organochlorines or heavy metals) or radioactive substances, concerns regarding the risk of residues in the animal's meat or milk may prevent affected animals from being allowed to enter the human or animal food chains. In situations where the economic value of an animal has been lost, an owner may elect humane euthanasia rather than proceeding with decontamination and subsequent management or medical treatment.

Some situations may involve requests to give special consideration to specific animals with high emotional, financial, and cultural value. Examples include children's pets, valuable breeding animals, and animals that are rare, endangered, or closely associated with a specific community or region (such as zoo, refuge, or circus animals). Other large animals have high value because of their training or function, such as mounted police equines and draft animals. Emergency responders must carefully consider the potential risks and benefits before committing personnel and resources to the retrieval and decontamination of any animal.

History dictates that pre-emergency and response plans and standard operating procedures and protocols must also address animal decontamination. The response to Hurricane Katrina in 2005 demonstrated the importance of established decontamination procedures to allow efficient triage and treatment of the thousands of animals brought to shelters, veterinary clinics, field hospitals, and onto public transportation as floodwaters rose. The evacuating public expects to be able to bring their affected animals with them and to accompany their animals through the decontamination process. Ultimately, the decision to decontaminate animals and to what extent is made on a case-by-case basis and requires input from all affected parties: emergency responders; local, state, and sometimes federal authorities; animal owners; humane and animal sheltering organizations; and veterinarians.

LAWS AND REGULATIONS GOVERNING ANIMAL DECONTAMINATION

At this time, there are not many laws in the United States that specifically require first responders to perform decontamination on animals unless the animals present a human health hazard. The Pets Evacuation and Transportation Standards Act of 2006 was signed into federal law on October 6, 2006, and requires jurisdictions to include pets and service animals in disaster and emergency planning; however, the act does not address the inclusion of large animals in such plans.

A review of hazardous materials incidents revealed a variety of animals affected in hazardous environments, including service animals, working animals, domesticated animals, farm animals that produce food or fiber products, farm animals intended for human consumption, and exotic animals housed in zoos and various other locations. Some of the aforementioned classifications of animals have been afforded special rights under current laws, specifically working and service animals, while others are provided limited to no rights. Therefore, local policies and procedures should be written to include the results of a multihazard analysis and risk assessment for animals in the planning and response jurisdiction and should include, at a minimum,

- the location of the various classifications and species of animals within the planning and response jurisdiction;
- the owner, responsible party, point of contact, etc. for each location;
- the agency identified as having the role of performing decontamination on these animals;
- the appropriate equipment; and,
- the appropriate training to provide an acceptable standard of care.

Farm Animals and Exotic Species

Farm animals and exotic animals housed in public accommodations should be handled with the assistance of or under the direction of the responsible party, depending on the predetermined level of knowledge the responsible party has concerning hazardous materials and animal decontamination. In most states, implied and informed consent for animals for emergency and/or medical care parallel the laws for implied and informed consent for humans. The animal is generally considered the property of the owner, who has the legal right to refuse or limit the level of care provided to the animal.

Working and Service Animals

Working and service animals are addressed in a category of the law separate from other animals. Working animals include, but are not limited to: police dogs specially trained in tactical operations, drug detection, explosives detection, and accelerant detection for arson investigation; police horses; and search-and-rescue animals. Many of these animals are also considered commissioned officers by the authority having jurisdiction (AHJ). Accordingly, these animals must be afforded all rights and protections to the same level as their handlers—including decontamination procedures and medical assistance (Figure 19.3).

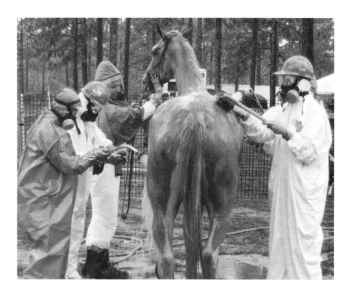

Figure 19.3 *Team members in full personal protective equipment practice technical wet decontamination of a police horse in a training scenario. Live animals should be used in training scenarios to allow the decontamination group to understand the handling challenges involved in the large animal decontamination procedure. Secondary containment or chemical restraint may be necessary for the safety of operational personnel. Courtesy of Tomas Gimenez.*

In most states, service animals are provided special rights and privileges within the law because they have typically received special training to assist their disabled owners/handlers. These service animals must often remain with their owner/handler and therefore may require decontamination to the same extent as the owner. Common examples of service animals include, but are not limited to, guide dogs for the sight or hearing impaired. There are also other service animals, such as monkeys and pigs, that have received training to provide assistance to paraplegics and to fulfill other special needs for the disabled. Title III of the Americans with Disabilities Act (42 U.S.C. § 12182[a]) requires that, *"No individual shall be discriminated against on the basis of disability in the full and equal enjoyment of the goods, services, facilities, privileges, advantages, or accommodations of any place of public accommodation."*

Service animals are generally considered the property of, and in some states, an extension of the disabled person. Therefore, the service animal is eligible to receive the legal rights as stated within the disability laws. Other service animals are considered therapy animals and visit hospitals, convalescent homes, and children's homes for mental and physical therapy of humans. There are significant numbers of equids (horses, mules, and donkeys) used in developed countries for mental and physical therapy provided by handicapped riding programs. Although these animals are considered valuable members of the medical treatment community and require unique dispositions and specialized training to perform these functions, their legal rights are unclear. It is recommended that local policies and procedures be established to address these animals to ensure the animals are decontaminated and determined to be safe and returned to their owners to fulfill their responsibilities.

Although no legal decisions have specifically addressed the need to decontaminate service animals, current federal and state laws define a clear responsibility to do so. Many of these same laws include provisions assessing penalties on those responsible for not providing an acceptable standard of care. Emergency response agencies should be aware of the applicable statutes in their jurisdictions and consult legal counsel on the rights of all animals, not only working and service animals, in emergency and disaster situations. They should also be aware of how such laws would apply in a mass casualty situation.

First response agencies must develop policies and procedures to address decontamination of animals, train the emergency responders in those techniques, and provide the appropriate equipment to perform those techniques as a part of their normal HazMat emergency response duties. The EPA and Occupational Safety and Health Administration (OSHA) requirements are distinct and separate. Generally speaking, the best management practice is to combine all HazMat training into the same session when agency requirements are similar; however, compliance with each rule should be assured.

CONTAMINANTS

The source and type of contaminants vary widely with the incident. This chapter addresses the most common sources and types of contaminants that are or could be present in any event involving HazMat.

Commonly Encountered Toxic Substances

Ultimately, the decision to decontaminate animals is made on a case-by-case basis, considering the number and species of animals affected and the personnel and resources required to safely and efficiently manage the incident. In addition, the nature of the specific toxic substance or substances involved (when known) will determine which decontamination techniques should be incorporated into an incident-specific decontamination plan. Table 19.1 lists some common chemical toxicants that may be encountered during incidents involving large animals, along with special considerations for decontamination. Similar considerations will be necessary following incidents involving biological (including zoonotic) and radioactive agents. Some infectious diseases and radioactive substances may require temporary isolation or prolonged quarantine of affected animals. The provision of appropriate and humane treatment of animals while ensuring human safety requires the coordinated efforts and prompt actions of emergency first responders, environmental health specialists, and veterinary professionals.

Sources of Contaminants

Criminal Event. A criminal event is any planned event that is intentionally initiated in violation of local, state, or federal law. These types of events may intentionally cause harm to the environment, property, animals, or humans. These events can generally be placed into two specific categories: (1) those incidents using chemical, biological, radiological, nuclear, and explosive (CBRNE) material or (2) incidents using materials of convenience.

Chemical, Biological, Radiological, Nuclear, and Explosive. This category generally refers to weapons of mass destruction (WMD) and will usually involve military-grade items or materials. An example of this type of event is the March 1995 sarin gas attack in several Tokyo subways carried out by a Japanese terrorist group. Twelve deaths occurred, over 50 people were severely injured, and thousands experienced temporary vision problems. Animals affected are unknown. In incidents where an attempt is made to replicate a military warfare agent for use as a WMD, the product used may be modified or unstable; it may not exhibit the same characteristics as the pure agent. Many variables may remain unknown for extremely long time periods following the initial attack; this could result in long-term health effects for animals and humans. Specific information must be provided to responders regarding the agent and dose involved to facilitate appropriate treatment and minimize exposure. Normally trained to identify one chemical or a combination of them, responders treat exposed victims in a logical manner; multiple chemicals or contaminants might explain disparities in symptoms of patients and confusion on the part of emergency responders. In these incidents, the decontamination methodologies used on animals will parallel those used on humans.

Materials of Convenience. Materials of convenience are those materials, both hazardous and nonhazardous, that could be used in a criminal method to cause harm and disruption of human's daily lives. Many examples have been described in textbooks on terrorism, in movies, and on the Internet. It is not the authors' intent to provide instruction on the implementation of these terrorist methods; the authors will simply state that this is a common hazard in and around most cities.

Many risk management software application systems are available for planning and response in chemical incidents. The EPA and the National Oceanic and Atmospheric Administration instituted a software program, Computer-Aided Management of Emergency

Table 19.1   Some common chemical toxicants that may be encountered in incidents affecting animals.

Toxicant Class	Sources	Special Considerations for Decontamination
Hydrocarbons	Diesel fuel Gasoline Motor oil Transmission fluid Stoddard solvents Mineral spirits Kerosene Jet fuel Benzene Toluene Xylene	Dermal decontamination generally consists of washing with liquid dish detergent and clipping hair that will not wash clean. Induction of emesis and gastric lavage are not recommended due to aspiration risk, and activated charcoal is unlikely to be of benefit.
Polychlorinated biphenyls	Electrical transformers and capacitors Lubricants in gas turbines Hydraulic systems	Animals should be washed multiple times if possible to reduce dermal absorption. Induction of emesis is contraindicated due to aspiration risk. Multiple doses of activated charcoal may prevent reabsorption of metabolites.
Toxic gases	Human and animal waste Refineries and smelters Food-processing plants Paper mills Combustion of various materials Refrigerants	Affected animals should be moved to fresh air, and no other decontamination may be needed. Signs due to exposure are generally treated with supportive care.
Detergents, acids, and alkalis	Household and industrial cleaning products Fire suppression foams Bleaches	Following bathing, animals should be monitored for at least 24 hours for signs of dermal irritation or ulceration. Oral dilution with water is recommended instead of inducing emesis or performing gastric lavage following ingestion.
Agricultural hazards	Fertilizers Herbicides Fungicides Insecticides Rodenticides	Concentrated solutions can cause severe burns of the eyes, skin, and mucous membranes. Antidotal treatment may be needed for anticholinesterase insecticides and anticoagulant rodenticides.

Sources: Murphy, Lisa et al. 2003. Toxicologic agents of concern for search-and-rescue dogs responding to urban disasters. *Journal of the American Veterinary Medical Association.* 222(3): 296–304; Wismer, Tina et al. 2003. Management and prevention of toxicoses in search-and-rescue dogs responding to urban disasters. *Journal of the American Veterinary Medical Association.* 222(3): 305–310; Langley, Rick, and Meggs, William. 2003. Farmers and farm personnel. In *Occupational, Industrial, and Environmental Toxicology,* Michael Greenburg, ed. pp. 154–161. Philadelphia, PA: Mosby.

Operations, to provide resources for planning and response. Available resources include "Area Locations of Hazardous Atmospheres" program; "Mapping Application for Response, Planning and Local Operational Tasks"; "Dense Gas Dispersion Model"; "Automated Resource for Chemical Hazard Incident Evaluation"; and "Risk Management Program Comprehensive (RMP*Comp) Modeling Program." These modeling programs allow offsite consequence analysis of worst case and alternate scenarios associated with chemical incidents.

One example is the intentional release of a hazardous or toxic substance, such as anhydrous ammonia or chlorine, on the upwind side of a major metropolitan community. When calculating the worst case and alternate scenarios for one railroad tank car of anhydrous ammonia or chlorine, the RMP*Comp program indicated that the area several miles downwind from the

release site could be affected in a very negative manner due to the toxicity of these materials.

Agricultural Event. Agricultural events include spills or releases of any of the myriad of substances that can be found in modern farming and agricultural communities. These events also include exposure to other HazMats that exist within the community, including biologic materials. In 2005, an animal response team from Nature's Way Animal Rescue and Rehabilitation in Indiana responded to a call for assistance from a fire department within their response jurisdiction for the rescue of two cattle that had fallen through the concrete roof of a confined manure pit (Figure 19.4).

The response required that several technical issues be addressed in order to safely rescue these animals, including assessment of the manure pit (confined space entry procedures); the use of air quality monitoring

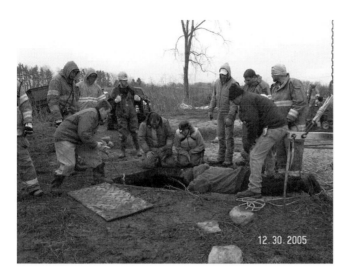

Figure 19.4 *Two cows fell through the roof of a manure pit in Indiana. Before lowering personnel into the tank, air monitoring equipment was inserted to ensure air quality for responders, especially when the animals' movements disturbed the 1 m (3 ft) deep manure. Courtesy of Dawn Slessman.*

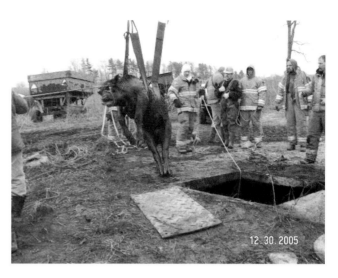

Figure 19.6 *A fire hose web sling is used to perform a vertical lift of the cattle from the manure pit approximately 10 m (33 ft) below. Responders noted that addition of a rear strap would have improved load balance and provided additional support. Courtesy of Dawn Slessman.*

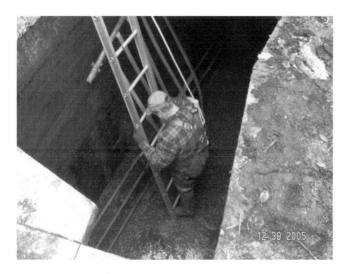

Figure 19.5 *Addressing fall protection and air quality as part of entry procedures, a responder enters the tank in waders to set up cattle panels for containment of the cattle. A veterinarian was on the scene to provide advice and sedation to the animals before attempting vertical lifts to remove the animals from the tank. Courtesy of Dawn Slessman.*

techniques to determine if hazardous levels of methane were present; fall protection and retrieval devices for the personnel who entered the restricted space; and stand-by rescue personnel for the entry team (Figure 19.5). All animals and rescue personnel were contaminated with cow manure. The animals were extricated from the tank using a web sling and a vertical lift procedure (Figure 19.6). Emergency animal decontamination primarily consisted of bathing the animals with water from a fire hose. Confined space entry procedures are relevant. In 2007 in Harrisonburg, Virginia, five

farmers were lost to methane poisoning in a similar cattle waste tank.

Industrial Accidents or Events

The December 3, 1984, incident at the Union Carbide India Ltd. pesticide plant in Bhopal, India, remains one of the worst industrial incidents in history. Water was introduced into a methyl isocyanate tank, initiating a reaction that liberated approximately 27 tons of methyl isocyanate gas into the atmosphere. Approximately 3,800 people died, and thousands others suffered partial or permanent disabilities. It is assumed, but was never documented, that there were many animal losses as well.

This incident, along with dozens of smaller events that have occurred, changed the way in which emergency response personnel plan, train, and respond to any incident that contains or may contain a hazardous substance. The Hazardous Waste Operations and Emergency Response standard regulation became effective on March 6, 1990. The regulation provides for the safety and health of employees and responders dealing with hazardous waste. Among other rights and responsibilities, the regulation allows emergency response agencies to identify the HazMats that are transported through, used, stored, or disposed of in their communities.

Non-Chemical Events

A non-chemical event is any event that results in the release of another class of materials that can cause harm to humans, animals, or the environment. Examples include exposure to naturally occurring bacteria or toxins, mud, or bodily fluids (from dead animals).

ROUTES OF EXPOSURE

Humans and animals can be exposed and affected by contaminants by inhalation, ingestion, or contact; the route of exposure is often dependent upon the physical state (liquid, solid, or gas) of the contaminant. Many contaminants (including biologic agents such as viruses, bacteria, and fungi) can produce exposure by more than one route, and the signs or symptoms observed may vary with the route of exposure.

Inhalation exposure results from breathing air contaminated with the agent. This is most commonly associated with gaseous contaminants but can also occur with aerosolized droplets of liquid contaminants.

Ingestion exposure refers to the intentional or accidental eating of the contaminant. This most commonly occurs with liquid or solid contaminants.

Contact exposure occurs when the contaminant is absorbed into the victim's body through the skin or mucous membranes (including the membranes of the mouth, nose, and eyes). This type of exposure can occur with any physical form of contaminant.

TYPES OF CONTAMINANTS

The types of contaminants and HazMats encountered generally fall into categories, as discussed next.

Highly Acutely Toxic

A single dose of or short duration of exposure to highly acutely toxic substances induces damage to the human body. These materials require only small doses to cause adverse effects. These substances are found in all physical states and have the ability to enter the victim by all routes of exposure. Examples include carbon disulfide, carbon tetrachloride, and potassium cyanide.

Moderately to Highly Chronically Toxic

Moderately to highly chronically toxic substances induce damage to the human body but generally require multiple exposures over a period of time. The substances are found in all three physical states and can enter the body by all routes of exposure. Examples include ethylene di-bromide and benzene (a component of gasoline).

Embryotoxic

Hazardous substances classified as embryotoxic cause damage to the fetus, including death, malformation, retarded growth, and postnatal functional deficits. Generally speaking, the fetus is most susceptible during the first trimester; however, with the increasing amounts and types of industrial and agricultural chemicals and pharmacological substances available, the fetus can potentially be affected throughout the entire prenatal period. Members of this group are also known as teratogens. Examples include lead compounds, for-mamide, and various alcohols (including ethanol, a component of beer, wine, and liquor).

Allergenic

Allergenic substances produce skin and respiratory hypersensitivities. The risk is most commonly posed by inhalation and direct skin contact with the material. Different animal species and subspecies exhibit varying degrees of sensitivity, which results in varying signs and symptoms. Examples include diazomethane, chromium, dichromates, formaldehyde, and isocyanides.

Flammable

Flammable contaminants are found in all three physical states and can enter the animal or human victim through any route or multiple routes of exposure. Flammable contaminants also include a wide range of secondary hazards, including local and systemic toxins and tertiary hazards (e.g., chemical irritants). This classification will generally present more than one contamination problem (i.e., local and systemic toxicity). Examples include hydrocarbon fuels, toluene, acetone, hydrogen, butane, and calcium carbide.

Highly Reactive or Explosive

Highly reactive or explosive substances are generally heat-, shock-, and friction-sensitive to the degree that some may react with the oxygen in the environment. The higher the concentration of the contaminant, the higher the risk involved in performing decontamination. Examples include peroxides, peroxide-forming compounds, and explosives.

Etiologic

This classification includes microorganisms (viruses, bacteria, fungi, etc.) that can cause illness, disease, or death in humans and/or animals. These microorganisms can enter the body through one or more routes. However, there are four factors that affect the ability of these organisms to cause negative effects:

- Virulence: the organism's ability to induce disease
- Dose: the number of organisms entering the body during exposure
- Physical environment: ambient temperature, humidity, etc.
- Health status of the victim: the ability of the victim's body to defend itself from infection

Examples include organisms found in infectious waste (e.g., *Escherichia coli*, *Salmonella*, *Cryptosporidium*, *Giardia*, *Leptospira*, etc.), avian influenza virus, etc.

Radioactive

Radiation energy includes nonionizing radiation (such as that associated with microwave ovens, sunlight, artificial ultraviolet light, etc.) and ionizing radiation (including alpha or beta particles and gamma rays).

Alpha particles are the largest particles and should not penetrate the skin; however, inhalation of these particles can result in a medical emergency. The use of proper personnel protective equipment (PPE) assists in avoiding contact with the material during rescue and decontamination operations. The next most common method of protection includes time, distance, and shielding.

Some radioactive materials, such as radiopharmaceuticals, have extremely short half-lives (the amount of time required for one-half of the particles to no longer be hazardous). In these types of incidents, isolation of the exposed animal for a specified time may be more successful than any other method of decontamination. After seven sequential half-lives, approximately 1% of the original amount remains. Examples include cesium-137, cobalt-60, radon-222, uranium hexafluoride, and plutonium.

Surface Contaminants

Surface contaminants are present on the outer surface of a material and have not been absorbed into the material. They are normally easily detected and removed. Examples include dusts, powders, and fibers.

Permeation Contaminants

Permeation contaminants are those that are absorbed into a material such as hair, fur, or tissue. They are very often difficult or impossible to detect and remove. However, if the contaminants are not removed, they may continue to permeate through the material. There are four factors that influence permeation:

- Contact time: the amount of time that the contaminant is in contact with the surface of the material. Increased contact time results in increased exposure doses.
- Concentration: the purity of the substance. Higher concentrations result in more rapid permeation breakthrough times and rates.
- Temperature: the temperature of the hazardous contaminant, the contaminated material, and the ambient temperature. In general, higher temperatures increase the permeation rate.
- Physical state: the form of the substance as a gas, liquid, or solid. The physical state of the hazardous contaminant directly affects the permeation breakthrough rate. Liquids generally have the most rapid permeation rates.

Direct Contamination

This method of contamination typically results from direct contact with the contaminant. There are various reasons for direct contamination occurring in the decontamination process: poor decontamination site management, selection of incompatible PPE, inadequate supply of good quality breathing air, and inadequate decontamination procedures.

Cross-Contamination

Cross-contamination results when an uncontaminated item comes into direct contact with a "dirty" (contaminated) item. This is also known as secondary contamination. Examples include the re-entry of successfully decontaminated personnel into a contaminated area or the use of a contaminated piece of equipment on a successfully decontaminated animal.

CONTROL ZONES TO LIMIT CONTAMINATION

Responders should immediately establish and enforce site control zones to limit spread of contamination, as follows:

- Hot zone: the area of primary contamination or where the air quality monitoring equipment first responded above the background levels.
- Warm zone: the area to which contaminated animal and human victims are brought for decontamination.
- Cold zone: the area where no hazard exists; all animals and humans have been successfully decontaminated. Triage and further treatment of victims is performed in this zone.

PERSONAL PROTECTIVE AND DECONTAMINATION EQUIPMENT

Personal Protective Equipment

In compliance with current OSHA and EPA standards, protection of emergency responders must be accomplished through the use of engineering controls, standard work practices, and administrative controls, or through the use of appropriate PPE.

PPE includes all clothing and other work accessories designed to create a barrier against workplace hazards. Examples include safety goggles, blast shields, hard hats, hearing protectors, gloves, respirators, aprons, and work boots. PPE should not be used as a substitute for engineering, work practice, and/or administrative controls to prevent exposure to hazardous chemicals. It is also important to note that PPE protects only the user and does not remove the hazard from the area. For example, a respirator may protect the wearer from toxic fumes, but does not protect others in the vicinity.

The specific level of PPE required is based in part on the following contributing factors: the type of tactical operation being performed (animal rescue or animal decontamination, or both); the necessity for triage, treatment, and transfer operations; and the identity, concentration, and physical state of the contaminant.

Levels of Personal Protective Equipment for Large Animal Rescue, Response, and Decontamination

Level A Response Personal Protective Equipment. Level A equipment is required when the greatest potential for exposure to hazards exists and when the greatest level of skin, respiratory, and eye protection is required. These fully encapsulating suits afford protection against petroleum products and halogenated hydrocarbons as well as nerve and blistering agents.

The following constitute Level A equipment:

1. Positive pressure-demand, full face-piece self-contained breathing apparatus (SCBA), or positive pressure supplied air respirator with escape SCBA, approved by the National Institute for Occupational Safety and Health (NIOSH)
2. Totally encapsulating vapor and chemical protective suit (meets National Fire Protection Association [NFPA] 1991)
3. Coveralls (as needed; safety officer [SO] determines use)
4. Long underwear (as needed; SO determines use)
5. Gloves, outer, chemical-resistant
6. Gloves, inner, chemical-resistant
7. Boots, chemical-resistant, steel toe and shank
8. Hard hat (under suit) (as needed; SO determines use)
9. Disposable protective suit, gloves, and boots (depending on suit construction, may be worn over totally encapsulating suit)
10. Two-way radio communication

Level B Personal Protective Equipment. Level B equipment is required under circumstances requiring the highest level of respiratory protection, with a lesser level of skin protection. It is recommended that teams have fully encapsulating suits when necessary for splash protection and coveralls for use in situations where splash hazards are not anticipated or expected.

The following constitute Level B equipment:

1. Positive-pressure, full face-piece SCBA, or positive-pressure supplied air respirator with escape SCBA (NIOSH approved)
2. Hooded chemical-resistant liquid splash-protective suit (meets NFPA 1992)
3. Coveralls (as needed; SO determines use)
4. Gloves, outer, chemical-resistant
5. Gloves, inner, chemical-resistant
6. Boots, outer, chemical-resistant, steel toe and shank
7. Boot covers, outer, chemical-resistant (disposable) (as needed; SO determines use)
8. Hard hat (as needed; SO determines use)
9. Face shield (as needed; SO determines use)

Level C Personal Protective Equipment. Level C protection equipment is used when the concentration(s) and type(s) of airborne substance(s) are known and the criteria for using air purifying respirators are met.

The following constitute Level C equipment:

1. Full-face or half-mask, air-purifying respirators (NIOSH approved)
2. Hooded chemical-resistant clothing (overalls; two-piece chemical splash suit; disposable chemical-resistant overalls)
3. Coveralls (as needed)
4. Gloves, outer, chemical-resistant
5. Gloves, inner, chemical-resistant
6. Boots (outer), chemical-resistant, steel toe and shank (as needed)
7. Boot-covers, outer, chemical-resistant (disposable) (as needed)
8. Hard hat (as needed)
9. Escape mask (as needed)
10. Face shield (as needed)

Level D Personal Protective Equipment. Protective equipment in this level includes work uniforms affording minimal protection, and is used for nuisance contamination (e.g., hair, dust, etc.) only. Most commercial animal facilities use this level of protection when working animals in daily management. No danger of chemical exposure exists, and the SO determines the use of equipment.

The following constitute Level D equipment:

1. Coveralls
2. Gloves (as needed)
3. Boots/shoes, chemical-resistant, steel toe and shank
4. Boots, outer, chemical-resistant (disposable) (as needed)
5. Safety glasses or chemical splash goggles (as needed)
6. Hard hat (as needed)
7. Escape mask (as needed)
8. Face shield (as needed)

Large Animal Specialty Decontamination Equipment

Large animal decontamination equipment could include, but is not limited to, the following items:

- Proper PPE for the decontamination team
- Large animal panels, commonly referred to as pig/hog panels or cattle panels, to provide containment of the animal during decontamination (Figure 19.7)

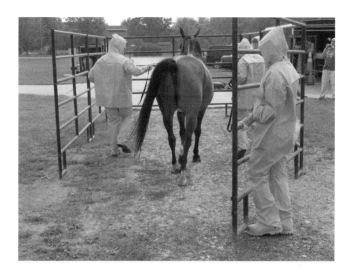

Figure 19.7 *Secondary containment of the animal allows responders to concentrate on their procedures and minimizes the chance of animal escape. Note the use of cross leads to maintain control of the horse. Courtesy of Bob Mauck.*

- Water supply with ability to control water temperature
- Ability to contain run off; if on soil, mark areas and build earthen dikes for later sampling and cleanup
- Buckets, brushes, sponges, long-handled brushes
- Garden hose
- Long-handled water wands
- Hand towels and washcloths for technical decontamination of the face and head
- Sterile lubricating eye ointment for the animal
- Halters and lead ropes

LARGE ANIMAL DECONTAMINATION

Specific decontamination procedures depend on a number of factors, but they primarily depend on the specific types of contaminants involved. Highly toxic materials and contaminants generally require more detailed and thorough decontamination procedures than do less toxic materials. A thorough understanding of the hazardous materials involved as well as the general principles of decontamination is essential to implementing effective procedures. Where applicable, the party responsible for the chemical incident will be held liable for the costs of replacement of decontamination equipment and supplies as well as the packaging, transportation, and proper disposal of all decontamination wastes (*US Code*, Title 42, Chapter 103: Comprehensive Environmental Response, Compensation and Liability Act [CERCLA]).

Despite proper PPE, personnel operating within the contaminated area should take precautions to avoid gross contamination. Measures include avoiding walking or kneeling in pooled liquids or other contamination sources such as spilled solids, splashed or

brushed contaminants, or saturated spills; avoiding unnecessary contact with contaminated containers or equipment; avoiding setting instruments or equipment down in pooled liquids, spilled solids, or saturated soils; minimizing the chance of a large animal injuring a person. Personnel in PPE often experience difficulty seeing and performing quick movements; in addition, the PPE can be frightening to the animals.

Personnel should avoid areas of vapor clouds, mists, gas release plumes, or windblown particulates and work from the upwind side whenever possible. To avoid splashing, responders must work methodically and carefully to handle animals, decontamination, or medical equipment.

FACTORS INFLUENCING THE DECONTAMINATION PROCESS

The decontamination process depends on many factors.

- The toxicity, corrosiveness, flammability, or reactivity of the contaminant
- The amount of contaminant to be cleaned and decontaminated
- The level of protective equipment required
- The species or subspecies involved, as well as the animal's individual tractability (willingness to be handled) and attitude
- The type of equipment used for the decontamination process
- The work function and training level of personnel on scene
- The location of the contamination (contamination of the upper areas of the animal present greater risk to the animal and the decontamination personnel)

TYPES OF DECONTAMINATION

Emergency Decontamination (Gross Decontamination)

The immediate threat to the animal's life and the potential for secondary contamination of other animals and humans determine the need for emergency decontamination procedures. Emergency decontamination procedures require minimal equipment, reduce secondary contamination (up to 80%), and do not require the establishment of formal contamination reduction corridors or formal decontamination processes. However, there are limitations to the emergency decontamination process: there may still be 20%–50% of the contaminant still present, and it will create contaminant runoff, necessitating considerations for runoff control.

Technical Decontamination

This method of decontamination is most commonly used because it primarily involves the use of water or soap and water solutions to physically wash the contaminant from the animal. The water reduces the concentration of the material through dilution, not by chemical alteration. There are several issues that must be addressed prior to initiating a dilution process. These include but are not limited to the following: the possibility that the contaminant is water-reactive, the water solubility of the contaminant, the possibility that the water runoff will increase the area of contamination, and the ability to properly contain and temporarily store the waste water. All runoff water is considered hazardous waste; therefore, the more water used, the more hazardous waste generated.

Dermal Decontamination. Compared to the conventional showering procedures used for decontaminating human victims and responders, dermal decontamination of large animals is typically a larger-scale, though not necessarily more complicated, operation. Large animals have thick hair coats and larger body sizes and surface areas; successful dermal decontamination of large animals by bathing requires adequate time, trained personnel, and sufficient resources, including access to large quantities of clean water. Appropriate drainage must be provided to avoid further exposure through drinking or prolonged contact with contaminated wastewater. This may be facilitated by providing slatted or perforated racks or rubber mats on which the animals can stand during bathing. Risks to personnel include injuries inflicted by the animals and prolonged exposure to potential toxins. Animals may be subject to injury, stress, and hypothermia.

In order to effectively decontaminate large animals, they must be confined to a relatively small area. Each animal should have sufficient area to stand and comfortably turn around in place. Adequate ventilation is also necessary in order to prevent the potentially hazardous buildup of gases and vapors from chemical contaminants or animal waste or pathogens. Individual animals may often be held in place by a head gate or one or more persons using a lead and halter, while groups may be able to be washed while confined in a small corral or herded through a narrow chute or similar setup (Figure 19.8). In order to prevent human and animal injury, chemical sedation may be necessary to calm nervous or aggressive animals, particularly those that are not accustomed to close contact with people (e.g., beef cattle or young horses). The judicious use of sedatives can also facilitate the process and reduce the risk of injury. However, the potential adverse effects of these drugs should be considered: stressed, injured, or debilitated animals may develop life-threatening hypotension, cardiac arrhythmias, or pulmonary conditions; animals may become unsteady or ataxic (uncoordinated); and these drugs may increase the unpredictability or aggressive nature of certain individuals. Only experienced personnel should handle

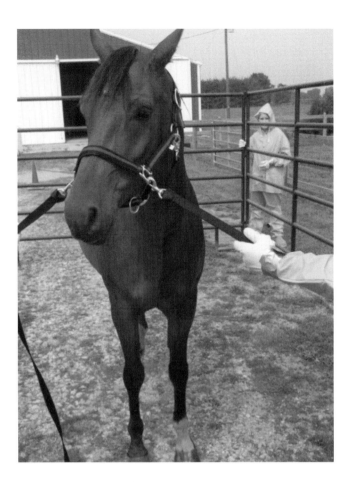

Figure 19.8 *Following gross and technical decontamination, a clean halter is placed and the horse is ready to go to the cold zone triage area. Courtesy of Bob Mauck.*

sedated or unsedated large animals. Administration of drugs for the purpose of chemical restraint should only be performed under the direct supervision of a licensed veterinarian.

The minimum PPE worn should include protective (preferably water-repellant) clothing, waterproof boots, chemical-resistant gloves, and safety goggles. Ideally, respiratory protection should be worn regardless of the contaminant involved because hair, dust, and aerosolized urine and fecal material have the potential to cause human illness.

The dermal decontamination process involves using brushes, scrapers, picks, and whatever tool fits the need without harming the animal in order to remove as much of the visible material as possible. Thorough cleaning of the hooves and feet of various species should be included.

Some dry, dusty, or powdery substances may be more easily removed using brushes or combs or by wiping them off with dry or slightly dampened towels; this may be better tolerated by some animals than bathing and decreases the quantity of water used. Some dusts or powders tend to clump when wet, making them more difficult to remove. Wetting dusty contaminants may also decrease the incidence of ocular (eye) and respiratory irritation from these agents. Potential disadvantages of this method include the time and close human contact that is required. Final decisions will be incident-specific, and procedures may need to be modified as the situation dictates.

Some well-trained animals may tolerate being vacuumed. The animal is cleaned with a specialized vacuum that uses high-efficiency particulate air (HEPA) filters on the discharge opening of the vacuum; personnel should be wearing respiratory protection as well. The HEPA filters physically capture particles 0.3 µm or larger in size. This procedure is effective for the removal of particulate or fibrous materials such as asbestos.

Liquid dishwashing detergent is economical and readily available, minimally irritating, and drying to animal and human skin, and readily removes most substances from the skin and hair of animals. Chemical solvents, such as degreasers and paint thinners, should not be used on animal skin. If tolerated by the animal, gauze, cotton swabs, or a soft toothbrush can be used to remove debris from the nostrils and ears. Towels or scrub brushes should be gently used to allow penetration of water and soap through the hair coat to the skin without causing abrasions or other injuries. Special attention should be given to skin folds and creases where contaminants or detergent might become trapped. Long or matted hair may need to be shaved or trimmed. Adequate rinsing is required to remove all residues and detergent from the skin and hair and should be repeated until the rinse water runs clear.

Planning must include a secure location where animals can be held after bathing. If animals cannot be safely housed nearby, a feasible means of transportation will need to be determined. During cold and inclement weather, special efforts should be made to protect animals from excessive winds or drafts.

Ocular Decontamination. Ocular exposure to chemical agents may cause problems ranging from mild irritation to irreversible damage and loss of vision, depending on the specific substance involved, its concentration, and the duration of the exposure. Many large animals, particularly horses, may not be considered salvageable if permanent ocular injury occurs.

The eyes should be repeatedly lavaged (flushed) with tepid water or sterile saline for 20–30 minutes (Osweiler, 1996). Ocular injuries can be very painful, and many large animal patients will not tolerate the necessary handling of their heads and eyes. If large numbers of animals require decontamination, time constraints render this strategy impractical. Since some beneficial rinsing of the eyes will probably occur during dermal decontamination of animals' heads, additional ocular flushing can be performed later on individual animals as needed. One unique strategy that has been

suggested is using a plastic cup to gently pour water directly over each eye (DeClementi, 2006). Even though some handling of the head is still required, this approach will likely be much less startling to most animals compared to a sudden pressurized stream of water.

Repeated lavage, diagnostic procedures such as fluorescein staining, and medical treatment (including ophthalmic ointments and systemic anti-inflammatory medications) may be required in affected animals. The animal handler and the veterinary professional treating the eyes should be especially cautious and attentive in order to avoid serious injury due to the sudden impact of a frightened, injured animal's swinging head.

Gastrointestinal Decontamination. Gastric evacuation is used to remove substances from the stomach when a potentially dangerous quantity has recently been ingested. It is usually most effective during the first two to four hours following the exposure (Osweiler, 1996). Vomiting is commonly induced in other animal species, such as dogs and cats, to evacuate the stomach, but this procedure cannot be safely or reliably performed on horses or ruminants. Swine may be the only livestock species in which vomiting can be induced.

Gastric lavage is another procedure used to remove foreign substances from the stomachs of animals. It is performed by repeated introduction of water and siphoning of the stomach contents via a large-bore nasogastric tube. The procedure typically requires sedation or anesthesia and is unlikely to be practical or useful in ruminants due to the large volume of the rumen. Neither induction of vomiting nor gastric lavage should be attempted with known ingestions of petroleum distillates or caustic substances due to the risks of aspiration and injury to the oral and esophageal mucosa (lining). Adsorbents such as activated charcoal (1–2 g/kg of body weight) are administered to physically adsorb (bind) a toxicant, which is then eliminated in the feces (Osweiler, 1996). Cathartics (laxatives) are often used alone or in conjunction with activated charcoal to more rapidly eliminate toxic substances from the gastrointestinal tract. Commonly used cathartics for large animals include sodium sulfate, magnesium sulfate, sorbitol, and mineral oil (Galey, 1996). Mineral oil may provide an added benefit of coating and soothing the gastrointestinal lining (Plumlee, 1996). Cathartics should be administered by a trained veterinary professional and administered via nasogastric intubation.

Surgical interventions such as gastrotomy and rumenotomy have been used in situations involving metallic objects and other persistent materials (Osweiler, 1996). While this may sometimes offer a viable option for highly valuable, individual animals, it is not practical in most field situations, especially when large numbers of animals are affected.

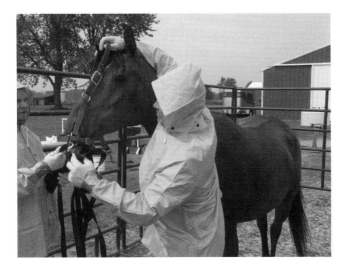

Figure 19.9 *In a practice scenario, a horse brought into the warm zone for decontamination is placed inside secondary containment. The contaminated (dirty) halter is exchanged for a clean one as a part of technical decontamination of the face. Courtesy of Bob Mauck.*

Isolation and Disposal

Isolation and disposal is normally a two-step process whereby contaminated articles are removed and isolated in a designated area/ or container prior to washing the animal. Contaminated articles are then properly packaged for later disposal in accordance with local, state, and federal laws. Halters, collars, leads, etc. are removed and replaced with clean, noncontaminated materials (Figure 19.9).

Chemical Degradation

Chemical degradation is the process of altering the chemical structure of the hazardous material by applying another chemical to the contaminated surface. Extreme care must be used when applying this method to an animal or human. As mentioned above, low-pressure water in large quantities serves as a primary cleaning solution that may be used for decontamination. Water not only dilutes and flushes away CBRNE agents and materials, but it will also chemically react with many chemical warfare agents (CWAs) to detoxify them. However, other substances may react with water to generate toxic products; the use of water as a decontamination solution should be based on knowledge of the contaminant involved.

Two other chemical decontamination processes easily used by first responders to neutralize CWAs and biological warfare agents have also been recommended for radioactive materials decontamination. These processes take advantage of common household materials that can easily be obtained from grocery stores, hardware stores, and swimming pool supply stores. These two methods are: (1) washing contaminated equipment with high pH (alkaline) soap solutions, and (2) washing or soaking contaminated equipment with

bleach (calcium hypochlorite or sodium hypochlorite) solutions.

Note: These methods and substances are not recommended for use directly on animals or unprotected people and preferably should not be used in their vicinity, due to the risk for oral, dermal, ocular, and respiratory exposures.

Disinfection

Disinfection is the destruction of microorganisms (viruses, bacteria, fungi, etc.). However, the process does not kill 100% of the microorganisms present. Disinfection is often achieved with solutions containing alcohols, phenols, iodine, or chlorine. The solutions induce physical or functional damage to the microorganisms. Disinfectant solutions are used on inanimate objects and surfaces, whereas antiseptics are used on living tissue. The use of bleach solutions, peroxide solutions, and hypochlorites is reserved for disinfectant use, and these solutions are not recommended for use directly on animals or humans.

Medical/Secondary Decontamination

Once appropriately trained and licensed veterinary care arrives on the scene or the animal is transported to a clinical setting, additional decontamination may be required. The chemical may have already begun to be systemically absorbed by the animal. The clinician may allow the animal to detoxify through normal metabolic processes or may choose to augment excretion and detoxification with various therapies such as intravenous fluids, activated charcoal, specific antidotes, gastric lavage, etc.

EVALUATING THE EFFECTIVENESS OF DECONTAMINATION

The effectiveness of the decontamination process can be evaluated using the following:

- Monitoring devices: This process uses HazMat monitoring devices to scan the area(s) of the animal(s) that were contaminated. Successful decontamination results in normal readings on the instrument; elevated readings indicate that additional decontamination is necessary (Figure 19.10). Electronic monitoring equipment is available for evaluating chemical and radiological contamination.
- Visual observation: The animal is visually observed for any unusual behavioral issues or physical conditions. The veterinarian should be closely involved with triage and observation.
- Medical monitoring: A variety of diagnostic laboratory tests can be used to detect increased liver enzymes, specific toxicants, etc., depending upon the hazardous substance to which the animal was exposed.

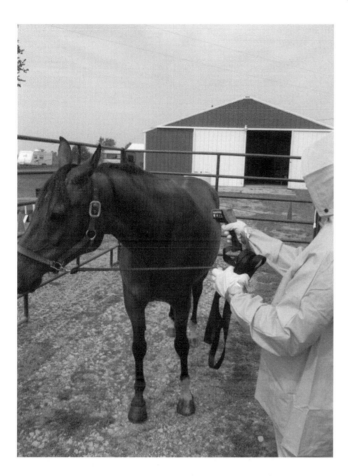

Figure 19.10 *After completing gross and technical phases of decontamination, a decontamination technician uses human electronic monitoring equipment to ensure that the animal has been decontaminated to the minimal level of contamination possible. Courtesy of Bob Mauck.*

SELECTING A DECONTAMINATION AREA

When selecting an appropriate site for animal decontamination, responders should consider the following:

- How much and what type of decontamination is necessary?
- To what extent will decontamination be accomplished in the field?
- Is the contaminant water-soluble?
- Is the contaminant water-reactive? If yes, what are the results when mixed with water?
- Can decontamination be conducted in a safe manner?
- Are the required resources immediately available?
- Can the equipment being used be properly decontaminated?

The Decontamination Group

The team of trained and adequately equipped personnel performing decontamination on animals is typically identified as the DECON or decontamination group. The team assigns a group leader who in turn answers to the hazardous materials branch manager within the incident command system/National Incident Management System structure for the incident. The decontamination group is responsible for the following issues:

- Determining the appropriate level and type of decontamination necessary for the situation
- Ensuring the decontamination area is established and operational prior to entry into the hot zone for rescue and/or removal of animals
- Ensuring proper decontamination procedures are used
- Coordinating decontamination operations with other branch, division, and group officers
- Coordinating the transfer of successfully decontaminated patients to the owner or veterinary triage/treatment and transport group
- Monitoring the overall effectiveness of the decontamination operations
- Controlling the operations, entry, and exit of all personnel within the decontamination area
- Ensuring that relief personnel are immediately available for the decontamination area
- Ensuring all supplies and support for the decontamination area are provided in a timely manner and through effective methods

Decontamination Area Site Selection Criteria

The HazMat branch manager, in consultation with the incident commander, SO, and decontamination team, is responsible for decontamination area site selection and designation. The decontamination area should meet the following criteria (Figure 19.11). It should:

1. be located upwind and uphill from the point of release.
2. be a reasonably flat, level area.
3. be sufficient size for anticipated operations.
4. be accessible from hard-surfaced roads.
5. have reasonable access from the incident scene (decontamination sites farther than 30 m [33 yd] from the incident scene will require transportation).
6. be away from rivers, streams, ponds, storm drains, or other environmentally sensitive areas (storm drains and manholes must be covered to prevent runoff from entering these systems).
7. offer natural or manmade depressions for directing and collecting decontamination run-off (lined with plastic sheeting and properly marked).

Indoors: Considerations. If the decontamination area chosen is indoors, the following should be considered:

DECONTAMINATION

Layout of A Typical Casualty Receiving Station

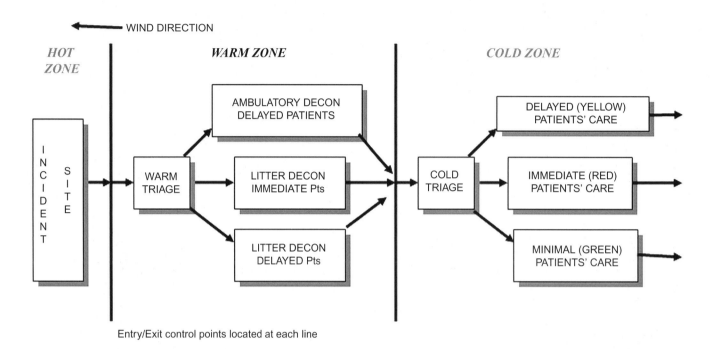

Entry/Exit control points located at each line

Figure 19.11 *This is a layout of a typical decontamination area. Although this layout reflects a typical arrangement for human decontamination, there is no justifiable reason that it cannot also be applied to a simplified version of animal decontamination. The concept of reducing the amount of contamination on the animals from the time they enter from the hot zone until they leave the decontamination reduction corridor remains the same. Courtesy of Bob Mauck.*

- Quick access and egress
- Adequate area for safe handling of large animals
- Nonslip, secure surfaces, and footing for animals
- Type and slope of floor
- Presence of floor drains
- Air flow to and from rooms and hallways

Outdoors: Considerations. If the decontamination area chosen is outdoors, the following should be considered.

- Access from a hard surface road or hard pack
- Sufficient clean, potable water supply
- Ability to address runoff
- Presence of or proximity to environmentally sensitive areas
- Presence of sanitary sewer or storm drains and consultation with the AHJ over the drains

Example Animal Decontamination Layout
The *decontamination corridor* is a pathway from the hot zone to the decontamination area and has clearly identified boundaries (Figure 19.12). Using signs for entrance and exit points is recommended, as well as plastic tarps with premarked stations for small animal decontamination operations. Large animals are often reluctant to walk over tarps or unfamiliar footing; concrete is the preferred surface for this use. The following are two examples of situations in which this layout is appropriate:

- Working dogs or police horses are led through decontamination with the assistance of the handler/rider, followed by decontamination of the handler/rider.
- The animal and owner have exited the hot zone together and can be decontaminated simultaneously at separate stations. They are reunited after decontamination is completed.

COMBINED DECONTAMINATION OPERATION

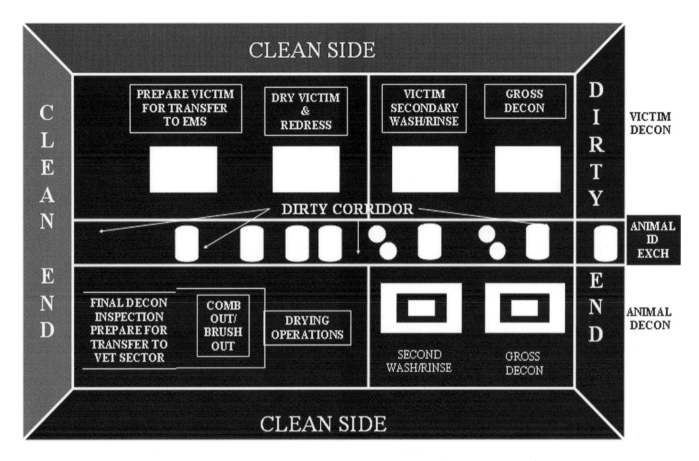

Figure 19.12 *This format for decontamination operations is recommended during the following circumstances: service animals and their owners are simultaneously decontaminated or the decontamination is of a precautionary nature. Courtesy of Bob Mauck.*

Sample to Determine Animal Decontamination Effectiveness

When decontamination procedures are activated because of high-risk contaminates (e.g., radiological, etiologic, pesticides, or other highly toxic materials), exposed animals should be triaged after decontamination and isolated for further medical evaluation and monitoring. This additional attention usually includes blood tests, urinalysis, and a minimum of 24-hour observation. In accordance with CERCLA, the expense of this required medical evaluation shall be the responsibility of the party liable for the spill or release.

DECONTAMINATION TERMINATION PROCEDURES FOR EQUIPMENT AND PERSONNEL

Equipment Procedures

Upon completion of the decontamination process, the decontamination area must be secured until the isolated clothing and equipment can be removed for proper cleaning and disposal. Items for disposal must be left in place for removal by a certified hazardous waste contractor, if possible. If the contaminated materials will likely remain at the site for an unacceptable period of time (i.e., more than a few hours, and/or will not be under the direct supervision of the AHJ), appropriate precautions must be taken, such as posted warning signs and labels attached to containers, to reduce the potential for additional personnel becoming contaminated. Law enforcement support and lighting may be necessary if the materials remain overnight. Chain of custody requirements must be maintained.

If it is determined that contaminated equipment can be safely and effectively decontaminated and is reusable, the HazMat branch manager and SO may direct that the equipment be recovered. Initial decontamination of equipment may be accomplished on site, with more thorough cleaning to be performed at an approved off-site location.

Personnel involved in collecting, decontaminating, and packaging equipment must wear appropriate PPE as determined by the HazMat branch manager, decontamination group, and/or SO. All equipment must be double-bagged and sealed in container(s) that contain appropriate identification for proper packaging and transport to an approved off-site location.

Waste solutions should be pumped or baled from the primary containments (e.g., wading pools, sumps, or secondary containment), and any waste accumulation within the secondary containment (liner) must be appropriately handled. This should be accomplished before removing the outer perimeter containment. If necessary, all decontamination equipment and wastes may be left on site and the site secured for cleanup and appropriate disposal by the hazardous waste removal contractor.

Personnel Procedures

When the decontamination group has completed decontamination of the affected animals and initiated protective equipment doffing procedures for the entry team, members of the decontamination group assist each other through the wash and rinse station. Team members also assist each other in doffing protective equipment and bagging of protective garments (as described in jurisdictional standard operating protocols). Decontamination personnel then report for medical evaluation on or off site.

When all steps of the decontamination procedures are activated because of high-risk contaminants (e.g., radiological, etiologic, pesticides, or other highly toxic materials) the decontamination group should be isolated for further medical evaluation and monitoring. This additional attention usually includes blood tests, urinalysis, and possibly an overnight stay. In accordance with CERCLA, the expense of this required medical evaluation shall be the responsibility of the party liable for the spill or release.

Swipe Tests

Swipe testing of protective clothing, SCBA, and other PPE equipment used at the scene may be required in some cases, especially in those incidents involving radiation, biologic agents, or highly toxic substances (e.g., pesticides). This is usually performed after decontamination procedures have been completed to determine if the decontamination process was effective in removing contaminants. Swipe tests detect only surface contamination, not chemical permeation into a given material.

Cloth or paper patches (swipes) are wiped over predetermined surfaces of a suspect object and submitted for analysis at a laboratory. Inner and outer surfaces of protective clothing should be swipe tested. Swipe tests should be performed by a qualified technician and processed at an appropriate laboratory. Area laboratories will include those as recommended by public health officials, department of environmental management or the state board of health.

Debriefing

A debriefing of decontamination and operational personnel should take place immediately after any decontamination operation to provide as much information about the contaminant as possible, including the following:

1. Material identification
2. Health effects
3. Signs and symptoms of exposure
4. Procedures required for follow-up medical evaluations
5. Exposure levels (when appropriate)

ACRONYMS USED IN CHAPTER 19

AHJ	Authority having jurisdiction
CBRNE	Chemical, biological, radiological, nuclear, and explosive
CERCLA	Comprehensive Environmental Response, Compensation and Liability Act
EPA	Environmental Protection Agency
HazMat	Hazardous materials
HEPA	High efficiency particulate air [filter]
NFPA	National Fire Protection Association
NIOSH	National Institute for Occupational Safety and Health
OSHA	Occupational Safety and Health Administration
PPE	Personal protective equipment
RMP*Comp	Risk Management Program Comprehensive
SCBA	Self-contained breathing apparatus
SO	Safety officer
WMD	Weapons of mass destruction

20 Special Veterinary Problems of Animals Requiring Technical Rescue

Dr. Janice Baker

INTRODUCTION

Conditions such as wounds, dehydration, and lameness are frequently observed after disasters and emergencies and are generally treated in routine manner by veterinarians. However, disasters and technical rescue situations can also present a special set of conditions in animals not commonly seen in everyday large animal veterinary practice. Near drowning, burns, smoke inhalation, environmental injury, toxicoses, and electrocution occur frequently in technical rescue situations. Veterinarians working with technical rescue teams should be familiar with diagnosis, mechanism of injury and treatment of these conditions (Figure 20.1).

Non-veterinary responders should be familiar with the basic physiologic mechanisms of these special problems, be able to recognize common clinical signs, and be able to perform basic first aid until veterinary care is available. Although this chapter is intended as an overview for non-veterinary responders, veterinarians new to technical rescue and disaster medicine may also find it beneficial. Information presented here is derived from veterinary scientific literature and the combined experience of several veterinarians involved closely in disaster response and large animal practice.

OVEREXERTION COMPLICATIONS

Animals entrapped, swimming for long periods, or fleeing capture can undergo an extreme amount of physiologic stress. Increased demands on the cardiovascular, respiratory, musculoskeletal, nervous, and thermoregulatory systems can lead to serious injury, illness, or death. Problems resulting from these conditions do not always present immediately during or following the stressful event. Complications from overexertion can develop hours to days after the initial physiological stress. This is one reason why successful extrication of a live animal does not always result in a successful outcome and provides further evidence why animals should not be chased on technical large animal emergency rescue (TLAER) scenes.

A prime example of delayed onset of a post-exertional complication is renal failure following successful extrication of an animal from entrapment in a confined space. During the time the animal is entrapped, it struggles causing sweat-induced loss of body water (leading to dehydration) and muscle stress. If the animal cannot drink, it cannot replenish the fluid lost to sweat evaporation. Myoglobin and other products of muscle breakdown are released from damaged muscle cells into the bloodstream, where they circulate to the kidneys. Myoglobin is a very large protein molecule that can accumulate in the kidney and lead to renal (kidney) insufficiency and failure. Dehydration enhances the renal damage by decreasing blood flow to and through the kidneys. The authors are aware of three recent rescue attempts where the animal died in its entrapment before the responders could even reach the animal. These animals were entrapped under trees, a barn, or in a trailer overturn for less than two hours, but succumbed to stress effects, not physical injuries.

TREATING THE INVISIBLE

Once the animal is freed from the situation, treatment is often focused on visible injuries such as lacerations and other open wounds. Non-veterinary personnel may be deceived by the observation that the animal is no longer struggling, sweating, or visibly stressed.

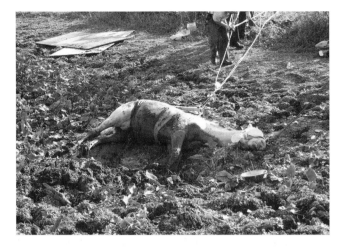

Figure 20.1 *Animals trapped in TLAER scenarios are subject to intense physiological and environmental stress that may cause detrimental medical conditions. For this reason, veterinary personnel should be on scene. This aged horse is being removed from mud entrapment and should be evaluated for possible hyperthermia (from sun exposure), hypothermia (body heat decreased by mud), lacerations (from obstacles in the mud), and myopathy (muscle damage from struggling). Courtesy Palm Beach County Fire/Rescue.*

Injured horses are commonly administered a non-steroidal anti-inflammatory drug (NSAID) (e.g., phenylbutazone or flunixin meglumine). NSAIDs can have toxic effects on the kidneys if the animal is dehydrated. Ideally, the hydration and cardiovascular status of the animal should be determined before the animal is extricated and a treatment plan devised to appropriately address dehydration and cardiovascular shock. When necessary and possible, treatment can be instituted prior to extrication.

Simple Treatment Options

A large animal veterinarian should be called to the scene to manage the animal's medical and physiologic conditions. It is critical to avoid focusing on the technical rescue effort to the detriment of the medical and physiologic well-being of the distressed animal. If the animal has been entrapped for a long period of time prior to extrication, responders should consider actions for supportive care as appropriate and practical. Examples include cooling (e.g., misting, fans, shade, etc.) or warming (e.g., blankets, warmed intravenous [IV] fluids, forced air heaters, etc.); providing shelter from wind; and administering IV fluids or offering a bucket of cool water. The use of common sense and basic human first aid is often appropriate. No TLAER scenario is exactly the same as another, and first responders should use good judgment and previously acquired knowledge to perform a good assessment and provide first aid care to the animal(s).

THE VETERINARIAN AS A TEAM MEMBER

The veterinarian on the scene of a technical rescue should focus on providing veterinary care as an operations team member and provide advice to the incident commander and other rescue personnel. If trained technical rescue personnel are on the scene, the veterinarian should avoid becoming involved in the actual extrication of the patient. Developing tunnel vision on an individual patient or technical aspect of the extrication can lead the medical personnel to overlook the physiologic change in the animal. This is especially true of incidents involving more than one animal, as the condition of an individual animal can change rapidly. An animal initially triaged as stable may begin to deteriorate, and if the veterinarian or other person providing veterinary care is distracted by the technical rescue efforts, he or she may overlook the change in the animal's condition.

Scene Management

A tenet of mass casualty management in humans is that the most experienced or senior medical provider is often located away from the actual treatment area guiding patient triage, movement, and transport while the medics, nurses, and other junior medical providers perform treatments and procedures as directed. This method allows the senior medical provider to focus on the overall operation, avoid focusing on one patient, and direct appropriate treatment of all patients relative to each other and the changing situation in their environment. Veterinarians and TLAER rescue teams should employ this method of scene management when possible. Most veterinarians are accustomed to direct contact with their patients and may initially be uncomfortable with this approach; however, the presence of adequately trained support personnel facilitates the veterinarian's duties by allowing him or her to focus on directing the assessment and treatment of animals.

PHYSIOLOGIC RESPONSES TO ENVIRONMENTAL CONDITIONS

Entrapment and injuries from struggling or avoiding capture can pose specific and unique medical problems. Entrapped animals cannot react to changes in environmental conditions around them and may be adversely affected by entrapment hazards (e.g., water, heat, mud, ice, obstacles). Veterinarians and other medical personnel participating in technical large animal emergency and disaster rescue should familiarize themselves with these problems and anticipate them when planning for and responding to technical rescue situations (Figure 20.2 and Figure 20.3).

An animal's physiology constantly attempts to maintain the internal homeostasis (physiologic equi-

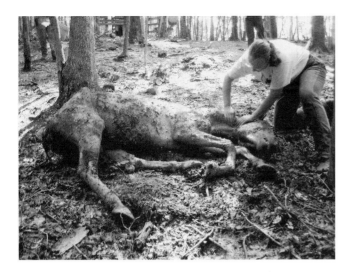

Figure 20.2 *In response to a dog chain placed around its neck, this horse struggled, asphyxiated, and fell down a hill. Responders are evaluating the animal and removing the chain. The animal did not survive. Courtesy Tomas Gimenez.*

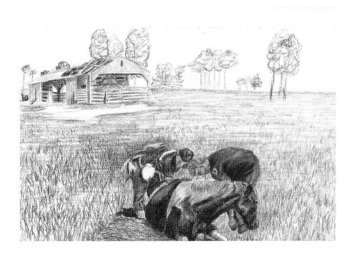

Figure 20.3 *Veterinary assistance team members deployed in response to Hurricane Katrina (2005) observed that most large animals left behind that were able to escape from structures survived. However, many had been impaled by flying debris. Others were forced to swim to escape their flooded pastures and became entangled in obstacles, trees, or fencing. These situations illustrate the wisdom of evacuating animals well ahead of impending disasters. Others, such as this animal, died of heat injuries and dehydration from lack of potable water. Courtesy of Julie Casil.*

librium) at certain optimum set points of body temperature, pH, oxygen and carbon dioxide saturation, glucose concentration, ion concentration, hydration, etc. The body addresses slight changes in either direction from optimum by changing detectable parameters such as heart rate, ion balance, and respiratory rate. The regulatory mechanisms and changes that are commonly expected in TLAER scenarios are discussed here.

Hyperthermia and Heat Injury

The term *hyperthermia* is defined as body temperature above normal. Specific normal ranges of body temperature are described in the literature for different species. An animal's temperature can be elevated for a variety of reasons, but two general categories include pyrogenic and nonpyrogenic causes. Pyrogenic hyperthermia is usually associated with infection or an inflammatory response, and nonpyrogenic hyperthermia is caused by overwhelmed or failed thermoregulatory mechanisms. Hyperthermia is sometimes used interchangeably with the terms *heat exhaustion, heatstroke,* and the more general term *heat injury.* This text will focus on nonpyrogenic hyperthermia as it applies to stressed, struggling, and exhausted animals in need of technical rescue or extrication. However, responders must assess the situation carefully for signs that an elevated temperature may be caused by infectious or inflammatory disease processes.

For example, an overturned livestock liner containing 680 market-weight hogs can be expected to be a stressful and frightful scenario as the pigs on the bottom of the pile are crushed by the weight of the animals above them or asphyxiated due to lack of oxygenated air. Other animals die of hyperthermia because they cannot adequately thermoregulate due to the crowded conditions.

An above-normal temperature is common following strenuous exercise, stress, and excitement and may not indicate a health problem. Following strenuous exercise, a horse's rectal temperature may reach 40–40.5°C (104–105° F) or higher without adverse affects. The animal's ability to recover to a normal body temperature following exercise is indicative of its health or potential health problems. For example, the body temperature of a horse that reaches 40.5°C (105° F) following exercise may not indicate a problem if the temperature is reduced within a few minutes of rest in a shaded area. However, if the temperature remains 40°C (104° F) after an hour of cooling, the animal shows little interest in drinking water, and it appears to be depressed, medical assessment is necessary.

The normal rectal temperature for a resting, adult horse ranges from 37.2–38.6°C (99–101.5° F). It is not uncommon for a horse's rectal temperature to reach 38.9°C (102° F) or higher on hot and humid days, especially if the animal is in direct sunlight or confined to a stall or trailer with poor ventilation. The rectal temperature of a horse following strenuous exercise or struggling in a hot, humid environment or confined in poorly ventilated space may easily reach 40.5–41.1°C (105–106° F); this rectal temperature may correspond to a muscle temperature of 45–46.1°C (113–115° F) or higher (Geor and McCutcheon, 1996). Core temperature, or the temperature of the innermost parts of the body, is considerably higher than the temperature at the skin or within the rectum. Hyperthermia induces a shift of blood from the viscera (organs) to the muscles and skin, resulting in hypovolemia (decreased blood volume), hypotension (decreased blood pressure), and hypoxemia (inadequate oxygen levels in the blood). High core temperatures can cause severe organ damage and blood clotting abnormalities, leading to severe illness or death. Each 1°C (1.8° F) increase in core temperature increases the body's oxygen demand by 10% (Auerbach, 2007). Temperatures in the nervous tissues, especially the brain, in excess of 41.1–42.2°C (106–108° F) can induce severe neural damage, swelling of the brain tissues, seizures, and other neurological problems.

Risk Factors for Hyperthermia and Heat Injury. Muscle tissue uses a large amount of metabolic energy, and conversion of this stored energy to the kinetic energy of muscle movement generates a large amount of heat. Compared to resting muscle, vigorous muscle movement can increase energy consumption by 40%–60%. Energy conversion from stored metabolic energy to kinetic energy of muscle movement is not efficient, with only 20%–25% of this energy going to muscle movement and the remaining 75%–80% lost as heat. Much of this heat is transferred from the muscle tissue to the bloodstream, where it must be dissipated from the body to prevent the animal from overheating (Geor and McCutcheon, 1996).

In most circumstances, normal thermoregulatory mechanisms are sufficient to dissipate excess heat, maintaining body temperature within a safe range and preventing damage to the body. When the amount of heat produced overwhelms the animal's ability to dissipate the heat, the animal is in danger of heat injury. The amount of heat produced by an animal depends on several factors. The degree of fitness and muscle mass, size of the animal, the speed or intensity of its struggle, and the duration of time over which the movement or struggle occurs all contribute to the amount of metabolic energy used and thus the amount of heat produced.

Heat Loss Methods. The ability of the animal to dissipate excess heat also depends on several factors. Heat loss from the body occurs by four main methods:

- Convection of heat occurs by transfer of heat down a temperature gradient in a gas or liquid (e.g., air or water). Heat produced by muscles is transferred to the lower-temperature bloodstream and carried to the lower-temperature body surfaces, then is transferred to the air (or water) from the skin surface. Convection accounts for a large amount of heat loss from the body under normal circumstances.
- Conduction of heat occurs by direct transfer of heat from one structure to another structure in direct

contact. An example of conduction is direct transfer of heat from muscle tissues to subcutaneous tissues and skin covering the muscle. Conduction accounts for a much smaller amount of heat loss than convection under normal circumstances, but it can play a significant role in heat loss during immersion in water.
- Evaporation of water from the skin (and as sweat) accounts for the majority of heat loss in certain species, especially horses, and in these species is the most important method of thermoregulation. In hot, dry environments, evaporation accounts for 55%–65% of heat loss from the body. In animals that do not sweat (e.g., swine), this is not an appreciable method of decreasing body temperature; however, they may evaporate temperature from their tongue by panting (pigs, ruminants). Sweating carries a large amount of heat from within the skin to the surface. As the water in the sweat evaporates, the heat is carried away from the body. Evaporation of water from the respiratory tract also significantly contributes to heat loss.
- Radiation is heat loss by emitting heat directly from the body into the environment (thermal radiation). As the animal generates heat from exercise, struggling, or other stressors, increased blood flow to the skin facilitates heat loss by convection, evaporation, and radiation.

Anything that impedes these innate cooling mechanisms can increase the risk of hyperthermia and heat injury. Hot, humid environments inhibit evaporation and convection. Prolonged exposure to direct or indirect sunlight increases radiant heat on the skin surface, impeding heat loss by conduction and further heating the body from an external heat source. Higher wind speed (including airflow generated by fans) increases convective heat loss.

Clinical Signs of Heat Exhaustion and Heatstroke. In human medicine, heat injury is generally divided into three categories of increasing severity: heat cramps, heat exhaustion, and heatstroke. In large animals, these conditions are generally broken into two categories, with muscle cramping (heat cramps) included in the category of heat exhaustion. Various texts and articles may categorize these conditions in a slightly different manner. Regardless of categorization, it is important to recognize mild to moderate or severe heat injury and to be aware of methods of prevention and treatment of these conditions.

For non-veterinary responders, the prevention and treatment are essentially the same. Understanding the severity of heat injury and the potential outcomes facilitates triage and prioritization of treatment, transport to veterinary care, and management of resources when multiple animals or other adverse conditions are involved.

Heat Exhaustion. The list of clinical signs below may occur with heat exhaustion. Animals may show varying signs, including one, a few, or all of these signs. None of these problems are specific to heat injury; each of these signs can also be observed with other conditions.

- Tachycardia (rapid heat rate)
- Tachypnea (rapid respiratory [breathing] rate)
- Increased rectal temperature (40–41.1°C [104–106° F])
- Dehydration, indicated by dry mucus membranes, prolonged capillary refill time (CRT) (more than two seconds), and poor skin turgor (tension), with rapid heart rate. Blood tests may reveal increased blood protein (7.5–9.0 gm/dl) and packed cell volume (PCV) (45–60%)
- Electrolyte abnormalities (detectable by blood tests)
- Depression
- Lack of interest in water, despite dehydration
- Lack of interest in food
- Reduced gastrointestinal motility, possible colic (abdominal pain)
- Muscle cramping or twitching, exertional rhabdomyolysis, (severe inflammation of the muscles; often called *tying up*)
- Loss of anal sphincter tone
- Prolapsed penis
- Cardiac arrhythmias (abnormal heart rhythms)
- Asynchronous diaphragmatic flutter (often called *thumps*)

Many of these signs occur due to electrolyte abnormalities, after a large amount of electrolytes are lost in sweat. Sodium, chloride, potassium, calcium, and magnesium are ions with important roles in muscle contraction, including cardiac muscle; electrolyte depletion can cause clinical signs ranging from muscle cramping to cardiac arrhythmias. Horses may lose as much as 10–15 l (2 1/2 to 4 gal) of sweat per hour while engaging in endurance-type exercise, resulting in severe electrolyte and fluid imbalances with prolonged exercise. Sweating loss of 40–50 l (10 1/2 to 13 gal) of water leaves a 500 kg (1,100 lb) horse 10% dehydrated (Carlson, 1983; Carlson, 1987). Similar fluid losses can be applied to the entrapped, struggling animal, or animals fleeing capture.

Heatstroke. In addition to the signs of heat exhaustion, animals with heatstroke may also exhibit several or all of the following clinical signs.

- Severe tachycardia (increased heart rate). The heart rate may decrease or become undetectable as the animal nears death.

- Severe tachypnea (rapid breathing). As the animal nears death, agonal breaths (irregular, gasping breaths) may be observed.
- Increased rectal temperature (more than 41.1°C [106° F]).
- Severe depression, collapse, coma, unconsciousness.
- Neurological signs, such as stumbling, collapse, convulsions.
- Severe dehydration, as indicated by dry mucous membranes, prolonged CRT (more than three seconds), abnormal mucous membrane color ("muddy" colored), cold extremities, PCV greater than 60%, and total protein levels in excess of 9.0 gm/dl.
- Blood clotting disorders, such as unusual bruising, bleeding from nose or mouth, or bloody diarrhea.

Clinical signs such as tachycardia, tachypnea, severe dehydration (poor skin turgor, pale or dark, dry mucus membranes, and prolonged CRT) indicate progression to shock and signal the need for immediate veterinary care regardless of the inciting cause.

Prevention and Treatment for Heat Injury

Preventive measures should begin as soon as possible on the TLAER scene. Even if the animal initially appears normal, responders should anticipate that problems may occur if the animal begins to struggle or if extrication is delayed. Animals that are recumbent from heatstroke should be triaged as *expectant* (death imminent).

Minimize Stress. Responders should remain calm and take measures to keep the animal calm to avoid inducing additional stress; such measures may include backing away from the animal and leaving it alone for a period of time, depending on the circumstances and temperament of the animal. The handling and movement of humans and other animals should be minimized. In some cases, the presence of another animal (usually an animal familiar to the animal victim) may help keep the entrapped animal calm. This is especially true for mares with foals or maternal–offspring pairs of other species, but responders should keep in mind that this can also aggravate the situation; the decision to use this method should be made on a case-by-case basis. The animal handler should simulate grooming behavior and use a calm voice.

Active Cooling Methods. Shade should be provided as soon as possible, using tarps, blankets, or other materials in a manner that does not further frighten or stress the animal. If the situation allows, misting, spraying, or sponging the animal with water will often cool it through convection of heat off the skin surface to the water, followed by evaporation. If possible, water should be sprayed or sponged on the body and immediately removed with a sweat scraper or other flat object; water that remains in contact with the body surface quickly absorbs heat and will no longer cool the animal. A small amount of isopropyl (rubbing) alcohol can be diluted in the water and sponged on the animal to speed evaporation. One pint of isopropyl alcohol in a 40 l (10 1/2 gal) bucket of cold water results in a dilution that does not irritate normal skin. The eyes, mucous membranes, and skin wounds (if present) should be protected, and the solution should be sponged on the animal liberally across its neck, back, abdomen, and chest.

If the animal is trapped in a collapsed barn or overturned trailer, doors and windows can be opened only if responders can be sure that the animal will not attempt to escape through the openings. Alternatively, fans can be placed to increase ventilation and facilitate skin cooling (convection). When large loads of animals (e.g., pig or cattle liner overturn, etc.) are affected, and individual animals cannot be treated, providing active cooling methods (e.g., hosing, shade, ventilation) will reduce losses and make entrapped animals more comfortable.

A trained individual should consider placing an IV catheter and administering fluids to lower the animal's body temperature and, more importantly, combat dehydration and shock. The types of fluids administered are often limited to what the veterinarian or other responder has in stock; any crystalloid fluid can be administered, but a 0.9% sodium chloride solution supplemented with potassium chloride is recommended. Hypertonic saline may also be administered, but must be followed by isotonic fluids.

If the situation permits, water should be offered in a soft water bucket (to prevent possible breakage or injury from metal or plastic if the animal begins to struggle). Animals suffering from heat exhaustion may appear disinterested in drinking water, despite severe dehydration; this should not be misinterpreted as disinterest due to adequate hydration. An unfortunate but relatively common mistake of well-intentioned responders is to force-feed the animal water orally using a garden hose; this commonly results in aspiration of the water into the upper airway and the lungs, causing serious and often fatal complications. With the exception of very small amounts of specific medications, water or other fluids should never be forced into an animal's mouth.

Monitoring Temperature. The animal's rectal temperature should be obtained every 15–30 minutes, depending on the surrounding conditions. If responders are unable to obtain a rectal temperature and the scenario suggests the animal may overheat, it should be assumed that the animal is overheating and measures should be undertaken to cool the animal. Skin temperature is not an appropriate method for determining the actual temperature of the animal.

When the animal's temperature is slightly above normal for that species, active cooling measures should be stopped. For horses, this corresponds to a rectal temperature of 38.9–39.4°C (102–103° F). Following hyperthermia, animals can sometimes develop hypothermia, or a below-normal body temperature; this is often due to aggressive cooling efforts and impairment of the body's thermoregulatory mechanisms. The animal's temperature should be monitored closely, and active cooling measures resumed if the temperature begins to rise again.

Aftercare. When the entrapped animal is freed from the situation, its external appearance is not an adequate indicator of the animal's medical status. Minor external injuries may mislead responders into assuming the animal is healthy because it is able to walk away; however, the animal may develop disease, injury, or adverse effects hours to days after the incident. Internal injuries in these animals can be far more serious than the obvious external ones. Responders should strive to get the animal out of the predicament in an efficient manner (Figure 20.4). As mentioned in the beginning of this chapter, the combination of muscle damage, dehydration, and the administration of NSAIDs generates a potentially dangerous combination of conditions. It is recommended that owners and responders avoid administering NSAIDs until the animal is rehydrated and veterinary follow-up care is available.

Animals suffering from heat exhaustion often return to normal after sufficient cooling, appropriate treatment, and rest, but they should be monitored closely

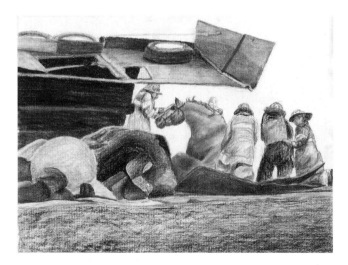

Figure 20.4 *Animals trapped in trailers and other confined spaces can be medically compromised despite the absence of obvious external injuries. Prolonged recumbency often results in skin, muscle, and nerve damage. In this case, the responders chose to cut away the trailer roof, increasing the time and effort required to rescue the animal. Courtesy of Julie Casil.*

for several days. Follow-up care by a veterinarian is important, including assessment of kidney and liver function. Animals suffering from heatstroke will likely require several days to weeks of critical care treatment by a veterinarian. Long-term complications such as permanent neurological disorders can occur, causing chronic problems after the initially successful rescue. Animals that have suffered a heat injury, especially as severe as heatstroke, are usually more prone to suffer heat injury again due to disruption of their thermoregulatory mechanisms. The severity of heatstroke and known long-term complications should be considered during triage of a large-scale incident.

Hypothermia

Hypothermia is defined as below-normal body temperature. A healthy animal can usually maintain its body temperature despite cold ambient conditions due to the thermoregulatory mechanisms and evolutionary adaptations of the species. Most large animals grow long hair coats during the colder months of the year. Shivering is a normal physiological mechanism in response to cold that helps increase the temperature of the muscles and dissipate the heat throughout the body to warm it. Blood vessels in extremities and closer to the skin constrict, preventing heat loss and diverting warm blood to the body core to maintain core and organ temperature. Heat loss still occurs by the methods described in the section on hyperthermia—convection, conduction, evaporation, and radiation—due to the large difference between body temperature and the outside environment. When heat loss exceeds the ability of the animal to produce and maintain body heat, hypothermia occurs (Figure 20.5).

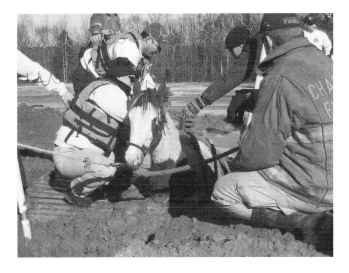

Figure 20.5 *The body temperature of a horse trapped in wet mud, even for a short demonstration period, will quickly begin to decrease. When brought out of the mud, this horse was decontaminated by the firefighters with warm water and large confined space blowers were used to dry the animal within minutes. Courtesy of Mary Gabriel.*

Risk Factors for Hypothermia. Severe damage to body tissues and functions can occur when the body temperature falls below 28.9–30.6°C (84–87° F) in most large animal species. However, a body temperature of 35.6°C (96° F), far above 30.6°C (87° F), can be an indication of a serious problem. It is important for responders to try to determine whether the hypothermia is the result of an otherwise healthy animal subjected to extreme cold conditions (such as a horse trapped in cold water or ice), or if it is an ill or injured horse that is not able to maintain its body temperature due to shock. Even in warm environments, an animal in shock may have a subnormal body temperature. Initially, treatment should be the same; warming the animal. However, treating the underlying cause of shock is important to prevent further deterioration of the animal's condition.

Another result of cold injury includes localized cold injury to specific parts of the body, such as the extremities, known as *frostbite*. Frostbite results from freezing of the body tissues. Humans are most commonly affected by frostbite on the fingers and toes; in contrast, the extremities of large animals are infrequently affected by frostbite. The ears and tails of newborns, and teats of lactating animals are most likely to be affected by frostbite. While not immediately life threatening, necrosis and infection can occur and cause systemic illness after the initial injury.

Factors contributing to cold injury of large animals include debilitating illness or injury; poor nutrition and poor body condition; age of the animal (very young and very old animals are more susceptible); entrapment in a confined space where movement (and movement-induced heat production by muscles) is limited; immersion in water, snow, or mud; or wetting of the coat from precipitation or transient submersion, followed by exposure to cold wind.

The temperature of the water is not critical; as long as the water temperature is less than the animal's body temperature, it can induce hypothermia. The body temperature of an animal or human begins to decrease toward the temperature of the water within 10 minutes after immersion. Body temperature will decrease approximately 30 times faster in water than in air of the same temperature (Auerbach, 2007). Although muscle activity and movement (e.g., struggling) in water produces heat, exercise or excessive movement in water greatly increases heat loss by conduction and convection (Auerbach, 2007). Once the body's energy stores are depleted, it does not require extremely cold water temperatures to induce hypothermia.

Clinical Signs of Hypothermia and Generalized Cold Injury. Cold injury occurs in stages and, as with heat injury, has no specific boundaries. The severity of cold injury can be staged partially on clinical signs, especially rectal temperature, as well as response to treatment. The following may be seen in animals with hypothermia:

- initial tachycardia (increased heart rate), followed by bradycardia (very slow heart rate)
- initial tachypnea (rapid respiratory rate), followed by bradypnea (very slow respiratory rate)
- low rectal temperature
- cool or cold feel to skin (in areas with minimal hair)
- lack of shivering
- pale mucus membranes, prolonged CRT (more than two seconds)
- depression, staggering, reluctance to move, collapse (especially in young or old animals)
- lack of interest in food and water
- hypoglycemia (low blood sugar; detectable by simple blood test)

Many commercial rectal thermometers do not read lowered body temperatures; the first aid kit should include a digital rectal thermometer made for reading extremely low body temperatures. Prolonged submersion in cool or cold water may cool the tissues of the anus and distal rectum by direct contact, causing a falsely low temperature reading.

Prolonged cold exposure can cause serious and irreversible damage to body tissues. Rectal temperatures below 28.9°C (84° F) cause severe tissue damage and organ failure. Coagulation (blood clotting) disorders are common following severe hypothermia in many species and can lead to excessive blood clotting, lack of blood clotting, or cardiac compromise. The heart is particularly sensitive to cold injury and prone to develop arrhythmias (abnormal heart rhythms) during the rewarming process. Sudden jerking or pulling may cause the heart to beat erratically and ineffectively with an arrhythmia such as ventricular tachycardia or ventricular fibrillation. This may easily occur as the animal is pulled or pushed, struggles, or is otherwise manipulated during a technical rescue and may explain the sudden death of some animals during or shortly after an otherwise successful extrication.

In humans and smaller animals such as dogs, resuscitation following extreme cold water submersion (for periods up to an hour or more) is sometimes successful. This is due to a physiologic reflex called the diving reflex, in which contact with the cold water (less than 5°C [41° F]) causes neurologic impulses from specific nerves in the face to travel rapidly to the central nervous system, slowing the heart rate, increasing blood pressure, and shunting blood to the brain and heart. Extremely cold water also decreases the body's metabolic requirements, reducing oxygen consumption and protecting the brain from damage. Once the human or small animal victim is rescued from the water, extensive medical emergency care and cardiopulmonary resuscitation (CPR) can occasionally revive them; an idiom in human medicine, "The patient isn't dead until they are warm and dead," refers to this phenomenon. The author was unable to find reports of this occurring in large animals or of successful revival of large animals in this manner. Realistically, the resuscitation of a large animal in this manner would require extensive and prolonged veterinary care in a critical care environment, which is impractical for most large animal emergencies and likely unavailable in a disaster or large-scale event.

NEONATAL ANIMAL EMERGENCY CONDITIONS

Very young animals will often develop hypoglycemia (low blood sugar) from increased metabolism by muscles in an attempt to maintain body temperature as well as lack of nutritional intake. Young animals have less glycogen and fat stores than adult animals, requiring more frequent feedings to maintain blood sugar levels. Separation from the dam or depression from concurrent illness or cold injury may lead to inability or unwillingness to nurse. If the dam is entrapped and the neonate is unable to access the udder to nurse, responders must address the condition of both animals.

If the neonate is unresponsive or unable to nurse on its own, it should not be force-fed milk or other fluids by syringe or other oral method. Neonates do not have a well-developed gag reflex and cannot protect their airways; incorrect administration of fluids can lead to aspiration of the fluid into the lungs and subsequent pneumonia. Intravenous fluids containing dextrose should be administered by veterinary personnel or human providers trained in animal medical response. Concentrated dextrose solutions can be caustic to tissues if accidentally administered outside the vein, and administration should not be attempted by untrained personnel. In smaller animals, such as lambs or goat kids, a small amount of dry sugar or Karo syrup placed underneath the tongue may help temporarily combat hypoglycemia as the sugar dissolves and is absorbed into the bloodstream through the mucus membranes. However, it can be aspirated if too much is applied. For weak but otherwise ambulatory neonatal animals, a 50% dextrose solution can also be used in this manner. The amount necessary for foals and calves is probably too large to be effective in this manner without causing aspiration. This method should only be used as a last resort, when a veterinary medical provider is not available. It should not be used as a substitute for veterinary assistance.

Treatment for Hypothermia

Like most emergency medical conditions in large animals, prevention of hypothermia is the best treatment. However, given the nature of technical rescue situations, it is likely that the animal will already be in a state of hypothermia when responders arrive and rescue efforts begin. Scene assessment and safety plays a major role in rescue efforts of the hypothermic animal. It is likely that the adverse conditions such as cold environmental temperature, a body of water or ice and snow, will pose a danger to human responders as well as the entrapped victim.

If possible while the animal is still entrapped, efforts should be made to keep it warm or warm the temperature of its surroundings. Using tarps or blankets to block wind, rain, or snow will decrease heat loss from the animal. The animal should be dried as much as possible and covered in blankets or field expedients. Hot packs can be applied near the neck and in the axillary region ("armpits" between the forelimbs and trunk) and groin, but the hot packs should be wrapped to prevent direct contact with the animal's skin.

If the animal is still in water, consider methods to pump warmer water into the immediate area. This may be effective in a small confined space such as a collapsed septic tank or small mud hole. Electric or kerosene heaters may be used to warm the immediate environment if they can be used safely in the situation, such as if the animal is on dry ground and away from flammable materials. If an animal is extricated but remains recumbent and unable to rise, responders should consider pulling it into a warmer area such as a barn by using a tarp, plywood sheet, or friction-reducing recumbent animal transport device such as the Rescue Glide (see Chapter 11). As mentioned elsewhere in this book, never attempt to drag or lift a large animal with a rope around the neck, as this will likely result in damage to the trachea or spinal column by choking the animal, or cause paralysis or death. Similarly, animals should not be dragged by ropes around their horns, tails, or extremities.

Straw or soft hay provides a great deal of insulation when used as bedding for hypothermic animals. It is especially good for situations where the animal cannot be moved indoors or to a warmer area. If it can be done safely, straw should be placed on the ground and the animal rolled or slid onto it so the animal is lying on the straw instead of having direct contact with the ground. Shavings can be used for this as well, but do not appear to provide the same degree of insulation as straw or hay. Blankets or tarps may also provide insulation. Thermal space blankets will help warm the animal by reflecting radiant heat back to the body and may be beneficial, especially for smaller or neonatal animals.

Dehydration can occur in hypothermic animals and must be addressed. The animal should be offered water in a soft bucket, although it will likely be disinterested in drinking. A trained individual (e.g., veterinarian or veterinary technician) should place an IV catheter (if this can be done safely) for the administration of warmed IV fluids. Fluids can be warmed by soaking IV fluid bags in hot water, placing them in a microwave for approximately one minute, or by placing them on the engine (and monitored carefully to ensure the heat of the engine does not melt the fluid bag) or dashboard heater of a running vehicle. The IV line tubing can be submerged in an insulated container of hot liquid; as the IV fluids pass through the submerged line, they are heated by the fluid before they enter the animal's vein. MRE (Meal, Ready-to-Eat) heaters work well for this purpose: the MRE heater is activated, wrapped in a towel or paper to protect the plastic IV tubing, and a section of the IV tubing is wrapped around the heater and taped in place. Additional warmed IV bags or hot water bottles can be placed around the animal's belly or trunk, first making sure to wrap the warmed materials in towels to prevent contact burns of the skin.

Rewarming a hypothermic animal is a difficult process, and as mentioned above, serious complications can arise as the animal's core temperature begins to rise. The hypothermic heart is extremely irritable and can convert to serious arrhythmias with sudden jerking movements or other stress. For this reason, vigorous massage of hypothermic humans is not recommended; although this has not been confirmed to occur in animal victims, it is similarly not recommended. Sudden death may occur during or shortly following a successful extrication. There is little that can be done for a large animal that develops cardiac arrest. Rapid changes in the animal's temperature should not be expected, but progressively warmer temperatures should be observed over a period of a few hours. Follow-up critical care with a veterinarian is essential.

IMMERSION AND SUBMERSION INJURIES (NEAR DROWNING)

Large animals frequently fall into natural bodies of water such as rivers, streams, and lakes; through ice or snow; or into mud holes and sink holes. It is not uncommon to see on the evening news a story of a bull in a swimming pool, a horse in a collapsed septic tank, a moose in an ice pond, or a similar situation. Despite the frequency with which these incidents occur, their presentations in the media are typically unscientific, anecdotal public interest entertainment rather than veterinary case reports.

Immersion and submersion injuries present separate specific problems and degrees of severity, although both can be fatal if not treated appropriately. *Immersion* is defined as being within the body of water or watery substance (e.g., mud, snow). *Submersion* (sometimes referred to as near drowning) means the animal has gone completely under the surface, or at a minimum the animal's head has gone under the surface, and its ability to breathe has been obstructed to the point where damage to the brain or other tissues has occurred from lack of oxygen. Immersion injuries may also include dermatologic conditions of the skin, hypothermia, and aspiration of water and other materials into the lungs. Submersion injuries may present the same problems associated with immersion, but they also include hypoxic (oxygen depletion) tissue damage.

There are several veterinary review articles on submersion injury and near drowning, but they are almost all derived from reports and studies of human submersion victims; treatment recommendations for animals are extrapolated from treatment of human victims. There are few reports in the veterinary literature on submersion injury in animals. One case report of a young gelding submersed in a swimming pool described the successful treatment of that animal, but was not sufficient to serve as the basis for a broad statement regarding treatment recommendations or prognosis.

Aspiration of Water and Other Materials. During immersion in water, mud, snow, or other material, the animal may be struggling, thrashing, or intermittently go underneath the surface of the liquid. It may gasp for air, and its breaths will likely be deeper and faster than usual. These conditions increase the risk of aspiration of water and other materials into the airways, causing potentially serious complications during or after the immersion event.

Aspiration during near drowning in humans can be associated with different complications, depending on the type of liquid involved in the incident. Aspirated salt water may contain bacteria, algae, sand, and other particulate matter. In addition, the osmotic effect of high salt concentration on the inside of the alveoli results in fluid movement from the pulmonary blood vessels and into the lung tissue (pulmonary edema). Freshwater from lakes, rivers, streams, and drainage canals may contain bacteria and protozoa, sand, silt, or other particulate matter. In any body of water with a dirt, silt, or sand bottom, the struggling animal will likely disturb this material, increasing the amount of debris floating in the water and the risk for aspiration of particles. A larger amount of particulate matter can be expected from aspiration in shallow water compared to deep water (Ender and Dolan, 1997). Chlorinated water, such as that found in swimming pools, should be relatively free of bacterial and other biological contaminants, but chlorine can be extremely irritating to tissues of the airway. Aspiration of mud can be much more serious due to physical obstruction of the lower airways by the viscous mud. Gastric contents may be regurgitated and aspirated during the struggle or after the animal loses consciousness, especially if it has swallowed large amounts of water into the stomach. These acidic gastric contents can induce further damage to the lung tissues.

Pneumonia and acute respiratory distress syndrome are common following aspiration, requiring intensive veterinary critical care. Research and data are minimal regarding aspiration of liquids in animals; extrapolation from human medical literature provides some information for the reader. For example, the type of liquid (mud, sewage, salt water, or freshwater) involved and microbial cultures taken from them have been categorized to help guide antimicrobial therapy (Humber, 1988). Additionally, in human drowning victims, 75%–90% aspirate materials into their lungs. Approximately 10%–30% of the drowned victims did not aspirate, but died due to asphyxiation secondary to the reflexive closure of their larynx; this is called *laryngospasm* and is a reflexive contraction of the laryngeal muscles to close the opening of the larynx to prevent the entry of liquid into the trachea and lungs (Humber, 1988; Ender and Dolan, 1997).

Immersion/Submersion Injury Treatment Considerations. The type of liquid involved in the immersion/ submersion incident has minimal effect on initial first aid unless the water is grossly contaminated (e.g., septic tank, hog manure lagoon, etc.) and gross decontamination is necessary (see Chapter 19).

The primary mechanism of injury associated with submersion is hypoxia. Oxygen depletion of the brain and other organs such as the heart, kidneys, and liver causes severe damage to these tissues. Cerebral edema, or swelling of the brain, and pulmonary edema are common following submersion injury. Seizures, coma, or other severe neurological dysfunction may occur during or shortly following rescue of the animal. Pneumonia from aspiration can worsen the tissue hypoxia and organ damage by impairing air exchange in the lungs. Kidney and liver failure can develop, further complicating treatment and worsening the prognosis. As with hypothermia, cardiac arrhythmias can occur, and the animal can die suddenly from cardiac arrest. Immediate critical care is necessary for survival of these animals; if it is not available, euthanasia should be considered.

Responders should follow the principles of ABC (airway, breathing, circulation; see Chapter 17) in the initial assessment and treatment. Airway and breathing are obviously important, but circulation (including the control of hemorrhage) may be the primary life-threatening issue if the animal was injured before or as it entered the water. It is important to remember that another injury or illness may have been the inciting cause for the immersion/submersion incident.

If a large animal is completely submerged and is unconscious at the time of rescue or shortly following rescue, it is unlikely that the animal will survive. Cardiopulmonary resuscitation is unlikely to be successful in horses and other large livestock due to their size; however, this should not deter efforts to revive the animal. Owners or bystanders may interpret the lack of resuscitation efforts as apathy, lack of concern for the animal's life, or incompetence on the part of technical rescue personnel. Smaller animals such as sheep, goats, foals, or calves may benefit from CPR (see Chapter 17).

If the animal is recumbent, its head should be positioned lower than its body to allow for fluid drainage from the airways and to decrease the risk of aspiration if the animal regurgitates or vomits. For smaller animals such as sheep and goats, responders may be able to carefully lift an animal's body above its head to allow drainage. The head should be supported and care should be taken to avoid pressure on the chest or abdomen (which may compromise the animal's respiratory ability and/or increase the risk of regurgitation).

Stimulation with minor pain or vigorous rubbing has been known to occasionally stimulate an animal to breathe. Gently twisting the ear or pinching the lip, muzzle, or eyelid may provide effective stimulation. Responders should remember to remain out of range of the limbs; seizure activity, struggling to rise, or other movement can occur without warning and cause injury.

If oxygen is available and can be safely used, it can be administered at a rate of 10–15 l/min using a mask held to the animal's nostril or tube pushed into the nostril approximately 15 cm (6 in.). For smaller animals, trained personnel should consider placing an endotracheal tube and providing positive-pressure ventilation.

If the animal is standing, it should be allowed to stand quietly, minimizing movement and other stress. If the animal is staggering, weak, or unsteady, personnel should avoid crowding the animal to provide physical support unless falling would put the animal back underneath the water (or other liquid). The animal should be allowed to lie down on dry ground if it is unstable, weak, or exhibits a willingness to lie down.

Animals surviving immersion or submersion in water require extensive veterinary care, including antibiotics, anti-inflammatory medications, IV fluid therapy, and supportive care. The administration of IV fluids following an immersion incident with aspiration or total submersion injury should be closely monitored; fluid therapy can worsen the effects of cerebral and pulmonary edema, and renal (kidney) damage may impair the animal's ability to excrete excess fluids. It is recommended that IV fluids be administered by trained veterinary personnel following a thorough evaluation of the animal's condition.

The intensive care often required to salvage submerged and immersed animals may be impractical based on economic restrictions or lack of appropriate resources. If treatment is to be pursued, and advanced veterinary resources are available, the animal should be immediately transferred to a veterinary facility capable of providing intensive care. If treatment will not be pursued, euthanasia should be performed (see Chapter 13).

Approximately 20% of human victims of immersion or submersion die from a condition known as circum-rescue collapse (sometimes called rewarming shock). Death may occur before, during, or after rescue and results from inadequate cardiac output, cardiac arrhythmia, or collapse of blood pressure (Auerbach, 2007). The frequency of this condition in large animals has not been determined, but is suspected to be similar.

Dermatologic Conditions Associated with Immersion. In 1999, heavy flooding following Hurricane Floyd trapped horses and other livestock across eastern North Carolina. Many animals were trapped in flooded barns or swept away in floodwaters. Others survived for days in deep water only to succumb to complications of aspiration pneumonia, hypothermia, and other infections in the days to weeks that followed. Perhaps the most common post-flood complication seen by veterinarians was severe dermatologic damage to the extremities and lower body from prolonged exposure to contaminated floodwater (Vivrette et al., 2001). Horses that were found in relatively clear, fast-moving water were less severely affected than those found in contaminated, stagnant water. The mildly to moderately affected horses were washed using basic decontamination techniques using a tincture of green soap (Simple Green) and were not administered antibiotics; all horses recovered well, with minimal scar formation. Horses that had been rescued from contaminated, stagnant water exhibited severe, necrotic (dying tissue) lesions of their limbs, resulting in skin sloughing and infection. Several horses developed *Pythium insidiosum* infections (pythiosis or "kunkers"), a severe and rapidly growing invasive fungal infection that necessitates surgical intervention or euthanasia. The most severely affected horse, rescued by helicopter sling load from contaminated, stagnant water to mid-chest level, exhibited severe skin sloughing, septicemia and endotoxemia, as well as a deep tendon laceration caused by barbed wire entrapment of a rear limb; the animal was humanely euthanatized. Similar immersion-related dermatologic conditions were seen in horses following Hurricane Katrina floods in Louisiana in 2005. Foot rot in cattle and thrush in horses are common following prolonged exposure of the feet to wet or damp conditions and are not limited to disasters or TLAER situations.

The conditions known as *trench foot*, *jungle rot*, or *immersion foot* are common problems of humans exposed to wet or damp conditions for prolonged periods; minimal dermatological research exists in animals, but related conditions occur. It has been frequently observed in military personnel after wearing wet boots for prolonged times and/or failing to remove their boots to allow their feet to dry and change their socks. In these conditions, the protective barrier of the epidermis is breached by water or sweat and small separations between the epidermis and dermis occur, causing blisters and sloughing of the skin. The protective skin barrier is compromised by the separation, increasing the risk of bacterial infection and cellulitis (infection and inflammation of the tissue layers underneath the skin). The nerves are damaged, and prolonged vasoconstriction (constriction of the blood vessels) occurs. The problem is generally worse in cold conditions, where constriction of cutaneous blood vessels contributes to the problem by decreasing the circulation of blood to the skin. However, it can occur in warm conditions, and is also often associated with fungal infection. Following Hurricane Floyd (1999), some horses and cattle that had been standing in contaminated water for 48–72 hours required treatment for immersion foot condition (Vivrette et al., 2001).

Treatment of Dermatologic Injuries. Thorough decontamination with mild soap and water is the most effective first aid treatment for dermatologic injury following prolonged immersion in water, mud, or severely contaminated material (such as septic tanks). Mild degreasing soaps and disinfectant soaps may be of benefit if material is difficult to remove from the skin surface and residual contamination is suspected. Hydrogen peroxide and undiluted iodine-based products should be avoided because they are caustic, damage tissues, and cause physical pain to the animal during application.

The animal should be relocated to clean, dry ground as soon as possible. If the animal is kept in a stall, wood shavings should be avoided if there are open wounds. Straw bedding is less likely to adhere to wounds, but generates dust that must be regularly removed. Topical medications (e.g., salves, ointments, or creams) should not be applied except as directed by a veterinarian.

Bandaging the limbs decreases swelling and edema, but it may maintain an excessively moist environment that adversely affects wound healing. Following initial cleansing and first aid, bandaging the limbs for transport to a veterinary hospital may protect the skin from further damage; if possible, the skin and hair should be allowed to dry before the bandages are placed. Excessive rubbing worsens the condition; minimal abrasion and pressure are recommended when the wounds are cleaned. Any areas of exposed tendon, joint, or bone should be covered with sterile bandages. Antibiotic therapy may be necessary but should be directed by a veterinarian. The administration of tetanus toxoid or tetanus antitoxin should only be performed on the direction of a veterinarian.

Complications may arise days to weeks following the initial event. Laminitis ("founder"), while not observed in the Hurricane Floyd animals studied, is a frequent complication following severe stress and/or injury and can be a life-threatening condition. Eye irritation, diarrhea from drinking contaminated water, and various other problems may occur and should be addressed by a veterinarian.

BURNS AND SMOKE INHALATION CONSIDERATIONS

Large animal burn victims present a challenge in TLAER, disaster response, and clinical veterinary medicine. Some burns are extremely painful for the victim, and many require extensive veterinary care to combat shock from fluid loss or septicemia from infection. The extent of care available for animal burn victims and projected poor quality of life issues make treatment of severely burned large animals generally impractical for financial and humane reasons. Severely burned large animal patients should be triaged as expectant (death imminent) in multiple animal or other large-scale incidents and humanely euthanatized as soon as possible.

Burns (Thermal Injury)

Burns are categorized as first, second, third, or fourth degree, with the depth of skin and tissue damage increasing with the number. The damage associated with first-degree burns (superficial burns) is limited to the outermost layers of the skin; these burns are painful, red, and swollen. Second-degree burns involve the dermis of the skin and are less painful. Third-degree burns are also called full-thickness burns, and they involve the skin and the underlying tissues. Fourth-degree burns involve loss of the skin and damage to the underlying tissues, bone, ligaments, and fat. Deeper burns induce nerve damage and are therefore less painful.

The severity of thermal injury depends on the temperature, duration of exposure, blood supply to the burned area, and wound environment. The depth of the injury correlates with morbidity (the severity of illness and damage produced by the burn), whereas the area of body surface burned correlates with mortality (death). In general, a "rule of 9" can be used to estimate the percentage of body surface affected by thermal injury: the forelimbs each represent 9% of body surface area; each hind limb represents 18%; the head and neck represent 9%; the thorax represents 18%; and the abdomen represents 18% of body surface area (Hanson, 2005).

Full-thickness burns (third and fourth degree) present the most overall threat to survival. Special scenarios in which friction burns occur, such as animals dragged behind or under trailers, are to be treated as below (Figure 20.6).

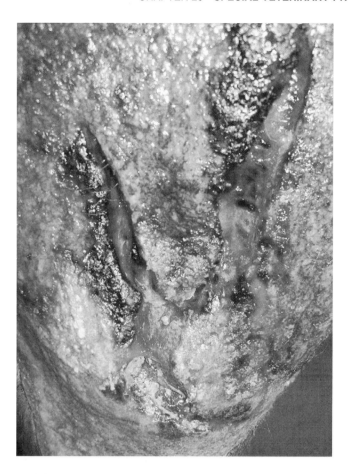

Figure 20.6 *This horse exhibits a burn injury obtained when it fell out of an unsecured horse trailer and was dragged approximately 300 m (1,000 ft) before the driver could stop. The horse is being rehabilitated and the injury is slowly healing. Courtesy of Debra Sedlmayer.*

Full-thickness burns over 10%–15% of the body; partial-thickness burns over greater than 30% of the body; burns to the face or head (especially those affecting the upper airways); severe burns exposing structures such as joints are all considered critical and carry a poor prognosis for survival. Burns covering 50% or more of the animal's body surface are usually fatal. The presence of a large laceration, bone fracture, or other large non-burn wound further complicates recovery due to the increased risk of infection and musculoskeletal complications.

Severe thermal injury produces local and systemic responses. In the local (skin) response, inflammation is the primary reaction, caused by damaged, leaking tissues and blood vessels. Tissue fluid and electrolyte shifts cause inflammation and fluid loss.

Systemic effects result from the loss of fluid, electrolytes, and protein. Hypovolemic shock, often called burn shock, is common. Pulmonary edema (swelling and fluid accumulation in the lung tissues) interferes with oxygen exchange in the lungs, resulting in tissue hypoxia (oxygen depletion) throughout the body.

Protein loss can result in additional fluid loss, delayed wound healing, and other complications associated with hypoproteinemia (inadequate levels of protein in the blood) and hypoalbuminemia (inadequate levels of albumin in the blood). Immune system depression occurs, increasing the animal's susceptibility to infection. The local and systemic responses to burns must be treated to increase the chance of survival for the animal (Geiser and Walker, 1984).

Cardiac output (a measure of the ability of the heart to circulate blood) can be dramatically reduced in response to thermal injury. Body heat is lost through the damaged skin, and the animal's metabolic rate increases. Burns involving 10% or more of the animal's body surface area increase the animal's core temperature by 1–2°C (2–4° F); this increases oxygen consumption, fat degradation, and protein and glucose utilization. If 30% or more of the body surface is burned, the animal's energy expenditures are doubled (Hanson, 2005).

When a thermal injury occurs, blistering may be observed. Damage to the blood vessels causes fluid extravasation (oozing) and swelling in the affected tissues. Tissue injury continues for 24–48 hours after the initial thermal injury; therefore, the burn will increase in severity over that period of time. Necrosis (tissue death) of the dermis and epidermis in full-thickness burns creates a hard, leathery, charred appearance to the skin; this is called *eschar* (Pascoe, 1999). As the eschar sloughs, it creates an increase in open wounds in addition to any partial-thickness wounds incurred during the thermal injury.

Complications are frequently encountered and include infection, self-mutilation, disfigurement, loss of function, and neoplasia (cancerous tissue growth). Skin grafting may be necessary to reestablish a functional skin cover of the injured areas. Several years may be required for recovery.

Smoke Inhalation

Many animals with thermal injury of the skin have concurrent smoke inhalation injury; the presence of inhalation injury and thermal skin injury is associated with a higher risk of pulmonary edema and infection. Many animals exposed to smoke do not have apparent burns of the skin, but they are still affected by inhalation injury (Figure 20.7). Smoke inhalation includes carbon monoxide (CO) poisoning, smoke poisoning, and thermal injury. The inhalation of smoke or hot gases during a fire severely irritates the mucosal (lining) tissue of the nasal passages, pharynx, larynx, and trachea. Damage can also occur in the lower airways of the lungs. Superheated air causes direct thermal injury to the upper airway, leading to edema and possible obstruction.

Carbon monoxide poisoning can occur if the animal is trapped in a barn or confined space during the fire.

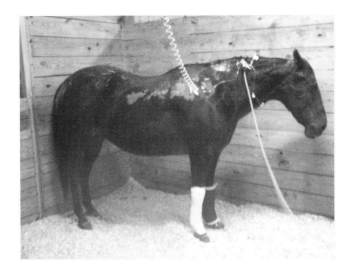

Figure 20.7 *This mare was one of two horses rescued from a barn fire. Although the skin burns do not appear severe, the mare suffered from smoke inhalation. Note the tan and clear lines providing oxygen via a tracheotomy and the coiled IV set delivering fluids and medications. This mare died from severe pneumonia and pulmonary edema due to lung injury induced by smoke inhalation. Courtesy Dr. Kimberly May.*

Carbon monoxide (CO) is an odorless, colorless, and tasteless gas with an affinity for hemoglobin that is 200 times that of oxygen (Auerbach, 2007). CO binds to the red blood cells' hemoglobin molecule in place of oxygen, reducing oxygen delivery to tissues and inducing tissue hypoxia and death.

In addition to the hot gasses emitted by the fire or initial blast, particulate matter (ash) can be forced or drawn into the airways and lungs, inducing severe inflammation and pulmonary edema and interfering with oxygen exchange in the lungs. More than 280 toxic products have been identified in burning, treated wood, including aldehydes, that can induce severe inflammation and damage when inhaled (Auerbach, 2007). Many different gasses may be produced during a fire (e.g., hydrogen cyanide, hydrochloric acid, aldehydes, phosgene, sulfuric acid, etc.), especially in a structural fire where a variety of synthetic materials burn; these gasses can cause severe inflammation of the trachea and bronchi when they mix with the water normally found in airway secretions. This will likely not change the treatment given by a first-responder, but should be kept in mind for longer-term care.

The inhalation of super-heated air can induce severe thermal injury of the upper airways, primarily the nasal passages and pharynx. Severe edema and swelling can occur, resulting in airway obstruction.

Terms frequently used to describe the lung injury observed with inhalation of smoke or gasses are *acute lung injury* (ALI) and, in a more severe form, *acute respiratory distress syndrome*. These terms signify a marked inflammatory response, decreased ability of the lungs to expand, and poor oxygen exchange from the lungs to the bloodstream. Affected animals exhibit dyspnea (difficulty breathing), coughing, or abnormal noise while breathing (stridor). Froth or foam may drip from the animal's nostrils or mouth; it may be pink or tinged with blood, mucus, ash, or other particulate material. This froth is the result of pulmonary edema.

Pseudomembranes may develop on the lining of the trachea and lower airways. These are sheets of inflammatory proteins, dead cells sloughing from the airway lining, and mucus, which forms a thick lining along airway tissues. This material can obstruct the airway and may need to be physically removed through a tracheotomy or bronchoscopy (Kemper et al., 1993). Severely affected human and small animal patients usually require hospitalization in a critical care setting and mechanical ventilation through an endotracheal tube. Mechanical ventilation is impractical in large animal patients because it requires general anesthesia, which cannot be safely maintained for extended periods of time (several days of mechanical ventilation may be necessary).

First Aid Treatment of Thermal Injuries. The immediate steps in treating burns include removing the animal from the source of the burn and stopping the burning process. Once the tissue becomes heated, the burn will continue to progress as the heat dissipates to adjacent tissues. Responders should not put themselves or others in danger when removing the animal from the source of the thermal injury (e.g., barn fire, wild fire, etc.).

Once the source of the thermal injury has been separated from the animal, responders should assess the animal's ABCs and address issues as necessary. If humidified oxygen is available, it should be administered by holding a human oxygen mask to the animal's nostril. Some animals may tolerate tubing placed within the nasal passage and secured to a halter. If the upper airway, nostrils, or face is burned, tissue swelling around the airway may obstruct breathing and an emergency tracheotomy may be necessary (see Chapter 17). If a tracheotomy is performed, the oxygen source should be held close to the tracheal opening without blocking it. The amount of oxygen that can be delivered through the tubing is very small compared with the total volume of oxygen and air the animal requires, and the administration of oxygen via the tubing provides only supplemental oxygen for the animal. The animal should be kept as calm as possible by limiting movement and minimizing the number of persons handling the animal. Bleeding should be controlled with direct pressure as with basic first aid, keeping in mind the animal's skin may be more fragile or painful due to the thermal injury.

Immediate steps should be taken to stop the burning process. Pouring water or saline over the affected area for several minutes is beneficial. Ice water is not recommended because it may induce hypothermia as heat is rapidly lost through the damaged skin. If the source of the burn is adhered to the skin, such as grease or melted objects (e.g., halters, blankets) it should not be removed, but should be cooled with water. Most horse halters and blankets are made of synthetic material; although the material is often flame resistant, it can melt and adhere to the skin. Any portions of the material adhered to the animal's skin should be left in place and cut away from the remaining material.

Pain control and restraint are critical. Administration of a NSAID such as phenylbutazone or flunixin meglumine decreases pain and inflammation. However, opioids (e.g., butorphanol tartrate, fentanyl, etc.) often provide more potent pain control. The administration of an opioid and compatible sedative/analgesic (e.g., xylazine, detomidine, medetomidine, etc.) is often necessary to provide optimal pain control and reduce anxiety and movement. Any animal patient suffering burns must be evaluated by a veterinarian if not already triaged as expectant (death imminent). Unless the ABCs are compromised, burn patients are often not treated further after initially stopping the burning process in a mass casualty situation.

Active cooling of the thermally injured area should continue for 10–15 minutes. Hypothermia occurs more easily in burned animals, especially in cold weather.

Salves, lotions, ointments, or creams should not be placed on injured areas except on the direction of a veterinarian. Most commercial salves and creams purchased at feed and tack stores are lanolin-based; they may increase heat retention (potentially worsening the injury) and can be difficult to remove from burned skin. These topical medications have minimal antibacterial properties and are likely to be contaminated from prior use.

If available, dry, sterile dressings should be placed over the burned areas. If sterile dressings are not available, disposable diapers or sanitary pads can be used for small burns. Cotton or similar materials are more likely to adhere to the injured skin or leave particulate material, and they should be avoided. For larger burns, a clean pillowcase or sheet may help prevent debris such as dust or soot from further contaminating the wound. Horse blankets and materials that have been kept outdoors in a barn, tack room, or horse trailer should be avoided because they are likely to contaminate the thermally injured area with dust or dirt.

Eye injuries, particularly corneal injuries, are commonly observed in association with thermal injury. The animal's eyes should be rinsed with saline or clean water to remove debris and to cool the sensitive tissues of the eyes. Eye injuries are often extremely painful, and many animals resent treatment of their eyes. The

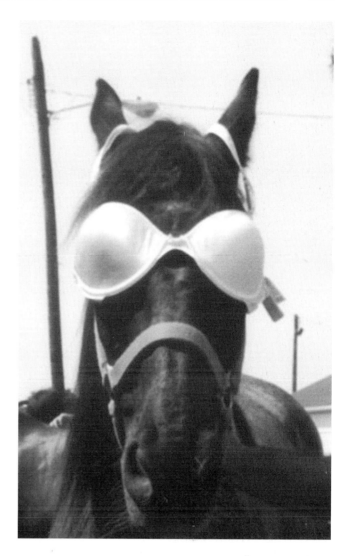

Figure 20.8 *A woman's brassiere can be used as a field expedient to protect the eyes of a horse that has sustained injury or as a blindfold for special situations. One cup may be cut out to allow the animal to see with the uninjured eye. Courtesy of Tomas Gimenez.*

importance of treatment should be weighed against the level of stress it induces in the animal; if the animal is markedly stressed by the procedure, treatment should be temporarily stopped. Triple antibiotic ointments (not containing steroids) or sterile ophthalmologic lubricant ointment may be applied if no major injury is noted to the eye. The eye should be covered; a brassiere serves as a good field-expedient eye protection (Figure 20.8). Obvious injuries should be evaluated by a veterinarian before any medications are applied.

Burn victims are at higher risk of developing tetanus. *Clostridium tetani*, the bacterial agent that causes tetanus, is present in soil. Thermal injuries compromise the skin barrier and increase the risk of invasion by pathogenic organisms. Appropriate tetanus prophylaxis should be considered.

First Aid Treatment for Smoke Inhalation. When the animal has been removed from the source of the smoke, it should be kept as calm as possible because increased stress increases the body's demand for oxygen. While acute lung injury and acute respiratory distress syndromes are common following burns and smoke inhalation, many animals will present with less-severe forms of ALI and can recover well with aggressive veterinary care.

If oxygen is available, it should be administered via an oxygen mask or nasal tube as described above. The animal's respiratory rate, respiratory effort, and breathing characteristics (e.g., noise) should be assessed. An emergency tracheotomy may be necessary for the reasons described above in the section on burns. However, a tracheotomy reduces the animal's ability to forcibly cough and clear mucus and other debris from its airway; this procedure should be performed only if the upper airway is obstructed. The animal should be allowed to lower its head; this may aid in draining particulate matter, mucus, and other material from its upper airway.

Immediate veterinary care is recommended; however, it may be best to delay transport until the animal is more stable, indicated by a decrease in respiratory rate and more relaxed respiratory effort. The stress of transportation may cause the animal's condition to deteriorate; this is especially true of livestock or horses that are not used to human handling or being trailered.

The prophylactic (preventive) administration of antibiotics to animals affected by thermal or inhalation injury is generally not performed. Several studies have shown that prophylactic antibiotic administration did not decrease the incidence of infection. In addition, the prophylactic use of antibiotics in these patients may increase the risk of infection with antibiotic-resistant bacteria (Hanson, 2005). If infection occurs, appropriate antibiotics are administered based on microbial culture results.

RECUMBENT, DOWNER ANIMALS

The majority of veterinarians and horse and livestock handlers have experienced the challenges presented by the animal that is recumbent (down) and cannot rise on its own. In TLAER scenarios this is a common problem and may be a primary or secondary event to the incident (Figure 20.9). Many conditions can result in weakness, ataxia (incoordination) and recumbency, including calving paralysis and metabolic disorders in cattle; equine protozoal myeloencephalitis, West Nile virus infection, equine herpes virus infection, and many other neurological problems in horses; fractured limbs, neck, or back; and severe malnutrition. Regardless of the initial cause, animals that are recumbent and

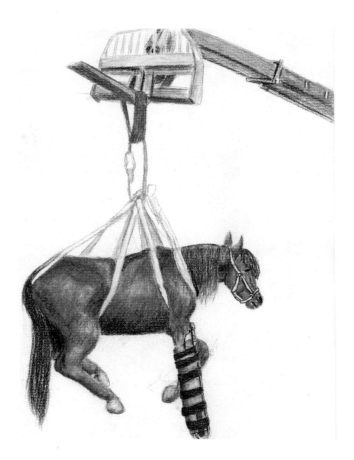

Figure 20.9 *A recumbent horse (secondary to falling into a ravine and exhausting itself) is supported in a modified figure eight sling and safely lifted to solid ground. Although this type of sling is considered to be old technology, it will work. The possible fracture is stabilized by a Kimzey splint placed over a modified Robert Jones bandage. Courtesy of Julie Casil.*

unable to rise present a challenge to responders and veterinarians.

The purpose of this section is to introduce the physiologic processes and problems that are associated with prolonged recumbency and struggling and initial first aid measures that should be implemented. In TLAER scenarios, recumbency may be commonly due to inability to maintain footing on a slick surface, entanglement or entrapment in or by an obstacle, cast against an object, or exhaustion. The underlying cause of the animal's recumbency must be addressed and treated, if possible. Unfortunately, many clinical problems resulting in recumbency cannot be quickly resolved on a single farm call, and treatment and recovery may be laborious processes. There are numerous methods for assisting the recumbent animal to rise (see Chapter 16).

Common Medical Problems Associated with Recumbency

Beyond assessment of the ABCs and stabilization of fractures or unstable soft tissue limb injuries, hypothermia and hyperthermia are immediate problems that

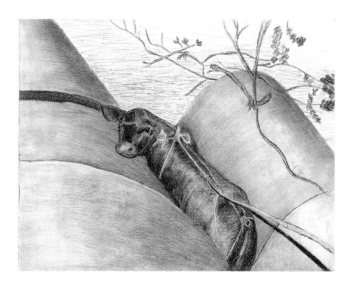

Figure 20.10 *This calf became entrapped between two large culverts in Mississippi in the middle of the night. The only equipment available to the two responders were a length of rope and a tractor with a boom. Using a modified Figure eight sling, the 175 kg (385 lb) calf was safely and efficiently rescued. The veterinarian was concerned about the crushing injuries to the animal's body and limbs, but the animal survived with treatment. Courtesy of Julie Casil.*

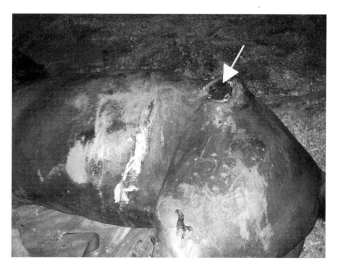

Figure 20.11 *This quarter horse gelding was recumbent due to equine protozoal myeloencephalitis, a parasite that can affect the brain and spinal cord. The animal was recumbent, with periodic support using a poorly improvised sling, for over three weeks prior to transport to a veterinary facility. Note the severe decubital ulcers (including the exposure and infection of the tuber coxae of the pelvis, as indicated by the white arrow) and the deep skin wound overlying the abdomen (packed with gauze), caused by pressure and poor placement of the sling. The gelding was euthanatized. Courtesy of Dr. Kimberly May.*

must be addressed. Animals recumbent and struggling in direct sunlight or hot, humid environments are especially susceptible. The animal should be kept cool using measures previously described, and its body temperature should be closely monitored.

Muscle movement generates body heat. Animals that have been recumbent for prolonged periods are often not able to produce muscle movement to generate sufficient heat. Shivering may be observed, but as the heat loss from the body surpasses the heat production, the animal becomes hypothermic and shivering may cease. This is especially true for young animals or very old, debilitated, or malnourished animals with reduced body fat or energy stores to combat the continued metabolic demand of keeping warm.

Prolonged struggling causes muscle breakdown and physical abrasions or other wounds to the skin. Muscle cell damage releases myoglobin into the tissues and bloodstream; this protein travels via the bloodstream to the kidneys, where it obstructs the filtration system of the kidneys and causes renal (kidney) damage. In combination with dehydration and the administration of certain NSAIDs, myoglobin can induce renal failure.

After long-term recumbency or entrapment between obstacles (Figure 20.10) or underneath a structure (as in a barn collapse), constant pressure on the skin decreases skin circulation and applies shear forces that produce abrasions or tearing of the skin (Figure 20.11). Scalding from urine or feces irritates the skin and worsens skin damage. These lesions are known as decu-

bitus ulcers (or bedsores when they are observed in human patients) and can present significant challenges to successful treatment.

The large size and weight of large animals such as horses and cattle present several challenges. First, it is often difficult to move or manipulate the animals to provide good nursing care and keep them clean. Second, their body weight facilitates skin breakdown by pressure necrosis.

The dependent, or down-side, lung of a recumbent large animal becomes partially collapsed as a result of incomplete chest expansion. This decreases the amount of oxygen delivered to the body tissues and causes consolidation of the dependent lung as fluids, mucus, and other materials collect within the alveoli and air passages.

The weight of the body on pressure points (bony prominences) of the trunk, head, and limbs can cause decreased circulation and pressure damage to muscles (pressure myopathy) and nerves (pressure neuropathy). Muscles and nerves bearing the weight of the body are, in effect, crushed between the weight of the body and the bone or nonexpandable structure (fascia) surrounding the muscles. The muscle tissue swells with fluid as the animal's weight inhibits lymphatic flow and blood circulation to and from the area, worsening damage to the muscle and nerves (Van Metre and Callan, 2003). The treatment of crushing and compartment injury is beyond the scope of this chapter; those interested in these subjects are encouraged to consult veterinary texts.

First Aid Treatment of Recumbent Animals. After assessing the scene for safety issues, responders should assess the animal for life-threatening injuries, using the principles of ABC. Airway obstruction, weakness due to blood loss, or other life-threatening issues must be addressed before a more thorough assessment is performed.

The animal's hydration status should be evaluated, and a trained individual should place an IV catheter and administer fluids appropriate for the animal's condition. If the animal is conscious and alert but unable to rise, it may be offered water in a soft rubber bucket and small amounts of food on the ground. Analgesic (pain relieving) and anti-inflammatory medications may be administered when the animal is sufficiently hydrated.

Although initial treatment in the field should not focus on assisting the animal to a standing position, this should be addressed as soon as the animal's medical condition permits. Rescuers should not attempt to keep the animal standing if it obviously intends to lie down or cannot support itself in a standing position. There is little benefit to keeping a horse with colic (horse exhibiting abdominal pain) or neurological problems standing other than trying to move it to a safer place to lie down. Once the animal is down, it should be allowed to maintain that position unless there is significant risk to the animal or responders.

Following assessment of the ABCs, the limbs should be evaluated for obvious deformities indicating the presence of fractures. If fractures are suspected or confirmed and treatment is to be pursued, the limb(s) should be bandaged and splinted as described in Chapter 17; euthanasia may be necessary for certain fractures that have poor prognoses.

Neurological problems that cause recumbency cannot usually be diagnosed in the field. With the exception of spinal cord or cranial (head) injuries, field diagnosis is not necessary. Rabies should always be considered a differential diagnosis for neurological disease despite the animal's rabies vaccination status (see Chapter 3).

If possible, the animal should be maintained in a sternal position (lying on its sternum and stomach) to allow expansion of both sides of the chest (and both lungs) during respiration (breathing). This is particularly of concern in ruminants (e.g., cattle, goats, llamas, etc.) to prevent a condition called bloat. If necessary, straw or hay bales can be used to support the animal in sternal recumbency. Soft bedding (e.g., straw) should be provided. When prolonged lateral recumbency (greater than one to two hours) is anticipated, the animal's position should be changed hourly (i.e., rolled so that the opposite side becomes the dependent, or down, side). Veterinary care should be sought as soon as possible. Due to varying medical reasons, large animals become recumbent and unable to rise, and veterinary assistance and consultation in their technical rescue is extremely important.

ACRONYMS USED IN CHAPTER 20

ABC	Airway, breathing, circulation
ALI	Acute lung injury
CO	Carbon monoxide
CPR	Cardiopulmonary resuscitation
CRT	Capillary refill time
IC	Incident commander
IV	Intravenous
MASCAL	Mass casualty
MRE	Meal, Ready-to-Eat
NSAID	nonsteroidal anti-inflammatory drug
PCV	Packed cell volume
TLAER	Technical large animal emergency rescue

21 Livestock Transport Emergency Response

Jennifer Woods

INTRODUCTION

Commercial livestock liners are consistently present on roadways, transporting animals to farms, auctions, stockyards, or slaughterhouses as part of the human food chain. Considering the large number of animals they may contain, these trailers represent a significant concern when they are involved in incidents. Commercial horse transporters and large farms may also use semi-tractor trailer configurations to haul animals. The approaches and considerations associated with incidents involving these vehicles are discussed in this chapter.

COMMERCIAL LIVESTOCK CARRIER WRECKS

In Alberta, Canada, wrecks of commercial livestock carriers, liners, or pot-belly trailers (also called possumbelly trailer) are common scenarios and are encountered by professional emergency responders in both small communities and metropolitan areas more than 20 times per year (Woods, 2006). A search of published incidents in online newspapers in North America over a four-year period yielded an average of 100 incidents reported annually (Woods, 2006). Similarly, 12 and 18 incidents were reported annually in the United Kingdom and Australia, respectively. Consulting emergency responders speculate those numbers represent less than 25% of the total annual number of incidents involving these vehicles (Gimenez and Gimenez, 2006b).

Hundreds of thousands of commercial large animals are transported inter- and intrastate each day in the United States and other countries. Due to the large number of animals present and special considerations associated with these vehicles, in this book livestock trailer incidents are treated separately from the issues of smaller trailer wrecks (see Chapter 9). This chapter will not attempt to exhaustively delineate each and every type of trailer construction, design, or accident scenario; rather, it is intended as a guideline to allow first responders to make informed decisions at incident scenes involving commercial livestock trailers.

OVERTURNED HORSE LINER CASE REPORT

On September 15, 2004, a local equine practitioner was asked by a client to respond to an overturned horse liner in Lawrenceburg, Indiana. The sheriff's department was contacted for assistance. Dr. John Nenni and a technician arrived on the scene approximately 20 minutes after the accident. A 16.15 m (53 ft) pot-bellied stock trailer carrying 52 horses was overturned down a steep embankment (an approximately 50-degree slope) and had pulled down electrical lines. The roof of the overturned trailer had been peeled back during the wreck, allowing over a dozen horses to escape. Bystanders had diverted the animals and several fatally injured horses into a corral. A nearby power company truck responded immediately to turn off the power to the electrical lines.

The veterinarian began triaging the animals confined in the corral. Nine animals were dead, and many more required euthanasia. The veterinarian's mobile unit was stocked with a supply of euthanasia solution sufficient to euthanatize six horses. A bystander lent the veterinarian a pistol to use to euthanatize the horses. One horse was euthanatized before the incident commander (IC) was able to discuss the situation with the veterinarian. The rescue effort became focused on the 18 horses that remained trapped in the lower deck of the trailer, standing on top of each other. Traffic was diverted to a side road for increased safety (Figure 21.1).

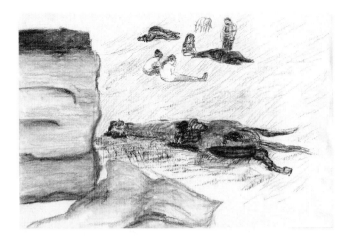

Figure 21.1 *In a 2004 incident, a livestock trailer containing 52 horses overturned and ejected numerous animals. It is abnormal for these prey animals to remain recumbent when approached unless they are fatally injured. Bystanders were visibly upset when a responding veterinarian performed emergency triage and was forced to euthanatize many of the animals on the scene. Courtesy of Julie Casil.*

The trailer was overturned on its right side at a steep angle, and the horses were crowded and standing on top of others. The local fire department cut apart a ramp at the neck of the trailer, and one horse had to be euthanatized before two others could be removed. At this point it was determined that it was too dangerous to allow the horses to walk across the trailer walls: the animal's hooves fell through the ventilation holes and the aluminum surface was too slick to provide traction for the scrambling horses.

The decision was made to sedate every horse on the lower deck of the trailer. In order to perform this task, the veterinarian was required to enter the confined space of the trailer, walking over recumbent horses to give them each a dose of a short-term anesthetic. The fire department provided protective equipment (e.g., jacket, gloves, and a helmet) for the veterinarian. Because further extrication of the animals proved difficult, the decision was made to upright the trailer. Wreckers were used to carefully winch the trailer upright while the veterinarian triaged the previously loose animals contained in the corral.

Wounds in the surviving horses varied from minor scratches and abrasions to broken limbs and a penetrating chest wound. Twelve horses were euthanatized after examination; because these animals were not inside the trailer, they were euthanatized using a pistol, and the euthanasia solution was reserved for euthanatizing injured animals still in the trailer.

After the trailer was righted, the veterinarian and veterinary technician volunteered to enter it and triage, catch, halter, and lead out the live horses that were able to walk out of the trailer. The cut surfaces of the trailer were extremely sharp, inducing additional injuries.

Dead animals were removed with a tractor, chains, and manual power.

Of the 52 animals, 21 were dead on the scene or were euthanatized. The remaining animals were loaded on trailers and continued their journey to Kentucky. The Kentucky State Veterinarian's office ensured that all of the animals were examined by a veterinarian upon arrival at their destination.

In a retrospective analysis of the incident, the veterinarian reported that he was considered by the emergency responders to be the "expert" on the scene, despite his recent graduation from veterinary school and his lack of experience with heavy rescue or livestock trailer extrication techniques. A safety officer was not designated, and all emergency services personnel assumed the veterinarian knew what to do. As has been recommended several times throughout this text, personnel should avoid entering confined spaces with the animals; there is significant risk of injury or death associated with this action. The veterinarian noted that having experienced horse handlers equipped with halters and lead ropes (none of the horses in the trailer were haltered) was crucial to handling the animals.

Since the incident, the veterinarian involved has attended technical large animal emergency rescue (TLAER) training, purchased protective gear, a pistol and 50 rounds of ammunition, rope for emergency halters, and additional first aid medical supplies. He communicated with his local emergency responders to make sure his contact information was updated in the regional 911 call center and has written educational articles to allow others to learn from his experience (Nenni, 2005b).

COMMERCIAL TRANSPORT

Livestock are transported in large aluminum trailers pulled by a semi-tractor unit (also known as live-haul trailers, cattle haulers, liners, and bullracks). The average size of a liner combination is 13.72–16.15 m (45–53 ft) in length, 2.59 m (102 in.) outside width, 2.51 m (99 in.) animal compartment width, and 4.11 m (13.5 ft) maximum height.

Loading

Commercial liners are loaded in accordance with animal transport standards, and special consideration is given to the distribution of weight; however, they carry large numbers of animals, which may be housed on two or three deck levels to increase the available floor space. To access the different levels, there are ramps and cut gates or dividers so that the load can be prevented from shifting as much as possible. Animals are manually driven into the different compartments of the trailer, and cut gates are closed to partition the load.

Load Size

Load size is normally determined by the following factors:

- Animal size
- Species
- Age of animals
- Size and design of trailers
- Weather conditions
- Condition of animals

Normal load sizes to be expected on incident scenes for each type of large animal include:

- Cattle (40–130 head)
- Swine (90–1,400 head)
- Sheep/goats (200–500 head)
- Poultry (1,700–30,000 head)
- Meat horses (25–50 head)
- Show horses (8–14 head)

SPECIAL CONSIDERATIONS ON THE SCENE

A loaded commercial livestock trailer involved in a motor vehicle accident or overturn is one of the most challenging and dangerous incidents for responders. The motor vehicle accident necessitates the implementation of safety procedures and proper scene management (see Chapter 5). The concurrent livestock incident often requires special equipment and personnel to be brought to the scene (e.g., secondary containment, cutting equipment, veterinarian, animal handlers). Handling skills by the on-scene personnel are crucial to preventing injuries when working with large animals. According to Jennifer Woods (2005), "overconfidence is the number one cause of injury to handlers."

What Is in the Trailer?

Few first responders have experience in handling commercial livestock. The extremely stressed animals present challenges to the most experienced handlers and can present significant risk to those with less or minimal experience. Millions of livestock (e.g., cattle, pigs) and poultry (e.g., chickens, turkeys) are transported in these vehicles every year. Less common, but more hazardous, are liners carrying zoo species, exotic circus or carnival animals (e.g., elephants, zebras, camels, etc.). Equids (e.g., horses, mules, donkeys) and specialty livestock (e.g., bison, elk) are less commonly transported in these vehicles.

From 1989–2006, over 2 million horses were slaughtered at U.S. Department of Agriculture-approved (USDA-approved) horse slaughter plants in the United States. Horse meat is a high-quality component of diets for carnivorous zoo animals and is exported to European countries for human consumption. U.S. horses have also been sent to slaughter in Mexico and Canada.

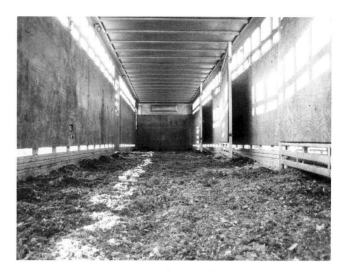

Figure 21.2 *An appropriate stock trailer for large numbers of horses should have sufficient head room, a single deck, and cut gate dividers to separate groups of animals and stallions. Animals of any species should be loaded to prevent injury to each other in transport, such as separating males and nursing mothers or horned animals from others. Courtesy of Tomas Gimenez.*

Horses destined for slaughter are generally sold at auctions and transported in straight-load trailers (Figure 21.2) to the only approved equine slaughter facilities in the United States.

Until June 2007, three U.S. facilities slaughtered horses; two plants located in Texas were closed in May 2007. The remaining facility, located in DeKalb, Illinois, was closed in June 2007 due to a state law prohibiting equine slaughter, but it was granted an injunction (and was allowed to reopen) pending appeal to a higher court. Proposed federal legislation (HR 503/ S 311) was introduced in the 110th Congress to prohibit shipping, transporting, moving, delivering, receiving, possessing, purchasing, selling, or donation of horses and other equids to be slaughtered for human consumption.

To ensure equids destined for slaughter are handled and transported in a humane manner, and in response to action taken by various humane organizations, the U.S. Congress included in the 1996 Farm Bill authority for the secretary of agriculture to issue guidelines to regulate the commercial transportation of equids to slaughter within the United States.

The purpose of the regulations was to establish minimum standards to ensure the humane movement of equids to slaughtering facilities via commercial transportation. They require the owner/shipper of the equids to take certain actions in loading and transporting them and require that the owner/shipper certify that the commercial transportation meets certain requirements. In addition, the regulations prohibit the commercial transportation to slaughtering facilities of equids considered to be unfit for travel, the use of electric prods on equines in commercial transportation to slaughter, and, as of February 5, 2007, the use of double-deck trailers for commercial transportation of U.S. equids to slaughtering facilities. This regulation applies only to equids shipped for slaughter and does not apply to the shipment of non-slaughter-bound horses in the United States (*Federal Register*, 2001).

Specialized Response

Livestock liner accidents commonly require lengthy on-scene response (4–12 hours) because the rescue of the live animals tends to become complicated, requiring specialized equipment and personnel. Triage and field euthanasia of mortally injured animals is required on most scenes. The carcasses of dead and euthanatized animals must be removed from the scene for proper disposal. Factors that increase the time and effort involved as well as the risk of injury include lack of preparedness and training, lack of access to resources, poor communication with animal-related resources in the local area, and the presence of too many people or media on the scene.

Trailer Design

Understanding the design of the inside of the animal compartment of the trailer is crucial to an effective response; without this knowledge, it can be difficult to effectively and efficiently cut access and egress openings. A liner trailer is manufactured as a series of compartments with decks, dividers, and gates that often become entangled with animal extremities when the trailer overturns. Animals will be pushed together in a maze of panels, gates, and ramp obstacles to create multiple confined spaces. Manure, urine, and blood from the animals make the surfaces slick and may represent minor biohazards to rescuers (Figure 21.3).

Communication Challenge

Noise from injured or excited animals or labored breathing of a large number of stressed animals hinders communication inside the trailer. Further complicating rescue efforts, the majority of liner wrecks and accidents occur in dark or during poor road conditions (e.g., ice, rain, snow). Commercial haulers often transport at night to avoid the environmental conditions of heat and sunlight that further stress animals, meet processing plant schedules, and to avoid delays in traffic on the roadways.

Valuable Load

Based on the ambient environmental conditions, measures to prevent heat exhaustion or hypothermia and frostbite may be necessary. Spraying the livestock with cool water on hot days or protecting them from the wind, freezing rain, and winter elements on cold days can prevent further losses. The large animals involved in these incidents can represent a significant financial

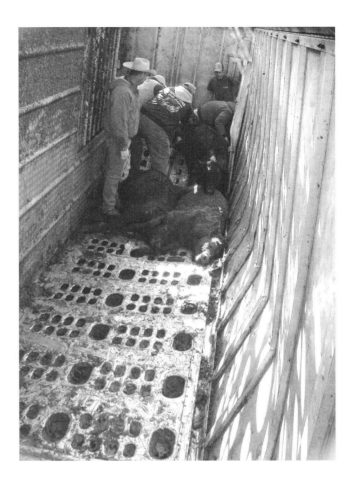

Figure 21.3 *A veterinarian assesses cattle on the bottom deck crushed by the weight of other animals when this trailer rolled on its side. It is important for responders to verify that animals that are fatally injured, crushed, or euthanatized are dead. Courtesy of Nathan Slovis.*

investment. Even if the animals are going to slaughter, losses and injury of live animals should be minimized. In one overturned trailer transporting bison in Montana, the load was valued at over $90,000. In another, a load of horses being shipped to quarantine in Kentucky was insured for over $250,000.

Quarantine Shipments

Animals slated for international shipment or delivery to quarantine facilities following international transport are subject to special regulatory restrictions intended to prevent the spread of animal disease. The state or provincial veterinarian and the appropriate federal agency (e.g., Canadian Food Inspection Agency; Department for Environment, Food and Rural Affairs; or USDA) should be notified as soon as possible of any incidents involving shipments of quarantined animals.

Specialty Event Horse Commercial Transport

The shipment of valuable show, race, and breedstock horses is a healthy industry in most countries around the globe and is completed via surface and air transportation. The air shipment of horses is not within the scope of this book. Most professional event horse commercial haulers use straight deck, solid-walled trailers that may feature air conditioning for their equine cargo. The value and insurance status of these animals are special considerations when responding to incidents involving these vehicles.

Many of these haulers will have one or several humans in the trailer to supervise the animals in transit or traveling as passengers to work at the next event. This may include a veterinarian, trainer, farrier, groom, rider, and stable hands. Regardless of the type of animal transport involved, responders should always check first for human victims when performing the assessment.

The inside of these trailers have rearrangable dividers, gates, and hide-away ramps to load and separate the animals. The animals are loaded through doors on the sides of the trailer and rarely from the back. Animals may be in separate stanchions tied in place with chains with snaps attached to both sides of the halter, or they may be loose in a small box stall compartment within the trailer. Often there will be hay nets and water buckets available for each animal. In an overturn, all of these pieces of equipment and dividers can become obstacles to accessing the animals and can contribute to injuries of the animals and responders (Figure 21.4).

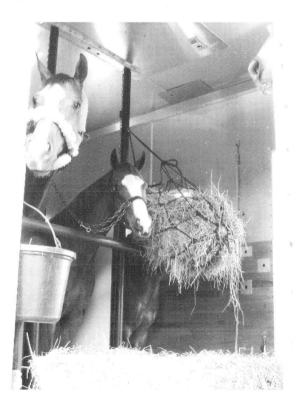

Figure 21.4 *Valuable racehorses and show horses are commonly transported nationwide and internationally via liners and airplanes. The interior of this trailer will become a confined space with obstacles if overturned. Courtesy of Rebecca Gimenez.*

OVERTURNED COMMERCIAL HORSE SHIPPER CASE REPORT

In February 2004, a commercial shipper transporting to quarantine 14 horses in a straight-deck, 16.15 m semi-trailer overturned the rig at 4 a.m. on a two-lane road in rural Lexington, Kentucky. These insured animals were recently imported from England. The nose of the trailer impacted a large tree at overturn, causing fatal injuries to two of the horses.

When local TLAER-trained responders and veterinarians arrived at the scene and started to divert traffic, a bystander was climbing into the trailer through the door on top to check on the horses. This person was removed while responders performed an assessment and stabilized the trailer, which was overturned on its right side and leaning against several large tree trunks (Figure 21.5). The state veterinarian was contacted in response to the quarantine seal, and alfalfa hay was thrown to the animals to keep them calm while responders developed a removal plan.

Because the trailer was approximately 1 m (3 ft) off the ground, responders were concerned that the legs of the animals would fall through the side walls. Also, access through the roof would have required the animals to jump down out of the trailer. Instead, access was made with a circular saw through the back of the trailer, the only part of the trailer with a clear path away from the incident (Figure 21.6).

As the entry opening was cut, another team of veterinarians and emergency services personnel established a fenced quarantine and triage station for the animals across the road in the riding arena of a local horse farm, using panels donated by local owners.

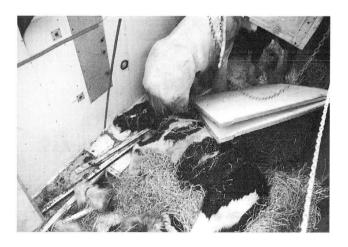

Figure 21.5 *After stabilizing the trailer, an assessment of the animals is required to determine progress of the rescue. This is the view from the top of an overturned equine transport en route to quarantine in Kentucky. Notice the large number of obstacles in the form of gates and dividers. One horse's legs are through the side of the trailer. Courtesy of Gary McFarland.*

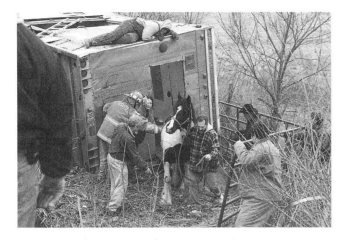

Figure 21.6 *After an assessment of the animals in the overturned trailer and removal of obstacles as possible through the top, responders are cutting the back of the trailer to allow the horses that are standing to walk out of the trailer and into the contained area. The firefighter on top of the trailer is communicating the reaction of the animals to the sound of cutting tools. Courtesy of Gary McFarland.*

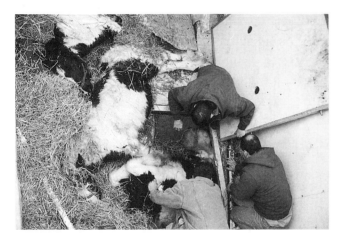

Figure 21.7 *Overturned liners and trailers can be expected to present numerous obstacles (e.g., dividers, water buckets, hay racks, horse clothing, sheared metal, etc.) for the animals and rescuers. This animal was sedated and remained in the trailer as the mobile animals were unloaded. The veterinarian can now thoroughly and safely assess the animal. Courtesy of Gary McFarland.*

Alternate transportation assets for the animals were dispatched to the scene by fire and rescue personnel.

A veterinarian entered the trailer and sedated some of the animals so that obstacles (e.g., dividers, gates) could be removed by personnel before attempting to release the horses. Animal handlers then entered the trailer and individually caught, haltered, and led the horses out of the back of the trailer, starting with the animals nearest the back and working slowly toward the front of the trailer (Figure 21.7). The two fatally wounded animals were euthanatized and slid out of the bottom of the trailer by cutting the hinges on the downside door and using it as a ramp.

Analysis of this incident highlighted the excellent relationship between the fire and rescue personnel and local veterinarians, who had met each other at a TLAER training event less than two months before. The IC commented that he could not have imagined a better-organized response or teamwork atmosphere to the incident (Slovis, 2004).

PREPAREDNESS

A plan is the first requirement of emergency preparedness for a commercial livestock trailer overturn, followed by access to available trained responders. A well-coordinated rescue effort minimizes costs for the transport owner, livestock producers, and livestock businesses. Planning and training for this specialty rescue niche allows the following:

- Fewer animals will need to be euthanatized.
- Traffic flow may be more quickly restored.
- Structural integrity of the trailer may be salvageable when it is cut properly.
- Duplication of effort and overlapping response services will be at a minimum.

Producer Involvement

The foundation of basic emergency response is the activation of local resources; this is a crucial part of response to incidents involving livestock. The tendency of first responders on liner wreck scenes is to rely on local livestock producers for assistance. Producers know how to handle livestock on their farms, but they will rarely have experience with large numbers of stressed and injured animals. In addition, they lack training in heavy rescue and specialty extrication techniques.

Animal Industry Resources

Assets that may be provided by local producers include

- facilities to hold animals,
- portable panels and penning materials,
- portable lighting,
- smaller trailers that can be maneuvered into tight spaces on roadsides,
- loading ramps,
- heavy equipment to clear the scene, and
- livestock or poultry handling specialists.

The local animal-owning community and first responders should communicate and establish a list of such resources for quick reference when an incident occurs. As stated previously, the presence of a veterinarian on the scene to triage the animals is recommended; effort should be made to identify local veterinarians who are willing and able to provide assistance. Personnel with special herding or handling skills for exotic

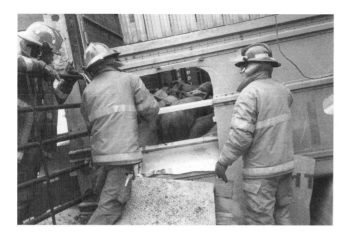

Figure 21.8 *Firefighters in Alberta, Canada, cut through the back of an overturned commercial pig liner to allow the live animals to escape into cattle panels set up as containment. The animals were then loaded onto an alternate transport. Courtesy of Jennifer Woods.*

and aggressive animals, producers or livestock professionals with experience handling various species, and brand inspectors can provide assistance. If a reciprocating saw or a circular saw with a metal-cutting, adjustable blade is not part of the local fire department's standard equipment, the resource list should include local assets who can supply the proper cutting tools (Figure 21.8).

Getting Local Emergency Planners Involved

Interested personnel and volunteers should approach their local law enforcement and fire departments to ask for a copy of its livestock emergency response plan; this plan may be a component of the county animal response team animal response plan. If there is not a plan available within the local emergency response agencies, they should be made aware of the specialty equipment, training, and services required for a response of this scope. A training session for first responders, law enforcement, veterinarians, and local commercial livestock producers can be organized. A regional approach is recommended because livestock emergency incidents often require a regional response. Model program examples include the funding of livestock emergency response courses by Canada's Alberta Farm Animal Care (AFAC) and the Saskatchewan Emergency Planners Association.

A Model for Preparedness. Alberta, Canada, has provided excellent leadership internationally in the area of livestock emergency preparedness and response. In 2005, AFAC, Hartford Insurance, and Canadian Farm Insurance established the Livestock Emergency Response (LER) hotline (1-866-684-3028). The province was divided into 12 regions, and each region was assigned a team leader trained in proper response techniques to coordinate a local response. Livestock haulers,

dispatchers from the 911 system, and producers have used the hotline, which dispatches trained personnel or assists callers with locating resources needed to respond to the incidents. Although Alberta is the only province in Canada currently regionalized with this plan, the hotline works throughout North America and can assist with livestock accident rescue advice and locating resources anywhere throughout Canada and the United States. The hotline staff are trained in TLAER procedures as well and have assisted with horse and small stock trailer accidents and barn fires.

Specialty Training

In 1997, the author developed a livestock emergency training program that specifically addresses traffic accidents involving large commercial livestock transporters. The program has been conducted throughout North America, providing instruction for trucking companies, fire departments, brand inspectors, and others involved in the livestock industry and emergency response services.

Professional instruction is available for livestock handling for all species of commercial livestock. Resources for locating this training in a local area include county extension agents, commercial food animal producers, and processing facilities in the local area. Various large animal rescue team and TLAER courses provide training to the Awareness level in response to livestock trailer incidents.

EUTHANASIA

Fatalities are relatively common in these incidents and may occur on impact or due to heat exhaustion, asphyxia, or crushing injuries (Figure 21.9). The lack of proper restraint of the animals will limit the veterinarian's ability to perform triage and provide treatment on the scene. It is unlikely that the attending veterinarian will have a sufficient amount of euthanasia solution to euthanatize more than a few animals, and the venous access necessary for intravenous injection may not be practical or possible. Projectile weapons are the most commonly employed method of field euthanasia in these incidents, even in the confined space of a trailer, because they allow the operator to maintain a safe distance from the animal (see Chapter 13).

For safety of responders or for animal welfare reasons, some animals may need to be immediately euthanatized. Regulations governing the euthanasia and transport of injured animals may vary from jurisdiction and state. Under the Alberta Animal Protection Act, for example, only peace officers (law enforcement, the Society for the Prevention of Cruelty to Animals, livestock investigators, and special constables) or the owner have the authority to euthanatize or give permission to euthanatize. The laws and regulations pertaining to the loading of compromised animals apply to

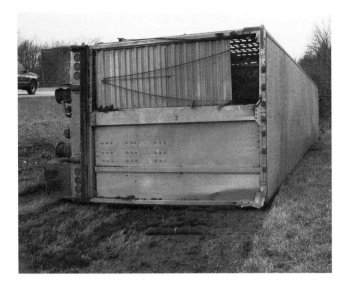

Figure 21.9 *This trailer overturned on a flat, straight interstate due to driver error. Many of the cattle inside are alive, but piled on top of each other. The animals at the bottom of the pile are suffocating. The driver fled the scene of the wreck. Courtesy of Nathan Slovis.*

these incidents. In Canada, the Handling of Unfit Animals guidelines provide information. Loading injured livestock is technically illegal in most countries, although some laws are relatively vague in regard to this subject. Additionally, for some transported large animals (bison, zoo animals) euthanasia may be the recommended plan for escaped individuals.

ACCIDENT STATISTICS

Based on a tracking database of commercial liner wrecks maintained by the author, 95% of liner incidents involve overturns. Of these, approximately 90% roll onto the right side (see Fig. 21.9). Liner wrecks tend to be single-vehicle accidents based on driver error or fatigue, and they most commonly occur between 12:00 midnight and 7:00 a.m. (Woods, 2006a). A large number of overturns occur on interstate exit ramps, and many of them involve escaped livestock.

An analysis of over 300 livestock trailer incidents has shown that trailers hauling cattle are the most likely to roll over, followed by those hauling pigs (Woods, 2006a). The most common explanation provided by the drivers is that the weight shifted; however, animals are loaded into these trailers to a specific density to prevent a weight shift that could destabilize the trailers. Discussions with law enforcement and industry personnel argue that a more probable explanation is driver error, impairment, inattention, excessive speed around corners, or driving too fast for road and traffic conditions.

TRAILER DESIGN

There are a variety of different livestock trailer designs available to commercial livestock haulers, and each design necessitates a different accident response scenario. A wide variety of cut gates, ramps, and deck levels within these trailers require separate considerations for extrication in each trailer.

Decking

Trailers with "bellies" or "pots" and multiple decking layers often require more difficult and timely extrication compared to straight haul trailers. "Fat" trailers (trailers designed to haul fat animals to slaughter) are usually the easiest to empty; they have limited gates and most often will have cargo doors on the back of trailers, allowing first responders to open the entire back end of the trailer without cutting an opening. Unfortunately, only a small percentage of commercial livestock trailers are fat trailers.

When trailers overturn, the available floor space is significantly reduced, especially if the trailer does not land flat on its side. When multi-deck trailers overturn, the floor space is further reduced, often leading to animals being piled up to eight layers deep on top of each other. This causes many animal deaths due to overheating or asphyxia.

Trailers with temporary decking are the most challenging because the decking is literally set on the "rails," a metal lip that extends outward several centimeters from the sides of the trailer halfway up the wall of the belly or the trailer wall and in the nose (front) of the trailer.

Rail decking relies on the weight of the animals to keep it in place; when the trailer overturns, the temporary decking falls away from the rails, removing the floor for one level of animal. The animals become tangled in the layers of decking, requiring the removal of decking and animals. Other trailers have permanent flooring to create decks, but the permanent decking creates a confined space in the bottom tier of the trailer.

Manufacturer

Although all commercial trailers are made of aluminum, the build and design vary with manufacturer. There may be one brand or model of livestock trailer that is extremely difficult to cut apart, whereas others are relatively easy to dismantle. For example, the size and thickness of the support beams and back panel may require specialty cutting techniques.

The Roof

The majority of livestock liner trailers have aluminum roofs, but there is an increasing trend in fiberglass roof construction, especially for swine haulers. Fiberglass roofs tend to shatter on impact, allowing the escape of animals on the top deck of the trailer. Aluminum roofs remain intact until cut open.

Side Walls

The side walls are constructed of a very thin sheet of aluminum. Ventilation holes are cut along the length of the side walls; the size and spacing of the holes may vary with the manufacturer. Although the ventilation holes are necessary to provide ventilation and reduce heat stroke, when a trailer overturns, the ventilation holes become holes in the floor through which the animal's hooves and legs can fall and become entrapped. The injuries sustained range from minor abrasions to limb fractures or traumatic limb amputation. Trapped animals must often be euthanatized because they cannot be safely extricated. If the overturned trailer is straddling a ditch or rests above ground or road level, removing live animals is extremely challenging.

Plywood, rubber mats, or loose decking within the trailer can be used for temporary flooring. It may be necessary to use dead animals as a stable base since they are in place and difficult to remove with live animals sharing the space.

EXTRICATION TOOLS

The aluminum used to manufacture these liners offers challenges to responders used to working with steel during extrication work.

Based on numerous reports from actual responses to liner accidents as well as training sessions with fire departments that have cut donated liners apart to try different techniques and tools, this chapter includes suggestions on extrication tools and cutting equipment that have been successfully used, as well as those tools that are not applicable to these scenarios.

Best Tools for Cutting a Trailer

- Reciprocating saw: This type of saw can efficiently cut apart the roof and the back end of a commercial liner trailer. The blade must be constantly lubricated with dish soap or a special blade lubricant while cutting the aluminum on these trailers. The blade on this saw will not hurt animals on the other side, and the noise generated is minimal. This saw is preferred for use on trailers containing swine. A 28 V cordless reciprocating saw is ideal for this function.
- Circular saw with an adjustable metal cutting blade: This saw provides the most rapid cutting action and can be used on the back end of a trailer as well as the roof. In order to lessen the chance of cutting the animals on the other side of the roof, the blade should be set at approximately 4 cm (1 1/2 in.) to allow it to cut through the "ribs" of the trailer. This saw may cut into the animals' skin, especially that of

pigs, when used to make roof cuts. For this reason, it is best to use the reciprocating saw on the roof of swine liners. The saw should be retracted slightly when cutting the roof and pushed deeper when cutting the aluminum ribs of the roof. *Note:* On certain trailer designs, the circular saw will not penetrate sufficiently to cut all the way through the back panel (it is approximately 1 cm [3/8 in.] too shallow.) To resolve this problem, the circular saw can be used to make the initial cut, and a reciprocating saw can be used to cut through the remaining 1 cm (3/8 in.) of metal.

Tools That Successfully Cut the Trailer

- Air chisel: This chisel cuts the roof but does not effectively cut the ribs of the roof or the back panel of the trailer. It is also extremely loud, elevating stress levels in the livestock and possibly inducing a panic response.
- Chop saw: This saw is very large and difficult to handle for overhead cuts. Two people are required to stabilize and lift the saw, potentially increasing the risk of injury. This saw cuts very deep, and it can injure or kill animals on the other side of the metal.
- Cutters: These tools will cut the aluminum, but do not create a smooth edge. Cutting efforts with these tools are often very time-consuming.

Tools That Will Not Successfully Cut the Trailer

- Hydraulic spreaders or jaws of life: These tools are not acceptable because they are designed to spread, not cut. They will tear the aluminum, and they do not create sufficient openings.
- Cutting torches: These tools are contraindicated on animal transports because they melt the aluminum and will burn the animals.
- Rescue circular saw (K-12): The use of a rescue circular saw (K-12) was aborted while cutting an opening on the back of a large horse van because the saw jammed on the aluminum, plywood, and rubber layers of the van wall. The cutting was finished with a reciprocating saw. There are many circumstances where this saw will make significant sparks.

OVERTURNED CATTLE LINER CASE REPORT

At 4 a.m. in Atlanta, Georgia, a cattle trailer driver fell asleep traveling at 70 mph (112 kph) on Interstate 75 and hit a barrier. The incident involved multiple lanes of traffic as parts of the engine and cab were thrown onto the other side of the barrier, causing secondary accidents. The trailer skidded along the barrier for over 200 m (655 ft), but the trailer was structurally intact

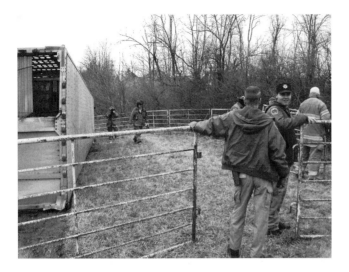

Figure 21.10 *Before unloading the live animals in this overturned trailer, cattle panels are set up for containment away from the road and are maneuvered to form a funnel shape for loading in alternate transport trailers called to the scene. Courtesy of Nathan Slovis.*

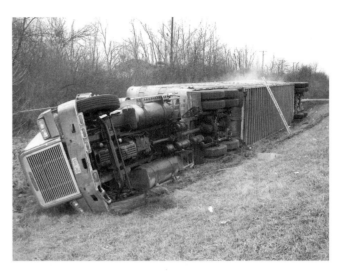

Figure 21.11 *First responders use a ladder to assess the condition of the animals inside the trailer while awaiting the arrival of cattle panels for containment before cutting a doorway in the roof. Note the steam rising from these stressed animals despite the low winter temperatures. Courtesy of Nathan Slovis.*

and contained numerous beef cattle that survived the impact.

The Georgia State Patrol contacted the Equine Inspection Division of the Georgia Department of Agriculture (GDA). Based on previous training provided across the state, the GDA had contact and resource lists of businesses and individuals from all over the state. Local livestock handling personnel were contacted, a police escort was coordinated to facilitate delivery of livestock panels, and a rescue cattle hauler trailer was escorted to the scene. A portable ramp was used to load the cattle from the destroyed trailer.

The cattle were not unloaded until containment was available and deployed to the scene (Figure 21.10). When the panels arrived, one team of responders set up containment while another cut the roof of the trailer to gain access and allowed the animals to slowly exit the trailer. A third team encouraged the cattle to load onto the rescue trailer.

In an analysis of this incident, the prearranged contact list significantly expedited the response effort. Attempting to locate equipment, cattle panels, and special assistance by searching phone books would have consumed great amounts of time and resources and decreased the likelihood of a successful response. Despite a model communications plan and readily available resources, the interstate was blocked for eight hours.

ROLLING DIRECTION

The incident scenario is very different when responding to a trailer that overturns onto its right side (which is common) compared to one that overturns onto its left side (rare), due to the configuration of compartments and gates.

BEFORE CUTTING OR RELEASE OF ANIMALS

Occasionally, responders or bystanders try to open the trailer to release the animals or open doors or windows to check the status of the animals, and some animals escape the trailer. An assessment should be made through the preexisting ventilation holes or openings in the trailer (Figure 21.11).

Under no circumstances should rescuers enter a capsized livestock trailer containing conscious animals. When interior gates must be cut, trained responders should enter only when the animals have been removed from the first compartment. Once the panels are in place outside and an escape route has been opened, mobile animals will usually exit the trailer on their own. Infrequently, one or more animals may resist exiting the trailer; minimizing the noise level and flashing lights and providing good lighting may encourage the animals to move into the holding area. Most species prefer moving toward brighter alleyways and trailers, but elk will load more easily if the trailer is darker than the outside area.

Lack of knowledge and experience in livestock incident response and in the rescue and handling of unpredictable and stressed stock has caused additional animal losses on past incident scenes. Animals should not be released and openings should not be made in the trailer until all containment is established and emergency services are on the scene.

Provide Containment

The trailer side walls or roof can be torn open by hitting an obstacle overhead or while overturning, allowing animals to escape. In several incidents, the pot or belly of the trailer was impacted by a vehicle or obstacle, compromising the structural integrity of the side walls and allowing animals to escape. If animals have escaped before responders arrive on the scene, a containment area should be established and the loose animals contained before they cause secondary incidents.

If the trailer has not been breached and all animals remain contained within the trailer, temporary containment (i.e., with livestock panels) should be established around the area where cutting and unloading will occur; this should be established before extrication begins. The corral must be sufficiently large to hold several animals away from the main extrication area and provide separation from the animals for the responders. It is not necessary to enclose the entire trailer; a funnel of fencing to the rear of the rescue trailer is sufficient and easily established. It is unsafe to cut the escape hole and back the rescue trailer directly to it without containment fencing; animals may escape between the trailers, and animal handlers can become trapped when they attempt to drive animals into the rescue trailer.

Animals should be released (unloaded) into a holding corral as small groups from each compartment as it is opened and reloaded on the rescue trailer as a group. Unloading one animal at a time from the wrecked trailer does not take advantage of their herd instincts. Isolation is a strong stressor of livestock, and they can become very unpredictable and dangerous when alone and stressed. Animals become and remain calm if they are allowed to gather in a herd outside the trailer, especially if there is alfalfa hay. If individual animals are loaded onto the rescue trailer alone, the isolated animal will often attempt to escape when the door is opened to load other animals.

Each animal species reacts differently to high levels of stress. Horses are inclined to panic and may kick, strike, rear, or bite. Cattle tend to appear stunned and will remain in place until an escape route is evident. Dairy bulls, elk, and bison are most likely to charge regardless of the location and situation. Pigs, horses, camelids (e.g., camels, llamas, alpacas, guanacos, vicunas) and elk are more likely to bite.

The corral paneling should be tarped if possible to block the animal's vision beyond the enclosure as they unload and to block access to the media and cameras. Animals will often unload more quickly and are less likely to charge the panels or responders if the walls of the enclosure appear solid. If there are only a few tarps available, the panels closest to the extrication point should be tarped.

Rescue/Recovery Trailers

Basic, open-configuration stock trailers are recommended for use as rescue/recovery trailers because they can accommodate all types of livestock, including poultry, and animal carcasses. Reloading animals into another commercial livestock trailer can be challenging for handlers, requires portable ramping, increases animal stress, and may not be possible based on the orientation of the overturned trailer. Stock trailers do not require loading ramps, can be more easily maneuvered into place, and provide a humane method of transport following an accident. The animals should be reloaded without overcrowding; several trailers may be necessary to accommodate all animals. Carcasses are more easily loaded into dump trailers or trucks with heavy equipment brought to the scene.

STARTING THE CUT

Accessing the Top Deck through the Roof

The first access cut should be made into the roof to allow emptying of the top deck of the trailer. A common mistake is to cut the access like a ramp and lay the cut piece down on the ground. Aluminum is very slippery; the animals will slip and fall on this makeshift ramp or refuse to walk over it, and it becomes a safety hazard for the personnel on scene who try to step on it. *Note:* When cutting, the opening should be approximately the size and shape of a house door.

It is easiest to start at the bottom of the door, with the saw traveling along the framing approximately 5 cm (2 in.) above ground level. The opening should begin at the inside aspect of a rib, traveling across the bottom and cutting through one rib (or two ribs depending on trailer design and rib spacing), arriving at the next rib, and turning the saw upward to cut along the inside of this rib. Cutting on the inside of the ribs preserves stability (structural strength) on each side of the opening and creates smoother edges. The cut is continued up the rib to approximately the same height as a household door. The saw is then turned, and a cut is made across the top toward the starting rib (passing through the middle rib[s] again at the higher level). The cut is stopped and the "door" created is opened only after personnel and equipment have been cleared away from the area and containment has been established. Creating the opening in this manner eliminates one sharp vertical edge. In addition, the door itself provides a visual barrier on one side (Figure 21.12). The remaining jagged edges can be effectively covered with pool noodles.

Emptying the Top Deck

The top deck is normally emptied first and does not require personnel to enter the trailer to unload the animals. The mobile animals will often exit readily on their own if personnel are not obstructing their path.

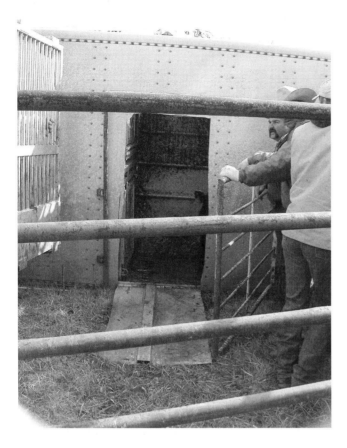

Figure 21.12 *A door is cut in the roof of the trailer to allow animals to exit the trailer into the containment area. It is preferable to cut the access point like a household door; the cut metal is an unacceptable ramp because of its slick surface and sharp edges. Sharp edges can be covered with pool noodles available from toy, pool, or discount stores. Courtesy of Nathan Slovis.*

When one animal exits, the remaining animals willingly follow. The animals can also be coaxed into leaving by positioning a handler on the top of the trailer, applying psychological or sometimes even physical pressure from above the animals' heads. After the mobile animals are unloaded from the upper compartment, it is safe for handlers to enter the trailer and assess the downed animals.

Animals that are fatally injured must be euthanatized in the trailer. They should not be dragged alive off the trailer unless euthanasia in place presents a safety risk to personnel. Livestock can safely be euthanatized inside the trailer using projectile weapons (see Chapter 13). Responders must ensure all animals are dead before they are removed from the trailer. Carcasses should be removed manually or with winches and placed outside the trailer, unless they cannot be removed from the scene and must be transported in the wrecked trailer.

Emptying the "Doghouse"

If the trailer has a "doghouse" compartment (located on the rear, right side of the top deck) and the trailer is overturned onto its right side, the gate to the doghouse often breaks open or can be easily opened. If this is the case, the animals in the doghouse can be encouraged to exit the trailer through the original hole cut in the roof. If rescuers are unable to open the gate on the doghouse, a second hole must be cut in the roof at that location.

If the trailer is overturned onto its left side, there is a good chance that there are animals trapped in the suspended doghouse. Ramps must be set up to unload the animals from this compartment. A hole can be cut in the back-end panel of the trailer (up high on the panel) to access this compartment. The pull-out ramp used to load the top deck of the trailer can be used as portable ramping to unload the animals.

Emptying the Neck/Nose

Due to trailer design and paneling, it is rarely possible to unload the neck (front portion) of the trailer through the hole cut in the top deck access area. There is usually a large panel between the neck and the top deck. Cutting an access hole into the neck area is generally more easily and quickly accomplished than removing the divider panel. If the trailer overturns on its left side, the gate on the left side of the top deck that is used to access the neck for loading may be used. The decisions made depend on individual trailer design and the severity of structural damage sustained during the incident.

Emptying the Back End and Lower Deck

After the top deck, doghouse, and neck/nose are emptied, animals can be unloaded from the back end and lower deck. The back end and belly are accessed through the rear of the trailer. If it is a straight haul trailer, the back end is cut open for unloading the animals in these compartments. If it is a pot belly or possum-bellied trailer, the back end compartment should be emptied first.

If the trailer overturns on its left side, extrication of animals in these compartments is relatively easy as no cutting is required on the back panels. The roller door will be at ground level and can easily be removed. Most animals, except large bulls, horses, and elk, will be able to exit through the roller door opening; the opening can be enlarged to accommodate the larger animals.

If the trailer is overturned on its right side, access to the back end and lower deck requires cutting an opening, unless the trailer has cargo doors. This area is more difficult to cut than the roof, and some brands of trailers are more challenging than others. The hinges on the alley sort gate may have to be cut separately because it is often welded to the inside of a panel, requiring cuts through the back panel and the alley gate. Once this panel is open, the back end of the trailer can be emptied.

Emptying the Belly

The final compartment emptied is the belly or pot. This compartment can be accessed through the back end of the trailer once it has been emptied, providing access to the gate and panels that separate the belly from the remaining compartments. The cutting configuration depends on whether the trailer has a three-quarter gate or a center gate. Three-quarter gates can be opened upward and should be tied to the top of the trailer; the live animals are then unloaded through the opening originally cut in the back end.

Center gates are more common. The gate is opened upward and secured, but the small panel to which the gate hinges or latches must be removed. The animals are then removed through the back end of the trailer.

What to Avoid

Responders should minimize their cutting efforts to maximize efficiency and reduce the risk of compromising the trailer's structural integrity. Based on field research and practical experience, professional responders have suggested the following approaches be avoided.

- Cutting through the floor/bottom of the trailer or through the solid top deck floor. Not only is this a very difficult and time-consuming area to cut, but it will also cause irreparable damage to the trailer. It is never necessary to cut through the floor, unless the roof and the back end of the trailer are simultaneously blocked. The entire trailer can be unloaded through the roof and/or back end.
- Cutting the opening larger than necessary. The opening should only be sufficiently large to release one animal at a time or allow safe access for handlers. The openings, on average, should approximate the size of a household door. By keeping the size of the exit only large enough for one animal, their exit from the trailer is controlled and human risk is minimized.
- Cutting too many openings in the trailer. This compromises the structural integrity and strength of the trailer, increasing the risk of collapse. When excessive cuts are made, it also increases the difficulty for towing recovery companies to upright the trailer because the weakened structure causes the trailer to twist.
- Allowing the use of winches or tow trucks to tear the trailer apart to make access. This equipment creates jagged and sharp edges and openings and is inefficient and dangerous for responders.
- Uprighting a trailer full of animals. First, the trailer will not hold up to the weight of the animals against the side walls as the trailer is uprighted, and it will

begin to tear apart. Second, it will further injure and kill animals.

POULTRY

Commercial poultry are grown in large commercial houses with 5,000–40,000 animals per house. They are transported to slaughter processing facilities on large trucks in open wire cages. These animals are usually transported at night to avoid heat stress. An individual turkey can weigh from 7 lb (3.2 kg) (poults) up to 35 lb (16 kg) (meat). Chickens range from 3–7 lb (1.4–3.2 kg). When loose, these animals are difficult to catch, manipulate, and carry. Most cannot fly due to their heavy weight (bred for meat), but they can still move faster on the ground than a human. Their tendency to flutter and make a lot of noise increases the stress and nervousness of the entire flock (Woods, 2006a). They may try to hide under objects, cages, or the overturned trailer. Poultry are extremely sensitive to heat and cold and can suffocate in their travel cages or die from stress and fear. When handled calmly, flocks can be easily herded and contained using portable fencing. Individual poultry can be trapped in hand nets and returned to the flock.

Poultry Transports

Commercial trailers hauling poultry differ from commercial livestock trailers in that most poultry haulers consist of a flat deck trailer with framing that holds individual crates full of poultry. Depending on trailer design and use, these crates can be metal cages welded onto the trailer or they can be heavy plastic crates placed into the framing of the trailer. The loose crates are often secured by only a small metal lip. These crates easily come off the trailer in an accident and can also be discharged from the trailer when the trailer corners sharply at excessive speed. A crate containing poultry can be a deadly road hazard. Small poults and hens are often transported in cube vans, buses, or specially designed tip trailers that can contain as many as 30,000 birds.

Loose Poultry

Because of the large numbers of animals involved, poultry trailer wrecks present challenges in containment. Some poultry become loose as the crates break open on impact, while others remain trapped in damaged crates. Loose poultry must be herded and grouped away from the incident. Although they cannot fly, poultry move quickly and are easily frightened by noises or fast movements. Portable snow fencing and construction fencing are acceptable options for temporary corral systems (see Chapter 8). Animals may then be individually caught and placed back in crates from a secondary trailer or loaded onto a stock trailer. For smaller poultry, a push broom can be used to gently herd them into containment. Poultry must be protected from extreme weather conditions to prevent heat or cold stress.

Crates

Overturned crates should be manually uprighted and placed flat on the ground during the initial response to the accident. Rescuers should ensure that all legs and wings of the poultry are inside the crates before uprighting them. Damaged but intact crates containing live animals should be loaded onto a secondary trailer and transported to the processing plant. The cages of some poultry trailers are welded to the trailer, and a cutting torch is necessary to disassemble the cages. It can be very difficult to extricate animals—particularly those located on the downside—from these trailers.

Poultry-Handling Specialists

Poultry-handling specialists may be located by contacting the producer or processing plant. These specialists are trained to properly and efficiently catch poultry and are skilled in the process of cervical dislocation (the preferred euthanasia method for most poultry under 7 lb [3.2 kg]). Turkeys are large and can be especially difficult to euthanatize; personnel trained in emergency euthanasia of turkeys should be on the scene as quickly as possible.

SWINE

Swine are grown in large, commercial houses with hundreds of animals per house. They are transported to slaughter processing facilities on large pot belly or multi-deck trailers, normally at night to avoid heat stress. Market weight pigs (approximately six months of age) commonly encountered in a slaughter trailer overturn are approximately 68–90 kg (150–200 lb); adult sows and some pet pigs can approach 272 kg (600 lb); and boars can reach 362 kg (800 lb). These animals can move faster than a human, and they may attack. Swine are extremely sensitive to heat and cold, and they can suffocate in transport or die from stress and fear. When handled calmly, pigs may be driven slowly, using pig boards or emergency medical services (EMS) backboards. Portable fencing provides adequate containment.

Formidable Animals

Pigs are intelligent animals. In addition, they are large, strong, and have low centers of gravity. Their teeth are large, and they will bite. They are difficult to restrain; the ears are not appropriate handles. These animals should be handled with respect and caution (Woods, 2006b).

Special Considerations

Swine are extremely sensitive to environmental temperatures, have very little insulating hair, and cannot sweat. They can die from heat exhaustion, frostbite, or wind chill. Pigs quickly suffocate inside an overturned trailer on a warm day. Overheating is a serious concern with pigs and commonly leads to animal losses in transport. They must be cooled off in warm weather by misting them inside and outside the trailer to prevent heat stress and death. A fire hose may be used to provide a fine spray to mist the animals on scene. Many swine trailers have sprinkler systems to cool the animals; if the system is functional, it can be used to keep the animals cool during extrication.

It is often difficult to determine if a pig is injured unless it is very obvious; pigs can die from cardiac arrest induced by stress. Caution is recommended when approaching a downed pig because it can rise and attack without warning. Swine should not be chased, as this increases the risk of stress and muscle injury. They should be driven slowly (Woods, 2006b).

Pigs can suffer from fatigue and can die from shock; they must be allowed time to recover from stress. Electric prods or forced movement can result in fatalities. Pigs that show no outward signs of injury must be segregated from mobile pigs and allowed time to recover. It is not unusual for a pig to be down for an hour or more before recovery. If a pig has not recovered from fatigue within two hours, recovery is unlikely and euthanasia should be considered.

Pig squeals can exceed 130 decibels (dB) (National Agriculture Safety Database, 2002), higher than noise levels encountered at rock concerts or while using a chainsaw. Sustained exposure to levels over 95 dB can result in permanent hearing loss. Animal handlers and rescuers should consider appropriate hearing protection, especially if entering the trailer to euthanatize animals.

Bribe Them with Food

When pigs escape an overturned trailer, they are easily bribed with food and do not tend to wander unless chased. Loose pigs can be herded with pig boards, plywood, EMS backboards, or police riot shields.

Note: Although lassoing loose cattle may be a necessary means of capture, this method is unacceptable for use on pigs. The anatomy of a pig's head and neck does not allow secure rope placement. In addition, many horses are frightened by the smells and sounds generated by pigs; riders may be injured as their horses react to the animals.

COMMERCIAL LIVESTOCK ACCIDENT RESPONSE PROTOCOL FOR DRIVERS

The condition and welfare of the driver is the primary concern in an accident. If the driver is uninjured and physically able, he or she should perform the following procedures:

1. Call 911 and advise the dispatcher of the accident location, the type of livestock on board, the number of animals, and the status of any loose livestock. Provide 911 with the number for the LER hotline at 1-866-684-3028 in North America. Suggest that police and fire approach the scene with sirens off if possible.

2. Light flares and set out warning signs to alert approaching traffic of the accident.

3. Phone the hauling company's dispatcher and/or insurance companies to advise them of the accident.

4. Slowly herd any loose livestock from the roadway and gather them in one area as far away from traffic as possible. Allow them to graze or provide hay to keep them calm. If available, use portable fencing or cattle panels to keep the animals contained.

5. Release statements only to persons in authority (i.e., emergency services personnel). Do not talk to media or bystanders about the accident or the load being transported.

6. When first responders (fire, police, ambulance) arrive on the scene, brief them on the following details:
   - Type of animals
   - Number of animals
   - Status of any loose animals
   - Known hazards
   - Hauling company or processing plant emergency plan and contact information
   - Resources en route
   - Resource contact numbers such as LER Hotline at 1-866-684-3028 in North America

7. Respect the accident scene chain of command; assist if needed.

8. Perform salvage, rescue, and recovery assistance as needed.

9. Arrange for removal of animal carcasses. Dead stock removal is a user-pay service, and the owner of the truck and/or the livestock is responsible for contacting a company to request pickup.

10. Document the incident. The IC should also assign a non-rescuer to take photographs of the incident at arrival on the scene and during the rescue and recovery operation.

ACRONYMS USED IN CHAPTER 21

AFAC	Alberta Farm Animal Care
dB	Decibels
EMS	Emergency medical services
GDA	Georgia Department of Agriculture
IC	Incident commander
LER	Livestock emergency response
SO	Safety officer
TLAER	Technical large animal emergency rescue
USDA	U.S. Department of Agriculture

22 Learning from Actual Incident Scenarios

Dr. Tomas Gimenez and Dr. Rebecca Gimenez

INTRODUCTION

Large animals end up in some of the most unbelievable circumstances imaginable, due to several factors: owner negligence, the animal's tendency to play, excitability, and herd dynamics. Although true accidents occasionally occur, the majority of these situations are preventable incidents. The examples in this chapter are provided as learning tools for the reader who may not realize the variety of incidents that have occurred.

Lack of knowledge in techniques for large animal extrication often prolongs the rescue time, potentially compromising the medical status of the animal victim and increasing the risk of secondary accidents. Each incident is unique: the solutions are never the same nor is there ever only one solution to an incident. Readers are encouraged to submit their own TLAER experiences to the authors at tlaer@bellsouth.net.

These scenarios are provided as learning opportunities for students of TLAER procedures and methodologies. The readers should imagine themselves in the scenario and consider options for an effective response. In the first section of scenarios, the authors prompt the readers with questions; in the last examples, there is only a short description of the incident.

PROBLEM-SOLVING SCENARIOS

Responders are encouraged to think through the following examples to determine how they might approach each rescue scenario, taking into account scene safety, management, and security concerns for responders, bystanders, and specialty personnel (e.g., veterinarians, etc.).

Horse in a Mobile Home

A pasture gate was left open by a county maintenance worker, and three horses escaped and ran across an open field. Two of the horses returned to their pasture, but the third fell into a ravine in the field where an old mobile home had been pushed and partially buried. The horse landed in the middle of the mobile home and severely lacerated his legs. The horse was found approximately three hours later. The owner called 911.

Simple solution? Firefighters cut the debris away to make an egress for the horse out of the wreckage, caught and haltered the animal, and walked it to safety by cutting a trail from the bottom of the ravine.

More complicated solution? Firefighters considered bringing in a crane and equipment for a vertical lift. However, the mobile home and horse were positioned 10 m (33 ft) below flat ground above.

Notes. The owner refused to allow the veterinarian on the scene to treat the horse's injuries, and walked the animal home one-half mile (0.8 km). The animal control officer on the scene could not intervene due to local regulations.

Lessons learned. The second solution (vertical lift) would have required responders entering the wrecked mobile home with a potentially dangerous animal to place the sling, increasing the risk of injury to the responders and animal. As stated numerous times throughout this book, responders should avoid entering confined spaces with animals. The first solution offers the advantages of simplicity and avoidance of responders entering the potentially dangerous wreckage in close proximity to a struggling, frightened animal.

Prevention. Secure fencing, common sense, and monitoring of gates can reduce the risk of animal escape from pastures. Posting signs instructing that gates should remain closed, and providing secure latch systems, increase the awareness that there are animals in the area and decrease the risk that gates will be left open.

Horse in a Hole

A 250 kg (550 lb) colt was covered with mud and fell into a hole underneath the small shed in which he was kept.

Solution? The owner placed a dog chain around the horse's neck to attempt to drag him out of the hole. The chain choked the struggling and terrified horse, and the owner was kicked in the face as the animal struggled. EMS was dispatched. The local animal control officer was dispatched to the scene. Upon arrival to the scene, the chain was still around the colt's neck.

Appropriate solution? The animal was placed on a Rescue Glide, hauled down the hill to a waiting equine ambulance, and transported to a veterinary facility.

Notes. The animal was in severe shock with neurological compromise, and was eventually euthanized.

Lessons learned. This case demonstrates the importance of avoiding use of the head and neck as anchors. Pressure of the chain around the colt's neck asphyxiated the animal, inducing a panic response and struggle that severely injured the owner. In addition, the chain can cause trauma to the trachea, spinal canal, esophagus, blood vessels (including the carotid arteries), and soft tissues of the neck; these injuries can result in fatal complications.

Prevention. The importance of maintaining a safe environment for animals, especially young animals, is critical to preventing incidents. All holes, particularly those large enough to entrap an animal, should be filled or the animal's access prevented by secure fencing.

Horse under Culvert

A horse was exploring a ditch in his pasture and became entrapped under a small culvert. The horse was trapped for almost 24 hours before the owners realized he was missing and began looking for him.

Solution? Webbing and a rope system were placed for a forward assist. Once removed from the entrapment, the exhausted horse was allowed to rest; he was allowed to lay quietly, and hay bales were used to support him in sternal recumbency.

Notes. Two days after the rescue, the skin and subcutaneous muscle of the horse's dependent (down) side sloughed. With medical treatment, the horse survived.

Lessons learned. Animals trapped in lateral recumbency for prolonged periods of time are at significant risk of skin, muscle, and nerve damage associated with pressure and limited movement. Pressure-induced skin damage may not be immediately evident.

In addition, animals entrapped for prolonged periods of time are usually exhausted and dehydrated. Cardiovascular shock may occur. A veterinarian should assess the animal on the scene; treatment to stabilize the animal may be necessary before it is extricated, and immediate veterinary care following extrication is extremely important.

Prevention. Animals should be checked at least once a day. One should not assume that because they have grass and water they can be left unsupervised for days. Animal access to potentially hazardous areas in fields or pastures should be prevented by secure fencing.

Horse Fallen Down a Mountainside

A Thoroughbred gelding slipped 75 m (250 ft) off a wet trail in the Smoky Mountains (Tennessee), 10 km (6 miles) from the trailhead. The animal was positioned in dorsal recumbency (on its back) between a rock and a tree. The owner removed the bridle and saddle, but was unable to contact authorities due to a lack of cell phone reception. The owner had no option but to leave the animal overnight. The temperature was 20°C (68° F), and it rained all night.

How would you approach this rescue, and what would you pack on your back to take to the site? Responders were concerned that the horse would be in shock and possibly dead from exposure. They arrived at the trailhead close to midnight, met with the park rangers and the owner, and developed a response plan. Items packed by the responders included rope system equipment, webbing for sling emplacement, and a portable A-frame in the event a vertical lift became necessary. A horse blanket was carried to the scene. The veterinarian transported emergency medications (e.g., antibiotics, anti-inflammatory drugs, euthanasia solution), hypertonic saline, 20 l of crystalloid intravenous (IV) fluids, supplies for IV catheterization, and basic wound care and bandaging supplies. All materials transported were packed in water-resistant materials to protect them from the rain.

At dawn, they hiked up the mountain in the rain to the site where the owner reported the horse had been trapped. As they arrived at the site, they discovered that the animal had extricated itself, found a side trail, and found its way back to the main trail. The gelding was dehydrated, hypothermic, and exhibiting signs of shock.

How does the focus of your rescue change at this point, and how can you use the five personnel you have available? Because the horse had extricated itself from the entrapment, the rescue focus changed to addressing the animal's medical condition and returning it to the trailhead. The horse was immediately blanketed to help warm him. The veterinarian assessed the animal, placed an IV catheter, and administered fluids to combat dehydration and shock. Responders assisted the veterinarian by restraining the animal, holding fluid bags, and ensuring that the return trail was clear. An anti-inflammatory medication was administered after the fluids to reduce the risk of renal (kidney) damage. When the animal's condition was sufficiently stable that it could walk, rescuers offered the animal opportunities to drink from puddles as it was walked to the trailhead. At the trailhead, the owner wanted to load the horse on her trailer and take him home (five-hour drive).

How do you handle this scenario to ensure appropriate veterinarian follow-up care? The veterinarian discussed the horse's condition with the owner and emphasized the risks associated with delaying additional treatment (e.g., shock, renal damage, death). The owner was informed that trailering the horse in its present condition for five hours could result in life-threatening conditions, and it was in the animal's best interest to hospitalize it for several days.

Notes. The horse was loaded on the equine ambulance, fed electrolytes, offered water to drink, and delivered to a local veterinary practitioner's facility. The horse was administered 45 l of fluids, treated for multiple contusions and minor lacerations, edema, and pain, and released four days later.

Lessons learned. Occasionally, animals are able to rescue themselves from entrapment; however, these animals are still at risk of developing medical conditions associated with the entrapment, struggle, and environmental conditions. Responders should prepare for a worst-case scenario and equip themselves properly.

Communication is key in ensuring that the animal's owner understands the medical conditions and risks associated with the entrapment and the rescue. It should be emphasized that an apparently normal animal can rapidly decompensate and that problems can be observed several days after the rescue.

Prevention. Common sense dictates that riders should remain in groups and develop emergency plans. Attention to weather conditions and trail safety can prevent many incidents.

Recumbent Neglect Case

A quarter horse mare was severely starved and unable to stand on her own for almost 36 hours. The mare was dehydrated, malnourished, hypoproteinemic (low blood protein), and immobile. Through the efforts of a dozen firemen and volunteers, the mare was manually lifted to her feet. In an attempt to improve circulation to the horse's limbs, those present began to rub her body furiously. The nearest veterinary hospital was two hours away.

How could this mare have been lifted using fewer personnel? Emplacement of a sling and the use of an A-frame or tractor boom are effective for lifting recumbent animals.

Is the "rescue" really over for this animal? Although the horse was easily loaded into the trailer, the mare collapsed during transport. The veterinarian assessed the mare on arrival at the facility. Nineteen liters of IV fluids were administered to address the mare's dehydration, and medication was applied to her bleeding sores. Over the following several days, the mare collapsed five times; a tow truck was called to lift the animal using a large homemade animal sling. The mare eventually recovered.

Lessons learned. Starved and neglected large animals can recover with long-term care, proper nutrition, exercise, and attention. Severely starved animals often require veterinary treatment and/or hospitalization to address medical issues (e.g., hypoproteinemia, parasitism, anemia, skin conditions, wounds, diarrhea, colic, etc.) and may require sling support until they have regained sufficient strength.

Horse in Iced-Over Pond

A 750 kg (1,650 lb) draft horse escaped from his stall and fell through the ice surface of a frozen pond in below-zero ambient temperatures. Within minutes, almost a hundred rescuers were on the scene. A large number of volunteers arrived on the scene to assist in the rescue efforts. Three news helicopters hovered overhead throughout the rescue; live coverage of the entire event was broadcast from the circling helicopters, and records were broken for the number of telephone calls received in response to a news event. Local horse specialists were contacted by the media to offer suggestions on how to attempt the rescue.

What are the scene safety and security concerns? The large number of bystanders and volunteers presents a significant safety risk. Although well-intentioned, bystanders can hinder the rescue effort by physically interfering with procedures, obstructing escape paths, distracting responders, and endangering themselves and responders by attempting procedures for which they have not been trained. Following proper incident command system structure, a safety officer and public information officer should be designated to establish a safe perimeter for responders and to communicate with bystanders.

Proper personal protective equipment (PPE) and training in ice rescue techniques are prerequisites for this type of rescue scenario. Ice rescue requires specialized training and equipment to ensure safe and effective rescue.

What about the media coverage? The media should be discouraged from interfering with the rescue. If the presence of the helicopters interferes with the rescue by frightening the animal, law enforcement may need to intervene in the situation.

Solution? All attempts failed to secure tow straps to the wet horse. Two tow trucks broke down when the cold temperatures froze the hydraulic fluid in their engines and booms. Rescuers decided to cut larger holes in the ice with chainsaws. One rescue worker without PPE slipped and fell into the water with the struggling horse. The animal rescue effort was postponed until the rescue worker could be rescued.

After two and a half hours of struggling, the horse was finally dragged out of the hole and over the surface of the frozen pond by a backhoe and dragged on a plywood board 400 m (1,300 ft) to a large indoor arena.

Alternative solutions. Cutting an egress path in the ice, using several chain saws would allow an exit without dragging the animal over the surface of the ice and the possibility that the animal would again fall through the frozen surface. Emplacement of forward assist webbing would allow rescuers to assist the horse during its exit from the water. All responders must wear PPE, and an Ice Path or similar system is recommended to prevent possible ice breakthrough by responders.

Alternatively, if the animal was entrapped too far from the shore to cut an egress path, the ice hole could be enlarged and a vertical lift could be performed (with the legs of the frame secured by Ice Paths to prevent surface breakthrough). Once the animal has been lifted, it can be packaged on a Rescue Glide and transported across an Ice Path to shore.

What are the medical concerns associated with this scenario, and how should they be addressed? Hypothermia and frostbite were significant concerns associated with this scenario, as well as aspiration pneumonia from submersion and dehydration from struggling. The animal should be assessed by a veterinarian as soon as possible, and steps should be taken (e.g., heaters, blankets, and warmed IV fluids) to warm the patient.

After the recumbent animal was dragged to the indoor arena, a large crowd gathered around the animal while construction workers with space heaters worked to warm him. People massaged the animal's legs and urged it to rise; the horse made several unsuccessful attempts to rise, but was unsteady and fell headfirst to the ground. The horse was finally able to rise, but it was unsteady and trembling. The veterinarian recommended that the horse remain in the heated barn for recovery. Hours later, the animal was still shivering despite being covered in several blankets.

Lessons learned. Scene safety is paramount in ensuring the safety of the animal victim, responders, and bystanders. A safety perimeter should be immediately established to allow responders ample area to assemble equipment, perform the rescue, and assess the animal without interference by bystanders. Proper communication with the animal owner, bystanders, and the media can prevent negative images by ensuring that the rescue conditions and procedures and the animal's condition are understood.

Allowing large numbers of bystanders to surround an animal after a rescue presents significant risk of injury. Responders should always have an escape route, and bystanders obstructing this safety route are not able to rapidly clear away in case of emergency. In addition, crowding an animal that is attempting to rise places everyone at risk of injury if the animal tramples them or falls; a falling animal can crush an individual, or it can kick an individual as it struggles.

Rescued animals should be allowed to rest and should not be forced to rise. In this case, the animal should have been allowed to remain recumbent until it was sufficiently strong enough to rise. Responders should become concerned about animals that remain recumbent for more than four hours, but ample time should be allowed for the animal to rest immediately after it is extricated.

Responders without proper training in ice rescue techniques and ice rescue equipment should not attempt these rescues unless there is no other option. Regardless of training, proper PPE is essential. Stopping an animal rescue to rescue a responder delays the rescue process, jeopardizes the safety of responders, and creates an impression of incompetence.

Same day, second scenario. Later that day, the roof of the barn sheltering the previously rescued horse and 29 others was collapsing due to the weight of the snow. The people present started catching and evacuating horses. The sirens and engines of the responding police and fire trucks frightened several horses, including the recovering draft horse; the horse dragged its handler, became loose, and ran away in the darkness. The owner was able to catch and lead the horse and others to the safety of another barn, while other horses were shipped to nearby farms.

Lessons learned. Personnel should remain calm as they catch and evacuate animals from a barn in an emergency situation; animals are very receptive to human emotion, and nervous personnel increase the nervousness and excitability of the animals. Emergency responders should not use sirens as they approach the facility to avoid inducing a panic response by the animals. As animals are removed from the barn, they should be placed in a contained area—even if they are restrained by a handler—to prevent loose animals.

Prevention. Secure stall latches and barn doors (or barriers to barn exit) reduce the risk of loose animals. In areas that receive heavy snowfall, roof design modifications and/or regular removal of snow and ice from the barn roof prevents collapse.

Panicked Horse in Trailer

A nine-year-old Arabian gelding was loaded on the left (driver's) side of a two-horse, straight load trailer. During transit, he kicked out with both hind feet and bent the latch to the trailer door. The animal continued kicking, but the trailer latch was jammed. The owner stopped on the roadside, called a veterinarian and some friends, and entered the tack compartment to locate a tranquilizer for the horse. The horse continued kicking. Its front limbs became entrapped in the manger, and its right hind limb kicked through and became entrapped in the solid trailer divider. Despite the entrapment, the horse continued struggling and kicking.

What are the safety considerations in this scenario? In these scenarios, the individual's first impulse is to enter the trailer and calm the animal. However, this puts the individual at a significant risk of injury as the animal struggles; in addition, the human's nervousness and fear may worsen the animal's panic and struggle.

The attempted solution. The veterinarian arrived, opened the trailer escape door, and administered an IV tranquilizer. A friend entered the trailer from the right side to calm the animal and attempt to free its leg. The horse never stopped kicking.

Local police were dispatched and closed the roadway. Although present, local emergency responders lacked the knowledge to respond to the scenario. Over 50 bystanders gathered to watch the event. Two hours elapsed as the horse continued to kick and the veterinarian administered tranquilizers every 15 minutes; the horse would appear sedated, but any noise aroused him and he would resume kicking. The person in the trailer finally freed the entrapped hindlimb and slowly removed the divider. The divider was passed through the right rear door of the trailer after the door latch was cut and spread with hydraulic spreaders (jaws of life). Firefighters cut open the other door. The horse fell down in the trailer; the center post (between the two back doors) was cut at the ceiling and bent down.

The horse was dragged out of the trailer by its tail and legs onto a lawn.

What are the medical concerns associated with this scenario? Entrapped and struggling animals are at high risk of bone fracture, tendon/ligament injury, skin wounds (including lacerations and degloving injuries), dehydration, and hypovolemic shock. The animal in this scenario sustained severe lacerations and was in shock. Following extrication, the animal was transported to a veterinary facility and provided IV fluid support and critical care. Long-term care was necessary for the wounds, but the animal recovered from its injuries.

Lessons learned. This scenario emphasizes the importance of an incident action plan (IAP) and training in TLAER techniques. Poor planning increases the probability of an unsuccessful outcome. Responders trained in TLAER techniques are better equipped to devise an effective IAP.

Although human injuries did not occur in this scenario, the risk was high. As stated previously, personnel should not be allowed to enter a confined space with an entrapped animal. Opening the escape doors of the trailer presented a significant risk of injury to the animal and personnel if the animal attempted to exit the trailer through the door (*Note:* The escape doors are designed for human exit, and animals that attempt to exit through these doors are often trapped or injured).

The animal's exaggerated response to noise negated the effects of the sedation. Measures should be taken to reduce stimulation (e.g., noise, sound, etc.) of sedated but excitable animals. Placement of ear plugs, and possibly a blindfold, may have facilitated restraint and calmed the animal.

Sedative and tranquilizer medications have a more rapid onset time when administered intravenously; although administration of the medication in this case was accomplished without injury, the safety risks were significant. Intramuscular administration of a higher dose, using a jab-stick if necessary, allows initial sedation from a safe distance and prevents the veterinarian from entering a confined space with an excited, struggling animal. If possible and available (depending on the scenario), the induction of general anesthesia may have facilitated this rescue effort.

Prevention. Animals should be trained to load and trailer safely and calmly. Some animals trailer more comfortably in stock-type trailers. Protecting the animal's limbs with good quality leg wraps or shipping bandages can reduce the risk of limb injury during transport. Animals may panic in response to foreign objects or insects entering the trailer during transport; open windows should be protected with screens.

Mule Down Embankment

A 23-year-old mule rolled approximately 100 ft (30 m) down a low-angle rock outcropping. Although conscious, the 500 kg (1,100 lb) animal was dehydrated and exhausted from trying to rise. It could lift its head, but its hindquarters appeared to be paralyzed. The owner requested transport to an equine hospital for testing and treatment.

How can this animal be extricated, and what complications can be expected? The mule was located approximately 200 m (660 ft) from the ambulance trailer. The ground was soft from previous rain showers, and there were no trees to serve as anchors for a mechanical advantage rope system in the direction needed to move the animal. Equine emergency rescue unit (EERU) staff carried the Rescue Glide, padded hood, two canes (for safe leg handling), and a 10 cm diameter, 7 m (23 ft) nylon strap.

The 10 cm strap was also put around the shoulders and chest of the mule into a forward assist position; it was anchored to the front of the glide to provide support to the animal during the ascent up the hill as well as to keep it from sliding off of the back of the Rescue Glide.

Since the hill was too soft for heavy equipment, a long tow strap was secured to a tractor at the top of the hill and attached to the Rescue Glide. Two 8 mm (5/16 in.), 5 ft (1.5 m) long Prusik loops were attached to the rear corners of the Rescue Glide to assist in steering as the mule was hauled to the trailer. After clearing several obstacles out of the path of the tractor, the patient was successfully moved to within 10 m (33 ft) of the trailer. Using the slip sheet to reduce drag friction on the Rescue Glide, the winch cable was secured to the leading edge of the glide, and the animal was pulled into the EERU trailer for transport.

Lessons learned. The rescue was effective and relatively efficient, despite the obstacles encountered. During retrospective evaluation of the rescue, the rescuers recommended providing support to the animal's rear in addition to chest and shoulder support. The rescuers now have a strong Cordura nylon tarp rigged to encapsulate the animal's hips and anchor to the glide; if the animal does slip backward on the Rescue Glide, the tarp provides additional support.

Barn Fires

Barn fires killed a total of 34 horses in Clifton, Virginia, and Elkton, Maryland, within a one-week period. The Clifton fire was reported at 2:40 a.m., when a neighbor observed flames and called 911. The extreme heat and intensity of the fire prevented the neighbor or firefighters from saving any of the horses inside the barn.

The Elkton fire was reported at 6:40 p.m. and burned the 14,000-square-foot barn to the ground. More than 100 firefighters from three states fought the fire for 90 minutes before bringing it under control. The barn was not equipped with fire alarms or a sprinkler system; the Maryland fire code doesn't require either system in a barn.

Lessons learned. As stated in Chapter 10, barns are often fully engulfed in flames when the fires are noticed; there is often little opportunity to rescue the horses, unless personnel are already present at the scene when the fire begins. Fire alarms can decrease response time if they are directly linked to emergency dispatch. Sprinkler systems are highly recommended and can be an effective means of suppressing fires.

Horses in Stalls as Floodwaters Rise

Horses were trapped in a barn as water rose quickly after a beaver dam collapsed. A passerby called 911 and attempted to rescue the animals by opening all the stall doors.

Solution? Firefighters arrived to find the animals running down the road after their release. They were able to stop traffic and catch the animals, and they called animal control for transport to a nearby farm.

Lessons learned. Animals should be caught and led separately from the structure to safety. The amount of time required to catch the loose animals likely exceeded the time it would have required for responders to catch and lead individual horses to safety. In addition, the risk of a secondary incident caused by the loose animals negates the benefit obtained by freeing them from the flooding structure.

Prevention. Animal owners located in potential or confirmed flood plains should consider the geography of the area when determining the site and construction of the barn and have flood emergency plans in place. Posted signs with emergency contact information and an emergency plan facilitate a rapid, efficient response.

Haltered Horse Recumbant in Stall

EERU staff was contacted by a local veterinarian to request transport for an injured horse down in a barn stall. Upon arrival, the team was advised that the two-year-old gelding had been left in the stall overnight wearing a nylon halter. The gelding's right hind hoof was caught in the halter underneath the chin strap. The horse had severe abrasions on its body from thrashing around the stall for an unknown amount of time. Severe swelling of the head and neck were observed;

the animal was unable to open its eyes due to the swelling and injuries.

How will you get the animal out of the stall and to the ambulance? The horse's size prevented extrication on a Rescue Glide through the existing stall door, so the owner cut a larger doorway with a chainsaw after EERU staff placed ear plugs (made of soft rags) and a blindfold on the horse. Hobbles were applied to all four legs, but the horse displayed signs of discomfort as attempts were made to "package" him on the Rescue Glide; the limbs were secured together with a large steel carabiner, but not flexed toward the body. The Rescue Glide was pulled out of the stall using an all-terrain vehicle and maneuvered into the ambulance trailer for transportation to the veterinary hospital. The horse was monitored via a wireless video surveillance system during transportation.

Notes. Approximately 30 minutes away from the veterinary hospital, the driver observed the horse had moved its head, and pulled over and adjusted the pad back underneath the horse's severely swollen head. The owner was present to help make the adjustment. Upon arrival to the equine hospital, the horse was dead. The veterinarian hypothesized that the horse may have fractured its neck during its struggle to free its foot from the halter, or head trauma may have caused severe brain swelling and additional internal injuries. The owner did not authorize a necropsy; therefore, the exact cause of death was not determined.

Lessons learned. This scenario demonstrates that animals can sustain life-threatening injuries and can rapidly decompensate and die after rescue. Although veterinary care was not provided on the scene, it is unlikely that it would have been successful because of the severity of the injuries.

Prevention. Only properly fitting halters should be used on animals; poorly fitted halters are more likely to become caught on objects or permit an extremity to become entrapped in them. Halters with breakaway leather straps are recommended for young, excitable horses. This case provides evidence for the assertion that horses should not be haltered while in box stalls.

Arthritic, Geriatric Horse Down

A 37-year-old gelding was found recumbent (down) and motionless near a paddock gate. The gelding's eyes were open and he was breathing normally, but he was recumbent on top of an ice patch and made no attempts to rise.

How can one or a few people address this scenario? Nearby, two construction workers noticed the predicament and offered to help. The owner asked them to help pull the horse off the icy area by its tail. The fence section near the horse was removed, and a sturdy rope was tied to the horse's tail. Despite their efforts, they could not move the animal.

Now what? A forklift was nearby at the construction site, and was brought to the paddock area. One end of a long rope was flossed underneath the horse's hindquarters and around its abdomen and the other end of the rope was passed around the horse's chest; the resulting configuration formed a "handle" over the horse's back. The forklift approached the horse from the back and lowered the forks. One person threaded the rope handle on the tines, and the operator raised the forks to lift the horse off of the ice and set it down on firm ground.

Alternate method. A forward assist, backward drag, or sideways drag using a web sling could be used to pull the horse off the ice to firm ground. If the horse was unable to stand, a vertical lift or forklift-assisted lift may be necessary if a forward assist is unsuccessful.

Lessons learned. This small on-farm rescue is a common scenario involving geriatric and cast animals. Simple methods are often successful in these situations.

Prevention. Geriatric animals or those likely to have difficulty rising from a recumbent position should only be turned out in areas with good quality footing and should be monitored. Arthritis is a common condition in geriatric horses; medical treatment of arthritis improves the animal's comfort, quality of life, and ability to provide the hind limb propulsion necessary to rise to a standing position.

Stuck in the Muck

A Paint gelding was being allowed to drink from a creek during a trail ride. As the horse crossed the creek, he sank into the river bottom past his knees and was exhausted when he made it to the opposite bank. Another horse, ridden by a child, became severely mired in the muddy river bottom.

What field-expedient equipment might be available to perform a rescue? The people on scene pulled on the horse's head using the bridle reins and with lead ropes attached to the other horses' saddles. All attempts were unsuccessful, serving only to destroy the equipment.

A tractor was brought to the scene, but its center of gravity was high, and the mechanical advantage of a forward pull was lost. A small backhoe arrived, and the mare was extricated by looping ropes underneath and around her body and pulling with the backhoe.

Notes. Although the mare initially collapsed on the bank after extrication from the mud, she was uninjured.

Lessons learned. This scenario demonstrates that using an animal's head and neck as anchors is not recommended. Strong tension on an animal's head is often met with struggling and resistance. In addition, an animal that does not have freedom of its head and neck is less able to maintain its balance and assist in its own rescue. If possible, any inflatable personal flotation device, inner tube, or other device will be capable of giving the animal support for its head in the water or mud.

Prevention. Although not all trail incidents are preventable, proper attention to trail safety (including assessment of surfaces underneath water) can prevent many situations.

Horse Fallen from Moving Trailer

A 14-year-old gelding was severely injured when he fell from the back of a moving horse trailer and was dragged by the lead rope (still anchored to the trailer). The horse sustained severe abrasions to its abdomen, hindquarters, and hind limbs. The accident was observed by a neighbor, who stopped and directed traffic to avoid a collision and flagged down an oncoming vehicle. Coincidentally, a veterinary student was a passenger in the vehicle; the student was able to slow the hemorrhage (bleeding), and the horse was taken to a veterinary hospital, where he spent the next two weeks in intensive care.

The horse's condition was initially considered very guarded, but improved as it responded to treatment. Extensive daily treatments and medications were required for several months, and a full recovery was expected to require more than 12 months.

Lessons learned. A prompt response by the neighbor reduced the risk of a secondary incident (vehicle collision). Abrasive injuries, such as those sustained when dragged across road surfaces, are very similar to thermal injuries (burns) and require significant healing time.

Prevention. Appropriate trailer maintenance includes routine inspection of all door and gate latches. Damaged or failing latches should be replaced prior to use of the trailer for transporting animals. The use of a breakable link between the trailer tie and the trailer (e.g., a loop of bailing twine) would have prevented the animal from being dragged, but would not have prevented the horse from being ejected from the trailer due to latch failure.

Trapped between Bridge and Tree

An Arabian horse was found pinned between a bridge and a large tree. He was dehydrated and bloodied from struggling.

Solution? A web sling was emplaced, and the horse was manually extricated following mild sedation. The horse was moved off the bridge, allowed to recover, and walked to the barn for further assessment and treatment.

Notes. The horse died nine days later from complications from the injuries sustained in the accident, despite rapid initiation of treatment and appropriate care. A necropsy was not done—the mechanism of injury was unknown.

Lessons learned. Animals can sustain life-threatening injuries during their struggles and may not survive despite appropriate treatment.

Prevention. Access to potentially dangerous areas in pastures and paddocks should be prevented by secure fencing.

Horse in a Hole

A yearling quarter horse was found in a hole, with only its front legs visible above the ground surface.

Solution? When the legs were tied together and the animal's head was protected, the horse was tranquilized by a veterinarian to prevent injury to itself and people assisting in the rescue. Attempts to extricate the horse manually with ropes were unsuccessful. A tractor was brought to the scene, and ropes were attached to the horse's halter and leg hobbles. The horse was successfully extricated from the hole, and it was uninjured.

Lessons learned. This case demonstrates a scenario where the animal's distal limbs must be used as anchors. Increasing the surface area of rope in contact with the skin, such as the use of Prusik loops on the distal limb, reduces the risk of injury to the distal limbs. Alternatively, padding inserted between the hobbles and skin increases protection of the soft tissues of the limb. Care must be taken to ensure the head and neck are supported.

Prevention. Although the hole was not in the animal's pasture, a weakness in the fence allowed access to the area and other hazards. Proper fence maintenance includes regular evaluation of the fence for weakness and prompt repair.

Filly Trapped in a Feed Bunk

The EERU responded to a 250 kg (550 lb) filly trapped upside down in a feed bunk built into the wall of a barn. (This type of incident is extremely common and includes feeders, hay racks, and water tubs.) The bunk measured approximately 1 m (3 ft) tall and 2.2 m (7 ft) long. The horse filled the volume of the feeder, with only its feet protruding above the edge. A veterinary assessment revealed the horse to be dehydrated and showing signs of shock. The owner stated the horse could potentially have been trapped in the feed bunk for up to 20 hours.

How can this horse be extricated? Given the location of the horse's head and the fact that its body filled most of the feed bunk, the option of cutting the horse out of it with a chain saw was deemed too dangerous.

Using 2.5 cm (1 in.) tubular webbing, EERU staff rigged an anchor point on a 15 cm (6 in.) wide structure post approximately 2 m (6 1/2 ft) above the ground, where the ground post and the roof struts were bolted together. It was positioned so that the horse would be raised at a 45-degree angle using a 4:1 mechanical advantage rope system.

The responders used a custom sewn lifting strap that measured 3 m (10 ft) in length and 30 cm (1 ft) in width as a back and shoulder support; it was passed underneath the horses head and flossed underneath the animal until it was located behind the withers. A 4:1 pull system was assembled and attached to the strap using a large steel carabineer. The horse was pulled up into a "sitting" position, using the horse's hindquarters as a fulcrum point. The horse then was able to lean forward and tip out of the bunk.

Notes. The horse was unable to stand, so it was put in a recumbent position, warmed with a blanket, and treated for a minor rectal prolapse that resulted from the strain of her struggle. The horse was eating within 15 minutes of the rescue. After 45 minutes of treatment, the filly was able to stand on her own.

Lessons learned. This scenario used the filly's hindquarters as a fulcrum for pulling the front end upward and tipping the horse out of the bunk. Although no responder injuries occurred, this scenario presents the risk of injury from the animal's limbs; proper head protection is recommended when performing TLAER.

Prevention. Stall hazards, such as the feed bunk encountered in this scenario, should be removed from stalls (especially stalls containing young or excitable animals) or modified to break apart when animals become entrapped.

Horse in the Mud

A mare was found mired to withers level in the mud of a dried-up farm pond. Several people had used shovels in an attempt to dig the mare out of the mud, but the mud refilled each hole created by the shovels.

Solution? Boards were placed on top of the mud to provide secure surfaces for humans to stand on around the horse. The animal had been in the mud for at least four hours and was exhausted from struggling. A leather Santa Barbara sling was emplaced around the mare's chest. Very few personnel were on the scene; therefore, a winch was attached to one of the sling buckles at a 90-degree angle to her body, and a plywood board was placed against the mare's back for leverage. The mare was rolled out of the mud using injected air to break the suction and onto her side on the plywood. The winch was used to pull the mare the remaining 25 m (82 ft) out of the pond.

Lessons learned. Although successful in this scenario, a winch should never be attached directly to an animal (or to a sling placed on the animal). Mechanical advantage rope systems are preferred for this method. However, this successful rescue demonstrates that the rescue plan must be adapted to the individual scenario and the personnel and equipment available.

Truck Tire Blowout

While talking on her cellular phone, an owner hauling two horses in a bumper-pull trailer at 110 kph (68 mph) lost control of the vehicle when the right front tire of her pickup truck blew out. Evaluation of the tire tracks showed the rig veered sharply to the right and jumped the entrance ramp toward the yield sign before the driver could stop the rig. The trailer did not overturn.

Solution? The horses were uninjured, appeared unconcerned, and were easily unloaded and reloaded into the ambulance trailer for transport to safe facilities while the tire was replaced and the vehicle was driven to a dealer for assessment and repairs.

Lessons learned. This scenario demonstrates the importance of driver attention and vehicle maintenance. Although not all tire failures can be predicted, proper vehicle maintenance and attention to the road eliminates the risks of excessive tire wear, inadequate tire inflation, bearing lubrication, and road hazard-induced tire damage.

Prevention. Appropriate speeds are recommended when trailering animals. In addition, distractions such as cellular phone conversations increase the risk of vehicular incidents.

Impaired Commercial Horse Van Driver

Fourteen draft-type horses were being hauled from New York to Kentucky for post-international importation quarantine. The driver was drinking beer while driving and veered off the road in the early morning hours on a two-lane, rural road. The trailer hit a tree and fell onto its right side, wedged on top of a dead tree trunk approximately 4 ft (1.2 m) above the ground. The preliminary scene assessment revealed horses with their legs through the trailer windows, horses trapped underneath others, and multiple injured horses.

What are the special considerations in this scenario? The animals were subject to federal quarantine restrictions, and communication with state and federal authorities was necessary before the rescue attempt could be initiated. The state veterinarian's office dispatched a representative to maintain federal quarantine restrictions on the shipment of horses.

A veterinarian with TLAER training responded within minutes of the accident, along with a team of trained firefighter rescue professionals. By the time responders arrived at the scene, a well-meaning bystander had already entered the horse compartment. The bystander was removed from the compartment, and responders provided alfalfa hay to keep the horses calm while they evaluated the situation and developed a response plan.

How can the animals be extricated? The decision was made to cut a hole in the back wall of the trailer and create a ramp to lead the ambulatory horses out of the trailer. The recumbent animals were sedated and allowed to slide out through a large defect in the lowest sidewall of the trailer (which was 4 ft off the ground on stumps). Two horses died as a result of injuries sustained in the accident, but the remaining 12 horses were triaged at a farm across the road and loaded on another trailer for transport to the quarantine station.

Lessons learned. This rescue is an example of the benefits of experienced, TLAER-trained personnel on the scene of an incident. Responder safety was preserved, and the response was efficient and successful.

Prevention. Driver impairment, and possibly speed, played an important causative role in this incident.

Horse Trapped in Trailer

A horse owner on her way to a show brought one horse to the show grounds early, before anyone there was available to help. She started to unload her horse, but when she opened the back door on the two-horse trailer, the horse attempted to back out of the trailer before the butt-bar was removed and before the trailer tie could be disengaged. The animal was bleeding from its mouth. One front limb was entrapped in the manger, and the other limb protruded from the window on the left side of the trailer. The horse's full weight was pulling on the trailer tie, and the horse's back limbs were underneath it in a sitting position. The horse was quiet and minimally responsive.

How should this situation be addressed? The horse's leg was gently pushed back into the trailer. The trailer tie was not cut for fear that the horse would fall over backward if it was cut. The divider was removed, and both trailer doors were opened. Rescuers startled the horse to urge it to a standing position. As soon as the tension of the animal's weight was released, the panic snap on the trailer tie disconnected, and the horse bolted backward off the trailer. The owner contained and caught the horse. The only injury sustained was a broken tooth, and the horse was shown successfully the same day.

Lessons learned. The presence of blood often instills panic in owners but is not necessarily associated with the severity of the injuries. Panic snaps, although designed to release in emergency situations, often fail to disengage when excessive tension is placed upon them. The horse in this incident demonstrated a prey species response commonly called *sulking*; after struggling unsuccessfully to free itself, the animal stops struggling and becomes minimally responsive to stimuli. Sulking animals present significant danger in that they can suddenly and explosively move without warning, increasing the risk of animal and responder injury. Retrospective evaluation of this incident suggests that the rear trailer doors should have been shut once the divider was removed and personnel exited the trailer, to allow the horse to be contained after it rose. Also, a second, longer lead rope attached to the horse's halter and held by a handler could have prevented the animal from becoming loose when the panic snap disengaged.

Horse Stuck in Mud

A Thoroughbred horse placed in a new pasture became trapped in the thick mud 20 ft (6 m) from shore. When discovered, the animal was exhausted and hypothermic.

Solution? The veterinarian attempted to extricate the animal by himself. After several hours of unsuccessful attempts, the horse was euthanatized, and the carcass was removed with a tractor.

Bottom line? It is extremely dangerous and unsafe for personnel to attempt rescues without assistance. In addition, rescue attempts by solitary individuals are often unsuccessful.

Cow in Farm Pond

A cow became trapped to the level of her abdomen in mud only 2 m (6 1/2 ft) from shore in a pond. Local farmers gathered to attempt to remove the cow from its predicament. A tractor, ropes, chain, and a winch were brought to the scene.

Solution? After wading into the mud to reach the cow, the owner placed the winch cable around the cow's neck. The winch was turned on, and the command to reel it in was given. When the cable tightened around her neck, the cow struggled against the tension. The operator turned off the winch, which slowly ceased tightening. By the time the winch stopped pulling on the cable, the animal had been decapitated.

What would have been an appropriate method for rescuing this cow? Using boards for secure footing, rescuers should have emplaced webbing for a forward assist using manual traction or a mechanical advantage rope system to extricate the animal. As stated in Chapter 7, the injection of air into the mud around the animal's limbs greatly facilitates extrication.

Lessons learned. Rescuers should avoid entering mud with entrapped animals because they may themselves become mired and require rescue. As previously stated numerous times, the head and neck of an animal are not acceptable anchor points unless no other options are available. Vehicles or winches should never be directly attached to an animal; rope systems allow controlled tension that can be easily applied and released.

Prevention. Animal access to potentially hazardous areas should be prevented by secure fencing.

Horse Caught over Wooden Fence

Several horses were playing in an arena at liberty when the youngest animal was chased by a dominant animal and attempted to escape by jumping the fence. The filly's front end cleared the fence panel, but her hind end was caught on the fence and she was suspended over the wooden fence board and electrified wire. The filly was quiet and allowed rescuers to approach and calm her.

What are the hazards and challenges associated with this situation? The primary hazards in this situation are the wooden fence, the electrical wire, and the presence of a large number of bystanders (including children). Young animals are often more excitable, and present handling challenges. After power to the electric fence was disconnected, the owner approached the horse and calmed it while another rescuer cut the wire and

fence board with a reciprocating saw. The horse was uninjured.

Lessons learned. This scenario is an example of the effectiveness of a well-designed plan. The hazards were addressed by disconnecting the power to the electric fence and cutting the board. The importance of a calm individual in control of the animal cannot be overstated.

Prevention. Placing groups of animals in small areas can increase dominant herd behavior and increase the risk of injuries and incidents. Subordinate animals should be provided with adequate escape areas.

Mare and Foal in Barn Fire

An Arabian foal was born after midnight, and the owner placed a heat lamp in the stall for the foal. The heat lamp fell into a feeder, initiating a fire at approximately 4 a.m. A passerby saw the fire, called 911, and alerted the owners of the farm. By the time the owners got to the fire, the barn was fully engulfed, and the horses were dead of smoke inhalation.

The horses inside are lost, but are there others? An Arabian stallion contained in a run near the burning barn was saved, and firefighters were able to control the fire and protect nearby livestock and structures.

Lessons learned. Wooden structures are fire hazards and become quickly engulfed. Prevention of barn fires is critical.

Prevention. Unprotected appliances should never be left unattended in barns. A fire alarm may have signaled the fire in time for a rescue to take place, and a sprinkler system may have suppressed the fire and prevented the animal losses. Modern barn materials are less flammable and safer.

INCIDENT OVERVIEWS

The following represents a small portion of recent incidents collected by the author that demonstrate various aspects of TLAER concepts, both good and bad, that have occurred. Responders attempting to provide justification to their department for funding training and equipment are encouraged to conduct an intensive Internet search for reported incidents.

TheHorse.com, 2007

A barn fire at Eureka Downs racetrack in southeast Kansas killed 43 horses, and only one horse survived the flames. The 90-stall barn was built in 1989 and required three hours and three fire engines to successfully extinguish the fire. The Kansas fire marshal is investigating the cause of the fire. The survivor suffered smoke inhalation and severe burns of 25% of his body. The horse is expected to survive the fire but its racing future is uncertain. Early estimates pegged the total damage at $1 million.

On-Scene Report, 2006

Three hundred goats on their way to a New Jersey slaughterhouse were killed in a rollover accident in Lampasas County. The next year over 240 goats were killed in a similar accident near San Francisco. Seven hundred goats were in a cattle trailer when the driver of the 18-wheeler hauling the goats swerved to avoid deer in the road, causing the truck to overturn on its right side.

The Anderson News, September 1, 2004

A Kentucky couple's horse was mired in mud up to its neck and withers, and the female owner, seeking to sooth the animal, also became trapped in the mud. Emergency responders extricated the woman, and firefighters from the Lexington Fire Department used air injection to break the suction of the mud while a vertical web sling was used to lift the animal with a large tractor. A local veterinarian on the scene treated the horse for minor injuries and exhaustion.

Las Vegas Review Journal, January 14, 2005

Ranchers and cowboys worked together to rescue over 600 cattle and calves trapped in mud and rising floodwaters in the Virgin River, Nevada. A National Guard helicopter was used to drop one day's ration of hay to them. The floodwaters were only 100 m wide, but extremely fast moving. As the cattle were driven across the water, one horse slipped into quicksand and briefly trapped her rider underneath her in the water. At least 10 stranded cattle were trapped in mud and could not be rescued; the animals died in place. Ranchers reported unsuccessful attempts to remove them by their tails from the mud.

The Miami Herald, April 6, 2004

Two girls were riding along a suburban neighborhood road when one was thrown from her horse. The horse ran down the road until it was hit by a pickup truck. The horse sustained a broken leg and was euthanatized on the scene by a veterinarian. This was the second incident involving a horse–vehicle collision; the horse in the previous incident was instantly killed on impact.

The Garden City Telegram, April 11, 2001

The rear wheels on a cattle liner trailer locked up, causing a fire that burned a hole in the rear of the aluminum trailer and killed four cows. The surviving cattle were transferred to another trailer via a separate ramp system before the ruined trailer could be removed from the highway.

BBC News World Edition, July 20, 1982

A car bomb in Hyde Park exploded as Blues and Royals troopers made their way to the Changing of the Guard ceremony. Four troopers and seven horses were killed in the IRA bomb blast, and several men and horses were severely injured.

theadvocate.com, June 24, 2004

A defectively designed westbound on-ramp to the I-10 bridge over the Mississippi River and a broken speed limit warning sign caused a 1994 cattle trailer wreck that killed one man, paralyzed another, and set a herd of 98 cattle loose on the freeway and in a neighborhood. The incident required almost 12 hours to capture all the cattle and clean up the scene. A judgment against the state of Louisiana Department of Transportation was ordered in the sum of $8.2 million dollars.

The Clarion Ledger, August 26, 2004

An overturned cattle trailer obstructed traffic for at least four hours on Interstates 20 and 55, and U.S. Highways 80 and 49 in Mississippi as over 50 head of loose cattle were rounded up by firefighters, police, and riders. The driver stated the load shifted at the curve on I-55. Nineteen cattle were killed in the initial overturn.

The Daily and Sunday Review, September 23, 2004

Eighteen cattle died on impact or had to be euthanatized on the scene of a cattle truck overturn. The crash sheared off the roof of the cattle trailer as it slid past several trees, allowing 31 animals to escape into a neighborhood for several hours. Bystanders chased the animals for over four hours.

Henry Herald, October 21, 2004

The cattle contained in an overturned cattle truck were cooled by fans brought by rescue workers while loose cattle were herded off the freeway. Thirteen cattle and the driver died in the incident on I-75.

The Grand Rapids Press, December 28, 2004

Firefighters in surface ice rescue gear, a veterinarian, and neighbors with heavy equipment arrived on the scene to rescue a draft horse trapped in ice. The ambient temperature was 3°C (37° F), and the horse's body temperature had dropped to 35°C (95° F) by the time she was successfully pulled to shore using ropes and a pickup. The horse was placed underneath a tarp and hot air from blowers powered by a generator, and warmed IV fluids were administered. The owner reportedly planned to fence off the pond to prevent future accidents.

The Star-Ledger, December 31, 2004

More than 100 people, including various emergency personnel, responded to assist with extricating two weanling horses from ice 33 ft (10 m) from shore on a frozen pond. A responder walked out onto the ice and roped each horse. The rope was attached to a pickup truck, and the horse pulled from the ice. A veterinarian treated the horses on the scene.

Rapid City Journal, April 12, 2004

A cattle truck containing 40 bison was driven at excessive speed for the weather and road conditions at midnight and overturned on a Montana highway. Fourteen hours elapsed as the rescue occurred. Four bison died during the overturn, and two were euthanatized due to the presence of severe injuries. Winches were used to remove live animals that refused to leave the trailer. The hooves of many of the bison penetrated the thin sidewalls of the trailer. Ten bison that escaped from the trailer were shot by patrolmen after being assessed by the insurance company because the animals could not be herded and reloaded in another trailer.

The Providence Journal, February 21, 2005

Firefighters and emergency medical technicians rescued a horse in a 3 m (10 ft) deep frozen pool in a backyard using ropes and fire hoses. A department of public works backhoe broke up the ice in the pool so that 15 people could free the horse within 25 minutes.

Nugget Newspaper, January 20, 2004

A horse caught in a ranch irrigation pond was rescued by his owners. They lassoed the horse from the bank and crawled out on the ice to place a halter on the horse. Using sledgehammers, they cracked an ice path to shore. The owner landed in the water next to the horse on at least one occasion as she was breaking the path, and she was not wearing PPE.

The Daily Record, April 13, 2005

A semi-trailer hauling 87 hogs to market near Benson, North Carolina, overturned at the I-40/I-95 interchange due to excessive speed. The rescue effort to save the animals inside the trailer was successful: only four sows died. Three smaller trailers were brought in with cattle panels to move the pigs. Local swine experts were called in to assist with moving the hogs. Firefighters used water to hose down and cool the animals while on the scene for over four hours.

The Daily Star, December 23, 2003

A horse fell through the ice of a pond, and rescuers used ropes tied to the tail to pull the horse onto the ice and then to solid ground using human power. Two firefighters donned wetsuits to break up the ice around the animal with sledgehammers. Heat packs and blankets were used to warm the animal successfully.

NBC17.com, April 22, 2005

Cowboys responded to an overturned cattle truck scene to assist with rounding up 13 loose cattle that fled into surrounding neighborhoods. Three animals were euthanatized on the scene by a veterinarian called to the accident. Traffic was stopped for two hours.

lol.com, April 14, 2005

In Lagos, Nigeria, nineteen people were killed and numerous more were injured when a cattle truck's tires blew out and it overturned in a ditch. The truck was hauling cattle and human passengers in the trailer.

Baldwin City Signal, April 21, 2005

A fully loaded cattle trailer overturned in a neighborhood. The roof had to be cut open to extricate over 50 cattle. Cattle panels were brought to the scene to contain the animals until local cattle farmers arrived with trailers to transport the cattle off site. The road was closed for five hours. A bull bit a person.

Personal report, North Wales, United Kingdom, 2005

In North Wales, United Kingdom, a young bull walked onto a pool cover, fell through into the pool, and was struggling in 4 ft of water. Firefighters got into the pool with the bullock and slung a makeshift fire hose sling around its rear end, allowing them to assist it to exit the pool by climbing stairs made of concrete blocks.

Personal report, Canterbury, United Kingdom, 2 November, 1998

In Canterbury, United Kingdom, a large tree fell onto a stable, trapping a horse underneath the branches and inside the crushed stable. Firefighters spent two hours cutting away the branches and metal; a veterinarian assisted by sedating the animal. A fire hose sling in forward assist configuration was fashioned around the horse's body, and the animal was pulled out from underneath the wreckage with minimal injuries.

Firehouse.com, April 11, 2005

A horse slipped into a concrete drainage ditch 1 m (3 ft) deep and 1 m wide and ended up on its back for several hours. Responders, including a veterinarian, unsuccessfully attempted to lift the animal with straps around all four legs using a small tractor. The veterinarian tranquilized the animal and attached a tractor chain to the animal's halter and pulled it out using the halter as an anchor point. The animal survived.

North Metro Fire Rescue, March 5, 2005

In Northglenn, Colorado, a horse fell into the owner's backyard pool and was trapped in the pool cover. Fire crews drained the pool, called for a crane and a veterinarian to harness the horse, and performed a vertical lift to remove the horse from the pool three hours later.

High Desert Star, April 27, 2005

A highly trained border collie and her owner, who worked with animal control, responded to assist police officers with a herd of 20 loose horses running away from a stable and out onto neighborhood streets. The dog was able to round up all of the horses and return them to their stable within minutes of arriving on scene.

Bedford Bulletin, April 13, 2005

A 6 ft sinkhole collapsed as a farmer was plowing his garden with two draft horses, and the animals disappeared into the 10 ft (3 m) deep hole with the plow attached. Two backhoes were called in by police to slowly remove the soil and walk the top horse out of the hole up a soil ramp. The second horse was sedated, straps were attached, and it was lifted by a backhoe to its feet.

Telegram and Gazette, July 12, 2001

A horse fell through an old bridge in Pisgah State Park, Vermont. Fire and rescue responders used webbing around the horse's chest to pull the sedated and blindfolded animal to safety on the bank out of the muddy marsh.

Times Dispatch, January 10, 2001

A horse trailer containing two horses was overturned by crosswinds on an Interstate 95 bridge in Virginia. Two veterinarians and fire rescue responded. Two lanes were closed for two hours while the horses were sedated, removed, and loaded in alternate transport.

The Saratogian, March 20, 2004

A horse wandered onto a frozen pond and fell through the ice. Fire department responders used axes to make a channel to the horse, placed a rope on its halter, and led it to dry ground. Cold water rescue suits were worn by the responders.

Inland Valley Daily Bulletin, March 22, 2004

A horse was mired in quicksand in the bottom of a floodwater debris basin; as it struggled, it sank to its withers in the mud. Rescuers supported the animal's head and kept its nostrils out of the muddy water while forward assist straps were emplaced. Firefighters manually pulled the animal out of the mud in minutes.

Sun Sentinel, January 27, 2004

Firefighters trained in equine rescue worked to save a horse accidentally ridden into a canal late in the day. Earlier, untrained rescuers had unsuccessfully attempted to extricate the animal using a tractor. Using a harness and rope systems, the trained responders were able to lift the animal out of the canal. This was the second horse in canal incident in a week in the area.

Sentinel, November 15, 2002

A sinkhole swallowed a barn and two horses into a mass of mud, trees, and barn parts. The first horse drowned soon after the collapse. Fire department personnel worked with a local veterinarian to attempt a rescue, including pumping water out of the hole as it filled to give them time to place rescue equipment on the animal. In the end, the second animal died as well, as the suction effect of the mud prevented rescuers from pulling the animal to safety. The animal died as it was removed with a winch and webbing around its body; it was asphyxiated by the equipment. This case demonstrates the importance of planning, training, and correct methods; a rescue attempt cannot be considered a success if the animal is killed by the rescue method.

LAFD News, May 30, 2005

Fire, EMS, heavy rescue, animal services and U.S. Search and Rescue (USAR) members responded to assist with a horse mired to chest level in mud. An individual became temporarily pinned underneath the struggling animal and was injured. Professional rescuers used webbing to quickly and successfully extricate the animal. A veterinarian responded to evaluate the animal and pronounced it healthy.

KSL News, May 12, 2005

A horse became entrapped in soggy ground while being ridden, and the owner contacted 911 after several hours of unsuccessful attempts to extricate the horse. Firefighters and animal control officers dug trenches on each side of the animal and scooped the excess mud and water out with buckets. The animal was able to walk out of the trench.

WSVN News, September 2, 2003

A horse trapped overnight in a mud hole was rescued by firefighters in Miramar, Florida, using heavy equipment and webbing; however, it was unable to rise due to exhaustion. Firefighters and EMS kept the animal stable with supplemental oxygen and cooled it with water until the veterinarian arrived to administer IV fluids and medications to support the animal. Eight hours later, the animal was pronounced to be recovered.

NBC10.com, July 7, 2004

A Belgian draft horse slipped and fell in 6 in. (15 cm) of mud and could not rise. Local firefighters and a crane company responded, using webbing to raise the animal. Although the webbing could have been placed more safely than it was, underneath the neck, the animal was lifted to its feet.

Sligo Weekender News, November 29, 2005

A cattle trailer containing three cows became unhitched and slid into the quay under the bridge in the UK. Two animals survived and fought for breath inside the almost submerged trailer for an hour while rescue crews in boats used cutters to remove the gate on the trailer. The cows jumped to freedom and swam to the opposite shore to safety. The animals were contained and loaded onto another trailer for transport.

Knoxville.com, September 11, 1984

A cattle truck loaded with 78 weanling and yearling foals overturned on Interstate 40 in Kentucky. Several horses had escaped the wrecked trailer, several were dead, and several more had severe injuries that necessitated euthanasia on the scene. Several others were euthanatized several days later due to their injuries. Twenty-one of the animals were loaded on another trailer and transported to a veterinary school for intensive treatment; the remaining animals were released for transport to their new homes.

Angus Fire.com, June 2000

A woman was trapped underneath her horse in a ditch for over an hour before a man walking his dog found her; the horse was on the woman's legs. Fire crews used air bags to lift the horse enough to free the woman's legs. Four hours later, using fire hoses to make a sling, the horse was pulled free of the ditch.

Manchester Online, November 28, 2002

Striking firefighters left their picket line to save a drowning horse trapped for six hours in a ditch near Manchester, United Kingdom. After the British Army said they could only respond to human emergencies, the owners pleaded for the firefighters to assist. The 90-minute operation involved muscle power, gentle persuasion, bales of hay, and a mechanical digger; the horse was successfully rescued.

Owner Report, August 22, 2004

The door of a trailer transporting 28 calves to a sale opened during transit. All 28 calves exited the trailer and fell onto the roadway. Four calves sustained fractured necks or backs and were euthanatized on the scene; four more were severely injured. The remaining animals were loaded back onto the trailer for delivery to the sale.

Owner Report, February 16, 2006

A horse fell out of the back of a horse trailer and was dragged 300 yards (900 ft) because it was still tied in the trailer. The horse, with severe skin injuries, was being rehabilitated at a local farm, and the veterinarian reported excellent success in the 30 days since the accident.

The New York Post, February 22, 2006

A mounted police horse bolted and threw its rider in rush hour traffic after being hit by two vehicles at a red light. The horse and rider suffered moderate but survivable injuries.

Kinston Free Press, February 15, 2006

A pony wandering in the road was hit and killed by a driver that left the scene of the accident. The driver's truck was found by police officers 1 km (1/2 mile) down the road and was towed. The owner called in later, told officers what happened and was cited for leaving the scene of the accident.

The Denver Channel.Com, January 23, 2006

A 31-year-old horse that had fallen into a shallow ditch was lifted to safety by emergency responders after it was lodged for two hours. Under the supervision of a veterinarian, rescuers used straps and rope systems to lift the horse.

Scotland Today, September 21, 2004

A veterinarian and a Coast Guard winchman were sent to the hospital after attempting to rescue a cow on a cliff side. The veterinarian fell off the cliff into the sea and was followed by the winchman, and both men were rescued by other members of the Coast Guard. Meanwhile, the cow got up and walked away unscathed.

Forbes.com, January 20, 2006

A man stopped for gas and suddenly noticed his four-month-old camel was no longer in the horse trailer he was hauling. He called police, which started a two-county search for the animal. The camel was found one hour later along the side of the road. The animal, which had jumped out of the trailer at 55 mph (88 kph), received only bumps and scratches for the effort.

CBS News, March 18, 2004

A male gorilla that had been teased by some youths scaled a wall in his exhibit at the Dallas Zoo and bit four people during his 30-minute rampage through the zoo. A Code One (dangerous animal escape) was issued, and zoo workers attempted to dart the animal; but when the gorilla confronted law enforcement officers, they shot the animal.

Boston Globe, September 9, 2004

The gate of a trailer transporting three bison opened, ejecting one bison on the I-495 freeway. The bison survived the fall, and a state trooper on scene had to order people in the stopped traffic back into their cars as they attempted to photograph the animal. The owner fired two darts into the animal to kill it before it could cause an accident.

The Prague Post, August 21, 2002
In the Czech Republic, the zoo director defended his order to shoot a bull elephant drowning during tremendous flooding in the Prague Zoo. Several other animals (a hippopotamus, a lion, and a bear) had to be shot to protect the public. Over 1,100 animals were successfully rescued and moved to high ground, including rhinos and other large mammals. The 100-year-flood plan was overwhelmed by a 500-year flooding event.

The Press Enterprise, June 19, 2003
After slipping off a trail on a ride at 1 a.m., a horse spent three days in a canyon while the owners attempted to extricate the animal themselves. On the third day, a large animal rescue team (Alta Loma, California) consisting of trained rescuers (i.e., firefighters, veterinarian, volunteers) were flown into the remote canyon and successfully helicopter-lifted the horse in an Anderson Sling. The horse was transported to animal control pursuant to an investigation into the scenario.

Equus, October 2002
A horse fell into an old septic tank in a neighbor's front yard. A tow truck and a veterinarian were called to the scene, and chains were wrapped around the horse's body to lift it out of the hole. The animal survived the incident and the rescue.

The Equine Showcase, January 2003
A veterinarian related his story of being lowered on the ball of a boom truck down into a 20 m (66 ft) deep well to assess a mare that had fallen into it. With a flashlight and a syringe of anesthetic, he was lowered to the mare, injected her in the vein, and performed triage. The mare had sustained an open fracture of her rear leg and was euthanatized in the well.

CU News, Fall 1998
A horse was missing at feeding time, and the manager found it with only one leg sticking out of a hole almost 8 ft (2.4 m) deep. Veterinarians responded and tranquilized the horse, then used hobbles to the legs to lift it out of the hole. The horse recovered uneventfully.

Gimenez and Gimenez, Summer 1999
A mare was caught in mud, and the owners spent two hours trying to dig her out. Using a Santa Barbara strap as a surcingle, trained rescuers pulled the mare almost 25 m (82 ft) to safety with a winch attached to the surcingle.

CU News, April 2000
Three mares owned by Clemson University Equine Farm with hot brands on their hips were stolen from a pasture. The Stolen Horse Information network and local media increased local awareness about the theft, and the mares were recovered almost one month later with altered and additional brands.

Gimenez and Gimenez, January 27, 2000
A horse fell through the rotten floor of a horse trailer and was dragged several hundred meters. The soft tissue of the legs was destroyed and the animal was euthanatized by a veterinarian.

On-Scene Report, November 19, 2001
A motorist noticed blood dripping from the cattle trailer in front of her and stopped the driver. A cow had fallen through the rotten floor of the trailer. Police and local rescuers were called to assist, moving the cow out of the hole and replacing the rotten flooring.

The Recorder, November 25, 2003
A Belgian horse fell through a cellar and was trapped for several hours before rescuers reached him. They removed all the boards and joists carefully and manually dug a ramp out of the cellar to walk him out. The horse remained calm as the obstacles were removed and quietly exited the cellar.

Lewa Wildlife Conservancy Newsletter, June 2005
The World Society for the Protection of Animals and Lewa Wildlife Conservancy coordinated an elephant rescue for a bull elephant that had fallen into a pit latrine on a farm in Africa and was now being approached by local farmers who wanted to kill the animal for its meat. Using slings, sedation, a tractor, and a Land Cruiser, the elephant was successfully pulled from its entrapment and disappeared into the forest.

Newsround, May 4, 2005
A baby elephant in India had slipped into a 10 m (33 ft) deep well, and its mother was frantically trying to free it. Villagers dug a sloping ramp into the well and walked the baby out. By this time, the wild mother had abandoned her calf; the calf had sustained a leg injury, and was taken to an elephant orphanage for treatment and care until the mother could be found.

Wetlands Wire, December 11, 2003
A three-year old endangered white rhinoceros was trapped in the mud of an African lake. Volunteers and game experts arrived to rescue the calf. The calf was darted with a tranquilizer (etorphine); using ropes placed around the chest of the animal, over 100 people pulled it to safety. As it approached shore and could assist with its own rescue, the antidote was administered and the rhinoceros walked out when urged by volunteers and the veterinarian.

BBC News, March 13, 2002

In Thailand, an elephant participating in a village celebration fell into a muddy hole and remained there for over 20 hours. Finally, rescue workers arrived, and within 3 hours were able to free the elephant using straps and a crane to lift it while simultaneously digging away the earth with a backhoe. The owner rode the animal out of the hole and gave it a well-deserved bath.

Wildlife Trust of India, October 25, 2004

An adult cow elephant slipped into a 2 ft (0.6 m) wide, 15 ft (4.5 m) deep trench trying to rescue her calf; when found, the cow's breathing was extremely labored; and when slightly tranquilized, the animal died. The calf was rescued from underneath the cow's front legs by digging out the earth, and the orphaned calf was transferred to an elephant refuge.

Voice of the TWH, June 2002

After trail riding in a pasture, a horse sank to its withers in a dried pond bed. Its owner and friends attempted to rescue him for two hours. As rain clouds threatened, a friend arrived with a backhoe and pulled the mud out from each side of the horse, making a ramp so it could walk to safety.

The Chronicle of the Horse, July 15, 2005

A six-week-old foal fell off a 20 ft (6 m) cliff in Wales. A volunteer lifeboat crew and a local diver swam into shore to catch the foal, using a length of kelp as a halter. The two men assisted the foal over the treacherous rocks and swam with the foal to the lifeboat, where it was lifted on board. The foal was transported to the shore and reunited with its owner and dam.

The Chronicle of the Horse, September 16, 2005

Horse owners with a preconceived evacuation plan for their horses coordinated the evacuation of over 80 horses from the city park and a private facility two days before Hurricane Katrina hit their farms in New Orleans. Satellite photos showed the initial floodwaters reached the rafters of the barn. The owner's enactment of an evacuation plan was credited with saving the lives of all these animals.

The Chronicle of the Horse, July 22, 2005

A cow with its head trapped between two trees was rescued from its predicament by a volunteer rescue squad and two concerned horseback riders. A variety of rescue methods (e.g., shoring, dropping one tree with a chainsaw, and lifting the animal) were considered, but what was effective was an air bag braced between the trees to move them apart a sufficient distance to free the animal's head.

The Simi Valley Acorn, July 16, 2004

A horse that fell down a 100 m (330 ft) cliff in Thousand Oaks, California, was injured and unable to walk out a trail cut by responders. The disaster animal response team, USAR, and fire departments implemented a joint rescue using a helicopter lift of the animal. This was the fourth sling load of a horse out of a similar predicament in a six-month period by these teams.

The Australian, January 23, 2006

A lost bottlenose whale swam 64 km (40 miles) up the Thames River and became trapped in the tidal shallows. A rescue team used inflatable air logs to support it for transport to a barge. Initially, lifting the animal with a Chinook helicopter was considered, but the barge option was considered safer for the conscious 4-ton animal. Unfortunately, the animal died before it could be released in the North Sea 48 hours later.

The Vail Daily, January 21, 2006

In a two-day operation, 25 moose cows and calves were relocated to Grand Mesa, Colorado, from Utah. Helicopters were used to remotely net gun the animals, and the animals were blindfolded and their legs hogtied for the lift. They were sling loaded from the capture locations to a staging area, loaded on road transport trailers, and delivered the next day to their release locations.

News.com.au, November 7, 2004

Five brumbies (wild horses) were shot by animal control officers when they escaped from a military compound and were standing next to the pasture fence. The officers were apparently concerned the animals would run into nearby traffic, but the officers made no effort to contain them or open the gate to return them to their pasture. The Royal Society for the Protection of Cruelty to Animals-Australia (RSPCA-A) launched an investigation into the incident after numerous citizens complained.

Calgary Herald, July 4, 2005

In a media event that turned tragic, 202 bucking horses intended for use in the annual Calgary Stampede rodeo were being driven by 12 professional cowboys and more than 20 urban residents through downtown Calgary (population 1 million) at the end of a six-day historic drive as part of Alberta's centennial celebration. A passing train spooked the horses; they stampeded over the Bonnybrook Bridge, and many of the animals jumped the sides of the bridge to fall to their deaths or drown in the river. Nine horses died, and the city expected an investigation by the Humane Society.

Santa Maria Times, October 13, 2005

A horse fell 150 ft (45 m) off a trail in a national forest and was trapped at the bottom of a canyon. Firefighters and rescuers spent two days cutting a trail to get the horse out. They considered rope and forward assist systems, but in the end the Humane Society decided to use a UC Davis-Anderson Sling and sedation to sling load the horse to safety underneath a fire service helicopter.

St. Augustine Record, April 10, 2007

A horse was trapped in mud, and his well-meaning owner tried to assist him by holding his head above water. The fire department had to rescue the woman first, while pumping the pond water out, then took three hours to rescue the horse with a modified web sling. The horse died one and a half hours after extrication from dehydration, exhaustion, and hypothermia.

HorseandHound.com, August 7, 2007

A horse is trapped to its shoulders in quicksand in the United Kingdom on the beach with approximately 45 minutes before the tide will overwhelm the stricken animal. A trained TLAER team extricates the animal with no injuries in just 20 minutes using a Nikopoulos needle, strop guide, webbing, and injected water and air.

ACRONYMS USED IN CHAPTER 22

EERU   Equine emergency rescue unit
EMS   Emergency medical services
IAP   Incident action plan
IV   Intravenous
PPE   Personal protective equipment
TLAER   Technical large animal emergency rescue
USAR   Urban Search and Rescue

Appendix 1

Some Common Communications Options

Equipment type	Initial Cost	Usage Fees (unit/month)	Range	Advantages	Disadvantages
Pagers	0–$50	$8–$18	Variable	Inexpensive, very portable	Variable reliability, variable range, No confirmation of reception
Wireless telephones (analog or digital)	0–$150	$35–$450	Variable	Universal usage, portable	May have high usage costs, no group coverage, variable reliability
Simplex VHF/UHF or owner operated UHF repeater two-way radio	$450–$600 per vehicle, $5000+ for base	0	Up to 32 km (20 mi)	Inexpensive operation costs after installation Allows good local group coverage, reliable	Requires FCC license Requires radio tower Requires transmitter, technician Simplex—poor mobile to mobile coverage
450 MHZ trunking two-way radio	$470–$600 per unit	$14–$25	Up to 80 km (50 mi)	Inexpensive, good range, good group coverage, reliable	Not available everywhere
900 MHZ two-way radio	$800-$1,000 per unit	$25–$37	Up to 56 km (35 mi)	Still inexpensive compared to wireless telephones, good group coverage, reliable	Not available everywhere Equipment and usage fees seem higher than 450 MHZ
Satellite two-way radio	$3,500–$5,400 per vehicle	$70–$100	Unlimited in North America	Very reliable, excellent range, good group coverage	Expensive installation, high usage fees, but comparable to wireless and Nextel
Nextel	About $150 per unit	$60–$80	Variable	Can combine pagers, wireless telephones, and interpersonal two-way type communication	Not available everywhere, poor group coverage (very expensive if group coverage is requested) Proprietary—will not work with other wireless systems

Technical Large Animal Emergency Rescue Equipment

This list is intended as a guide, not as an all-inclusive or exhaustive list of equipment that responders may want to purchase or cache for a TLAER incident. Many of these recommendations may be purchased commercially off the shelf or manufactured locally.

Note: The equipment listed below is intended for use by personnel with certified training in technical large animal emergency rescue. Use of this equipment without adequate training can result in serious injury or death. Certified webbing and shackles that meet NFPA standards may be purchased instead of using locally acquired gear (fire hose slings, etc.).

Personal Gear

Gloves
Reflective jacket or shirt
Boots (with or without steel toe)
Protective headwear (heavy duty helmet with chinstrap)
Goggles
Ear protection
Protective clothing
Level C HazMat suits, gloves, goggles, or mask
Swiftwater/floodwater rescue gear (personal flotation device, wet and/or dry suit, boots, helmet) certification required
Surface ice rescue gear (personal flotation device, surface ice rescue suit, boots, helmet) certification required
Body harness

Necessary Basic Rescue Equipment

This list includes equipment and supplies that TLAER rescuers will use most often and that represent a minimal investment to produce effective rescues.

3 – Emergency rope halter (7 m Prusik cord or Kernmantle rescue rope)
2 – 30 m of 2 cm Kernmantle static rope
1 – 10 m × 10 cm nylon webbing with sewn loops on each end
1 – Santa Barbara sling (leather or nylon)
4 – 2 m of 10 cm wide fire hose web with sewn loops on each end
4 – 1.2 m of 10 cm wide fire hose web with sewn loops on each end
1 – Spread bar for vertical lift (aluminum or steel)
1 – Fleece-lined breast collar (with sturdy hardware)
2 – Set of fleece-lined hobbles
3 – 4 l (1 gal) jug of water-based lubricant or liquid soap
Various sizes and lengths cribbing (lumber)
6 – 2 m Prusik loops of 2 cm static Kernmantle rope
12 – 30 cm Prusik loops of 0.7 cm cord
1 – Horse head protection (towel, pillow, human life vest)
12 – Large steel carabiners (4 cm gate opening)
1 – Leg-handling cane
1 – Boat hook
1 – King size bed sheet (dark color)
1 – Simple vertical lift web sling (Becker, Large Animal Lift, etc.)
1 – Nikopoulos needle
1 – Strop guide
1 – Large animal field first aid kit (consult a veterinarian)
Assorted general hand tools (shovels, saws, chain saw, etc.)
1 – Cordless reciprocating saw
1 – Long painters' poles with interchangeable accessories (cutters, carabiner hold open, S-hook, etc.)
1 – Insulated horse blanket

2 – Duct tape rolls
1 – 50 l water source (nonpressurized) in containers
1 – Containment portable fence (1.2 m × 33 m plastic fence)

Recommended Equipment

This list represents considerably greater monetary investment for equipment to perform more technical rescues.

1 – Kimzey aluminum leg splint
9 – Leg splints of different sizes made of 10 cm PVC pipe
Various padding and wraps for bandaging
1 – Portable winch (minimum 1,500 kg)
1 – 9:1 1/2 in. rope anchor system (with two double pulleys and assorted Prusik loops)
2 – 100 m of 2 cm Kernmantle static rope
24 – Large carabiners (steel)
1 – Tube brake (friction system)
2 – Low pressure air bags
1 – High pressure air bag
1 – Mud lance with pressurized air and/or pressure water source
1 – Rescue Glide set (with accessories)
1 – 5 m supply air-inflatable fire hose with Storz caps
1 – A-frame (steel or aluminum) and/or tripod
1 – Large animal (veterinary quality) first aid kit
Liquid detergent and long-handled brushes

1 – 33 m water hose
1 – Portable power generator
2 – Portable floodlights on stands
Various sizes of halters, lead ropes, animal tack
Large animal physical restraint (twitch, Stableizer, etc.)
12 – Steel cattle panels

May Be Necessary

This list includes equipment that may be used rarely by a TLAER-trained team and represents a significant investment.

1 – UC Davis-Anderson Sling (with accoutrements)
1 – All-terrain vehicle with winch
1 – Large animal ambulance (trailer and truck)

Miscellaneous Equipment

Rope and gear identification labels
Inventory tags
Backpack-type rescue storage bags
Car-size tire inner tubes with can of air
Waterproof canvas tarps
Disposable camera
Video camera
Transport boxes for equipment
Chemical capture equipment (consult with a veterinarian)

Large Animal Emergency Rescue Equipment Vendors

In addition to the manufacturers listed, there are other manufacturers that sell similar equipment used in human/large animal rescue. TLAER instructors have found the companies listed below to provide appropriate equipment. We do not have a vested or financial interest in any of these companies.

Some equipment items designed specifically for large animal emergency rescue, such as the Nikopoulos needle and strop guide, are not manufactured commercially. These items can be custom-made by a steel/aluminum welding shop.

Acute blood loss treatment
QuikClot
Z-Medica, LLC
Newington, CT
860-667-2222
www.z-medica.com
info@z-medica.com

Aluminum leg splint
Kimzey Veterinary Products
www.kimzeymetalproducts.com
(888) 454-6039

Boat hooks
Westport Marina, Inc.
Part No. DAV4132
(877)744-7786
www.shipstore.com

Custom web slings
New Haven Moving Equipment
2490 Verna Court
San Leandro, CA 94577-4223
800-624-7950 (Jena)
510-562-1927 (fax)
www.newhaven-usa.com

Discount dealer for all brands of rescue equipment
Technicalrescue.Com
(800)771-5342
www.technicalrescue.com

Equine skid stretcher (Rescue Glide)
L.A.R.G.E.
www.rescueglides.com
Greenville, SC

Rescue Glide
Ben McCracken
benmccracken@rescueglides.com
(864)270-1344

Helicopter sling (UC Davis-Anderson Sling)
CDA Products, CA
(707) 743-1300
(707) 743-2530 fax

Horse halters (rope halters and lead ropes)
www.parelli.net
www.clintonanderson.com
www.johnlyons.com

Human rapid extrication harness
MAST
www.sling-link.com

Large hooks, shackles, steel rods, etc,
McMaster-Carr Industrial Supply Company
(404) 346-7000
Atlanta, GA
www.mcmaster.com

Light steel animal containment panels
Darwin Kell
800-863-3211
Carlisle, PA
info@bentpinealpacas.com
www.bentpinealpacas.com

Miscellaneous
www.armysurpluswarehouse.com

Portable fencing
Polygrid Ranch Fence
Jerry B. Leach Co.
(800)845-9005
www.jerrybleach.com

Protective clothing
Cascade Fire Equipment
1-800-654-7049
www.cascadefire.com

Protective clothing and rescue equipment
Forestry Suppliers, Inc.
(800) 647-5368
www.forestry-suppliers.com

Public safety clothing and equipment
Galls
1-800-477-7766
www.galls.com

Rescue rope and hardware
CMC Rescue Equipment
1-800-235-5741
www.cmcrescue.com

Rescue rope and hardware
Karst Sports, Shinnston, WV
www.mgmtsys.com
1-800-734-2851

Rescue rope and hardware
PMI-Petzl Distribution, Inc.
(800) 282-7673
www.pmi-petzl.com

Rescue rope and hardware
Rock-n-Rescue
1-800-346-7673
http://www.rocknrescue.com

Safety personal protection equipment
Tychem SL
Lakeland Industries, Inc.
Steve McCully
stevem@lakeland-ind.com
Decatur, AL
800-645-9291
http://www.lakeland.com

Sea Catch
www.seacatch.com

Simple vertical lift Becker sling
Dr. Kathleen Becker, DVM
becker@hast.net
http://www.hast.net/rescue-equipment.htm

Snap shackles
Catamaran Sailor
www.catsailor.com

STOR-IT
Horse first aid storage system
Perfect World Luggage
15415 Triple Creek
San Antonio, TX 78247
877-487-4677
www.madewithhorsesense.com

Water-based lubricant
OB Lube
HAR-VET
www.har-vet.com
800-872-7741

Water rescue and other rescue equipment
The Rescue Source
(800) 45-RESCUE
www.rescuesource.com

Technical Large Animal Emergency Rescue Training: Recommendations for Student Competency Goals for Operational Certification (24) Hours

- "Large animal" is intended to include equine, bovine, swine, caprine, and camelid animals. TLAER training has relevance to exotics and wild animals, but they require specialized training and preparation not covered in depth in this course.
- Students taking TLAER courses should consider certification in basic rope rigging and ICS—100 level first.
- Students completing TLAER courses should consider certification in 40-hour first responder and cpr, swift/flood water/surface ice rescue, ICS series courses, and agro-terrorism prevention, and intermediate rope rigging as follow-on.
- TLAER courses should combine didactic classroom instruction with a variety of audio visual, demonstration, and hands-on laboratory work emphasizing teamwork. Laboratory should include live animal demonstrations and procedure practice with hands-on work for each student.

Rescuer Safety—Risk Assessment, Teamwork, Personal Protective Equipment, Incident Command System, Personal Planning

Large Animal Handling—Basic (Hands-On Approach, Haltering, Leading, Holding under Controlled Conditions)

Large Animal Handling—Intermediate (Hands-On Approach, Haltering, Leading, Holding under Uncontrolled Conditions; Reacting to Scary Event; Loading under Stressful Conditions)

Large Animal Handling—Advanced (Hands-On Physical Restraint for Veterinary Procedures; Hands-On Approach, Haltering, Holding, Restraint under Uncontrolled or Simulated Rescue Conditions)

Large Animal Behavior and Senses—Normal (Video, Live Animal Demonstration)

Large Animal Behavior—Under Stressful and Rescue Conditions (Video)

Understanding the Special Weapons That Large Animals can Wield (Video, Live Animal Demonstration)

Coordination with Veterinary Assets Prior to and On-Scene

Coordination with Emergency Management Prior to and On-Scene

Coordination with Volunteers, the Public, Bystanders and the Animal Owner

Understanding Flight Mechanisms and Flight Distance—Awareness, Alertness, and Action Zones

Understanding the Herd Instinct and Fear of Being Alone (Live Animal Demonstration)

Understanding Basic Prey and Predatory Animal Behavior (Video, Live Animal Demonstration)

Containment Strategies for Loose Large Animals (Hands-On Singles and Multiples, Multiple Species, Live Animal Demonstration)

Suitable and Unsuitable Anatomical Structures for Rescue Equipment Emplacement

Employment of the Hampshire Slip (Hands-On Practice with Live Animal)

Employment of the Forward Assist (Hands-On Practice, Live Animal Demonstration)

Employment of the Backwards Drag (Person Demonstration, Live Animal Demonstration)

Incident Command System Applicable to TLAER Incidents—Basic Awareness (ICS-100)

Overview of Trailer Configurations, Sizes, Types

Structural Integrity and Trailer Construction Aspects

Common Causes of Trailer Wrecks or Accidents

Response to Trailer Wrecks, Accidents, Overturned Trailers and Semi-Trailers/Liners

Livestock Liner Overturn in TLAER Response

Trailer Overturn and Cutting Considerations for Extrication (Hands-On Trailer Overturn)

Personal Protective Equipment Applicable to TLAER Incidents (Demonstration)

Special Applications of Rope Rescue Techniques to TLAER Incidents (Demonstration and Hands-On)

Harnessing of Large Animals for Simple Web Vertical Lift Sling (Hands-On Practice with Becker Sling, Large Animal Lift; Live Animal Demonstration)

Choosing Appropriate Lifting Equipment for Vertical Lift (Demonstration—Crane and/or Helicopter)

Confined Space/Structural Collapse Issues in LAR Incidents (Video, Demonstration)

Trench Issues in LAR Incidents (Video, Demonstration)

Common Causes of Barn Fires

Wildfire Evacuation Planning

Review of Horse Barn Fire and Wildfire Response Considerations

Comparison of Barn Fire Incidents Demonstrating Importance of Prevention (Video)

Mud/Floodwater/Swiftwater/Ice Rescue Issues in TLAER

Appropriate Prioritization of Rescue Attempts in TLAER (RETHROG-H)

Review of Special Mud Rescue Techniques (Hands-On Practice with Nikopolous Needle, TLAER Air/Water Injection Systems, Santa Barbara Sling, Hampshire Slip; Live Animal Demonstration)

Swiftwater and Floodwater Training Requirements and Safety—Basic Awareness

Review of Rescue Barge Loading and Equine Floatation Device Employment

Surface Ice Rescue Training Requirements and Safety—Basic Awareness

Weapons of Mass Destruction and Agro-Terrorism Considerations in TLAER Response

Hazardous Materials Issues in TLAER (Floodwater, Septic Tanks, Manure Pits, Agricultural Chemicals)

Intentional Foreign Animal Disease Considerations in TLAER Incidents—Basic Awareness

Introduction to Large Animal Decontamination (Demonstration)

Decontamination of Large Animals—Set Up for Gross Decon (Hands-On And Demonstration)

Public Health and Food Safety Issues in TLAER—Basic Awareness

Legal Considerations in TLAER Incidents

Financial Considerations in TLAER Incidents

Basic Search and Rescue Considerations (Practical Exercise)

Handling and Transport of Recumbent Animals (Rescue Glide, Tarp, Hands-On and Live Animal Demonstration)

Helicopter Operations and Safety Related to TLAER Incidents—Basic Awareness

Review of Handling and Transport Considerations of Large Animals in Airlift Rescue

Basic Field First Aid Considerations for TLAER Incidents

Intermediate Field First Aid Considerations for TLAER Incidents

Awareness of Chemical Immobilization Issues Related to TLAER Incidents (Video)

Introduction to Sedative/Tranquilizer Protocols and Effects Related to TLAER Incidents

Basic Humane Considerations for Physical and Chemical Restraint of Large Animals

Emergency Humane Destruction/Field Euthanasia (Chemical Euthanasia, Projectile Weapons, Captive Bolt, Exsanguination, Video)

Review of 911 Dispatch Flow Sheet in Response to TLAER Calls

The 911 Dispatcher—Keys to Increased Communication and Better Response Assets

Review of On-Scene Responder Behavior and Safety

How to Conduct an After-Rescue Review and Documentation (Practical Exercise)

Basic Overview of TLAER in Disaster Scenarios and Review of Lessons Learned in TLAER Situations

Basic Overview of Prevention, Mitigation, Preparation, Response and Planning Cycles in TLAER Disasters

Glossary

AAEP: American Association of Equine Practitioners, with over 6,000 member veterinarians that specialize in equids (horses, mules, donkeys).

AAVDM: American Academy for Veterinary Disaster Medicine.

ABC: Airway, breathing, and circulation; as promoted in first aid training for primary assessment of a large animal victim.

AC officer: Animal control officer.

Agonal: The last reflexive breaths stimulated by the central nervous system in a dying mammal.

AHA: American Humane Association.

Animal control: Division of county government responsible for enforcement of county, state, and federal laws and regulations involving animals.

Animal handler: Member of the operations section responsible for handling and directing movement or restraint of a large animal.

Animal rescue: A term commonly used to denote assistance, adoption, and/or rehabilitation of abused, starved, neglected, or abandoned animals. Does not necessarily refer to technical procedures used in rescue.

ASPCA: American Society for the Prevention of Cruelty to Animals.

AVMA: American Veterinary Medical Association.

BEVA: British Equine Veterinary Association.

Bombproof anchor: The strong, nonmoving point used to attach one end of the rescue system. A bombproof anchor must be several times stronger/heavier than the victim to which it is connected. Examples of bombproof anchors include fire engines, other large trucks, heavy construction equipment, large trees, buildings, etc. Examples of unsuitable anchors include cars, small trucks, small trees, fence posts, power or telephone poles.

Bovine: Cattle of the *Bos indicus* (zebu, Brahman cattle) and *Bos taurus* species.

Camelids: Includes South American camelids (llama, alpaca, guanaco, vicuna) and Asian (dromedary and Bactrian) camels.

Caprine: Goats.

Captive bolt: Euthanasia device that has a rod that penetrates the animal's skull and stuns its brain. This method must be followed by a secondary method of euthanasia.

Carabiner: Steel or aluminum device used to join two rescue components in line.

CART: County animal response team; a part of the state animal response team model for animal disaster planning.

CBRNE: Chemical, biological, radiological, nuclear, and explosive.

Chemical capture: The use of drug darts or other injectors to immobilize an animal.

Colic: Pain originating from the abdomen.

Consequence management: Term adopted by the Department of Homeland Security to denote the response to events including terrorism, natural disasters, and similar incidents. This term replaces the term emergency management.

Cord: Nylon rescue rope with a diameter of 10 mm (3/8 in.) or less.

Cribbing: Any type of lumber used in a technical rescue.

Critical distance: The distance at which an animal may choose to attack instead of flee from a perceived threat or person.

CVT: Certified veterinary technician.

DART: Disaster animal response team.

DECON: Decontamination of CBRNE materials from a living thing.

DEHFR: Days End Horse Farm Rescue (Lisbon, Maryland).

DEMHS: Department of Emergency Management Homeland Security. This designation is used by some states (i.e., Connecticut) for the state emergency management agency/division.

DHS: Department of Homeland Security at the federal level.

Dispatch: Public-safety emergency telecommunications that ensure citizens in need of emergency, health, and social services are matched safely, quickly, and effectively with the most appropriate resource.

DMAT: Disaster medical assistance team.

DMORT: Disaster mortuary operations team.

Dynamic: Also known as high stretch. Nylon rope that stretches 15%–30% when loaded. The rope used in rock climbing is dynamic, intended to reduce the impact force of a sudden stop of the load after a fall. This has minimal application in TLAER.

EERU: Equine Emergency Response Unit.

EMS: Emergency medical services personnel; may be paramedics, EMTs, or nurse/doctor volunteers trained for human medical response.

EMT: Emergency medical technician.

EOP: Emergency operations plan.

EPA: Environmental Protection Agency.

Equine: Horses, mules, donkeys, and exotic equids (such as zebras) of the genus *Equus*.

ESA: Endangered Species Act. Promulgates laws related to endangered species protection and management.

ESF: Emergency support function. A group of organizations that perform similar or like functions are consolidated into a single, cohesive unit to allow better management of emergency response functions.

Euthanasia: The process of humanely killing an animal without causing pain or suffering.

Expectant: A triaged victim that is lowest priority for first aid; the victim has fatal injuries, and death is imminent.

FARAD: Food Animal Residue Avoidance Database. Developed to prevent chemical residues from entering the human food chain.

FEMA: Federal Emergency Management Agency.

Flake: Mode of storage of rescue rope in a bag. The rope is "flaked" into the bag by stacking, not coiling, short sections of rope into the bag with one hand while holding the edge of the bag with the other hand.

Flight distance: The distance to which a prey animal will move to feel safe when presented with a predator or frightening object.

Fomite: Inanimate objects such as boots, clothing, equipment, vehicles, crates, and packaging that can carry an agent and/or spread disease through mechanical transmission.

Gibbs ascender: Metal device that grabs 25 mm (1 in.) rope, and serves the same function as a Prusik hitch.

GIS: Global information system.

GPS: Global positioning system. The device uses reference satellites to determine an exact point position on the face of the earth.

HazMat: Hazardous materials.

Head-to-head: Horses are loaded in-line facing each other, as in large commercial haulers.

HEART: Humane Equine Aid and Rapid Transport.

HSA: Humane Slaughter Association.

HSUS: Humane Society of the United States.

Humane: Characterized by tenderness, compassion, and sympathy for people and animals; treating an animal with respect and minimizing pain and stress during handling and/or euthansia.

IC: Incident commander. The member of the response team who is assigned overall responsibility for directing response activities, including developing strategies, managing resources, and planning operations.

ICS: Incident command system. The nationally used, standardized, on-scene emergency management concept designed to allow users to adopt an integrated organizational structure equal to the complexity and demands of single or multiple incidents without being hindered by jurisdictional boundaries.

IFAW: International Fund for Animal Welfare.

ILPH: International League for the Protection of Horses.

Infected premises: A defined area, which may be all or part of a property, in which an infectious disease or disease agent exists or is believed to exist.

In-line loading: The horses are located in a trailer facing the towing vehicle.

Kernmantle: Rescue rope consisting of parallel nylon fibers (kern,) held together and covered by a sheath (mantle) of woven nylon strands.

LART: Large animal rescue team or large animal rescue training.

Latitude: The angular distance north or south from Earth's equator, expressed in degrees of measurement. Locations north of the equator are assigned a positive value. Locations south of the equator are assigned a negative value. The entire United States is assigned a positive latitude coordinate.

Lifeline: Name given to the rescue rope being used in a rescue that suspends or pulls the live victim.

Liner: A livestock commercial hauler.

Logistics: That section of an incident response in charge of planning the delivery and disposition of equipment, personnel and supply.

Longitude: The angular distance from the Prime Meridian, which is an imaginary line located near Greenwich, England, that bisects both poles and is expressed in degrees of measurement. Locations east of the Prime Meridian are in the positive range. Locations west of the Prime Meridian are in the negative range. The entire United States is assigned a negative longitude coordinate.

Low-stress livestock handling: Livestock are handled and moved using low stress and often passive methods, which are becoming popular for safety reasons.

LVT: Licensed veterinary technician.

Mechanical advantage: The ratio of output force (acting on a load) produced by a machine or system to the applied effort (input force). When the term is applied to the use of a rope system, it implies the ability of a rope system to allow the rescuer to move a load by pulling only a fraction of the load's weight.

MSPCA: Massachusetts Society for the Prevention of Cruelty to Animals.

MWD: Military working dog.

NAIS: National Animal Identification System.

Natural horsemanship: Handling, riding, and training methods based on knowledge of horse behavior and instincts, instead of using force.

NDMS: National Disaster Medical System. It includes disaster medical assistance team, national medical response team, disaster mortuary operations team, and veterinary medical assistance team personnel under the jurisdiction of the U.S. Department of Health and Human Services.

NEMA: National Emergency Management Association.

NFIRS: National Fire Incident Reporting System. A central database for the tracking of fire/rescue incidents. It does not track specific TLAER-related incidents such as horse trailer accidents or horse barn fires.

NFPA: National Fire Protection Association.

NIMS: National Incident Management System.

NMRT: National medical response team.

NRP: National Response Plan.

NVRT: National Veterinary Response Team

Operations: Section personnel of the incident command system directly involved in performing a rescue or responding to an incident.

OSHA: Occupational Safety and Health Administration.

PAO: Public Affairs Officer

PETA: People for the Ethical Treatment of Animals.

PIO: Public information officer.

PPE: Personal protective equipment. Each type of specialty rescue requires specialized or general safety equipment.

Premises: A defined area or structure, which may include all or part of a farm, enterprise, or other private or public land, building, or property.

Prey animal: An animal hunted or seized for food, especially by carnivorous animals (predators).

Prusik hitch: A Prusik loop wrapped around a rescue rope on one end, and attached to an item of rescue hardware (e.g., pulley, etc.) by a carabiner on the other end. To grab effectively on the rope, the diameter of the Prusik cord should be 70% or less than the diameter of the rope to which it is attached.

Prusik loop: Loop made with 7–9 mm (3/8 in.) nylon rescue cord with both ends connected with two fisherman's knots.

Quarantine: Legal restrictions limiting movement imposed on a place, animal, vehicle, personnel, etc.

RCMP: Royal Canadian Mounted Police.

Rendering: Processing by heat to inactivate infective agents. Rendered material may be used in various products according to particular disease circumstances.

Responders: Those individuals who, in the early stages of an incident, are responsible for the protection and preservation of life, property, evidence, and the environment. Includes emergency response providers, emergency management, public health, clinical care, public works, and other skilled support personnel that provide immediate support services during prevention, response, and recovery operations.

Restricted area: A declared area surrounding an infected premises that is subject to intense surveillance and movement controls; smaller than a control area.

RETHROG-H: A mnemonic for remembering the priority of rescuing a victim in water: Reach, throw, row, go, then helo.

Risk enterprise: A livestock or livestock-related enterprise with a high potential for disease spread, for example, an abattoir, milk factory, artificial breeding center, or livestock market.

Rope protector: Section of canvas or webbing placed between a lifeline and any abrasive surface during a rescue. Fire hose sections are commonly used for rope protection.

RSPCA: Royal Society for the Prevention of Cruelty to Animals.

RVT: Registered veterinary technician.

Safety buddy: A person whose only responsibility is to look after the safety of a responder directly involved in a dangerous activity such as a rescue or fire suppression.

Salvage: Recovery of all or a portion of the market value of animals by treatment and use of products, according to disease circumstances.

SAR: Search and rescue.

SART: State animal response team.

SCBA: Self-contained breathing apparatus.

SEMS: Standardized Emergency Management System.

Shock load: A sudden, unplanned, heavy impact placed upon a rescue rope during an incident. Rescue rope and hardware that has been subjected to a shock load should not be used again for live rescues.

Slant-load: The horses are located in the trailer at a 30–35-degree angle to the tow vehicle.

Sling load: Use of a helicopter to suspend a live animal under the aircraft using an appropriate sling device.

Snap shackle: A shackle designed to be released under load. The snap shackle allows rapid and safe disconnection of the webbing from the spread bar as soon as the animal touches safe ground.

SO: Safety officer.

SOG: Standard operating guidance.

SOP: Standard operating procedure or protocol.

SPCA: Society for the Prevention of Cruelty to Animals.

Spread bar: Section of metal used to maintain the vertical alignment of the sling webbing during a simple vertical lift system, maintaining the weight distribution and balancing the load during the lift.

Staging area: Location where rescue personnel are located on standby during an incident.

Staging tarp: Tarp used to lay out rescue equipment during an incident response.

Static: More appropriately called low stretch; the physical characteristic of rope. Rescue rope that stretches approximately 5% while loaded. All ropes used in rescue efforts should be low stretch.

Susceptible animals: Animals that can be infected with a disease.

Suspect animals: Animals that may have been exposed to an exotic or serious infectious disease such that quarantine and intensive surveillance are warranted; or an animal not known to have been exposed to a disease agent but showing clinical signs requiring differential diagnosis.

Suspect premises: Premises containing suspect animals.

Swine: Pigs of all species (includes *Sus scrofa* and *Sus scrofa domestica*).

Tandem Prusiks: Two Prusik hitches, one shorter than the other, placed next to each other as a brake in a rope system.

TAR: Technical Animal Rescue; course designed by Code-3 Associates and American Humane Association in the early 1990s.

Technical large animal emergency rescue (TLAER): The use of any procedure that will free or remove a large animal from a harmful environment without causing death or injury to the animal or the rescuers.

Tracing: The process of locating animals, persons, or things that may be implicated in the spread of disease so that appropriate action can be taken.

USAR: Urban search and rescue. Certified team members work with a variety of trained dogs and specialty equipment to find survivors after disasters trapped in homes, buildings, and debris.

USDA: United States Department of Agriculture.

USFWS: United States Fish and Wildlife Service.

Vector: A living organism, frequently an arthropod, that transmits an infectious agent from one host to another. A biological vector is one in which the infectious agent must develop or multiply before becoming infective to a recipient host. A mechanical vector is one that transmits an infectious agent from one host to another but is not essential to the life cycle of the agent.

VERT: Veterinary emergency response team.

VETS: Veterinary Emergency Treatment Service (University of Florida College of Veterinary Medicine).

VMAT: Veterinary medical assistance team; has been replaced by NVRT.

VMO: Veterinary medical officer.

WMD: Weapons of mass destruction.

WSPA: World Society for the Protection of Animals.

Zoonosis: A disease of animals that can be transmitted to humans.

References

Advanced Rescue Technology (ART). 2004. April/May, p. 18. www.advancedrt.com.

Amass, Keith. 1999. Personal communication.

American Academy on Veterinary Disaster Medicine (AAVDM). 2002. Dr. Ole H.V. Stalheim. Original Documentation Forming the Academy Is Archived at Iowa State University. AAVDM Newsletter, 7(4).

American Association of Equine Practitioners (AAEP) Welfare Committee. 2004. "AAEP Care Guidelines for Equine Rescue and Retirement Facilities." http://www.aaep.org/pdfs/rescue_retirement_guidelines.pdf.

American Veterinary Medical Association (AVMA), 2002. *U.S. Pet Ownership Demographic Sourcebook.* www.avma.org.

American Veterinary Medical Association (AVMA), 2002. Is your state emergency management agency doing all it can to get you the help you need in a disaster? February 15, 2002, in the Online version of the *Journal of the American Veterinary Medical Association* available at: http://www.avma.org/onlnews/javma/feb02/s021502i.asp.

American Veterinary Medical Association (AVMA). 2007. AVMA Guidelines on Euthanasia. http://www.avma.org/issues/animal_welfare/euthanasia.pdf.

Anderson, Charles. 2004. Personal communication.

Anderson, I. 2002. *Foot and mouth disease 2001: Lessons To Be Learned Inquiry.* London: Stationery Office.

APHIS. 2002. "Animal Health Hazards of Concern During Natural Disasters." http://www.aphis.usda.gov/vs/ceah/cei/taf/emerginganimalhealthissues_files/hazards.pdf.

Aronson, H., and Tough, S.C. 1993. Horse-related fatalities in the province of Alberta, 1975–1990. *American Journal of Forensic Medical Pathology.* 14(1): 28–30.

Askew, Tammy. 2001. Personal communication.

Askew, Tammy. 2001. Have you seen Bunny? *Equine and Bovine Magazine.* Fair Play, SC: Leisure Media Publishers.

Auer, J.A. 2005. *Equine Surgery*, 3rd ed. Phildelphia, PA: W.B. Saunders Co.

Auerbach, P.S., Ed. 2007. *Wilderness Medicine*, 5th ed. Philadelphia, PA: Mosby Elsevier.

AVA (Australian Veterinary Association). 1987. Guidelines on humane slaughter and euthanasia. *Australian Veterinary Journal.* 64: 4–7.

Baker, Janice. 2000. Personal communication.

Baker, Janice. 2004. Emergency euthanasia of horses. From the *Proceedings of the National Disaster Medicine System Conference*, Dallas, TX.

Baker, Janice. 2005a. Scene safety and security in veterinary emergency response. In *Proceedings of the National Disaster Medicine System Conference*, Orlando, Florida.

Baker, Janice. 2005b. Personal communication.

Baker, Janice. 2006. Personal communication.

Baker, Paul. 2005. Personal communication.

Baker, Paul. 2006. Personal communication.

Ball C.G., Ball J.E., Kirkpatrick A.W., et al. 2007. Equestrian injuries: Incidence, injury patterns, and risk factors for 10 years of major traumatic injuries. *American Journal of Surgery.* 193: 636–640.

Bazzarre, Al. 2006. Personal communication.

Berger, J., Kock, M., Cunningham C., and Dodson, N. 1983. Chemical restraint of wild horses: Effects on reproduction and social structure. *Journal of Wildlife Disease.* 19(3): 265–8.

Bevan, Laura. 2002. Personal journal of the HSUS Hurricane Katrina response.

Bevan, Laura. 2005. Personal communication.

Bixby-Hammett, D., and Brooks, W.H. 1990. Common injuries in horseback riding (review). *Sports Medicine.* 9(1): 36–47.

Blackburn, Captain. 2004. Personal communication.

Booth, N.H. 1988. Drug and chemical residues in the edible tissues of animals. In *Veterinary Pharmacology and Therapeutics*, 16th ed. pp 1149–1205. Ames: Iowa State University Press.

Bopp, S.B. 2001. Feeling the HEAT. *Bovine Veterinarian.* May/June 30: 4–8.

Brebner, J.T. 1980. Reaction time in personality theory. In A. T. Welford (ed.), *Reaction Times.* pp. 309–320. New York: Academic Press.

Brebner, J.T., and Welford, A.T. 1980. Introduction: An historical background sketch. In A.T. Welford (ed.), *Reaction Times.* pp. 1–23. New York: Academic Press.

Brison, R.J., and Pickett, C.W. 1991. Nonfatal farm injuries in eastern Ontario: A retrospective survey. *Accident Analysis and Prevention.* 23(6): 585–94.

Brown, Kimberly S. 2008. Lessons from Barbaro. Article 11536. *THE HORSE.* March 23, 2008.

Bukowski, R.W., Budnick, E.K., and Schemel, C.F. 2002. Estimates of the operational reliability of fire protection systems. In *Proceedings of the Society of Fire Protection Engineers.* pp. 111–124.

Bureau of Justice Statistics, 2007. http://www.ojp.usdoj.gov/bjs/pub/press/csllea04pr.htm.

Busch, H.M. Jr., Cogbill, T.H., Landercasper, J., and Landercasper, B.O. 1986. Blunt bovine and equine trauma. *Journal of Trauma.* 26(6): 559–60.

Carlson, G.P. 1983. Thermoregulation and fluid balance in the exercising horse. In S.G. Persson, and R.J. Rose, eds., *Equine Exercise Physiology.* pp 291–309. Cambridge, England: Granata Publications.

Carlson, G.P. 1987. Hematology and body fluids in the equine athlete. In Davis, ed., *Equine Exercise Physiology.* pp 393–425. CA: ICEEP Publications.

Carrillo E.H., Varnagy, D., Braga, S.M., et al. 2007. Traumatic injuries associated with horseback riding. *Scand J Surg.* 96: 79–82.

Carroll, J., Murphy, C.J., Neitz, M., Hoeve, J.N., and Netz, J. 2001. Photopigment basis for dichromatic color vision in the horse. *Journal of Vision.* 1(2): 80–87.

Cattet, M.R.L., Caulkett, N.A., Streib, K.A., et al. 1999. Cardiopulmonary response of anesthetized polar bears to suspension by net and sling. *Journal of Wildlife Diseases.* 35(3): 548–556.

Caulkett, N.A., and Cattet, M.R.L. 2002. Anesthesia of bears. *Zoological Restraint and Anesthesia.* D. Heard, ed. International Veterinary Information Service.

CDC. 2006. "Interim Guidelines for Animal Health and Control of Disease Transmission in Pet Shelters." http://www.bt.cdc.gov/disasters/hurricanes/katrina/animalhealthguidelines.asp.

CDC. 2007. "Bioterrorism Agents/Disease." http://www.bt.cdc.gov/agent/agentlist.asp.

Chapa, Sergio. 2005. "Bill would stiffen penalties against owners of highway roaming cattle." *The Brownsville Herald.* April 24, 2005.

Chitnavis, J.P., Gibbons, C.L., Hirigoyen, M., Lloyd, Parry J., and Simpson, A.H. March, 1996. "Accidents with horses: What has changed in 20 years?" *Injury.* 27(2): 103–5.

Coates, L. 1999. Flood fatalities in Australia, 1788–1996. *Australian Geographer.* 30(3): 391–408.

Cobb, Jim, and Currens, Jim. May 2001. Karst: The Stealthy hazard. *Geotimes.* http://www.agiweb.org/geotimes/may01/feature2.html.

Cole, Mark. 2005. Personal communication.

Cole, Mark. 2006. Personal communication.

Collins, T. 2003. "Equine Slings." California Department of Food and Agriculture, Animal Health Branch. http://www.cdfa.ca.gov/ahfss/ah/equine_slings.htm.

Collins, Timothy B. 2003. Pulling a horse during a rescue: Is there a wrong end? *Search and Rescue Magazine.* 1(1): 10–12.

Cooke, Sandra. 2004. Rescue Glide: 10 Years of helping horses. *Practical Horseman.* December, 80–83.

Cordes, Timothy. 2000. Equine identification—The State of the art. In *Proceedings of the American Association of Equine Practitioners.* 46: 300–301.

Cordes, Timothy. 2001. *Federal Register.* 66(236): 63587–63617. 9 CFR Parts 70 and 88 [Page 63588] 9 CFR, Parts 70 and 88 [Docket No. 98-074-2] RIN 0579-AB06 EFFECTIVE DATE: February 5, 2002. Dr. Timothy Cordes, Senior Staff Veterinarian, National Animal Health Programs, VS, APHIS, 4700 River Road Unit 43, Riverdale, MD 20737-1231; (301) 734-3279.

Creiger, Sharon. 2005. Personal communication.

Culver, Anne. 2006a. *Proceedings of the HSUS National Conference on Animals in Disaster.* Arlington, VA, June 2, 2006.

Culver, Anne. 2006b. Personal communication.

DART Valley Horse Owners Association. 2004. *The Hoof Beat.* June 2004. http://www.vhoa.org/newsletter/articles/200406_newsletter_01.htm.

DeClementi, Camille. 2006. Personal communication.

Dennis, Melinda. 2003. Personal communication.

Durak, Carolyn. 2006. Personal communication.

Dwyer, R. 1999. Horse barn fires. *Lloyd's Equine Disease Quarterly* (8): 1

Dwyer, Roberta. 2006. Personal communication.

Dzurak, Michael. 2006. Personal communication.

Edge, Erik. 1989. Personal communication.

Ender, P.T., and Dolan, M.J. 1997. Pneumonia associated with near-drowning. *Clinical Infectious Disease.* 27: 896–907.

Exadaktylos, A.K., Eggli, S., Inden, P., and Zimmermann, H. 2002. Hoof kick injuries in unmounted equestrians. Improving accident analysis and prevention by introducing an accident and emergency based relational database. *Emergency Medicine Journal.* 19: 573–575.

FARAD. Food Animal Residue Avoidance Databank Homepage. http://www.farad.org/.

Farm Bill Forum Comment Summary & Background. 2006. U.S. Department of Agriculture. http://www.usda.gov/documents/ANIMAL_WELFARE.doc.

Federal Register. 2001. Commercial Transportation of Equines to Slaughter; Final Rule. 66(236): 9 CFR Parts 70, 88: pp. 63587–63617. wais.access.gpo.gov.

FEMA, Emergency Management Institute. 1998. "IS-195 Incident Command System Basic." Washington, D.C.: Department of Homeland Security.

FEMA. 2007. "U.S. Fire Administration/U.S. Department of Homeland Security Report on Firefighter Fatalities in the United States in 2006." Washington, D.C.: Department of Homeland Security.

Ferris, K.K., Berschnieder, Hudson, L.C., and Vivrette, S.L. 2001. Disaster relief management of companion animals affected by the floods of Hurricane Floyd. *Journal of the American Veterinary Medical Association.* 218(3): 354–9.

Ferris, Kelley. 2000. Personal communication.

Fire Services Guides. 1998. HMSO: Fire Risk Assessment http://www.fire.org.uk/risk/risk2-5.htm and www.fsiuk.co.uk/fire_risk_assessment_guide.htm.

Fox, John. 2005. Personal communication.

Fox, John. 2006. Personal communication.

Fox, John, and Fox, Debra. 2000. *Large Animal Rescue Course Manual.* Felton, CA.

French, J., Ing, R., von Allmen, S., and Wood, R. 1983. Mortality from flash floods: A review of the national weather service reports, 1969–1981. *Public Health Report.* 98(6): 584–588.

Galey, Francis D. 1996. Disorders caused by toxicants. In *Large Animal Internal Medicine,* 2nd ed. Bradford P. Smith, ed. St. Louis: Mosby-Year Book, Inc.

Galloway, Jeff. 2006. Personal communication.

Galton, F. 1899. On instruments for (1) testing perception of differences of tint and for (2) determining reaction time. *Journal of the Anthropological Institute.* 19: 27–29.

Geiser, D.R., and Walker, R.D. 1984. Management of thermal injuries in large animals. *Veterinary Clinics of North American Large Animal Practice.* 6(1): 91–105.

Geor, R.J., and McCutcheon, J.L. 1996. Thermoregulation and clinical disorders associated with heat stress and exercise. *Compendium of Clinical Veterinarian Education.* 18(4): 436–444.

Giebel, G., Braun, K., and Mittelmeier, W. 1993. Equestrian accidents in children. *Der Chirurg.* 64(11): 938–47.

Gilchrist, J., Thomas, K.E., Wald, M., et al. 2007. Nonfatal traumatic brain injuries from sports and recreational activities—United States, 2001–2005. *Morbid Mortal Weekly Rep.* July, (56): 733–737.

Gilchrist, M.J. 2000. A national laboratory network for bioterrorism: Evolution from a prototype network of laboratories performing routine surveillance. *Military Medicine.* 165: 28–31. (7 Suppl 2).

Gilman, Mark. 2003. Personal communication.

Gimenez, Rebecca. 2000. "Using the Rescue Glide in Technical Large Animal Rescue." Presentation to the SC Association of Veterinary Technicians, Columbia, SC.

Gimenez, Rebecca M. 2004a. "Large animal water rescue." In *Proceedings of the National Disaster Medicine System Conference.* Dallas, Texas.

Gimenez, Rebecca. 2004b. "Using the Rescue Glide in technical large animal rescue." In *Proceedings of the 2004 National Disaster Medicine System Conference*. Dallas, TX.

Gimenez, Rebecca M. 2005. "Behavior challenges: Large animals, the owner and the unwanted volunteer." In *Proceedings of the 2005 National Disaster Medicine Conference*. Orlando, FL.

Gimenez, Rebecca M. 2006a. "Cutting edge review—Large animal technical emergency rescue techniques." In *Proceedings of the US Army Force Health Protection Conference*. Albuquerque, NM.

Gimenez, R. 2006b. "Improving large animal treatment in the field—Patient transportation within the golden hour." In *Proceedings of the US Army Force Health Protection Conference*. Albuquerque, NM.

Gimenez, Rebecca. 2006c. Unpublished data at Pendleton, SC.

Gimenez, R., and Gimenez, T. 2002a. Personal communication.

Gimenez, Rebecca, and Gimenez, Tomas. 2002b. Personal communication.

Gimenez, Rebecca, and Gimenez, Tomas. 2006a. Unpublished data of horse trailer undercarriage concerns. Pendleton, SC.

Gimenez, Rebecca, and Gimenez, Tomas. 2006b. Unpublished database and research on incidents involving horse trailers. Pendleton, SC.

Gimenez, Rebecca M., Gimenez, Tomas, and Mark Gilman. 2003. "Emerging answers to technical large animal rescue problems." From the Poster Presentation, *International Veterinary Emergency Critical Care Conference Proceedings*. (9): 785.

Gimenez, Tomas, 1998. Unpublished accident report at Clemson, SC.

Gimenez, Tomas. 2000. Unpublished data. Clemson, SC.

Gimenez, Tomas. 2005. "Hurricane Katrina—lessons learned." Presentation to PEARL on 29 June, 2006.

Gimenez, Tomas, and Gimenez, Rebecca M. 2000. "Large Animal rescue techniques." In *Proceedings, 5th Annual North Carolina Veterinary Conference*, p. 173–177. Raleigh, NC.

Gimenez, Tomas, and Gimenez, Rebecca M. 2002. "Introduction to large animal emergency rescue." In *30th Annual NASAR Conference Proceedings*, Section Six, 1–13.

Gimenez, Tomas, Gimenez, Rebecca M., Stafford, Keith B., Reece, Venaye P., and Johannessen, Douglas T. "How to safely manage a potentially rabid equine." In *Proceedings of the 49th American Association of Equine Practitioners Convention*. 49: 274–279.

Goldblum, D., Frueh, B.E., and Koerner, F. 1999. Eye injuries caused by cow horns. *Retina*. 19(4): 314–7.

Grandin, Temple. 1999. Safe handling of large animals (cattle and horses). *Occupational Medicine: State of the Art Reviews*. 14(2). Philadelphia, PA: Hanley & Belfus, Inc.

Grandin, Temple. 2004. Personal communication.

Grandin, Temple, and Johnson, C. 2005. *Animals in Translation—Using the Mysteries of Autism to Decode Animal Behavior*. New York, NY: Scribner.

Graper, Mike. 2005. Personal communication.

Green, Jim. 2005. Personal communication.

Haertel, Kandee. 1999. Equine Rescue Techniques—An Introduction for Emergency Response. Training manual.

Haertel, Kandee. 2000. Emergency on the highway. *The Sentinel*. Libertyville, IL: Libertyville Saddle Shop.

Haertel, Kandee. 2004. Personal communication.

Hafen, B.Q., Kareen, K.J., and Mistovich, J.J. 1996. *Prehospital Emergency Care*, 5th ed. Upper Saddle River, NJ: Prentice Hall.

Hamilton, James. 2003. "Small/large animal decontamination and processing domestic animals" In *Proceedings of the 2003 National Disaster Medicine System Conference*. Reno, NV.

Hamilton, Vonda. 2006. Personal communication.

Hanson, R.R. 2005. Management of burn injuries in the horse. *Vet Clin North Am Equine Pract*. 21(1): 105–23.

Haven, John, DVM. 2006. Personal communication.

Hawthorne, T., and Manley, B. 2004. NFPA 150: New life for an old document. *NFPA Journal*. November/December.

HEART. 2006. "Humane Equine Aid and Rapid Transport." Representative Carissa Grimm. Personal communication.

Heath, S.E. 1998. "Animals in Disaster IS-010—Module A Awareness and Preparedness." Emergency Management Institute, FEMA.

Heath, S.E. 1998. "Animals in Disaster IS-011—Module B Community Planning." Emergency Management Institute, FEMA.

Heath, S.E. 1999. *Animal Management in Disasters*. St. Louis, MO: Mosby, Inc.

Heath, S.E. 2002. "Animals in Disaster IS-306—Module C Livestock in Disasters." Emergency Management Institute, FEMA.

Hendrick, W., and Zaferes, A. 1999. *Surface Ice Rescue*. 1st ed. Fire Engineering Books.

Henneke, D.R., Potter, G.D., Kreider, J.L., and Yeates, B.F. 1984 Relationship between condition score, physical measurements and body fat percentage in mares. *Equine Veterinary Journal*. 15: 371–372.

Herbert, Kimberly. 2006. "Thoughts on Barbaro." # 7118. THE HORSE.com.

Hides, Sue. 2002. "Agriculture Notes, AG 1065 Humane Destruction of Non-Viable Calves less than 24 Hours." Australia State of Victoria, Department of Primary Industries.

Higdon, Michelle. 1998. Personal communication.

Hill, D.J., Langley, R.L., and Morrow, W.M. 1998. Occupational injuries and illnesses reported by zoo veterinarians in the United States. *Journal of Zoological Wildlife Medicine*. 29(4): 371–85.

Horse & Hound, 2006. Police and fire review emergency protocols. Horse and Hound online, 2 March, 2006. http://www.horseandhound.co.uk/news/article.php?aid=81176&cid=397.

Howard-Smith, L., and Reynolds-Scott, J.F. 1912. *The History of Battery A*. pp 142–158. Philadelphia: The John C. Winston Co.

HSE (Health and Safety Executive). 2003. "Police Officer Injuries." www.hse.gov.uk/foi/internalops/sectors/public/7_03_15.pdf.

Hubert, Jeremy. 2006. Personal communication.

Hudson, Lola C., Berschneider, Helen M., Ferris, Kelli K., and Vivrette, Sally L. 2001. Disaster relief management of companion animals affected by the floods of Hurricane Floyd. *Journal of the American Veterinary Medical Association*. 218(3): 354–359.

Humber, K.A. 1988. Near drowning of a gelding. *Journal of American Veterinary Medical Association*. 192(3): 377–378.

Iba, K., Wada, T., Kawaguch, S., Fujisaki, T., Yamashita, T., Ishii, S. 2001. Horse-related injuries in a Thoroughbred stabling area in Japan. *Archives of Orthopaedic and Trauma Surgery*. (9): 501–4.

Jagodzinski, T., and DeMuri, G.P. 2005. Horse-related injuries in children: A review. *Wisconsin Medical Journal*. 104(2): 50–4.

Johnson, Kelly. 2002. The FAD Operational Annex to the National Response Plan. Unpublished.

Jones, R.S., Knottenbelt, D.K., Mason, K., and O'Donnell, E. 1992. Euthanasia of horses. *The Veterinary Record: Journal of the British Veterinary Association*. 130(24): 544.

Jones, Shawn. 2002. Personal communication.

Jonkman, Ir. 2003. "Loss of Life Caused by Floods: An Overview of Mortality Statistics for Worldwide Floods." Delft Cluster at http://www.library.tudelft.nl/delftcluster/theme_risk.html.

Kastner, Leslie. 2005. Personal communication.

Kellogg, Barry, and Ho, Ben. 2002. "Urban search and rescue and veterinary care." *Proceedings of the 2002 National Disaster Medical System Conference*. Reno, NV.

Kemp, B.J. 1973. Reaction time of young and elderly subjects in relation to perceptual deprivation and signal-on versus signal-off condition. *Developmental Psychology*. 8: 268–272.

Kemper, T., Spier, S., Barratt-Boyes, S.M., and Hoffman, R. 1993. Treatment of smoke inhalation in five horses. *Journal of American Veterinary Medical Association*. 202(1): 91–4.

Keulemans, Helen, 2006. Personal communication.

Kiessler, L. 2004. The hoofed animals. In *Crisis Management for Non-Domestic Animals*. NC State Animal Response Team Zoo Day.

King, J.M. 1989. Cardiac muscle spasms after euthanasia. *Veterinary Medicine*. 84(1): 28.

Kinsey, Mike. 2003. Personal communication.

Kock, M.D., Clark, R.K., Franti, C.E., and Jessup, D.A. 1987a. Effects of capture on biological parameters in free-ranging bighorn sheep (*Ovis Canadensis*): Evaluation of drop-net, drive-net, chemical immobilization and the net-gun. *Journal of Wildlife Diseases*. 23(4): 641–51.

Kock, M.D., Clark, R.K., Franti, C.E., Jessup, D.A., and Weaver, R.A. 1987b. Capture methods in five subspecies of free-ranging bighorn sheep: An evaluation of drop-net, drive-net, chemical immobilization and the net-gun. *Journal of Wildlife Diseases*. 23(4): 634–40.

Kock, M.D., Clark, R.K., Franti, C.E., Jessup, D.A., and Wehausen, J.D. 1987c. Effects of capture on biological parameters in free-ranging bighorn sheep (*Ovis Canadensis*): Evaluation of normal, stressed and mortality outcomes and documentation of post-capture survival. *Journal of Wildlife Diseases*. 23(4): 652–62.

Landercasper, J., Cogbill, T.H., Strutt, P.J., and Landercasper, B.O. 1988. Trauma and the veterinarian. *Journal of Trauma*. 28(8): 1255–9.

Lane, David. 2004. Rescues from Mud, Ice and Unstable Ground—the Watersafe Conference. July 2004.

Langley, R. 1999. Physical hazards of animal handlers. *Occupational Medicine*. 14(2): 181–94.

Langley, R.L., and Hunter, J.L. 2001. Occupational fatalities due to animal-related events. *Wilderness Environmental Medicine*. 12(3): 168–74.

Lauze, Roger. 2006. Personal communication.

Leavitt, E.S., and Halverson, D. 1990. "Animals and their Legal Rights: A Survey of American Laws from 1641 to 1990." APHIS-USDA. pp.52–65. Washington, DC: Animal Welfare Institute.

LeBlanck, P.R., Fahy, R.F., and Molls, J. Annual Firefighter Fatality Statistics Reports, NFPA. 1997–2006. www.nfpa.org.

Loveman, L., and Bernard, R. 2005. "Making the Horse Barn Fire Safe." p. 1–24. New York: Humane Society of the United States.

Lovern, Cindy. 2005. Personal communication.

LSU. 2001. "LSU veterinarians help Coast Guard in rescue of stranded horses." *VCS NEWS* 2(3).

LSU (Louisiana State University). 2004. *Preparedness and Response to Agricultural Terrorism—Participant Manual*. Version 1.0. National Center for Biomedical Research and Training.

Lyons, John. 1992. Personal communication.

Madigan, John E. 2005. Personal communication.

Madigan, John E. 2005. The Large Animal Rescue Team, UC Davis Center for Equine Health, VERT (Veterinary Emergency Rescue Team). UC-Davis School of Veterinary Medicine. http://www.vetmed.ucdavis.edu/ceh/HR17-2Disaster.html.

Margentino, M.R., and Malinowski, K. 2004. "Safety Recommendations for the Stable, Barn Yard, and Horse/Livestock Structures." From the National Agricultural Safety Database. Rutgers Cooperative Extension. www.cdc.gov/nasd/docs/d000901-d001000/d000958/d000958.html.

Marshall, W.H., Talbot, S.A., and Ades, H.W. 1943. Cortical response of the anaesthesized cat to gross photic and electrical afferent stimulation. *Journal of Nerophysiology*. 6: 1–15.

Mayberry, Sandy. 2005. Personal communication.

McBride, Mary Ann T. 2000. "Safety issues and policies important to disaster response." In *Proceedings of the 5th Annual North Carolina Veterinary Conference*. Raleigh, NC.

McDonnell, Sue. 2003. *A Practical Field Guide to Horse Behavior. The Equine Ethogram*. Lexington, KY: The Blood-Horse.

McGinn, Thomas. 2004. "Growing national integrated animal disaster response capabilities one county, one state, one team at a time." In *Proceedings of the 2004 National Disaster Medicine System Conference*. Dallas, TX.

McGinn, Thomas. 2004. Personal communication.

McKee, S. 2005. "Coping In The Wake of Fair Hill Barn Fire." November, 2005. TheHorse.com. www.thehorse.com/viewarticle.aspx?ID=6324.

Merrick, Cindy. 2004. Personal communication.

Metcalf, Debi. 2006. Personal communication.

Miller, J.O., and Low, K. 2001. Motor processes in simple, go/no-go, and choice reaction time tasks: A psychophysiological analysis. *Journal of Experimental Psychology: Human Perception and Performance*. 27: 266.

Miller, Robert, Lamb, R., and Downs, H. 2005. *The Revolution in Horsemanship: What It Means to Mankind*. New York, NY: Lyons Press.

MMWR. 1990. Alcohol use and horseback-riding-associated fatalities—North Carolina, 1979–1989. *Morbidity and Mortality Weekly Report*. 41(19): 335,341–342. http://www.cdc.gov/mmwr/preview/mmwrhtml/mm4917a3.htm.

MMWR. 2000. Morbidity and mortality associated with hurricane Floyd—North Carolina, September–October 1999. *Morbidity and Mortality Weekly Report*. 49(17): 369–372.

Monti, Dean J. May 15, 2000. Disaster conference gives animal issues a "seat at the table." *American Veterinary Medical Association*. www.avma.org/onlnews/javma/may00/s051500a.asp.

Mooney, L.E. 1983. Applications and implications of fatality statistics to the flash flood problems. In *Proceedings of the 5th Conference on Hydrometeorology*. Tulsa, TX.

Morris, D.D. 1988. *Equine Internal Medicine*. S.M. Reed and W.M. Bayly, eds. pp. 562, 593. Philadelphia, PA: W.B. Saunders Company.

Moxley, Rick. 2004. Disaster response and exotic cats. In *Crisis Management for Non-Domestic Animals*. p. 37–42. NC State Animal Response Team Zoo Day.

Murphy, Lisa. 2004. Personal communication.

Murphy, Lisa. 2005. Personal communication.

Murphy, Lisa. 2006. Personal communication.

Nasci, R.S., and Moore, C.G. 1998. Vector-borne disease surveillance and natural disasters. *Emerging Infectious Diseases*. 4: 333–334.

National Agriculture Safety Database, 2002. http://www.cdc.gov/nasd/.

National Agricultural Statistics Service, 2007. http://www.nass.usda.gov/.

National Fire Protection Association (NFPA). 2000. "NFPA 150: Standard on Fire Safety in Racetrack Stables." Quincy, MA: National Fire Protection Association.

Nenni, John. 2005a. Personal communication.

Nenni, John. January 2005b. "Be Prepared for the Worst." In TheHorse.Com, Article 5328. www.thehorse.com/viewarticle.aspx?ID=5328.

Nenni, John. 2006. "Playtime Is Over." Unpublished report. Clemson, SC.

NGB (National Guard Bureau). 2005. "Guard Attempts Rescue of 100 Trapped Cattle." September, 22, 2005. www.ngb.army.mil/news/story.asp?id=1935.

Nixon A.J. 1996. *Equine Fracture Repair*. Philadelphia, PA: W.B. Saunders Co.

Nixon, Melissa. 2006. Personal communication.

North Carolina Department of Agriculture and Consumer Services (NCDA&CS). 1999. "North Carolina Floodplain Mapping Hurricane Floyd and 10-Year Disaster Assistance Report." http://www.ncfloodmaps.com/pubdocs/historicdata.htm.

Norwood, S., McAuley, C., Vallina, V.L., Fernandez, L.G., McLarty, J.W., and Goodfried, G. 2000. Mechanisms and patterns of injuries related to large animals. *Journal of Trauma*. 48(4): 740–4.

NSW. 2005. "Draft—Horse Management Plan for Guy Fawkes River National Park." http://www.nationalparks.nsw.gov.au/npws.nsf/Content/guy_fawkes_horses_draft_plan.

NSW. 2006. "Oxley Wild Rivers National Park—Draft Feral Horse Management Plan." http://www.nationalparks.nsw.gov.au/PDFs/draft_pom_feral_horses_oxley.pdf.

OAS (Office of Aircraft Services). 2000. *Operational Procedures Manual*. United States Department of the Interior. www.oas.gov/library/opm/06-32.PDF and www.oas.gov/library/dm/acetahb.pdf.

ODMP. 2006. "The Officer Down Memorial Page Remembers Officer Dana Everett Paladini." The Officer Down Memorial Page, Inc. www.ODMP.org/officer.php?oid=10320.

Ok, E., Deneme, M.A., Kucuk, C., Sozuer, E.M., and Ylmaz, Z. 2004. Large animal-related abdominal injuries. *Journal of Trauma*. 57(4): 877–80.

Olari, Bob. 2006. Personal communication.

O'Rourke, Kate. 2002. News. *Journal of American Veterinary Medical Association*. January 15, 2002. www.avma.org/onlnews/javma/jan02/s011502d.asp.

Orsini, J.A., and Divers, T.J. 2002. *Manual of Equine Emergencies*. 2nd ed. Philadelphia, PA: W.B. Saunders.

Osweiler, Gary D. 1996. *Toxicology*. Philadelphia, PA: Williams and Wilkins.

Otten D.R. 2001. Advisory on proper disposal of euthanatized animals. 1. *Journal of the American Veterinary Medical Association*. 219(12): 1677–8.

Parelli, Pat. 2000. *America's Lost Mustangs, National Geographic Explorer*. Produced and written by Bryan Armstrong. National Geographic Channel. Washington, D.C.

Parelli, Pat. 2004. Savvy Seminar. T. Ed. Garrison Arena, Clemson, SC.

Parelli, Pat. 2005. Savvy Seminar. Arden, N.C.

Parelli, Pat. 2006. Personal communication.

Park, Houston. 2004. Personal communication.

Park, Houston. 2006. Personal communication.

Pascoe, R.R. 1999. *Manual of Equine Dermatology*. D.C. Knottenbelt, ed. San Diego, CA: Sanders, Hartcourt and Brace.

Pasquini, Chris, Spurgeon, Tom, and Pasquini, Susan. 1996. *Anatomy of Domestic Animals, Systemic & Regional Approach,* 7th ed. Pilot Point, TX: Sudz Publishing.

Petridou, E., Kedikoglou, S., Belechri, M., Ntouvelis, E., Dessypris, N., and Trichopoulos, D. 2004. The mosaic of equestrian-related injuries in Greece. *The Journal of Trauma*. 56(3): 643–7.

Pettifer, G., Hubert, J., Latimer, F., McConnico, R., and Smith, J. 2002. Airlifting horses by helicopter: Sedation requirements. *Veterinary Anesthesia and Analgesia*. (29)2: 97–112.

Plumlee, Konstanze H. 1996. Metals and other inorganic compounds. Bradford P. Smith, ed. *Large Animal Internal Medicine*, 2nd ed. St Louis: Mosby-Year Book, Inc.

Puelo, Steve. 2003. *Dark Tide: The Great Boston Molasses Flood of 1919*. Boston, MA: Beacon Press.

Randles, Matt. 2004. Disaster response in carnivores. In *Crisis Management for Non-Domestic Animals*. p. 31–37. NC State Animal Response Team Zoo Day.

Ranson, J. 2002. Personal communication.

Ranson, John. 2006. Personal communication.

Rasin, Beth. 2005. Roger Lauze gives injured horses a fighting chance. *Chronicle of the Horse*. July, 15, 2005: 36–42.

Rathfelder, F.J., Klever, P., Nachtkamp, J., and Paar, O. 1995. Unfallchirurgie der RWTH Aachen. [Injuries in horseback riding—incidence and causes]. *Sportverletz Sportschaden*. 9(3): 77–83.

Ray, Slim. 1999. *Animal Rescue in Flood and Swiftwater Incidents*. Asheville, NC: CFS Press.

Ray, Slim. 2006. Personal communication.

Regan, P.J., Feldberg, L., Roberts, A.H., and Roberts, J.O. 1991. Hand injuries from leading horses. *Injury*. 22(2): 124–6.

Rigg, Nancy. 2005. Response to the Letter to the Editor. *Advanced Rescue Technology*. 8(4).

Robinson, E.S. 1934. Work of the integrated organism. C. Murchison, ed., In *Handbook of General Experimental Psychology*. Worcester, MA: Clark University Press.

Sanders, A.F. 1998. *Elements of Human Performance: Reaction Processes and Attention in Human Skill*. Mahwah, New Jersey: Lawrence Erlbaum Associates.

Santoni, Rosa L., and Tingle, Jeb, S. 2002. "Building Roads on Soft and Sandy Soils." U.S. Army Logistics Management College. http://www.almc.army.mil/alog/issues/JanFeb02/MS698.htm.

SCEF Equine Ambulance. 2006. Southern California Equine Foundation, Inc. www.scef-inc.com/about.html.

Scheve, Neva. 2005. Personal communication.

Seal, U.S., Siniff, D.B., Tester, J.R., and Williams, T.D. 1985. Chemical immobilization and blood analysis of feral horses (Equus caballus). *Journal of Wildlife Disease*. 21(4): 411–6.

Segerstrom, Jim. 2002. Advanced rescue techniques, search and rescue part II: A primer. In *Advanced Rescue Technology*. http://www.advancedrt.com/articles/rtarticles/RTSARII.html.

Shariat, Sheryll. 1996. "Injury Update—Horseback Riding Related Drownings 1988–1994." Oklahoma, Injury Prevention Service. Oklahoma State Department of Health.

Sharp, T., and Saunders, G. 2004. "Development of an Agreed Code of Practice and Standard Operating Procedures for the Humane Capture, Handling or Destruction of Feral Animals in Australia." NSW. Department of Primary Industries, Orange, NSW.

Shearer, J.K., and Nicoletti, Paul. 2002. "Procedures for Humane Euthanasia: Humane Euthanasia of Sick, Injured or Debilitated Livestock." University of Florida Extension Service.

Slessman, Dawn. 2006. Personal communication.

Slovis, Nathan. 2004. Personal communication.

Slusher, Bill. 2006. Personal communication.

Smythe, Joanne. 2006. Personal communication.

Sorli, J.M. 2000. Equestrian injuries: A five year review of hospital admissions in British Columbia, Canada. *Injury Prevention*. 6: 59–61.

South Dakota OEM. 1997. "Listing of Past Natural Hazards Occurrences and Disasters—Livestock Losses." South Dakota. http://www.oem.sd.gov/Mitigation/hmgp/past_1.htm.

Spadavecchia, Claudia, Arendt-Nielsen, Lars, Andersen, Ole K., Spadavecchia, Luciano, Doherr, Marcus, and Schatzmann, Urs. 2003. Comparison of nociceptive withdrawal reflexes and recruitment curves between the forelimbs and hind limbs in conscious horses. *American Journal of Veterinary Research*. 64(6): 700–707.

Spruill, A. 2004. Handling birds in a crisis. In *Crisis Management for Non-Domestic Animals*. NC State Animal Response Team Zoo Day.

Stafford, Keith. 2006. Personal communication.

Stashak, T. 1991. *Equine Wound Management*. Philadelphia: Lea & Febiger.

State of Michigan. 2004. Plaintiff-*Appelle vs. Stephen R. Fennell*, Defendant-Appellant. State of Michigan, Court of Appeals. Final Court Opinion. January 08, 2004. http://courtofappeals.mijud.net/documents/OPINIONS/FINAL/COA/20040108_C241339_44_1O.241339.OPN.COA.PDF.

Taglionc, Ray. 2004. Personal communication.

Taylor, Erin L., Galuppo, Larry D., Madigan, John E., Scarlett, Christine, and Steffey, Eugene P. 2005. Use of the Anderson Sling suspension system for recovery of horses from general anesthesia. *Veterinary Surgery*. 34(6): 559.

Thompson, Eric. 2006. Personal communication.

Thurmon, J.C. 1986. Euthanasia of food animals. *The Veterinary Clinic of North America: Food Animal Practice*. 2(3): pp 743–756.

Timney, B., and Keil, K. 1992. Visual acuity in the horse. *Vision Research.* 32(12): 2289–2293.

Ueeck, B.A., Dierks, E.J., Homer, L.D., and Potter, B. 2004. Patterns of maxillofacial injuries related to interaction with horses. *Journal of Oral Maxillofacial Surgery.* 62(6): 693–6.

UK Guide to Risk Assessment (GRA). *Rescues of Animals.* London: The Stationery Office Ltd, The Publications Centre.

Ullah, F., Masoodurchman Aslam M., and Tahir, M. 2005. Mammalian bite injuries to the head and neck region. *Journal of College of Physicians and Surgeons Pakistan.* 15(8): 485–8.

U.S. Army Engineer Research and Development Center (ERDC). 2006. Personal communication.

USDA, 2004. "The National Animal Identification System (NAIS)." APHIS Program Aid No. 1797.

USDA. 2004. "Docket No. 04–013N– Humane Handling and Slaughter Requirements and the Merits of a Systematic Approach. *Federal Register.* 69(174) Thursday, September 9, 2004. http://www.fsis.usda.gov/OPPDE/rdad/FRPubs/04-013N.pdf.

USDOI. 1998. *Aerial Capture, Eradication and Tagging of Animals (ACETA) Handbook.* (351 DM 2–351 DM 3). Department of the Interior Departmental Manual. Washington, D.C.

USFWS (U.S. Fish and Wildlife Service). 2002. Krueger, Betsy W. DVM. "Secondary Pentobarbital Poisoning of Wildlife." http://cpharm.vetmed.vt.edu/USFWS/USFWSFPentobarbFactSheet.pdf.

USGS (U.S. Geological Survey). 2001. "The Universal Transverse Mercator Grid." Fact Sheet 077-01 (August). http://erg.usgs.gov/isb/pubs/factsheets/fs07701.html

Van Metre, D.C., and Callan, R.J. 2003. Downer cows: Prognostic indicators and treatment options. In *Proceedings of the American College Veterinary Internal Medicine.*

Vivrette, S.J., Baker, J.L., Hudson, C.C., Woods, R.V., and Kuhn, L.J. 2001. Dermatitis and pythiosis in North Carolina horses following Hurricane Floyd. In *Proceedings, World Conference on Veterinary Dermatology.*

von Fieandt, K., Huhtala, A., Kullberg, P., and Saarl, K. 1956. Personal tempo and phenomenal time at different age levels. *Reports from the Psychological Institute,* No. 2, University of Helsinki.

Watson, J.T., Gayer, M., and Connolly, M.A. 2007. Epidemics after natural disasters. *Emerg Infect Dis* [serial on the Internet]. 2007 Jan [July 31, 2007]. http://www.cdc.gov/EID/13/1/06-0779.htm.

Welford, A.T. 1980. Choice reaction time: Basic concepts. In A. T. Welford (ed.), *Reaction Times.* New York: Academic Press. pp. 73–128.

WHO (World Health Organization), Food Safety Department. 2002. "Terrorist Threats to Food: Guidance for Establishing and Strengthening Prevention and Response Systems."

Wilson, Latonna. 2006. Personal communication.

Witte, Jodi. 2005. Personal communication.

Wolfe, B. 2004. Introduction. In *Crisis Management for Nondomestic Animals.* NC State Animal Response Team Zoo Day.

Woods, Jennifer. 2005. Personal communication.

Woods, Jennifer. 2006a. North American Livestock Incident Tracking Database. Unpublished data.

Woods, Jennifer. 2006b. Personal communication.

Woodworth, R.S., and Schlosberg. H. 1954. *Experimental Psychology.* New York: Henry Holt.

Wren, G. 1997. Preparing the feedlot for heat stress. *Bovine Veterinarian.* 4–6.

Wright, Bob. 2005. "Euthanasia of Horses." Ontario Ministry of Agriculture, Food and Rural Affairs.

Zajackowski, J.S., and Wheeler, E. 2002. "Fire Safety in Horse Stables." Pennsylvania State College of Agricultural Sciences, Agricultural Research and Cooperative Extension. www.age.psu.edu/extension/factsheets/g/G100.pdf

Index